## FOURTH EDITION

# NURSING INFORMATICS

## and the Foundation of Knowledge

# The Pedagogy

***Nursing Informatics and the Foundation of Knowledge, Fourth Edition*** drives comprehension through a variety of strategies geared toward meeting the learning needs of students, while also generating enthusiasm about the topic. This interactive approach addresses diverse learning styles, making this the ideal text to ensure mastery of key concepts. The pedagogical aids that appear in most chapters include the following:

## Key Terms

| | | |
|---|---|---|
| » Artificial intelligence | » Connectionism | » Intuition |
| » Brain | » Decision making | » Knowledge |
| » Cognitive informatics | » Empiricism | » Logic |
| » Cognitive science | » Epistemology | » Memory |
| » Computer science | » Human Mental Workload (MWL) | » Mind |
| | » Intelligence | » Neuroscience |
| | | » Perception |

*Key Terms*  Found in a list at the beginning of each chapter, studying these terms will create an expanded vocabulary.

*Objectives*  Providing a snapshot of the key information encountered in each chapter, the objectives serve as a checklist to help guide and focus study. Objectives can also be found within the text's online resources.

## Objectives

1. Trace the evolution of nursing informatics from concept to specialty practice.
2. Relate nursing informatics metastructures, concepts, and tools to the knowledge work of nursing.
3. Explore the quest for consistent terminology in nursing and describe terminology approaches that

## Introduction

Those who followed the actual events of Apollo 13, or who were entertained by the movie (Howard, 1995), watched the astronauts strive against all odds to bring their crippled spaceship back to Earth. The speed of their travel was incomprehensible to most viewers, and the task of bringing the spaceship back to Earth seemed nearly impossible. They were experiencing a crisis never imagined by the experts at NASA, and they made up their survival plan moment by moment. What brought them back to Earth safely? Surely, credit must be given to the technology and the spaceship's ability to withstand the trauma it experienced. Most amazing, however, were the traditional nontechnological tools, skills, and supplies that were used in new and different ways to stabilize the spacecraft's environment and keep the astronauts safe while traveling toward their uncertain future.

This sense of constancy in the midst of change serves to stabilize experience in many different life events and contributes to the survival of crisis and change. This rhythmic process is also vital to the healthcare system's stability and survival in the presence of the rapidly changing events of the Knowledge Age. No one can dispute the fact that the Knowledge Age is changing health care in ways that will not be fully recognized and understood for years. The change is paradigmatic, and every expert who addresses this change reminds healthcare professionals of the need to go with the flow of rapid change or be left behind.

As with any paradigm shift, a new way of viewing the world brings with it some of the enduring values of the previous worldview. As health care continues its journey into digital communications, telehealth, and wearable technologies, it brings some familiar tools and skills recognized in the form of **values**, such as **privacy, confidentiality**, autonomy, and nonmaleficence. Although these basic values remain unchanged, the **standards** for living out these values will take on new meaning as health professionals confront new and different moral dilemmas brought on by the adoption

*Introductions*  Found at the beginning of each chapter, the introductions provide an overview highlighting the importance of the chapter's topic. They also help keep students focused as they read.

**Research Briefs** These summaries encourage students to access current research in the field.

**RESEARCH BRIEF**

Using an online survey of 1,227 randomly selected respondents, Bodkin and Miaoulis (2007) sought to describe the characteristics of information seekers on e-health websites, the types of information they seek, and their perceptions of the quality and ethics of the websites. Of the respondents, 74% had sought health information on the Web, with women accounting for 55.8% of the health information seekers. A total of 50% of the seekers were between 35 and 54 years of age. Nearly two thirds of the users began their searches using a general search engine rather than a health-specific site, unless they were seeking information related to symptoms or diseases. Top reasons for seeking information were related to diseases or symptoms of medical conditions, medication information, health news, health insurance, locating a doctor, and Medicare or Medicaid information. The level of education of information seekers was related to the ratings of website quality, in that more educated seekers found health information websites more understandable, but were more likely to perceive bias in the website information. The researchers also found that the ethical codes for e-health websites seem to be increasing consumers' trust in the safety and quality of information found on the Web, but that most consumers are not comfortable purchasing health products or services online.

The full article appears in Bodkin, C., & Miaoulis, G. (2007). eHealth information quality and ethics issues: An exploratory study of consumer perceptions. *International Journal of Pharmaceutical and Healthcare Marketing, 1*(1), 27–42. Retrieved from ABI/INFORM Global (Document ID: 1515583081).

**Summaries** Summaries are included at the end of each chapter to provide a concise review of the material covered, highlighting the most important points and describing what the future holds.

nence granted physicians.

## Summary

In this chapter, we have traced the development of informatics as a specialty, defined nursing informatics, and explored the DIKW paradigm central to informatics. We also explored the need for and the development of standardized terminologies to capture and codify the work of nursing and how informatics supports the knowledge work of nursing. This chapter advanced the view that every nurse's practice will make contributions to new nursing knowledge in dynamically interactive CIS environments. The core concepts associated with informatics will become embedded in the practice of every nurse, whether administrator, researcher, educator, or practitioner. Informatics will be prominent in the knowledge work of nurses, yet it will be a subtlety because of its eventual fulsome integration with clinical care processes. Clinical care will be substantially supported by the capacity and promise of technology today and tomorrow.

Most importantly, readers need to contemplate a future without being limited by the world of practice as it is known today. Information technology is not a panacea for all of the challenges found in health care, but it will provide the nursing profession with an unprecedented capacity to generate and disseminate new knowledge at rapid speed. Realizing these possibilities necessitates that all nurses understand and leverage the informatician within and contribute to the future.

**BOX 6-3 CASE STUDY: CASTING TO THE FUTURE**

In the year 2025, nursing practice enabled by technology has created a professional culture of reflection, critical inquiry, and interprofessional collaboration. Nurses use technology at the point of care in all clinical settings (e.g., primary care, acute care, community, and long-term care) to inform their clinical decisions and effect the best possible outcomes for their clients. Information is gathered and retrieved via human–technology biometric interfaces including voice, visual, sensory, gustatory, and auditory interfaces, which continuously monitor physiologic parameters for potentially harmful imbalances. Longitudinal records are maintained for all citizens from their initial prenatal assessment to death; all lifelong records are aggregated into the knowledge bases of expert systems. These systems provide the basis of the artificial intelligence being embedded in emerging technologies. Smart technologies and invisible computing are ubiquitous in all sectors where care is delivered. Clients and families are empowered to review and contribute actively to their record of health and wellness. Invasive diagnostic techniques are obsolete, nanotechnology therapeutics are the norm, and robotics supplement or replace much of the traditional work of all health professions. Nurses provide expertise to citizens to help them effectively manage their health and wellness life plans, and navigate access to appropriate information and services.

**THOUGHT-PROVOKING QUESTIONS**

1. Imagine you are in a social situation and someone asks you, "What does a nurse do?" Think about how you will capture and convey the richness that is nursing science in your answer.
2. Choose a clinical scenario from your recent experience and analyze it using the Foundation of Knowledge model. How did you acquire knowledge? How did you process knowledge? How did you generate knowledge? How did you disseminate knowledge? How did you use feedback, and what was the effect of the feedback on the foundation of your knowledge?

**Case Studies** Case studies encourage active learning and promote critical thinking skills. Students can ask questions, analyze situations, and solve problems in a real-world context.

**Thought-Provoking Questions** Students can work on these critical thinking assignments individually or in a group. In addition, students can delve deeper into concepts by completing these exercises online.

# Dee McGonigle, PhD, RN, CNE, FAAN, ANEF

Director, Virtual Learning Experiences (VLE) and Professor
Graduate Program, Chamberlain College of Nursing
Member, Informatics and Technology Expert Panel (ITEP) for the
American Academy of Nursing

# Kathleen Mastrian, PhD, RN

Associate Professor and Program Coordinator for Nursing
Pennsylvania State University, Shenango
Sr. Managing Editor, *Online Journal of Nursing Informatics (OJNI)*

**FOURTH EDITION**

# NURSING INFORMATICS

## and the Foundation of Knowledge

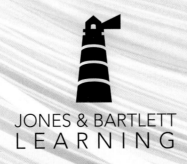

JONES & BARTLETT
LEARNING

*World Headquarters*
Jones & Bartlett Learning
5 Wall Street
Burlington, MA 01803
978-443-5000
info@jblearning.com
www.jblearning.com

Jones & Bartlett Learning books and products are available through most bookstores and online booksellers. To contact Jones & Bartlett Learning directly, call 800-832-0034, fax 978-443-8000, or visit our website, www.jblearning.com.

Substantial discounts on bulk quantities of Jones & Bartlett Learning publications are available to corporations, professional associations, and other qualified organizations. For details and specific discount information, contact the special sales department at Jones & Bartlett Learning via the above contact information or send an email to specialsales@jblearning.com.

12268-8

**Production Credits**
VP, Executive Publisher: David D. Cella
Executive Editor: Amanda Martin
Editorial Assistant: Christina Freitas
Production Manager: Carolyn Rogers Pershouse
Senior Marketing Manager: Jennifer Scherzay
Product Fulfillment Manager: Wendy Kilborn
Composition: S4Carlisle Publishing Services
Cover and Text Design: Michael O'Donnell
Rights & Media Specialist: Wes DeShano
Media Development Editor: Shannon Sheehan
Cover Image (Title Page, Part Opener, Chapter Opener): © fotomak/Shutterstock
Printing and Binding: LSC Communications
Cover Printing: LSC Communications

**Library of Congress Cataloging-in-Publication Data**
Names: McGonigle, Dee, editor. | Mastrian, Kathleen Garver, editor.
Title: Nursing informatics and the foundation of knowledge/[edited by]
   Dee McGonigle, Kathleen Mastrian.
Description: Fourth edition. | Burlington, MA: Jones & Bartlett Learning,
   [2018] | Includes bibliographical references and index.
Identifiers: LCCN 2016043838 | ISBN 9781284121247 (pbk.)
Subjects: | MESH: Nursing Informatics | Knowledge
Classification: LCC RT50.5 | NLM WY 26.5 | DDC 651.5/04261--dc23

LC record available at https://lccn.loc.gov/2016043838

6048

Printed in the United States of America
21 20 19 18     10 9 8 7 6 5 4

# Special Acknowledgments

We want to express our sincere appreciation to the staff at Jones & Bartlett Learning, especially Amanda, Christina, and Carolyn, for their continued encouragement, assistance, and support during the writing process and publication of our book.

# Contents

## SECTION VI: RESEARCH APPLICATIONS OF NURSING INFORMATICS     459

### 21   Nursing Research: Data Collection, Processing, and Analysis     463
*Heather E. McKinney, Sylvia DeSantis, Kathleen Mastrian, and Dee McGonigle*

### 22   Data Mining as a Research Tool     477
*Dee McGonigle and Kathleen Mastrian*

### 23   Translational Research: Generating Evidence for Practice     495
*Jennifer Bredemeyer, Ida Androwich, Dee McGonigle, and Kathleen Mastrian*

# Preface

The idea for this text originated with the development of nursing informatics (NI) classes, the publication of articles related to technology-based education, and the creation of the *Online Journal of Nursing Informatics (OJNI)*, which Dee McGonigle cofounded with Renee Eggers. Like most nurse informaticists, we fell into the specialty; our love affair with technology and gadgets and our willingness to be the first to try new things helped to hook us into the specialty of informatics. The rapid evolution of technology and its transformation of the ways of nursing prompted us to try to capture the essence of NI in a text.

As we were developing the first edition, we realized that we could not possibly know all there is to know about informatics and the way in which it supports nursing practice, education, administration, and research. We also knew that our faculty roles constrained our opportunities for exposure to changes in this rapidly evolving field. Therefore, we developed a tentative outline and a working model of the theoretical framework for the text and invited participation from informatics experts and specialists around the world. We were pleased with the enthusiastic responses we received from some of those invited contributors and a few volunteers who heard about the text and asked to participate in their particular area of expertise.

In the second edition, we invited the original contributors to revise and update their chapters. Not everyone chose to participate in the second edition, so we revised several of the chapters using the original work as a springboard. The revisions to the text were guided by the contributors' growing informatics expertise and the reviews provided by textbook adopters. In the revisions, we sought to do the following:

- Expand the audience focus to include nursing students from BS through DNP programs as well as nurses thrust into informatics roles in clinical agencies.
- Include, whenever possible, an attention-grabbing case scenario as an introduction or an illustrative case scenario demonstrating why the topic is important.
- Include important research findings related to the topic. Many chapters have research briefs presented in text boxes to encourage the reader to access current research.
- Focus on cutting-edge innovations, meaningful use, and patient safety as appropriate to each topic.
- Include a paragraph describing what the future holds for each topic.

New chapters that were added to the second edition included those focusing on technology and patient safety, system development life cycle, workflow analysis, gaming, simulation, and bioinformatics.

In the third edition, we reviewed and updated all of the chapters, reordered some chapters for better content flow, eliminated duplicated content, split the education and research content into two sections, integrated social media content, and added two new chapters: *Data Mining as a Research Tool* and *The Art of Caring in Technology-Laden Environments*.

In this fourth edition, we reviewed and updated all of the chapters based on technological advancements and changes to the healthcare arena, including reimbursement mechanisms for services. We have pared this edition down to 26 chapters from the previous edition's 29; one chapter each was deleted from Sections II, V, and VII. Section I includes updates to the same five chapters on the building blocks of nursing informatics, with extensive changes to Chapter 3, *Computer Science and the Foundation of Knowledge Model*. To improve flow, we combined content. In Section II, the previous four chapters were narrowed to three. New Chapters 6, *History and Evolution of Nursing Informatics* and 7, *Nursing Informatics as a Specialty,* were developed and appropriate material from previous Chapters 6, 7, and 8 were assimilated. This section ends with an updated Chapter 8, *Legislative Aspects of Nursing Informatics: HITECH and HIPAA* (formerly Chapter 9). Section III contains the same five chapters, although all were updated and Chapter 13, *Workflow and Beyond Meaningful Use* (formerly Chapter 14) now reflects the payment models and reimbursement issues that we are adjusting to after meaningful use has gone away. Section IV contains the same five chapters with updated content and some name changes to reflect the current status of informatics and healthcare. Chapter 15 was renamed to *Informatics Tools to Promote Patient Safety and Quality Outcomes,* and Chapter 16 has been changed to *Patient Engagement and Connected Health.* Section V went from three chapters to two chapters: Chapter 19 (formerly Chapter 20) was updated, while the new Chapter 20, *Simulation, Game Mechanics, and Virtual Worlds in Nursing Education,* had content from former Chapters 21 and 22 integrated during its development. Section VI was renamed to Research Applications of Nursing Informatics. It still has the same four chapters, which have been updated, but the first chapter in this section, 21, was renamed to reflect nursing research; its new name is *Nursing Research: Data Collection, Processing, and Analysis.* Section VII went from three chapters to two chapters. Because emerging technologies are discussed throughout the text, the chapter focusing specifically on that was removed. The two chapters that remain are Chapter 25, *The Art of Caring in Technology-Laden Environments,* and the new Chapter 26, *Nursing Informatics and Knowledge Management.* In addition, the ancillary materials have been updated and enhanced to include competency-based self-assessments and mapping the content to the current NI standards.

We believe that this text provides a comprehensive elucidation of this exciting field. Its theoretical underpinning is the Foundation of Knowledge model. This model is introduced in its entirety in the first chapter (*Nursing Science and the Foundation of Knowledge*), which discusses nursing science and its relationship to NI. We believe that humans are organic information systems that are constantly acquiring, processing, and generating information or knowledge in both their professional and personal lives. It is their high degree of knowledge that characterizes humans as extremely intelligent, organic machines. Individuals have the ability to manage knowledge—an ability that is learned and honed from birth. We make our way through life interacting with our environment and being inundated with information and knowledge. We experience our environment and learn by acquiring, processing, generating, and disseminating knowledge. As we interact in our environment, we acquire knowledge that we must process. This processing effort causes us to redefine and restructure our knowledge base and generate new knowledge. We then share (disseminate) this new knowledge and receive feedback from others. The dissemination and feedback initiate this cycle of knowledge over again, as we acquire, process, generate, and disseminate the knowledge gained from sharing and re-exploring our own knowledge base. As others respond to our knowledge dissemination and we acquire new knowledge, we engage in rethinking and reflecting on our knowledge, processing, generating, and then disseminating anew.

The purpose of this text is to provide a set of practical and powerful tools to ensure that the reader gains an understanding of NI and moves from information through knowledge to wisdom. Defining the demands of nurses and providing tools to help them survive and succeed in the Knowledge Era remains a major challenge. Exposing nursing students and nurses to the principles and tools used in NI helps to prepare them to meet the challenge of practicing nursing in the Knowledge Era while striving to improve patient care at all levels.

The text provides a comprehensive framework that embraces knowledge so that readers can develop their knowledge repositories and the wisdom necessary to act on and apply that knowledge. The text is divided into seven sections.

- Section I, *Building Blocks of Nursing Informatics,* covers the building blocks of NI: nursing science, information science, computer science, cognitive science, and the ethical management of information.
- Section II, *Perspectives on Nursing Informatics,* provides readers with a look at various viewpoints on NI and NI practice as described by experts in the field.

- Section III, *Nursing Informatics Administrative Applications: Precare and Care Support,* covers important functions of administrative applications of NI.
- Section IV, *Nursing Informatics Practice Applications: Care Delivery,* covers healthcare delivery applications including electronic health records (EHRs), clinical information systems, telehealth, patient safety, patient and community education, and care management.
- Section V, *Education Applications of Nursing Informatics,* presents subject matter on how informatics supports nursing education.
- Section VI, *Research Applications of Nursing Informatics,* covers informatics tools to support nursing research, including data mining and bioinformatics.
- Section VII, *Imagining the Future of Nursing Informatics,* focuses on the future of NI, emphasizes the need to preserve caring functions in technology-laden environments, and reviews the relationship of nursing informatics to organizational knowledge management.

The introduction to each section explains the relationship between the content of that section and the Foundation of Knowledge model. This text places the material within the context of knowledge acquisition, processing, generation, and dissemination. It serves both nursing students (BS to DNP/PhD) and professionals who need to understand, use, and evaluate NI knowledge. As nursing professors, our major responsibility is to prepare the practitioners and leaders in the field. Because NI permeates the entire scope of nursing (practice, administration, education, and research), nursing education curricula must include NI. Our primary objective is to develop the most comprehensive and user-friendly NI text on the market to prepare nurses for current and future practice challenges. In particular, this text provides a solid groundwork from which to integrate NI into practice, education, administration, and research.

Goals of this text are as follows:

- Impart core NI principles that should be familiar to every nurse and nursing student
- Help the reader understand knowledge and how it is acquired, processed, generated, and disseminated
- Explore the changing role of NI professionals
- Demonstrate the value of the NI discipline as an attractive field of specialization

Meeting these goals will help nurses and nursing students understand and use fundamental NI principles so that they efficiently and effectively function as current and future nursing professionals to enhance the nursing profession and improve the quality of health care. The overall vision, framework, and pedagogy of this text offer benefits to readers by highlighting established principles while drawing out new ones that continue to emerge as nursing and technology evolve.

# Acknowledgments

We are deeply grateful to the contributors who provided this text with a richness and diversity of content that we could not have captured alone. Joan Humphrey provided social media content integrated throughout the text. We especially wish to acknowledge the superior work of Alicia Mastrian, graphic designer of the Foundation of Knowledge model, which serves as the theoretical framework on which this text is anchored. We could never have completed this project without the dedicated and patient efforts of the Jones & Bartlett Learning staff, especially Amanda Martin, Emma Huggard, and Christina Freitas, all of whom fielded our questions and concerns in a very professional, respectful, and timely manner.

Dee acknowledges the undying love, support, patience, and continued encouragement of her best friend and husband, Craig, and her son, Craig, who has made her so very proud. She sincerely thanks her cousins Camille, Glenn, Mary Jane, and Sonny, and her dear friends for their support and encouragement, especially Renee.

Kathy acknowledges the loving support of her family: husband Chip; children Ben and Alicia; sisters Carol and Sue; and parents Robert and Rosalie Garver. She dedicates her work on this edition to her dad, Robert, who died September 17, 2016. Kathy also acknowledges those friends who understand the importance of validation, especially Katie, Lisa, Kathy, Maureen, Anne, Barbara, and Sally.

# Authors' Note

This text provides an overview of nursing informatics from the perspective of diverse experts in the field, with a focus on nursing informatics and the Foundation of Knowledge model. We want our readers and students to focus on the relationship of knowledge to informatics and to embrace and maintain the caring functions of nursing—messages all too often lost in the romance with technology. We hope you enjoy the text!

# Contributors

Ida Androwich, PhD, RN, BC, FAAN
Loyola University Chicago
School of Nursing
Maywood, IL

Emily Barey, MSN, RN
Director of Nursing Informatics
Epic Systems Corporation
Madison, WI

Lisa Reeves Bertin, BS, EMBA
Pennsylvania State University
Sharon, PA

Brett Bixler, PhD
Pennsylvania State University
University Park, PA

Jennifer Bredemeyer, RN
Loyola University Chicago
School of Nursing
Skokie, IL

Steven Brewer, PhD
Assistant Professor, Administration of Justice
Pennsylvania State University
Sharon, PA

Sylvia M. DeSantis, MA
Pennsylvania State University
University Park, PA

Judith Effken, PhD, RN, FACMI
University of Arizona
College of Nursing
Tucson, AZ

Nedra Farcus, MSN, RN
Retired from Pennsylvania State University, Altoona
Altoona, PA

Kathleen M. Gialanella, JD, RN, LLM
Law Offices
Westfield, NJ
Associate Adjunct Professor
Teachers College, Columbia University
New York, NY
Adjunct Professor
Seton Hall University, College of Nursing &
    School of Law
South Orange & Newark, NJ

Denise Hammel-Jones, MSN, RN-BC, CLSSBB
Greencastle Associates Consulting
Malvern, PA

Nicholas Hardiker, PhD, RN
Senior Research Fellow
University of Salford
School of Nursing & Midwifery
Salford, UK

Glenn Johnson, MLS
Pennsylvania State University
University Park, PA

June Kaminski, MSN, RN
Kwantlen University College
Surrey, British Columbia, Canada

Julie Kenney, MSN, RNC-OB
Clinical Analyst
Advocate Health Care
Oak Brook, IL

Margaret Ross Kraft, PhD, RN
Loyola University Chicago
School of Nursing
Maywood, IL

Wendy L. Mahan, PhD, CRC, LPC
Pennsylvania State University
University Park, PA

Heather McKinney, PhD
Pennsylvania State University
University Park, PA

Nickolaus Miehl, MSN, RN
Oregon Health Sciences University
Monmouth, OR

Lynn M. Nagle, PhD, RN
Assistant Professor
University of Toronto
Toronto, Ontario, Canada

Ramona Nelson, PhD, RN-BC, FAAN, ANEF
Professor Emerita, Slippery Rock University
President, Ramona Nelson Consulting
Pittsburgh, PA

Nancy Staggers, PhD, RN, FAAN
Professor, Informatics
University of Maryland
Baltimore, MD

Jeff Swain
Instructional Designer
Pennsylvania State University
University Park, PA

Denise D. Tyler, MSN/MBA, RN-BC
Implementation Specialist
Healthcare Provider, Consulting
ACS, a Xerox Company
Dearborn, MI

The Editors also acknowledge the work of the following first edition contributors (original contributions edited by McGonigle and Mastrian for second edition):

Kathleen Albright, BA, RN
Strategic Account Manager at GE Healthcare
Philadelphia, PA

Schuyler F. Hoss, BA
Northwest Healthcare Management
Vancouver, WA

Audrey Kinsella, MA, MS
Information for Tomorrow
Telehealth Planning Services
Asheville, NC

Peter J. Murray, PhD, RN, FBCS
Coachman's Cottage
Nocton, Lincoln, UK

Susan M. Paschke, MSN, RN
The Cleveland Clinic
Cleveland, OH

Sheldon Prial, RPH, BS Pharmacy
Sheldon Prial Consultance
Melbourne, FL

Jackie Ritzko
Pennsylvania State University
Hazelton, PA

Marianela Zytkowsi, MSN, RN
The Cleveland Clinic
Cleveland, OH

# Building Blocks of Nursing Informatics

**Nursing professionals are information-dependent knowledge workers.** As health care continues to evolve in an increasingly competitive information marketplace, professionals—that is, the knowledge workers—must be well prepared to make significant contributions by harnessing appropriate and timely information. Nursing informatics (NI), a product of the scientific synthesis of information in nursing, encompasses concepts from computer science, cognitive science, information science, and nursing science. NI continues to evolve as more and more professionals access, use, and develop the information, computer, and cognitive sciences necessary to advance nursing science for the betterment of patients and the profession. Regardless of their future roles in the healthcare milieu, it is clear that nurses need to understand the ethical application of computer, information, and cognitive sciences to advance nursing science.

To implement NI, one must view it from the perspective of both the current healthcare delivery system and specific, individual organizational needs, while anticipating and creating future applications in both the healthcare system and the nursing profession. Nursing professionals should be expected to discover opportunities to use NI, participate in the design of solutions, and be challenged to identify, develop, evaluate, modify, and enhance applications to improve patient care. This text is designed to provide the reader with the information and knowledge needed to meet this expectation.

Section I presents an overview of the building blocks of NI: nursing, information, computer, and cognitive sciences. Also included in this section is a chapter on ethical applications of healthcare informatics. This section lays the foundation for the remainder of the book.

The *Nursing Science and the Foundation of Knowledge* chapter describes nursing science and introduces the Foundation of Knowledge model as the conceptual framework for the book. In this chapter, a clinical case scenario is used to illustrate the concepts central to nursing science. A definition of nursing science is also derived from the American Nurses Association's definition of nursing. Nursing science is the ethical application of knowledge acquired through education, research, and practice to provide services and interventions to patients to maintain, enhance, or restore their health, and to acquire, process, generate, and disseminate nursing knowledge to advance the nursing profession. Information is a central concept and health care's most valuable resource. Information science and systems, together with computers, are constantly changing the way healthcare organizations conduct their business. This will continue to evolve.

To prepare for these innovations, the reader must understand fundamental information and computer concepts, covered in the *Introduction to Information, Information Science, and Information Systems* and *Computer Science and the Foundation of Knowledge Model* chapters, respectively. Information science deals with the interchange (or flow) and scaffolding (or structure) of information and involves the application of information tools for solutions to patient care and business problems in health care. To be able to use and synthesize information effectively, an individual must be able to obtain, perceive, process, synthesize, comprehend, convey, and manage the information. Computer science deals with understanding the development, design, structure, and relationship of computer hardware and software. This science offers extremely valuable tools that, if used skillfully, can facilitate the acquisition and manipulation of data and information by nurses, who can then synthesize these resources into an ever-evolving knowledge and wisdom base. This not only facilitates professional development and the ability to apply evidence-based practice decisions within nursing care, but, if the results are disseminated and shared, can also advance the profession's knowledge base. The development of knowledge tools, such as the automation of decision making and strides in artificial intelligence, has altered the understanding of knowledge and its representation. The ability to structure knowledge electronically facilitates the ability to share knowledge structures and enhance collective knowledge.

As discussed in the *Introduction to Cognitive Science and Cognitive Informatics* chapter, cognitive science deals with how the human mind functions. This science encompasses how people think, understand, remember, synthesize, and access stored information and knowledge. The nature of knowledge, including how it is developed, used, modified, and shared, provides the basis for continued learning and intellectual growth.

The *Ethical Applications of Informatics* chapter focuses on ethical issues associated with managing private information with technology and provides a framework for analyzing ethical issues and supporting ethical decision making.

The material within this book is placed within the context of the Foundation of Knowledge model (shown in Figure I-1 and periodically throughout the book, but more fully introduced and explained in the *Nursing Science and the Foundation of Knowledge* chapter). The Foundation of Knowledge model is used throughout the text to illustrate how knowledge is used to meet the needs of healthcare delivery systems, organizations, patients, and nurses. It is through interaction with these building blocks—the theories, architecture, and tools—that one acquires the bits and pieces of data necessary, processes these into information, and generates and disseminates the resulting knowledge. Through this dynamic exchange, which includes feedback, individuals continue the interaction and use of these sciences to input or acquire, process, and output or disseminate generated knowledge. Humans experience their environment and learn by acquiring, processing, generating, and disseminating knowledge. When they then share (disseminate) this new knowledge and receive feedback on the knowledge they have shared, the feedback initiates the cycle of knowledge all over again. As individuals acquire, process, generate, and disseminate knowledge, they are motivated to share, rethink, and explore their own knowledge base. This complex process is captured in the Foundation of Knowledge model. Throughout the chapters in the *Building Blocks of Nursing Informatics* section, readers are challenged to think about how the model can help them to understand the ways in which they acquire, process, generate, disseminate, and then receive and process feedback on their new knowledge of the building blocks of NI.

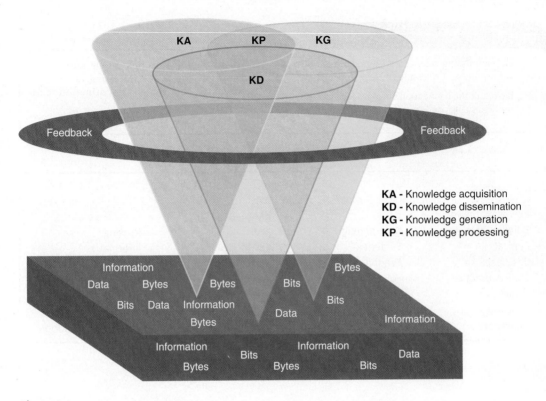

KA - Knowledge acquisition
KD - Knowledge dissemination
KG - Knowledge generation
KP - Knowledge processing

**Figure I-1** Foundation of Knowledge Model
Designed by Alicia Mastrian

# CHAPTER 1

# Nursing Science and the Foundation of Knowledge

Dee McGonigle and Kathleen Mastrian

## Introduction

**Nursing informatics** has been traditionally defined as a specialty that integrates **nursing science**, computer science, and information science to manage and communicate data, information, knowledge, and wisdom in nursing practice. This chapter focuses on nursing science as one of the **building blocks** of nursing informatics. As depicted in **Figure 1-1**, the traditional definition of nursing

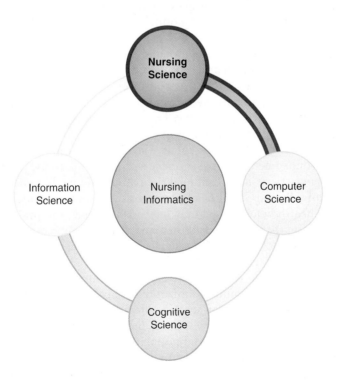

**Figure 1-1** Building Blocks of Nursing Informatics

informatics is extended to include cognitive science. The **Foundation of Knowledge model** is also introduced as the organizing **conceptual framework** of this text, and the model is tied to nursing science and the practice of nursing informatics. To lay the groundwork for this discussion, consider the following patient scenario:

> *Tom H. is a registered nurse who works in a very busy metropolitan hospital emergency room. He has just admitted a 79-year-old man whose wife brought him to the hospital because he is having trouble breathing. Tom immediately clips a pulse oximeter to the patient's finger and performs a very quick assessment of the patient's other vital signs. He discovers a rapid pulse rate and a decreased oxygen saturation level in addition to the rapid and labored breathing. Tom determines that the patient is not in immediate danger and that he does not require intubation. Tom focuses his initial attention on easing the patient's labored breathing by elevating the head of the bed and initiating oxygen treatment; he then hooks the patient up to a heart monitor. Tom continues to assess the patient's breathing status as he performs a head-to-toe assessment of the patient that leads to the nursing diagnoses and additional interventions necessary to provide comprehensive care to this patient.*

Consider Tom's actions and how and why he intervened as he did. Tom relied on the immediate **data** and **information** that he acquired during his initial rapid assessment to deliver appropriate care to his patient. Tom also used technology (a pulse oximeter and a heart monitor) to assist with and support the delivery of care. What is not immediately apparent, and some would argue is transparent (done without conscious thought), is the fact that during the rapid assessment, Tom reached into his **knowledge** base of previous learning and experiences to direct his care, so that he could act with **transparent wisdom**. He used both **nursing theory** and **borrowed theory** to inform his practice. Tom certainly used nursing process theory, and he may have also used one of several other nursing theories, such as Rogers's science of unitary human beings, Orem's theory of self-care deficit, or Roy's adaptation theory. In addition, Tom may have applied his knowledge from some of the basic sciences, such as anatomy, physiology, psychology, and chemistry, as he determined the patient's immediate needs. Information from Maslow's hierarchy of needs, Lazarus's transaction model of stress and coping, and the health belief model may have also helped Tom practice professional nursing. He gathered data, and then analyzed and interpreted those data to form a conclusion—the essence of science. Tom has illustrated the practical aspects of nursing science.

The American Nurses Association (2016) defines nursing in this way: "Nursing is the protection, promotion, and optimization of health and abilities, prevention of illness and injury, facilitation of healing, alleviation of suffering through the diagnosis and treatment of human response, and advocacy in the care of individuals, families, groups, communities, and populations" (para. 1). Thus the focus of nursing is on human responses to actual or potential health problems and advocacy for various clients. These human responses are varied and may change over time in a single case. Nurses must possess the technical skills to manage equipment and perform procedures, the interpersonal skills to interact appropriately with people, and the cognitive skills to observe, recognize, and collect data; analyze and interpret data; and reach a reasonable conclusion that forms the basis of a decision. At the heart of all of these skills lies the management of data and information. This definition of nursing science focuses on the ethical application of knowledge acquired through education, research, and practice to provide services and interventions to patients to maintain, enhance, or restore their health and to acquire, process, generate, and disseminate nursing knowledge to advance the nursing profession.

Nursing is an information-intensive profession. The steps of using information, applying knowledge to a problem, and acting with wisdom form the basis of nursing practice science. Information is composed of data that were processed using knowledge. For information to be valuable, it must be accessible, accurate, timely, complete, cost-effective, flexible, reliable, relevant, simple, verifiable, and secure. Knowledge is the awareness and understanding of a set of information and ways that information can be made useful to support a specific task or arrive at a decision. In the case scenario, Tom used accessible, accurate, timely, relevant, and verifiable data and information. He compared that data and information to his knowledge base of previous experiences to determine which data and information were relevant to the current case. By applying his previous knowledge to data, he converted those data into information, and information into new knowledge—that is, an understanding of which nursing interventions were appropriate in this case. Thus information is data made functional through the application of knowledge.

Humans acquire data and information in bits and pieces and then transform the information into knowledge. The information-processing functions of the brain are frequently compared to those of a computer, and vice versa (see a discussion of cognitive informatics for more information). Humans can be thought of as organic information systems that are constantly acquiring, processing, and generating information or knowledge in their professional and personal lives. They have an amazing ability to manage knowledge. This ability is learned and honed from birth as individuals make their way through life interacting with the environment and being inundated with data and information. Each person experiences the environment and learns by acquiring, processing, generating, and disseminating knowledge.

Tom, for example, acquired knowledge in his basic nursing education program and continues to build his foundation of knowledge by engaging in such activities as reading nursing research and theory articles, attending continuing education programs, consulting with expert colleagues, and using **clinical databases** and **clinical practice guidelines**. As he interacts in the environment, he acquires knowledge that must be processed. This processing effort causes him to redefine and restructure his knowledge base and generate new knowledge. Tom can then share (disseminate) this new knowledge with colleagues, and he may receive **feedback** on the knowledge that he shares. This dissemination and feedback builds the knowledge foundation anew as Tom acquires, processes, generates, and disseminates new knowledge as a result of his interactions. As others respond to his **knowledge dissemination** and he acquires yet more knowledge, he is engaged to rethink, reflect on, and re-explore his **knowledge acquisition**, leading to further processing, generating, and then disseminating knowledge. This ongoing process is captured in the Foundation of Knowledge model, which is used as an organizing framework for this text.

At its base, the model contains bits, bytes (a computer term used to quantify data), data, and information in a random representation. Growing out of the base are separate cones of light that expand as they reflect upward; these cones represent knowledge acquisition, **knowledge generation**, and knowledge dissemination. At the intersection of the cones and forming a new cone is **knowledge processing**. Encircling and cutting through the knowledge cones is feedback that acts on and may transform any or all aspects of knowledge represented by the cones. One should imagine the model as a dynamic figure in which the cones of light and the feedback rotate and interact rather than remain static. Knowledge acquisition, knowledge generation, knowledge dissemination, knowledge processing, and feedback are constantly evolving for nurse scientists. The transparent effect of the cones is deliberate and is intended to suggest that as knowledge grows and expands, its use becomes more transparent—a person uses this knowledge during practice without even being consciously aware of which aspect of knowledge is being used at any given moment.

Experienced nurses, thinking back to their novice years, may recall feeling like their head was filled with bits of data and information that did not form any type of cohesive whole. As the model depicts, the processing of knowledge begins a bit later (imagine a timeline applied vertically) with early experiences on the bottom and expertise growing as the processing of knowledge ensues. Early on in nurses' education, conscious attention is focused mainly on knowledge acquisition, and beginning nurses depend on their instructors and others to process, generate, and disseminate knowledge. As nurses become more comfortable with the science of nursing, they begin to take over some of the other Foundation of Knowledge functions. However, to keep up with the explosion of information in nursing and health care, they must continue to rely on the knowledge generation of nursing theorists and researchers and the dissemination of their work. In this sense, nurses are committed to lifelong learning and the use of knowledge in the practice of nursing science.

The Foundation of Knowledge model (**Figure 1-2**) permeates this text, reflecting the understanding that knowledge is a powerful tool and that nurses focus on information as a key building block of knowledge. The application of the model is described to help the reader understand and appreciate the foundation of knowledge in nursing science and see how it applies to nursing informatics. All of the various nursing roles (practice, administration, education, research, and informatics) involve the science of nursing. Nurses are **knowledge workers**, working with information and generating information and knowledge as a product. They are knowledge acquirers, providing convenient and efficient means of capturing and storing knowledge. They are knowledge users, meaning individuals or groups who benefit from valuable, viable knowledge. Nurses are knowledge engineers, designing, developing, implementing, and maintaining knowledge. They are knowledge managers, capturing and processing collective expertise and distributing it where it can create the largest benefit. Finally,

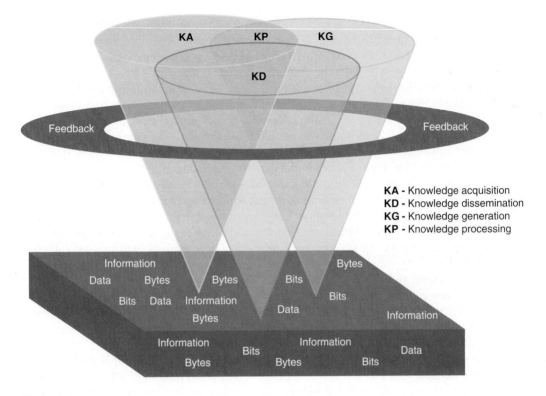

**Figure 1-2** Foundation of Knowledge Model
Designed by Alicia Mastrian

they are knowledge developers and generators, changing and evolving knowledge based on the tasks at hand and the information available.

In the case scenario, at first glance one might label Tom as a knowledge worker, a knowledge acquirer, and a knowledge user. However, stopping here might sell Tom short in his practice of nursing science. Although he acquired and used knowledge to help him achieve his work, he also processed the data and information he collected to develop a nursing diagnosis and a plan of care. The knowledge stores Tom used to develop and glean knowledge from valuable information are generative (having the ability to originate and produce or generate) in nature. For example, Tom may have learned something new about his patient's culture from the patient or his wife that he will file away in the knowledge repository of his mind to be used in another similar situation. As he compares this new cultural information to what he already knows, he may gain insight into the effect of culture on a patient's response to illness. In this sense, Tom is a knowledge generator. If he shares this newly acquired knowledge with another practitioner, and as he records his observations and his conclusions, he is then disseminating knowledge. Tom also uses feedback from the various technologies he has applied to monitor his patient's status. In addition, he may rely on feedback from laboratory reports or even other practitioners to help him rethink, revise, and apply the knowledge about this patient that he is generating.

To have ongoing value, knowledge must be viable. Knowledge viability refers to applications (most technology based) that offer easily accessible, accurate, and timely information obtained from a variety of resources and methods and presented in a manner so as to provide the necessary elements to generate new knowledge. In the case scenario, Tom may have felt the need to consult an electronic database or a clinical guidelines repository that he has downloaded on his tablet or smartphone, or that resides in the emergency room's networked computer system, to assist him in the development of a comprehensive care plan for his patient. In this way, Tom uses technology and **evidence** to support and inform his practice. It is also possible in this scenario that an alert might appear in the patient's electronic health record or the clinical information system (CIS) reminding Tom to ask about influenza and pneumonia vaccines. Clinical information technologies that support and inform nursing practice and nursing administration are an important part of nursing informatics.

This text provides a framework that embraces knowledge so that readers can develop the wisdom necessary to apply what they have learned. Wisdom is the application of knowledge to an appropriate situation. In the practice of nursing science, one expects actions to be directed by wisdom. Wisdom uses knowledge and experience to heighten common sense and insight to exercise sound judgment in practical matters. It is developed through knowledge, experience, insight, and reflection. Wisdom is sometimes thought of as the highest form of common sense, resulting from accumulated knowledge or erudition (deep, thorough learning) or enlightenment (education that results in understanding and the dissemination of knowledge). It is the ability to apply valuable and viable knowledge, experience, understanding, and insight while being prudent and sensible. Knowledge and wisdom are not synonymous: Knowledge abounds with others' thoughts and information, whereas wisdom is focused on one's own mind and the synthesis of experience, insight, understanding, and knowledge. Wisdom has been called the foundation of the art of nursing.

Some nursing roles might be viewed as more focused on some aspects rather than other aspects of the foundation of knowledge. For example, some might argue that nurse educators are primarily knowledge disseminators and that nurse researchers are knowledge generators. Although the more frequent output of their efforts can certainly be viewed in this way, it is important to realize that nurses use all of the aspects of the Foundation of Knowledge model regardless of their area of practice. For nurse educators to be effective, they must be in the habit of constantly building and rebuilding their foundation of knowledge about nursing science. In addition, as they develop and implement curricular innovations, they must evaluate the effectiveness of those changes. In some cases, they use formal research techniques to achieve this goal and, therefore, generate knowledge about the best and most effective teaching strategies. Similarly, nurse researchers must acquire and process new knowledge as they design and conduct their research studies. All nurses have the opportunity to be involved in the formal dissemination of knowledge via their participation in professional conferences, either as presenters or as attendees. In addition, some nurses disseminate knowledge by formal publication of their ideas. In the cases of conference presentation and publication, nurses may receive feedback that stimulates rethinking about the knowledge they have generated and disseminated, in turn prompting them to acquire and process data and information anew.

All nurses, regardless of their practice arena, must use informatics and technology to inform and support that practice. The case scenario discussed Tom's use of various monitoring devices that provide feedback on the physiologic status of the patient. It was also suggested that Tom might consult a clinical database or nursing practice guidelines residing on a tablet or smartphone, in the cloud (a virtual information storage system), or on a clinical agency network as he develops an appropriate plan of action for his nursing interventions. Perhaps the CIS in the agency supports the collection of data about patients in a **relational database**, providing an opportunity for **data mining** by nursing administrators or nurse researchers. In this way, administrators and researchers can glean information about best practices and determine which improvements are necessary to deliver the best and most effective nursing care (Swan, Lang, & McGinley, 2004).

The future of nursing science and nursing informatics is closely associated with nursing education and nursing research. Skiba (2007) suggested that techno-savvy and well-informed faculty who can demonstrate the appropriate use of technologies to enhance the delivery of nursing care are needed. Along those lines, Whitman-Price, Kennedy, and Godwin (2012) conducted research among senior nursing students to determine perceptions of personal phone use to access healthcare information during clinical. Their study indicated that ready access to electronic resources enhanced clinical decision making and confidence in patient care. Girard (2007) discussed cutting-edge operating room technologies, such as nanosurgery using nanorobots, smart fabrics that aid in patient assessment during surgery, biopharmacy techniques for the safe and effective delivery of anesthesia, and virtual reality training. She made an extremely provocative point about nursing education: "Educators will need to expand their knowledge and teach for the future and not the past. They must take heed that the old tried-and-true nursing education methods and curriculum that has lasted 100 years will have to change, and that change will be mandated for all areas of nursing" (p. 353). Bassendowski (2007) specifically addressed the potential for the generation of knowledge in educational endeavors as faculty apply new technologies to teaching and the focus shifts away from individual to group instruction that promotes sharing and processing of knowledge.

Several key national groups continue to promote the inclusion of informatics content in nursing education programs. These initiatives include the Vision Series by the National League for Nursing (NLN; 2015); recommendations in the *Quality and Safety Education for Nurses (QSEN)* learning modules (2014a); the Technology Informatics Guiding Education Reform (TIGER) Initiative (Healthcare Information and Management Systems Society, 2016); and Nursing Informatics Deep Dive by the American Association of Colleges of Nursing (AACN; 2016). These organizations focus on the need to integrate informatics competencies into nursing curricula to prepare future nurses for the tasks of managing data, information, and knowledge; alleviating errors and promoting safety; supporting decision making; and improving the quality of patient care. Nurse educators are challenged to prepare informatics-competent nurses who can practice safely in technology-laden settings.

The TIGER (2007) initiative identified steps toward a 10-year vision and stated a key purpose: "to create a vision for the future of nursing that bridges the quality chasm with information technology, enabling nurses to use informatics in practice and education to provide safer, higher-quality patient care" (p. 4). The pillars of the TIGER vision include the following:

- *Management and Leadership*: Revolutionary leadership that drives, empowers, and executes the transformation of health care.
- *Education*: Collaborative learning communities that maximize the possibilities of technology toward knowledge development and dissemination, driving rapid deployment and implementation of best practices.
- *Communication and Collaboration*: Standardized, person-centered, technology-enabled processes to facilitate teamwork and relationships across the continuum of care.
- *Informatics Design*: Evidence-based, interoperable intelligence systems that support education and practice to foster quality care and safety.
- *Information Technology*: Smart, people-centered, affordable technologies that are universal, useable, useful, and standards based.
- *Policy*: Consistent, incentives-based initiatives (organizational and governmental) that support advocacy and coalition-building, achieving and resourcing an ethical culture of safety.
- *Culture*: A respectful, open system that leverages technology and informatics across multiple disciplines in an environment where all stakeholders trust each other to work together toward the goal of high quality and safety (p. 4).

*The Essentials of Baccalaureate Education for Professional Nursing Practice* (AACN, 2008, pp. 18–19) includes the following technology-related outcomes for baccalaureate nursing graduates:

1. Demonstrate skills in using patient care technologies, information systems, and communication devices that support safe nursing practice.
2. Use telecommunication technologies to assist in effective communication in a variety of healthcare settings.
3. Apply safeguards and decision-making support tools embedded in patient care technologies and information systems to support a safe practice environment for both patients and healthcare workers.
4. Understand the use of CIS to document interventions related to achieving nurse-sensitive outcomes.
5. Use standardized terminology in a care environment that reflects nursing's unique contribution to patient outcomes.
6. Evaluate data from all relevant sources, including technology, to inform the delivery of care.
7. Recognize the role of information technology in improving patient care outcomes and creating a safe care environment.
8. Uphold ethical standards related to data security, regulatory requirements, confidentiality, and clients' right to privacy.
9. Apply patient care technologies as appropriate to address the needs of a diverse patient population.
10. Advocate for the use of new patient care technologies for safe, quality care.

11. Recognize that redesign of workflow and care processes should precede implementation of care technology to facilitate nursing practice.
12. Participate in the evaluation of information systems in practice settings through policy and procedure development.

The report suggests the following sample content for achieving these student outcomes (AACN, 2008, pp. 19–20):

- Use of patient care technologies (e.g., monitors, pumps, computer-assisted devices)
- Use of technology and information systems for clinical decision making
- Computer skills that may include basic software, spreadsheet, and healthcare databases
- Information management for patient safety
- Regulatory requirements through electronic data-monitoring systems
- Ethical and legal issues related to the use of information technology, including copyright, privacy, and confidentiality issues
- Retrieval information systems, including access, evaluation of data, and application of relevant data to patient care
- Online literature searches
- Technological resources for evidence-based practice
- Web-based learning and online literature searches for self and patient use
- Technology and information systems safeguards (e.g., patient monitoring, equipment, patient identification systems, drug alerts and IV systems, and bar coding)
- Interstate practice regulations (e.g., licensure, telehealth)
- Technology for virtual care delivery and monitoring
- Principles related to nursing workload measurement and resources and information systems
- Information literacy
- Electronic health record and physician order entry
- Decision support tools
- Role of the nurse informaticist in the context of health informatics and information systems

The Informatics and Healthcare Technologies Essentials of Master's Education in Nursing includes the following elements:

### Essential V: Informatics and Healthcare Technologies
*Rationale*

Informatics and healthcare technologies encompass five broad areas:
- Use of patient care and other technologies to deliver and enhance care
- Communication technologies to integrate and coordinate care
- Data management to analyze and improve outcomes of care
- Health information management for evidence-based care and health education
- Facilitation and use of electronic health records to improve patient care (AACN, 2011, pp. 17–18)

# Quality and Safety Education for Nurses

As nursing science evolves, it is critical that patient care improves. Sometimes, unfortunately, patient care is less-than-adequate and is unsafe. Therefore, quality and safety have become paramount. The QSEN Institute project seeks to prepare future nurses who will have the knowledge, skills, and attitudes (KSAs) necessary to continuously improve the quality and safety of the healthcare systems within which they work.

Prelicensure informatics KSAs include the following (QSEN Institute, 2014c):

| INFORMATICS | | |
| --- | --- | --- |
| **Knowledge** | **Skills** | **Attitudes** |
| Explain why information and technology skills are essential for safe patient care | Seek education about how information is managed in care settings before providing care<br><br>Apply technology and information management tools to support safe processes of care | Appreciate the necessity for all health professionals to seek lifelong, continuous learning of information technology skills |
| Identify essential information that must be available in a common database to support patient care<br><br>Contrast benefits and limitations of different communication technologies and their impact on safety and quality | Navigate the electronic health record<br><br>Document and plan patient care in an electronic health record<br><br>Employ communication technologies to coordinate care for patients | Value technologies that support clinical decision making, error prevention, and care coordination<br><br>Protect the confidentiality of protected health information in electronic health records |
| Describe examples of how technology and information management are related to the quality and safety of patient care<br><br>Recognize the time, effort, and skill required for computers, databases, and other technologies to become reliable and effective tools for patient care | Respond appropriately to clinical decision-making supports and alerts<br><br>Use information management tools to monitor outcomes of care processes<br><br>Use high quality electronic sources of healthcare information | Value nurses' involvement in design, selection, implementation, and evaluation of information technologies to support patient care |

**Definition:** Use information and technology to communicate, manage knowledge, mitigate error, and support decision making.

Graduate-level informatics KSAs include the following (QSEN Institute, 2014b):

| INFORMATICS | | |
|---|---|---|
| Knowledge | Skills | Attitudes |
| Contrast benefits and limitations of common information technology strategies used in the delivery of patient care<br><br>Evaluate the strengths and weaknesses of information systems used in patient care | Participate in the selection, design, implementation, and evaluation of information systems<br><br>Communicate the integral role of information technology in nurses' work<br><br>Model behaviors that support implementation and appropriate use of electronic health records<br><br>Assist team members to adopt information technology by piloting and evaluating proposed technologies | Value the use of information and communication technologies in patient care |
| Formulate essential information that must be available in a common database to support patient care in the practice specialty<br><br>Evaluate benefits and limitations of different communication technologies and their impact on safety and quality | Promote access to patient care information for all professionals who provide care to patients<br><br>Serve as a resource for how to document nursing care at basic and advanced levels<br><br>Develop safeguards for protected health information<br><br>Champion communication technologies that support clinical decision making, error prevention, care coordination, and protection of patient privacy | Appreciate the need for consensus and collaboration in developing systems to manage information for patient care<br><br>Value the confidentiality and security of all patient records |
| Describe and critique taxonomic and terminology systems used in national efforts to enhance interoperability of information systems and knowledge management systems | Access and evaluate high quality electronic sources of healthcare information<br><br>Participate in the design of clinical decision-making supports and alerts<br><br>Search, retrieve, and manage data to make decisions using information and knowledge management systems<br><br>Anticipate unintended consequences of new technology | Value the importance of standardized terminologies in conducting searches for patient information<br><br>Appreciate the contribution of technological alert systems<br><br>Appreciate the time, effort, and skill required for computers, databases, and other technologies to become reliable and effective tools for patient care |
| **Definition:** Use information and technology to communicate, manage knowledge, mitigate error, and support decision making. | | |

This text is designed to include the necessary content to prepare nurses for practice in the ever-changing and technology-laden healthcare environments. Informatics competence has been recognized as necessary in order to enhance clinical decision making and improve patient care for many years. This is evidenced by Goossen (2000), who reflected on the need for research in this area and believed that the focus of nursing informatics research should be on the structuring and processing of patient information and the ways that these endeavors inform nursing decision making in clinical practice. The increased use of technology to enhance nursing practice, nursing education, and nursing research will open new avenues for acquiring, processing, generating, and disseminating knowledge.

In the future, nursing research will make significant contributions to the development of nursing science. Technologies and translational research will abound, and clinical practices will continue to be evidence based, thereby improving patient outcomes and decreasing safety concerns. Schools of nursing will embrace nursing science as they strive to meet the needs of changing student populations and the increasing complexity of healthcare environments.

## Summary

Nursing science influences all areas of nursing practice. This chapter provided an overview of nursing science and considered how nursing science relates to typical nursing practice roles, nursing education, informatics, and nursing research. The Foundation of Knowledge model was introduced as the organizing conceptual framework for this text. Finally, the relationship of nursing science to nursing informatics was discussed. In subsequent chapters the reader will learn more about how nursing informatics supports nurses in their many and varied roles. In an ideal world, nurses would embrace nursing science as knowledge users, knowledge managers, knowledge developers, knowledge engineers, and knowledge workers.

### THOUGHT-PROVOKING QUESTIONS

1. Imagine you are in a social situation and someone asks you, "What does a nurse do?" Think about how you will capture and convey the richness that is nursing science in your answer.
2. Choose a clinical scenario from your recent experience and analyze it using the Foundation of Knowledge model. How did you acquire knowledge? How did you process knowledge? How did you generate knowledge? How did you disseminate knowledge? How did you use feedback, and what was the effect of the feedback on the foundation of your knowledge?

# References

American Association of Colleges of Nursing (AACN). (2008, October 20). The essentials of baccalaureate education for professional nursing practice. Retrieved from http://www.aacn.nche.edu/education-resources/BaccEssentials08.pdf

American Association of Colleges of Nursing (AACN). (2011, March 21). The essentials of master's education in nursing. Retrieved from http://www.aacn.nche.edu/education-resources/MastersEssentials11.pdf

American Association of Colleges of Nursing (AACN). (2016). Background and overview: Nursing informatics Deep Dive. Retrieved from http://www.aacn.nche.edu/qsen-informatics/background-overview

American Nurses Association. (2016). What is nursing? Retrieved from http://www.nursingworld.org/EspeciallyForYou/What-is-Nursing

Bassendowski, S. (2007). NursingQuest: Supporting an analysis of nursing issues. *Journal of Nursing Education, 46*(2), 92–95. Retrieved from Education Module database [document ID: 1210832211].

Cronenwett, L., Sherwood, G., Barnsteiner J., Disch, J., Johnson, J., Mitchell, P., . . . Warren, J. (2007). Quality and safety education for nurses. *Nursing Outlook, 55*(3), 122–131.

Girard, N. (2007). Science fiction comes to the OR. Association of Operating Room Nurses. *AORN Journal, 86*(3), 351–353. Retrieved from Health Module database [document ID: 1333149261].

Goossen, W. (2000). Nursing informatics research. *Nurse Researcher, 8*(2), 42. Retrieved from ProQuest Nursing & Allied Health Source database [document ID: 67258628].

Healthcare Information and Management Systems Society. (2016). The TIGER initiative. Retrieved from http://www.himss.org/professional-development/tiger-initiative

National League for Nursing (NLN). (2015). A vision for the changing faculty role: Preparing students for the technological world of health care. Retrieved from https://www.nln.org/docs/default-source/about/nln-vision-series-(position-statements)/a-vision-for-the-changing-faculty-role-preparing-students-for-the-technological-world-of-health-care.pdf?sfvrsn=0

Quality and Safety Information for Nurses (QSEN) Institute. (2014a). Courses: Learning modules. Retrieved from http://www.qsen.org/courses/learning-modules

QSEN Institute. (2014b). Graduate KSAs. Retrieved from http://www.qsen.org/competencies/graduate-ksas

QSEN Institute. (2014c). Pre-licensure KSAs. Retrieved from http://www.qsen.org/competencies/pre-licensure-ksas

Skiba, D. (2007). Faculty 2.0: Flipping the novice to expert continuum. *Nursing Education Perspectives, 28*(6), 342–344. Retrieved from ProQuest Nursing & Allied Health Source database [document ID: 1401240241].

Swan, B., Lang, N., & McGinley, A. (2004). Access to quality health care: Links between evidence, nursing language, and informatics. *Nursing Economic$, 22*(6), 325–332. Retrieved from Health Module database [document ID: 768191851].

Technology Informatics Guiding Education Reform. (2007). Evidence and informatics transforming nursing: 3-year action steps toward a 10-year vision. Retrieved from http://www.aacn.nche.edu/education-resources/TIGER.pdf

Whitman-Price, R., Kennedy, L., & Godwin, C. (2012). Use of personal phones by senior nursing students to access health care information during clinical education: Staff nurses' and students' perceptions. *Journal of Nursing Education, 51*(11), 642–646.

## Objectives

1. Reflect on the progression from data to information to knowledge.
2. Describe the term information.
3. Assess how information is acquired.
4. Explore the characteristics of quality information.
5. Describe an information system.
6. Explore data acquisition or input and processing or retrieval, analysis, and synthesis of data.
7. Assess output or reports, documents, summaries, alerts, and outcomes.
8. Describe information dissemination and feedback.
9. Define information science.
10. Assess how information is processed.
11. Explore how knowledge is generated in information science.

## Key Terms

- » Acquisition
- » Alert
- » Analysis
- » Chief information officers
- » Chief technical officers
- » Chief technology officers
- » Cloud computing
- » Cognitive science
- » Communication science
- » Computer-based information systems
- » Computer science
- » Consolidated Health Informatics
- » Data
- » Dissemination
- » Document
- » Electronic health records
- » Federal Health Information Exchange
- » Feedback
- » Health information exchange
- » Health Level Seven
- » Indiana Health Information Exchange
- » Information science
- » Information systems
- » Information technology
- » Input
- » Interfaces
- » Internet2
- » Internet of Things (IoT)
- » Knowledge
- » Knowledge worker
- » Library science
- » Massachusetts Health Data Consortium
- » National Health Information Infrastructure
- » National Health Information Network
- » New England Health EDI Network
- » Next-Generation Internet
- » Outcome
- » Output
- » Processing
- » Rapid Syndromic Validation Project
- » Report
- » Social sciences
- » Stakeholders
- » Summaries
- » Synthesis
- » Telecommunications

# CHAPTER 2

# Introduction to Information, Information Science, and Information Systems

*Kathleen Mastrian and Dee McGonigle*

## Introduction

This chapter explores information, information systems (ISs), and information science as one of the building blocks of informatics. (Refer to Figure 2-1.) The key word here, of course, is *information*. Information and information processing are central to the work of health care. A healthcare professional is known as a **knowledge worker** because he or she deals with and processes information on a daily basis to make it meaningful and inform his or her practice.

Healthcare information is complex, and many concerns and issues arise with healthcare information, such as ownership, access, disclosure, exchange, security, privacy, disposal, and dissemination. The widespread implementation of **electronic health records** (EHRs) has promoted collaboration among public- and private-sector stakeholders on a wide-ranging variety of healthcare information solutions. Some of these initiatives include **Health Level Seven** (HL7), the eGov initiative by **Consolidated Health Informatics** (CHI), the **National Health Information Infrastructure** (NHII), the **National Health Information Network** (NHIN), **Next-Generation Internet** (NGI), **Internet2**, and iHealth record. There are also **health information exchange** (HIE) systems, such as Connecting for Health, the eHealth initiative, the **Federal Health Information Exchange** (FHIE), the **Indiana Health Information Exchange** (IHIE), the **Massachusetts Health Data Consortium** (MHDC), the **New England Health EDI Network** (NEHEN), the State of New Mexico **Rapid Syndromic Validation Project** (RSVP), the Southeast Michigan e-Prescribing Initiative, and the Tennessee Volunteer eHealth Initiative (Goldstein, Groen, Ponkshe, & Wine, 2007). Many of these were sparked by the HITECH Act of 2011, which set the 2014 deadline for implementing EHRs and provided the impetus for HIE initiatives.

It is quite evident from the previous brief listing that there is a need to remedy healthcare **information technology** (IT) concerns, challenges, and issues faced today. One of the main issues deals with how healthcare information is managed to make it meaningful. It is important to understand

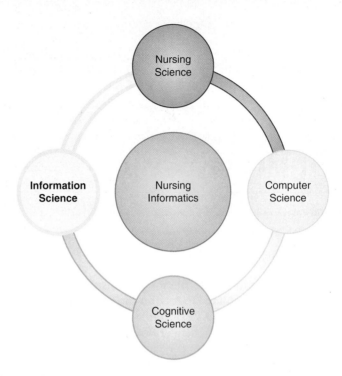

Figure 2-1 Building Blocks of Nursing Informatics

how people obtain, manipulate, use, share, and dispose of information. This chapter deals with the information piece of this complex puzzle.

## Information

Suppose someone states the number 99.5. What does that mean? It could be a radio station or a score on a test. Now suppose someone says that Ms. Howsunny's temperature is 99.5°F—what does that convey? It is then known that 99.5 is a person's temperature. The data (99.5) were processed to the information that 99.5° is a specific person's temperature. **Data** are raw facts. Information is processed data that has meaning. Healthcare professionals constantly process data and information to provide the best possible care for their patients.

Many types of data exist, such as alphabetic, numeric, audio, image, and video data. Alphabetic data refer to letters, numeric data refer to numbers, and alphanumeric data combine both letters and numbers. This includes all text and the numeric outputs of digital monitors. Some of the alphanumeric data encountered by healthcare professionals are in the form of patients' names, identification numbers, or medical record numbers. Audio data refer to sounds, noises, or tones—for example, monitor alerts or alarms, taped or recorded messages, and other sounds. Image data include graphics and pictures, such as graphic monitor displays or recorded electrocardiograms, radiographs, magnetic resonance imaging (MRI) outputs, and computed tomography (CT) scans. Video data refer to animations, moving pictures, or moving graphics. Using these data, one may review the ultrasound of a pregnant patient, examine a patient's echocardiogram, watch an animated video for professional development, or learn how to operate a new technology tool, such as a pump or monitoring system. The data we gather, such as heart and lung sounds or X-rays, help us produce information. For example, if a patient's X-rays show a fracture, it is interpreted into information such as spiral, compound, or hairline. This information is then processed into knowledge and a treatment plan is formulated based on the healthcare professional's wisdom.

The integrity and quality of the data, rather than the form, are what matter. Integrity refers to whole, complete, correct, and consistent data (**Figure 2-2**). Data integrity can be compromised through human error; viruses, worms, or other computer bugs; hardware failures or crashes; transmission errors; or hackers entering the system. **Figure 2-3** illustrates some ways that data can be compromised. Information technologies help to decrease these errors by putting into place safeguards, such as backing up files on a routine basis, error detection for transmissions, and user **interfaces** that help people enter the data correctly. High-quality data are relevant and accurately represent their corresponding concepts. Data are dirty when a database contains errors, such as duplicate, incomplete, or outdated records. One author (D.M.) found 50 cases of tongue cancer in a database she examined for data quality. When the records were tracked down and analyzed, and the dirty data were removed, only one case of tongue cancer remained. In this situation, the data for the same person had been entered erroneously 49 times. The major problem was with the patient's identification number and name: The number was changed or his name was misspelled repeatedly. If researchers had just taken the number of cases in that defined population as 50, they would have concluded that tongue cancer was an epidemic, resulting in flawed information that is not meaningful. As this example demonstrates, it is imperative that data be clean if the goal is quality information. The data that are processed into information must be of high quality and integrity to create meaning to inform assessments and decision making.

To be valuable and meaningful, information must be of good quality. Its value relates directly to how the information informs decision making. Characteristics of valuable, quality information include accessibility, security, timeliness, accuracy, relevancy, completeness, flexibility, reliability, objectivity, utility, transparency, verifiability, and reproducibility.

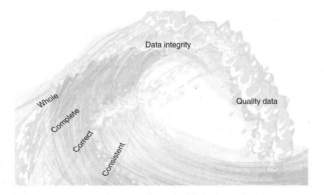

**Figure 2-2**  Data Integrity

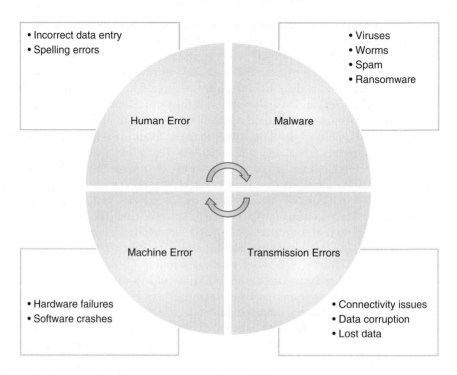

- Incorrect data entry
- Spelling errors

Human Error

- Viruses
- Worms
- Spam
- Ransomware

Malware

Machine Error

Transmission Errors

- Hardware failures
- Software crashes

- Connectivity issues
- Data corruption
- Lost data

**Figure 2-3** Threats to Data Integrity

Accessibility is a must; the right user must be able to obtain the right information at the right time and in the right format to meet his or her needs. Getting meaningful information to the right user at the right time is as vital as generating the information in the first place. The right user refers to an authorized user who has the right to obtain the data and information he or she is seeking. Security is a major challenge because unauthorized users must be blocked while the authorized user is provided with open, easy access (see the *Electronic Security* chapter).

Timely information means that the information is available when it is needed for the right purpose and at the right time. Knowing who won the lottery last week does not help one to know if the person won it today. Accurate information means that there are no errors in the data and information. Relevant information is a subjective descriptor, in that the user must have information that is relevant or applicable to his or her needs. If a healthcare provider is trying to decide whether a patient needs insulin and only the patient's CT scan information is available, this information is not relevant for that current need. However, if one needed information about the CT scan, the information is relevant.

Complete information contains all of the necessary essential data. If the healthcare provider needs to contact the only relative listed for the patient and his or her contact information is listed but the approval for that person to be a contact is missing, this information is considered incomplete. Flexible information means that the information can be used for a variety of purposes. Information concerning the inventory of supplies on a nursing unit, for example, can be used by nurses who need to know if an item is available for use for a patient. The nurse manager accesses this information to help decide which supplies need to be ordered, to determine which items are used most frequently, and to do an economic assessment of any waste.

Reliable information comes from reliable or clean data gathered from authoritative and credible sources. Objective information is as close to the truth as one can get; it is not subjective or biased, but rather is factual and impartial. If someone states something, it must be determined whether that person is reliable and whether what he or she is stating is objective or tainted by his or her own perspective.

Utility refers to the ability to provide the right information at the right time to the right person for the right purpose. Transparency allows users to apply their intellect to accomplish their tasks while the tools housing the information disappear into the background. Verifiable information means that one can check to verify or prove that the information is correct. Reproducibility refers to the ability to produce the same information again.

Information is acquired either by actively looking for it or by having it conveyed by the environment. All of the senses (vision, hearing, touch, smell, and taste) are used to gather input from the surrounding world, and as technologies mature, more and more **input** will be obtained through the senses. Currently, people receive information from computers (output) through vision, hearing, or touch (input); and the response (output) to the computer (input) is the interface with technology. Gesture recognition is increasing, and interfaces that incorporate it will change the way people become informed. Many people access the Internet on a daily basis seeking information or imparting information. Individuals are constantly becoming informed, discovering, or learning; becoming reinforced, rediscovering, or relearning; and purging what has been acquired. The information acquired through these processes is added to the personal knowledge base. **Knowledge** is the awareness and understanding of a set of information and ways that information can be made useful to support a specific task or arrive at a decision. This knowledge building is an ongoing process engaged in while a person is conscious and going about his or her normal daily activities.

# Information Science

Information science has evolved over the last 50 or so years as a field of scientific inquiry and professional practice. It can be thought of as the science of information, studying the application and usage of information and knowledge in organizations and the interface or interaction between people, organizations, and ISs. This extensive, interdisciplinary science integrates features from **cognitive science, communication science, computer science, library science,** and the **social sciences.** Information science is primarily concerned with the input, processing, output, and feedback of data and information through technology integration with a focus on comprehending the perspective of the **stakeholders** involved and then applying IT as needed. It is systemically based, dealing with the big picture rather than individual pieces of technology.

Information science can also be related to determinism. Specifically, it is a response to technologic determinism—the belief that technology develops by its own laws, that it realizes its own potential, limited only by the material resources available, and must therefore be regarded as an autonomous system controlling and ultimately permeating all other subsystems of society (Web Dictionary of Cybernetics and Systems, 2007, para. 1).

This approach sets the tone for the study of information as it applies to itself, the people, the technology, and the varied sciences that are contextually related depending on the needs of the setting or organization; what is important is the interface between the stakeholders and their systems, and the ways they generate, use, and locate information. According to Cornell University (2010), "Information Science brings together faculty, students and researchers who share an interest in combining computer science with the social sciences of how people and society interact with information" (para. 1). Information science is an interdisciplinary, people-oriented field that explores and enhances the interchange of information to transform society, communication science, computer science, cognitive science, library science, and the social sciences. Society is dominated by the need for information, and knowledge and information science focus on systems and individual users by fostering user-centered approaches that enhance society's information capabilities, effectively and efficiently linking people, information, and technology. This impacts the configuration and mix of organizations and influences the nature of work—namely, how knowledge workers interact with and produce meaningful information and knowledge.

# Information Processing

**Information science** enables the processing of information. This processing links people and technology. Humans are organic ISs, constantly acquiring, processing, and generating information or knowledge in their professional and personal lives. This high degree of knowledge, in fact, characterizes humans as extremely intelligent organic machines. The premise of this text revolves around this concept, and the text is organized on the basis of the Foundation of Knowledge model: knowledge **acquisition**, knowledge processing, knowledge generation, and knowledge dissemination.

**Information** is data that are processed using knowledge. For information to be valuable or meaningful, it must be accessible, accurate, timely, complete, cost-effective, flexible, reliable, relevant, simple, verifiable, and secure. Knowledge is the awareness and understanding of an information set and ways that information can be made useful to support a specific task or arrive at a decision. As an example, if an architect were going to design a building, part of the knowledge necessary for developing a new building is understanding how the building will be used, what size of building is needed compared to the available building space, and how many people will have or need access to this building. Therefore, the work of choosing or rejecting facts based on their significance or relevance to a particular task, such as designing a building, is also based on a type of knowledge used in the process of converting data into information. Information can then be considered data made functional through the application of knowledge. The knowledge used to develop and glean knowledge from valuable information is generative (having the ability to originate and produce or generate) in nature. Knowledge must also be viable. Knowledge viability refers to applications that offer easily accessible, accurate, and timely information obtained from a variety of resources and methods and presented in a manner so as to provide the necessary elements to generate knowledge.

Information science and computational tools are extremely important in enabling the processing of data, information, and knowledge in health care. In this environment, the hardware, software, networking, algorithms, and human organic ISs work together to create meaningful information and generate knowledge. The links between information processing and scientific discovery are paramount. However, without the ability to generate practical results that can be disseminated, the processing of data, information, and knowledge is for naught. It is the ability of machines (inorganic ISs) to support and facilitate the functioning of people (human organic ISs) that refines, enhances, and evolves nursing practice by generating knowledge. This knowledge represents five rights: the right information, accessible by the right people in the right settings, applied the right way at the right time.

An important and ongoing process is the struggle to integrate new knowledge and old knowledge so as to enhance wisdom. Wisdom is the ability to act appropriately; it assumes actions directed by one's own wisdom. Wisdom uses knowledge and experience to heighten common sense, and uses insight to exercise sound judgment in practical matters. It is developed through knowledge, experience, insight, and reflection. Wisdom is sometimes thought of as the highest form of common sense, resulting from accumulated knowledge or erudition (deep, thorough learning) or enlightenment (education that results in understanding and the dissemination of knowledge). It is the ability to apply valuable and viable knowledge, experience, understanding, and insight while being prudent and sensible. Knowledge and wisdom are not synonymous, because knowledge abounds with others' thoughts and information, whereas wisdom is focused on one's own mind and the synthesis of one's own experience, insight, understanding, and knowledge.

If clinicians are inundated with data without the ability to process it, the situation results in too much data and too little wisdom. Consequently, it is crucial that clinicians have viable ISs at their fingertips to facilitate the acquisition, sharing, and use of knowledge while maturing wisdom; this process leads to empowerment.

# Information Science and the Foundation of Knowledge

Information science is a multidisciplinary science that encompasses aspects of computer science, cognitive science, social science, communication science, and library science to deal with obtaining, gathering, organizing, manipulating, managing, storing, retrieving, recapturing, disposing of, distributing, and broadcasting information. Information science studies everything that deals with information and can be defined as the study of ISs. This science originated as a subdiscipline of computer science, as practitioners sought to understand and rationalize the management of technology within organizations. It has since matured into a major field of management and is now an important area of research in management studies. Moreover, information science has expanded its scope to examine the human–computer interaction, interfacing, and interaction of people, ISs, and corporations. It is taught at all major universities and business schools worldwide.

Modern-day organizations have become intensely aware of the fact that information and knowledge are potent resources that must be cultivated and honed to meet their needs. Thus information science or the study of ISs—that is, the application and usage of knowledge—focuses on why and how technology can be put to best use to serve the information flow within an organization.

Information science impacts information interfaces, influencing how people interact with information and subsequently develop and use knowledge. The information a person acquires is added to his or her knowledge base. Knowledge is the awareness and understanding of an information set and ways that information can be made useful to support a specific task or arrive at a decision.

Healthcare organizations are affected by and rely on the evolution of information science to enhance the recording and processing of routine and intimate information while facilitating human-to-human and human-to-systems communications, delivery of healthcare products, dissemination of information, and enhancement of the organization's business transactions. Unfortunately, the benefits and enhancements of information science technologies have also brought to light new risks, such as glitches and loss of information and hackers who can steal identities and information. Solid leadership, guidance, and vision are vital to the maintenance of cost-effective business performance and cutting-edge, safe information technologies for the organization. This field studies all facets of the building and use of information. The emergence of information science and its impact on information have also influenced how people acquire and use knowledge.

Information science has already had a tremendous impact on society and will undoubtedly expand its sphere of influence further as it continues to evolve and innovate human activities at all levels. What visionaries only dreamed of is now possible and part of reality. The future has yet to fully unfold in this important arena.

## Introduction to Information Systems

Consider the following scenario: You have just been hired by a large healthcare facility. You enter the personnel office and are told that you must learn a new language to work on the unit where you have been assigned. This language is used just on this unit. If you had been assigned to a different unit, you would have to learn another language that is specific to that unit, and so on. Because of the differences in various units' languages, interdepartmental sharing and information exchange (known as interoperability) are severely hindered.

This scenario might seem far-fetched, but it is actually how workers once operated in health care—in silos. There was a system for the laboratory, one for finance, one for clinical departments, and so on. As healthcare organizations have come to appreciate the importance of communication, tracking, and research, however, they have developed integrated **information systems** that can handle the needs of the entire organization.

Information and IT have become major resources for all types of organizations, and health care is no exception (see **Box 2-1**). Information technologies help to shape a healthcare organization, in conjunction with personnel, money, materials, and equipment. Many healthcare facilities have hired **chief information officers** (CIOs) or **chief technical officers** (CTOs), also known as **chief technology officers**. The CIO is involved with the IT infrastructure, and this role is sometimes expanded to include the position of chief knowledge officer. The CTO is focused on organizationally based scientific and technical issues and is responsible for technological research and development as part of the organization's products and services. The CTO and CIO must be visionary leaders for the organization, because so much of the business of health care relies on solid infrastructures that generate potent and timely information and

## BOX 2-1 EXAMPLES OF INFORMATION SYSTEMS

| Information System | How It Is Used |
|---|---|
| *Clinical Information System (CIS)* | Comprehensive and integrative system that manages the administrative, financial, and clinical aspects of a clinical facility; a CIS should help to link financial and clinical outcomes. An example is the EHR. |
| *Decision Support System (DSS)* | Organizes and analyzes information to help decision makers formulate decisions when they are unsure of their decision's possible outcomes. After gathering relevant and useful information, develops "what if" models to analyze the options or choices and alternatives. |
| *Executive Support System* | Collects, organizes, analyzes, and summarizes vital information to help executives or senior management with strategic decision making. Provides a quick view of all strategic business activities. |
| *Geographic Information System (GIS)* | Collects, manipulates, analyzes, and generates information related to geographic locations or the surface of the earth; provides output in the form of virtual models, maps, or lists. |
| *Management Information Systems (MIS)* | Provides summaries of internal sources of information, such as information from the transaction processing system, and develops a series of routine reports for decision making. |
| *Office Systems* | Facilitates communication and enhances the productivity of users needing to process data and information. |
| *Transaction Processing System (TPS)* | Processes and records routine business transactions, such as billing systems that create and send invoices to customers, and payroll systems that generate employees' pay stubs and wage checks and calculate tax payments. |
| *Hospital Information System (HIS)* | Manages the administrative, financial, and clinical aspects of a hospital enterprise. It should help to link financial and clinical outcomes. |

knowledge. The CTO and CIO are sometimes interchangeable positions, but in some organizations the CTO reports to the CIO. These positions will become critical roles as companies continue to shift from being product oriented to knowledge oriented, and as they begin emphasizing the production process itself rather than the product. In health care, ISs must be able to handle the volume of data and information necessary to generate the needed information and knowledge for best practices, because the goal is to provide the highest quality of patient care.

## Information Systems

ISs can be manually based, but for the purposes of this text, the term refers to **computer-based information systems** (CBISs). According to Jessup and Valacich (2008), CBISs "are combinations of hardware, software and telecommunications networks that people build and use to collect, create, and distribute useful data, typically in organizational settings" (p. 10). Along the same lines, ISs are also defined as "a collection of interconnected elements that gather, process, store and distribute data and information while providing a feedback structure to meet an objective" (Stair & Reynolds, 2016, p. 4). ISs are designed for specific purposes within organizations. They are only as functional as the decision-making capabilities, problem-solving skills, and programming potency built in and the quality of the data and information input into them. The capability of the IS to disseminate, provide feedback, and adjust the data and information based on these dynamic processes is what sets them apart. The IS should be a user-friendly entity that provides the right information at the right time and in the right place.

An IS acquires data or inputs; processes data through the retrieval, **analysis**, or **synthesis** of those data; disseminates or outputs information in the form of reports, documents, summaries, alerts, prompts, or outcomes; and provides for responses or feedback. Input or data acquisition is the activity of collecting and acquiring raw data. Input devices include combinations of hardware, software, and **telecommunications**, including keyboards, light pens, touch screens, mice or other pointing devices, automatic scanners, and machines that can read magnetic ink characters or lettering. To watch a pay-per-view movie, for example, the viewer must first input the chosen movie, verify the purchase, and have a payment method approved by the vendor. The IS must acquire this information before the viewer can receive the movie.

**Processing**—the retrieval, analysis, or synthesis of data—refers to the alteration and transformation of the data into helpful or useful information and outputs. The processing of data can range from storing it for future use; to comparing the data, making calculations, or applying formulas; to taking selective actions. Processing devices consist of combinations of hardware, software, and telecommunications and include processing chips where the central processing unit (CPU) and main memory are housed. Some of these chips are quite ingenious. According to Schupak (2005), the bunny chip could save the pharmaceutical industry money while sparing "millions of furry creatures, with a chip that mimics a living organism" (para. 1). The HµREL Corporation has developed environments or biologic ISs that reside on chips and actually mimic the functioning of the human body. Researchers can use these environments to test for both the harmful and beneficial effects of drugs, including those that are considered experimental and that could be harmful if used in human and animal testing. Such chips also allow researchers to monitor a drug's toxicity in the liver and other organs.

One patented HµREL microfluidic "biochip" comprises an arrangement of separate but fluidically interconnected "organ" or "tissue" compartments. Each compartment contains a culture of living cells drawn from, or engineered to mimic the primary functions of, the respective organ or tissue of a living animal. Microfluidic channels permit a culture medium that serves as a "blood surrogate" to recirculate just as in a living system, driven by a microfluidic pump. The geometry and fluidics of the device are fashioned to simulate the values of certain related physiologic parameters found in the living creature. Drug candidates or other substrates of interest are added to the culture medium and allowed to recirculate through the device. The effects of drug compounds and their metabolites on the cells within each respective organ compartment are then detected by measuring or monitoring key physiologic events. The cell types used may be derived from either standard cell culture lines or primary tissues (HµREL Corporation, 2010, para. 2–3). As new technologies such as the HµREL chips continue to evolve, more and more robust ISs that can handle a variety of biological and clinical applications will be seen.

Returning to the movie rental example, the IS must verify the data entered by the viewer and then process the request by following the steps necessary to provide access to the movie that was ordered. This processing must be instantaneous in today's world, where everyone wants everything *now*. After the data are processed, they are stored. In this case, the rental must also be processed so the vendor receives payment for the movie, whether electronically, via a credit card or checking account withdrawal, or by generating a bill for payment.

Output or **dissemination** produces helpful or useful information that can be in the form of reports, documents, summaries, alerts, or outcomes. A **report** is designed to inform and is generally tailored to the context of a given situation or user or user group. Reports may include charts, figures, tables, graphics, pictures, hyperlinks, references, or other documentation necessary to meet the needs of the user. A **document** represents information that can be printed, saved, emailed, or otherwise shared, or displayed. **Summaries** are condensed versions of the original information designed to highlight the major points. An **alert** is comprised of warnings, feedback, or additional information necessary to assist the user in interacting with the system. An **outcome** is the expected result of input and processing. **Output** devices are combinations of hardware, software, and telecommunications and include sound and speech synthesis outputs, printers, and monitors.

Continuing with the movie rental example, the IS must be able to provide the consumer with the movie ordered when it is wanted and somehow notify the purchaser that he or she has, indeed, purchased the movie and is granted access. The IS must also be able to generate payment either electronically or by generating a bill, while storing the transactional record for future use.

**Feedback** or responses are reactions to the inputting, processing, and outputs. In ISs, feedback refers to information from the system that is used to make modifications in the input, processing actions, or outputs. In the movie rental example, what if the consumer accidentally entered the same movie order three times, but really wanted to order the movie only once? The IS would determine that more than one movie order is out of range for the same movie order at the same time and provide feedback. Such feedback is used to verify and correct the input. If undetected, the viewer's error would result in an erroneous bill and decreased customer satisfaction while creating more work for the vendor, which would have to engage in additional transactions with the customer to resolve this problem. The *Nursing Informatics Practice Applications: Care Delivery* section of this text provides detailed descriptions of clinical ISs that operate on these same principles to support healthcare delivery.

## Summary

Information systems deal with the development, use, and management of an organization's IT infrastructure. An IS acquires data or inputs; processes data through the retrieval, analysis, or synthesis of those data; disseminates or outputs in the form of reports, documents, summaries, alerts, or outcomes; and provides for responses or feedback. Quality decision-making and problem-solving skills are vital to the development of effective, valuable ISs. Today's organizations now recognize that their most precious asset is their information, as represented by their employees, experience, competence or know-how, and innovative or novel approaches, all of which are dependent on a robust information network that encompasses the information technology infrastructure.

In an ideal world, all ISs would be fluid in their ability to adapt to any and all users' needs. They would be Internet oriented and global, where resources are available to everyone. Think of **cloud computing**—it is just the beginning point from which ISs will expand and grow in their ability to provide meaningful information to their users. As technologies advance, so will the skills and capabilities to comprehend and realize what ISs can become. As wearable tracking technologies and other health-related mobile applications expand, more robust and timely health data will be generated, and this data will need to be processed into meaningful information. "Practitioners and medical researchers can look forward to technologies that enable them to apply data analysis to develop new insights into finding cures for difficult diseases. Healthcare CIOs and other IT leaders can expect to be called upon to manage all the new data and devices that will be transforming healthcare as we know it" (Schindler, 2015, para. 2). Devices with sensors communicating with each other is known as the **Internet of Things (IoT)** and the future possibilities for health care are tremendous. "The IoT raises the bar—enabling connection and communication from anywhere to anywhere—and allows analytics to replace the human decision-maker" (Glasser, 2015, para. 3). Essentially, the sensor-collected data are transmitted to another technology, triggering an action or an alert that prompts feedback for an action. For example, "imagine a miniaturized, implanted device or skin patch that monitors a diabetic's blood sugar, movement, skin temperature and more, and informs an insulin pump to adjust the dosage" (para. 8).

It is important to continue to develop and refine functional, robust, visionary ISs that meet the current meaningful information needs while evolving systems that are even better prepared to handle future information and knowledge needs of the healthcare industry.

## THOUGHT-PROVOKING QUESTIONS

1. How do you acquire information? Choose 2 hours out of your busy day and try to notice all of the information that you receive from your environment. Keep diaries indicating where the information came from and how you knew it was information and not data.
2. Reflect on an IS with which you are familiar, such as the automatic banking machine. How does this IS function? What are the advantages of using this system (i.e., why not use a bank teller instead)? What are the disadvantages? Are there enhancements that you would add to this system?
3. In health care, think about a typical day of practice and describe the setting. How many times does the nurse interact with ISs? What are the ISs that we interact with, and how do we access them? Are they at the bedside, handheld, or station based? How do their location and ease of access impact nursing care?
4. Briefly describe an organization and discuss how our need for information and knowledge impacts the configuration and interaction of that organization with other organizations. Also discuss how the need for information and knowledge influences the nature of work or how knowledge workers interact with and produce information and knowledge in this organization.
5. If you could meet only four of the rights discussed in this chapter, which one would you omit and why? Also, provide your rationale for each right you chose to meet.

# References

Cornell University. (2010). Information science. Retrieved from http://www.infosci.cornell.edu

Goldstein, D., Groen, P., Ponkshe, S., & Wine, M. (2007). *Medical informatics 20/20*. Sudbury, MA: Jones and Bartlett.

Glasser, J. (2015). How the Internet of Things will affect health care. *Hospitals and Health Networks*. Retrieved from http://www.hhnmag.com/articles/3438-how-the-internet-of -things-will-affect-health-care

HµREL Corporation. (2010). Human-relevant: HµREL. Technology overview. Retrieved from http://www.hurelcorp.com/overview.php

Jessup, L., & Valacich, J. (2008). *Information systems today* (3rd ed.). Upper Saddle River, NJ: Pearson Prentice Hall.

Schindler, E. (2015). Healthcare IT: Hot Trends for 2016, Part 1. *InformationWeek*. Retrieved from http://www.informationweek.com/healthcare/leadership/healthcare-it-hot-trends-for -2016-part-1/d/d-id/1323722

Schupak, A. (2005). Technology: The bunny chip. *Forbes*. Retrieved from http://www.forbes .com/forbes/2005/0815/053.html

Stair, R., & Reynolds, G. (2016). *Principles of information systems* (12th ed.). Boston, MA: Cengage Learning.

Web Dictionary of Cybernetics and Systems. (2007). Technological determinism. Retrieved from http://pespmc1.vub.ac.be/ASC/TECHNO_DETER.html

1. Describe the essential components of computer systems, including both hardware and software.

2. Recognize the rapid evolution of computer systems and the benefit of keeping up-to-date with current trends and developments.

3. Analyze how computer systems function as tools for managing information and generating knowledge.

4. Define the concept of human–technology interfaces.

5. Assess how computers can support collaboration, networking, and information exchange.

## Key Terms

» Acquisition
» AMOLED (Active Matrix Organic Light-Emitting Diode)
» Applications
» Arithmetic logic units
» Basic input/output system (BIOS)
» Binary system
» Bit
» Bus
» Byte
» Cache memory
» Central processing unit (CPU)
» Cloud computing
» Cloud storage
» Communication software
» Compact disk read-only memory (CD-ROM)
» Compact disk-recordable (CD-R)
» Compact disk-rewritable (CD-RW)
» Compatibility
» Computer
» Computer science
» Conferencing software
» Creativity software

» Database
» Desktop
» Digital video disk (DVD)
» Digital video disk-recordable (DVD-R)
» Digital video disk-rewritable (DVD-RW)
» Dissemination
» Dots per inch (DPI) switch
» Double data rate synchronous dynamic random-access memory (DDR SDRAM)
» Dynamic random access memory (DRAM)
» Email
» Email client
» Electronically erasable programmable read-only memory (EEPROM)
» Embedded device
» Exabyte (EB)
» Executes
» Extensibility
» FireWire
» Firmware
» Flash memory
» Gigabyte (GB)
» Gigahertz

» Graphical user interface
» Graphics card
» Haptic
» Hard disk
» Hard drive
» Hardware
» High-definition multimedia interface (HDMI)
» Information
» Information Age
» Infrastructure as a service (IaaS)
» Instant message (IM)
» Integrated drive electronics (IDE)
» Internet browser
» IPS LCD (In-Plane Switching Liquid Crystal Display)
» Keyboard
» Knowledge
» Laptop
» Main memory
» Mainframes
» Megabyte (MB)
» Megahertz
» Memory
» Microprocessor
» Microsoft Surface
» Millions of instructions per second (MIPS)

» Mobile device
» Modem
» Monitor
» Motherboard
» Mouse
» MPEG-1 Audio Layer-3 (MP3)
» Networks
» Office suite
» Open source
» Operating system (OS)
» Parallel port
» Peripheral component interconnection (PCI)
» Personal computer (PC)
» Petabytes (PB)
» Platform as a service (PaaS)
» Plug and play
» Port
» Portability
» Portable operating system interface for UNIX (POSIX)
» Power supply
» Presentation
» Private cloud
» Processing
» Processor
» Productivity software

# CHAPTER 3

# Computer Science and the Foundation of Knowledge Model

Dee McGonigle, Kathleen Mastrian, and June Kaminski

| | | | |
|---|---|---|---|
| » Professional development | » Read-only memory (ROM) | » Synchronous dynamic random-access memory (SDRAM) | » User interface |
| » Programmable read-only memory (PROM) | » Security | | » Video adapter card |
| | » Serial port | | » Virtual memory |
| » Public cloud | » Small Computer System Interface (SCSI) | » Technology | » Wearable technology |
| » Publishing | | » Terabytes (TB) | » Wi-Fi |
| » Quantum bits (Qubits) | | » Throughput | » Wisdom |
| | » Software | » Touch pad | » Word processing |
| » Quantum computing | » Software as a service (SaaS) | » Touch screen | » World Wide Web (WWW) |
| » QWERTY | » Sound card | » Universal serial bus (USB) | » Yottabyte (YB) |
| » Random-access memory (RAM) | » Spreadsheet | » USB flash drive | » Zettabyte (ZB) |
| | » Supercomputers | » User friendly | |

## Introduction

In this chapter, the discipline of computer science is introduced through a focus on computers and the hardware and software that make up these evolving systems; computer science is one of the building blocks of nursing informatics (refer to **Figure 3-1**). **Computer science** offers extremely valuable tools that, if used skillfully, can facilitate the **acquisition** and manipulation of data and **information** by nurses, who can then synthesize these into an evolving knowledge and **wisdom** base. This process can facilitate **professional development** and the ability to apply evidence-based practice decisions within nursing care, and if the results are disseminated and shared, can also advance the professional knowledge base.

This chapter begins with a look at common computer hardware, followed by a brief overview of operating, productivity, creativity, and communication software. It concludes with a glimpse at how computer systems help to shape knowledge and collaboration and an introduction to human–technology interface dynamics.

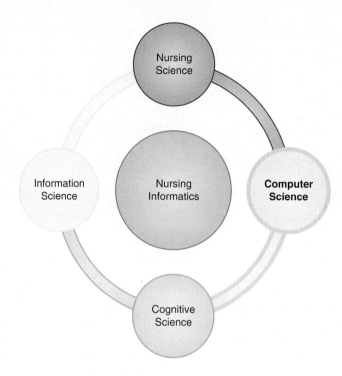

**Figure 3-1**  Building Blocks of Nursing Informatics

# The Computer as a Tool for Managing Information and Generating Knowledge

Throughout history, various milestones have signaled discoveries, inventions, or philosophic shifts that spurred a surge in **knowledge** and understanding within the human race. The advent of the computer is one such milestone, which has sparked an intellectual metamorphosis whose boundaries have yet to be fully understood. Computer **technology** has ushered in what has been called the **Information Age**, an age when data, information, and knowledge are both accessible and able to be manipulated by more people than ever before in history. How can a mere machine lead to such a revolutionary state of knowledge potential? To begin to answer this question, it is best to examine the basic structure and components of computer systems.

Essentially, a **computer** is an electronic information-processing machine that serves as a tool with which to manipulate data and information. The easiest way to begin to understand computers is to realize they are input–output systems. These unique machines accept data input via a variety of devices, process data through logical and arithmetic rendering, store the data in memory components, and output data and information to the user.

Since the advent of the first electronic computer in the mid-1940s, computers have evolved to become essential tools in every walk of life, including the profession of nursing. The complexity of computers has increased dramatically over the years, and will continue to do so. "Computing has changed the world more than any other invention of the past hundred years, and has come to pervade nearly all human endeavors. Yet, we are just at the beginning of the computing revolution; today's computing offers just a glimpse of the potential impact of computers" (Evans, 2010, p. 3). Major computer manufacturers and researchers, such as Intel, have identified the need to design computers to mask this growing complexity. The sophistication of computers is evolving at amazing speed, yet ease of use or **user-friendly** aspects are also increasing accordingly. This is achieved by honing hardware and software capabilities until they work seamlessly together to ensure user-friendly, intuitive tools for users of all levels of expertise. **Box 3-1** provides information about **haptic** technology, computing surfaces, and multi-touch interfaces, which are evolving technologies.

## BOX 3-1 IMMERSION, MICROSOFT, AND PQ LABS INTERFACES

### Dee McGonigle

Do not get too attached to your mouse and keyboard, because they will be outdated soon if Immersion, Microsoft, and PQ Labs have their way. From Immersion's (2016) haptic technology, the **Microsoft Surface** (Microsoft Corporation, 2016), and PQ Labs (2016) multi-touch capabilities, have you ever thought of digital information you can touch and grab? The sense of touch is a powerful sense that we use daily. Haptic technology continues to advance and "brings the sense of touch to digital content" (Immersion, 2016, para. 4). Haptic technology combined with a visual display can be used to prepare users for tasks necessitating hand–eye coordination, such as surgical procedures. Microsoft and PQ Labs are leading us into and evolving the next generation of computing, known as surface or table computing. Surface or table computing consists of a multi-touch, multiuser interface that allows one to "grab" digital information and then collaborate, share, and store that information, without using a mouse or keyboard—just the hands and fingers and devices such as a digital camera or smartphone. These interfaces can actually sense objects, touch, and gestures from many users.

We can enter a restaurant and interact with the menu through the surface of the table where you sit to eat. Once you have completed your order, you can begin computing by using the capabilities built into the surface or using your own device, such as a smartphone. You can set a smartphone on the table's surface and download images, graphics, and text to the surface. You can even communicate with others using full audio and video while waiting for your order. When you have finished eating, you simply set your credit card on the surface and it is automatically charged; you pick up your credit card and leave. This is a different kind of eating experience—but one that will become commonplace for the next generation of users. You can routinely experience this in Las Vegas, as well as in selected casinos, banks, restaurants, and hotels throughout the world.

You should seek to explore this new interface, which will forever change how we interact and compute. Think of the ramifications for health care especially as it relates to the haptic experience and wearables. Explore the Immersion reference provided for you.

**REFERENCES**

Immersion. (2016). Touch. Feel. Engage. Retrieved from http://www.immersion.com
    /wearables
Microsoft Corporation. (2016). Designed on Surface: A global art project. Retrieved from
    https://www.microsoft.com/surface/en-us/art
PQ Labs. (2016). Introducing G5: 4K Touch Fidelity. Retrieved from http://multitouch
    .com/product.html

As our capabilities evolve, so does the complexity of computer operations. The goal for vendors that provide computer systems and software is to decrease the learning curve for the user while enhancing the user's capacity to manipulate the system to meet their computing needs. Therefore, the complexity of the operation is concealed by the ease of use.

One example of this type of complexity masked in simplicity is the evolution of "**plug and play**" computer add-ons, where a peripheral, such as an iPod or game console, can be simply plugged into a serial or other **port** and instantly used.

Computers are universal machines, because they are general-purpose, symbol-manipulating devices that can perform any task represented in specific programs. For instance, they can be used to draw an image, calculate statistics, write an essay, or record nursing care data. In a nutshell, computers can be used for data and information storage, retrieval, analysis, generation, and transformation.

Most computers are based on scientist John Von Neumann's model of a processor–memory–input–output architecture. In this model, the logic unit and control unit are parts of the processor, the **memory** is the storage region, and the input and output segments are provided by the various computer devices, such as the keyboard, mouse, monitor, and printer. Recent developments have provided alternative configurations to the Von Neumann model—for example, the parallel computing model, where multiple processors are set up to work together. Nevertheless, today's computer systems share the same basic configurations and components inherent in the earliest computers.

# Components

## Hardware

Computer **hardware** refers to the actual physical body of the computer and its components. Several key components in the average computer work together to shape a complex yet highly usable machine that serves as a tool for knowledge management, communication, and creativity.

## Protection: The Casing

The most noticeable component of any computer is the outer case. **Desktop** personal computers have either a desktop case, which lies horizontally (flat) on a desk, often with the computer monitor positioned on top of it; or a tower case, which stands vertically, and usually sits beside the monitor or on a lower shelf or the floor. Most cases come equipped with a case fan, which is extremely critical for keeping the computer components cool when in use. **Laptop** and surface computers combine the components into a flat rectangular casing that is attached to the hinged or foldable monitor. Smartphones also have a protective outer plastic or metal case with a display screen.

## Central Processing Unit (CPU)/Processor

The **central processing unit (CPU)** is an older term for the **processor** and **microprocessor**. Sometimes conceptualized as the "brain" of the computer, the processor is the computer component that actually **executes**, calculates, and processes the binary computer code (which consists of various configurations of 0s and 1s), instigated by the **operating system (OS)** and other **applications** on the computer. The processor and microprocessor serve as the command center that directs the actions of all other computer components, and they manage both incoming and outgoing data that are processed across components. Some of the best processors include the AMD FX-9590, AMD FX-8320, AMD FX-6300, Intel Core i7-5820K, Intel Core i7- 4930K, Intel Core i7-5960X, Intel Core i5-6600K, and Intel Xeon processor (Futuremark, 2016).

The processor contains specific mechanical units, including registers, **arithmetic logic units**, a floating point unit, control circuitry, and cache memory. Together, these inner components form the computer's central processor. Registers consist of data-storing circuits whose contents are processed by the adjacent arithmetic and logic units or the floating point unit. **Cache memory** is extremely quick memory that holds whatever data and code are being used at any one time. The processor uses the cache to store in-process data so that it can be quickly retrieved as needed. The processor is protected by a heat sink, a copper or aluminum metal block that cools the processor (often with the help of a fan) to prevent overheating (refer to Figure 3-2).

In the past, the speed and power of a processor were measured in units of **megahertz** and was written as a value in MHz (e.g., 400 MHz, meaning the microprocessor ran at 400 MHz, executing 400 million cycles per second). Today, it is more common to see the speed measured in **gigahertz** (1 GHz is equal to 1,000 MHz); thus a processor that operates at 4 GHz is 1,000 times faster than an older one that operated at 4 MHz. The more cycles a processor can complete per second, the faster computer programs can run. However, according to Anderson (2016),

> Intel has said that new technologies in chip manufacturing will favour better energy consumption over faster execution times—effectively calling an end to "Moore's Law," which successfully predicted the doubling of density in integrated circuits, and therefore speed, every two years. (para. 1)

For example, the Intel Xeon processor E5-2699 v4 has a speed of 2.20 Ghz with 55 MB cache (Intel Corporation, 2016), making it more efficient at a lower speed.

In recent years, processor manufacturers, such as Intel, have moved to multicore microprocessors, which are chips that combine two or more processors. In fact, multiple microprocessors have become a standard in both personal and professional-level computers. Minicomputers were replaced by servers using microprocessors and multi-processors have replaced most **mainframes**.

As **mobile devices** and **embedded devices** are being integrated into our daily routines, mainframes can create secure transactions with the analytics necessary for organizations

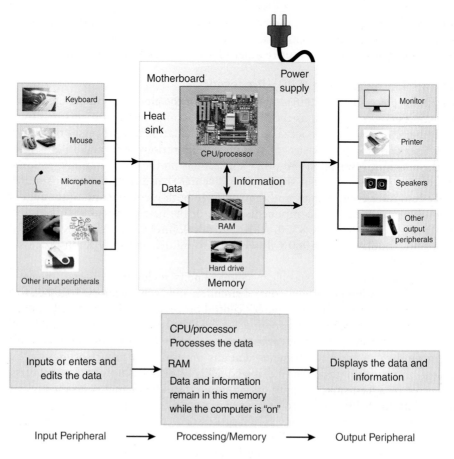

**Figure 3-2** Computer Components

to improve their business processes. IBM has found its niche and continues to build mainframes. According to Alba (2015),

> The concept of a "mobile transaction" is a bit of marketing-speak. Tons of transactions take place via mobile devices, and the mainframe is good at transaction processing. Put them together, and voilà: a computer the size of a backyard shed becomes a mobile product. (para. 6)

Powerful **supercomputers** are also using collections of microprocessors.

## Motherboard

The **motherboard** has been called the "central nervous system" of the computer because it facilitates communication among all of the different computer components. This makes it a key foundational component because all other components are connected to it in some way (either directly via local sockets, attached directly to it, or connected via cables). This includes **universal serial bus (USB)** controllers, Ethernet network controllers, integrated graphics controllers, and so forth. The essential structures of the motherboard include the major chipset, Super Input/Output chip, basic input/output system read-only memory, **bus** communications pathways, and a variety of sockets that allow components to plug into the board. The chipset (often a pair of chips) determines the computer's CPU type and memory. It also houses the north bridge and south bridge controllers that allow the buses to transfer data from one to another.

## Power Supply

The **power supply** is a critical component of any computer, because it provides the essential electrical energy needed to allow a computer to operate. The power supply unit converts the 120-volt AC main power (provided via the power cable from the wall socket into which the computer is plugged) into low-voltage DC power. Computers depend on a reliable, steady supply of DC power to function properly. The more devices and programs used on a computer, the larger the power supply should be to avoid damage and malfunctioning. Power supplies normally range from 160 to 700 watts, with an average of 300 to 400 watts. Most contemporary power supply units come equipped with at least one fan to cool the unit under heavy use. The power supply is controlled by pressing the on and off switch, as well as the reset switch (which restarts the system) of a computer.

Laptop and other portable computing machines, such as electronic readers and tablet computers, are equipped with a both rechargeable battery power supply and the standard plug-in variety.

## Hard Disk

This component is so named because of the rigid hard disks that reside in it, which are mounted to a spindle that is spun by a motor when in use. Drive heads (most computers have two or more heads) produce a magnetic field through their transducers that magnetizes the disk surface as a voltage is applied to the disk. The **hard disk** acts as a permanent data storage area that holds gigabytes (GB) or even terabytes (TB) worth of data, information, documents, and programs saved on the computer, even when the computer is shut off. Disk drives are not infallible, however, so backing up important data is imperative.

The computer writes binary data to the hard drive by magnetizing small areas of its surface. Each drive head is connected to an actuator that moves along the disk to hover over any point on the disk surface as it spins. The parts of the hard disk are encased in a sealed unit. The hard drive is managed by a disk controller, which is a circuit board that controls the motor and actuator arm assembly. The **hard drive** produces the voltage waveform that contacts the heads to write and read data, and handles communications with the motherboard. It is usually located within the computer's hard outer casing. Some people also attach a second hard drive externally, to increase available memory or to back up data.

## Main Memory or Random-Access Memory

**Random-access memory (RAM)** is considered to be volatile memory because it is a temporary storage system that allows the processor to access program codes and data while working on a task. The contents of RAM are lost once the system is rebooted, is shut off, or loses power.

The memory is actually situated on small chip boards, which sport rows of pins along the bottom edge and are plugged into the motherboard of the computer. These memory chips contain complex arrays of tiny memory circuits that can be either set by the processor during write operations (puts them into storage) or read during data retrieval. The circuits store the data in binary form as either a low (on) voltage stage, expressed as a 0, or a high (off) voltage stage, expressed as a 1. All of the work being done on a computer resides in RAM until it is saved onto the hard drive or other storage drive. Computers generally come with 2 GB of RAM or more, and some offer more RAM via **graphics cards** and other expansion cards.

A certain portion of the RAM, called the **main memory**, serves the hard disk and facilitates interactions between the hard disk and central processor. Main memory is provided by **dynamic random access memory (DRAM)** and is attached to the processor using specific addresses and data buses.

**Synchronous dynamic random-access memory (SDRAM)** (also known as static dynamic RAM) protects its data bits. The newer chip is **double data rate synchronous dynamic random-access memory (DDR SDRAM)** that allows for greater bandwidth and twice the transfers per the computer's internal clock's unit of time.

### Read-Only Memory

**Read-only memory (ROM)** is essential permanent or semipermanent nonvolatile memory that stores saved data and is critical in the working of the computer's OS and other activities. ROM is stored primarily in the motherboard, but it may also be available through the graphics card, other expansion cards, and peripherals. In recent years, rewritable ROM chips that may include other forms of ROM, such as **programmable read-only memory (PROM)**, erasable ROM, **electronically erasable programmable read-only memory (EEPROM)**, and **flash memory** (a variation of electronically erasable programmable ROM), have become available.

### Basic Input/Output System

The **basic input/output system (BIOS)** is a specific type of ROM used by the computer when it first boots up to establish basic communication between the processor, motherboard, and other components. Often called boot firmware, it controls the computer from the time the machine is switched on until the primary OS (e.g., Windows, Mac OS X, or Linux) takes over. The **firmware** initializes the hardware and boots (loads and executes) the primary OS.

### Virtual Memory

**Virtual memory** is a special type of memory that is stored on the hard disk to provide temporary data storage so data can be swapped in and out of the RAM as needed. This capability is particularly handy when working with large data-intensive programs, such as games and multimedia.

### Integrated Drive Electronics Controller

The **integrated drive electronics (IDE)** controller component is the primary interface for the hard drive, **compact disk read-only memory (CD-ROM)**, **digital video disk (DVD)** drive, and the floppy disk drive (found largely on pre-2010 computers).

## Peripheral Component Interconnection Bus

This component is important for connecting additional plug-in components to the computer. It uses a series of slots on the motherboard to allow **peripheral component interconnection (PCI)** card plug-in.

## Small Computer System Interface

The **Small Computer System Interface (SCSI)** component provides the means to attach additional devices, such as scanners and extra hard drives, to the computer.

## DVD/CD Drive

The CD-ROM drive reads and records data to portable CDs, using a laser diode to emit an infrared light beam that reflects onto a track on the CD using a mirror positioned by a motor. The light reflected on the disk is directed by a system of lenses to a photodetector that converts the light pulses into an electrical signal; this signal is then decoded by the drive electronics to the motherboard. There are **compact disk-recordable (CD-R)** and **compact disk-rewritable (CD-RW), digital video disk-recordable (DVD-R),** and **digital video disk-rewritable (DVD-RW)** drives. A DVD drive can do everything a CD drive can do, plus it can play the content of disks and, if it is a recordable unit, can record data on blank DVDs.

## Flash or USB Flash Drive

This portable memory device uses electronically erasable programmable ROM to provide fast permanent memory. The **USB flash drive** is typically a removable and rewritable device that includes flash memory and an integrated USB interface. They are easily portable due to their small size and are durable and dependable, and obtain their power from the device they are connected to via the USB port.

## Modem

A **modem** is a component that can be situated either externally (external modem) or internally (internal modem) relative to the computer and enables Internet connectivity via a cable connection through network adapters situated within the computer apparatus.

## Connection Ports

All computers have connection ports made to fit different types of plug-in devices. These ports include a monitor cable port, keyboard and mouse ports, a network cable port, microphone/speaker/auxiliary input ports, USB ports, and printer ports (SCSI or parallel). These ports allow data to move to and from the computer via peripheral or storage devices. Specific ports include the following:

- **Parallel port:** Connects to a printer
- **Serial port:** Connects to an external modem
- USB: Connects to a myriad of plug-in devices, such as portable flash drives, digital cameras, **MPEG-1 Audio Layer-3 (MP3)** players, graphics tablets, and light pens, using a plug-and-play connection (the ability to add devices automatically). The development of the USB Type-C–to–**high definition multimedia interface (HDMI)** adapter (Sexton, 2016) has expanded connectivity and transfer. HDMI is replacing analog video standards as an audio/video interface that can transfer

compressed and uncompressed video and digital audio data from any device that is HDMI-compliant to compatible monitors, televisions, video projectors, and audio devices.
- FireWire (IEEE 1394): Often used to connect digital-video devices to the computer
- Ethernet: Connects networking apparatus, such as Internet and modem cables

## Graphics Card

Most computers come equipped with a graphics accelerator card slotted in the microprocessor of a computer to process image data and output those data to the monitor. These in situ graphic cards provide satisfactory graphics quality for two-dimensional art and general text and numerical data. However, if a user intends to create or view three-dimensional images or is an active game user, one or more graphics enhancement cards are often installed.

## Video Adapter Cards

Video adapter cards provide video memory, a video processor, and a digital-to-analog converter that works with the processor to output higher quality video images to the monitor.

## Sound Card

The sound card converts digital data into an analog signal that is then output to the computer's speakers or headphones. The reverse is also accomplished by inputting a signal from a microphone or other audio recording equipment, which then converts the analog signal to a digital signal.

## Bit

A bit is the smallest possible chunk of data memory used in computer processing and is depicted as either a 1 or a 0. Bits make up the binary system of the computer.

## Byte

A byte is a chunk of memory that consists of 8 bits; it is considered to be the best way to indicate computer memory or storage capacity. In modern computers, bytes are described in units of megabytes (MB); gigabytes (GB), where 1 GB equals 1,000 MB; or terabytes (TB), where 1 TB equals 1 trillion bytes or 1,000 GB. Box 3-2 discusses storage capacities.

### BOX 3-2 STORAGE CAPACITIES

*Dee McGonigle and Kathleen Mastrian*

Storage and memory capacities are evolving. In the past few decades, there have been great leaps in data storage. It all begins with the bit, the basic unit of data storage, composed of 0s and 1s, also known as binary digits. A byte is generally considered to be equal to 8 bits. The files on a computer are stored as binary files. The software that is used translates these binary files into words, numbers, pictures, images, or video. Using this binary code in the binary numbering system, measurement is counted by factors of 2, such as 1, 2, 4, 8, 16, 32, 64, and 128. These multiples of the binary system in computer usage are also prefixed based on the metric system. Therefore, a kilobyte (KB) is actually 2 to the 10th power (210) or 1,024 bytes, but is typically considered to be 1,000 bytes. This is why one sees 1,024 or multiples of that number instead of an even 1,000 mentioned at times in relation to kilobytes.

In the early 1980s, kilobytes were the norm as far as computer capacity went, and 128 KB machines were launched for personal use. Subsequent decades, however, have seen advanced computing power and storage capacity. As capabilities soared, so did the ability to save and store what was used and created. Megabytes (MB) emerged as a common unit of measure; 1 megabyte is 1,048,576 bytes but is considered to be roughly equivalent to 1 million bytes. The next leap in computer capacity was one that some people could not even imagine: gigabytes (GB). A gigabyte is 1,073,741,824 bytes but is generally rounded to 1 billion bytes. Some computing experts are very concerned that valuable bytes are lost when these measurements are rounded, whereas hard drive manufacturers use the decimal system so their capacity is expressed as an even 1 billion bytes per gigabyte.

Computer capacity has moved into and beyond the range of terabytes, with capacities moving into the range of **petabytes (PB)**, **exabytes (EB)**, **zettabytes (ZB)**, and **yottabytes (YB)**. These terms for storage capacity are defined as follows:

1 TB = 1,000 GB
1 PB = 1,000,000 GB
1 EB = 1,000 PB
1 ZB = 1,000 EB
1 YB = 1,000 ZB

To put all of this in perspective, Lyman and Varian describe the data powers of 10:

 2 KB: A typewritten page
2 MB: A high-resolution photograph
10 MB: A minute of high-fidelity sound *or* a digital chest X-ray
50 MB: A digital mammogram
1 GB: A symphony in high-fidelity sound *or* a movie at TV quality
1 TB: All the X-ray films in a large, technologically advanced hospital
2 PB: The contents of all U.S. academic research libraries
5 EB: All words ever spoken by human beings

We have not even addressed ZB and YB. Stay tuned . . .

## REFERENCE

Lyman, P., & Varian, H. R. (2003). How much information? Retrieved from http://groups .ischool.berkeley.edu/archive/how-much-info-2003/

## Software

**Software** comprises the application programs developed to facilitate various user functions, such as writing, artwork, organizing meetings, surfing the Internet, communicating with others, and so forth. For the purposes of this overview, the various types of software have been divided into four categories: (1) OS software, (2) productivity software, (3) **creativity software**, and (4) communication software.

User friendliness is a critical condition for effective software adoption. The easier and more intuitive a software package seems to be to a user influences that user's perception of how clear the package is to understand and to use. The rapid evolution of hardware mentioned previously has been equally matched by the phenomenal development in software over the past three or four decades.

### Commercial Software

Several large commercial software companies, such as Apple, Microsoft, IBM, and Adobe, dominate the market for software, and have done so since the advent of the **personal computer (PC)**. Licensed software has evolved over time; hence, most products have a long version history. Many software packages, such as office suites, are expensive to purchase; in turn, there is a "digital divide" as far as access and affordability go across societal spheres, especially when viewed from a global perspective.

### Open Source Software

The **open source** initiative began in the late 1990s and has become a powerful movement that is changing the software production and consumer market. In addition to commercially available software, a growing number of open source software packages are being developed in all four of the categories addressed in this chapter. The open source movement was begun by developers who wished to offer their creations to others for the good of the community and encouraged them to do the same. Users who modify or contribute to the evolution of open source software are obligated to share their new code, but essentially the software is free to all. Apache OpenOffice, Google Docs, and NeoOffice are examples of open source productivity software (refer to Figure 3-3).

### OS Software

The OS is the most important software on any computer. It is the very first program to load on computer start-up and is fundamental for the operation of all other software and the computer hardware. Examples of commonly used OSs include the Microsoft Windows family, Linux, and Mac OS X. The OS manages both the hardware and the software and provides a reliable, consistent interface for the software applications to work with the computer's hardware. An OS must be both powerful and flexible to adapt to the myriad of types of software available, which are made by a variety of development companies. New versions of the major OSs are equipped to deal with multiple users and handle multitasking with ease. For example, a user can work on a word processing document while listening for an "email received" signal, have an **Internet browser** window open to look for references on the Internet as needed, listen to music in the CD drive, and download a file—all at the same time.

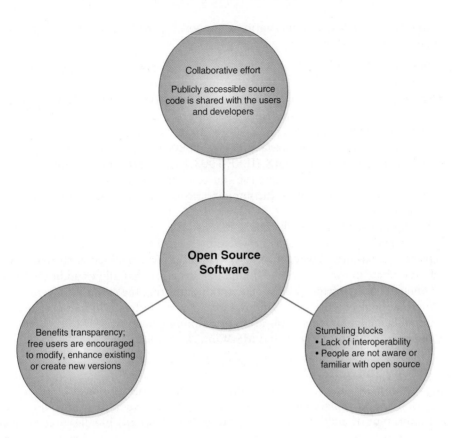

**Figure 3-3** Open Source Software

OS tasks can be described in terms of six basic processes:

- Memory management
- Device management
- Processor management
- Storage management
- Application interface
- **User interface** (usually a **graphical user interface** [GUI])

A GUI (pronounced "gooey") is used by OSs to display a combination of graphics and text such as icons, drop-down menus, and buttons; it allows you to use input and output devices as well as icons that represent files, programs, actions, and processes.

OSs should be convenient to use, easy to learn, reliable, safe, and fast. They should also be easy to design, implement, and maintain and should be flexible, reliable, error free, and efficient. For example, Silbershatz, Baer Galvin, and Gagne (2013) described how "Microsoft's design goals for Windows included security, reliability, Windows and POSIX application compatibility, high performance, extensibility, portability, and international support" (p. 831). The following goals were established by Microsoft:

- **Portability:** The OS can be moved from one hardware architecture to another with few changes needed.
- **Security:** The OS incorporates hardware protection for virtual memory and software protection mechanisms for OS resources, including encryption and digital signature capabilities.
- **Portable operating system interface for Unix (POSIX)** compliance: Applications designed to follow the POSIX (IEEE 1003.1) standard can be compiled to run on Windows without changing the source code. Windows OSs have varying levels of compatibility with the applications that ran on earlier versions of Windows OSs.
- Multiprocessor support: The OS is designed for symmetrical multiprocessing.
- **Extensibility:** This capability is provided by using a layered architecture with a protected executive layer for basic system services, several server subsystems that operate in user mode, and a modular structure that allows additional environmental subsystems to be added without affecting the executive layer.
- International support: The Windows OS supports different locales via the national language support application programming interface (API).
- **Compatibility** with MS-DOS and MS-Windows applications.

## Productivity Software

**Productivity software,** such as an **office suite,** is the type of software most commonly used both in the workplace and on personal computers. Several software companies produce this type of multiple-program software, which usually bundles together **word processing, spreadsheet, database, presentation,** Web development, and **email** programs.

The intent of office suites is generally to provide all of the basic programs that office or knowledge workers need to do their work. The bundled programs within the suite are organized to be compatible with one another, are designed to look similar to one another for ease of use, and provide a powerful array of tools for data manipulation, information gathering, and knowledge generation. Some office suites add other programs, such as database creation software, mathematical editors, drawing, and desktop **publishing** programs. Table 3-1 summarizes the application of programs included in some of the popular office suites: Microsoft Office, Apache OpenOffice, NeoOffice, Corel WordPerfect Suite, and Apple iWork.

## Creative Software

Creative software includes programs that allow users to draw, paint, render, record music and sound, and incorporate digital video and other multimedia in professional aesthetic ways to share and convey information and knowledge (Table 3-2).

## Communication Software

Networking and **communication software** enable users to dialogue, share, and network with other users via the exchange of email or **instant message (IM),** by accessing the World Wide Web, or by engaging in virtual meetings using **conferencing** software (Table 3-3)

Table 3-1 Office Suite Software Features and Examples

| Office Suite Software | | |
|---|---|---|
| **Program** | **Application** | **Examples** |
| Word processing | Composition, editing, formatting, and producing text documents | Microsoft Word, Open Office Writer, KOffice KWord, Corel WordPerfect or Corel Write, Apple Pages |
| Spreadsheets | Grid-based documents in ledger format; organizes numbers and text; calculates statistical formulae | Microsoft Excel, Open Office Calc, KOffice KSpread, Corel Quattro Pro, Apple Numbers |
| Presentations | Slideshow software, usually used for business or classroom presentations using text, images, graphs, media | Microsoft PowerPoint, Open Office Impress, KOffice KPresenter, Corel Show, Apple Keynote |
| Databases | Database creation for text and numbers | Microsoft Access (in elite packages), Open Office Base, KOffice Kexi, Corel Calculate, Corel Paradox |
| Email | Integrated email program to send and receive electronic mail | Microsoft Outlook, Corel WordPerfect Mail, Mozilla Thunderbird |
| Drawing | Graphics and diagram drawing | Open Office Draw, Corel Presentation Graphics, KOffice Kivio, Karbon, Krita |
| Math formulas | Inserts math equations in word processing and presentation work | Open Office Math, KOffice KFormula |
| Desktop publishing | Page layouts and publication-ready documents | Microsoft Publisher (in elite packages), Apple Pages |

## Acquisition of Data and Information: Input Components

Input devices include the keyboard; mouse; joysticks (typically used for playing computer games); game controllers or pads; Web cameras (webcams); stylus (often used with tablets or personal digital assistants); image scanners for copying a digital image of a document or picture; touch pads; or other plug-and-play input devices, such as digital cameras, digital video recorders (camcorders), MP3 players, electronic musical instruments, and physiologic monitors. These devices are the origin or medium used to input text, visual, audio, or multimedia data into the computer system for viewing, listening, manipulating, creating, or editing. The primary input devices on a computer are the keyboard, mouse, touch pad, and touch screen.

### Keyboard

A computer **keyboard** is very similar to the typewriter keyboards of earlier days and usually serve as the prime input device that enables the user to type words, numbers, and commands into the computer's programs. Standard computer keyboards have 110 keys and are organized to facilitate Latin-based languages using a **QWERTY** layout (so named because these letters appear on the first six keys in the first row of letters).

Table 3-2 Creative Software Features and Examples

| Creative Software | |
|---|---|
| **Program and Application** | **Software Examples** |
| **Raster graphics programs** | |
| Draw, paint, render, manipulate, and edit images, fonts, and photographs to create pixel-based (dot points) digital art and graphics. | Adobe Photoshop and Fireworks, Ulead PhotoImpact, Corel Draw, Painter, and Paint Shop Pro, GIMP (open source), KOffice Krita (open source) |
| **Vector graphics programs** | |
| Mathematically rendered, geometric modeling is applied through shapes, curves, lines, and points and manipulated for shape, color, and size. Ideal for printing and three-dimensional (3D) modeling. | Adobe Flash, Freehand, and Illustrator; CorelDraw and Designer, Open Office Draw (open source), Mirosoft Visio, Xara Xtreme, KOffice Karbon14 (open source) |
| **Desktop publishing programs** | |
| Page layout and publishing preparation for printed and Web documents, such as magazines, journals, books, newsletters, and brochures. | Adobe InDesign, Corel PageMaker, Microsoft Publisher, Scribus (open source), QuarkXPress, Apple Pages (note that many of the graphics programs can also be used for DTP) |
| **Web design programs** | |
| Create, edit, and update webpages using specific codes, such as XML, CSS, HTML, and Java. | Adobe Dreamweaver, Coffee Cup, Microsoft FrontPage, Nvu (open source), W3C's Amaya (open source) |
| **Multimedia programs** | |
| Combines text, audio, images, animation, and video into interactive content for electronic presentation. | Adobe Flash, Microsoft Movie Maker, Apple QuickTime and FinalCut Studio, Corel VideoStudio, Ulead VideoStudio, Real Studio, CamStudio (open source), Audacity (open source) |

Certain keys are used as command keys, particularly the control (CTRL), alternate (Alt), delete (Del), and shift keys, which can all be used to activate useful commands. The escape (ESC) key allows the user instantly to exit a process or program. The F keys, numbered F1 through F12, are function keys. They are used in different ways by particular programs. If a program instructs users to press the "F8" key, they would do so by pressing F8. The print screen (PrtSc) key sends a graphical picture or screen shot of a computer screen to the clipboard. This copied screen shot can then be pasted in any graphic program that can work with bitmap files.

Some keyboards have a wire and plug in, while others are wireless or cordless. Touch screen or virtual keyboards are those being incorporated into the touch screens of phones, gaming machines, and tablets, and they are also available through ease-of-access tools on laptops.

Table 3-3 Communication Software Features and Examples

| Communication Software | |
|---|---|
| **Email client** | |
| Allows user to read, edit, forward, and send email messages to other users via an Internet connection. The software can be resident on the computer or accessed via the World Wide Web. | **Resident programs**<br><br>Microsoft Outlook and Outlook Express, Eudora, Pegasus, Mozilla Thunderbird, Lotus Notes<br><br>**Web-based programs**<br><br>Gmail, Yahoo Mail, Hotmail |
| **Internet browsers** | |
| Enables user to access, browse, download, upload, and interact with text, audio, video, and other Web-based documents. | Mozilla Firefox, Microsoft Internet Explorer, Google Chrome, Apple Safari, Opera, Microbrowser (for mobile access) |
| **Instant messaging (IM)** | |
| Real-time text messaging between users, can attach images, videos, and other documents via personal computer, cell phone, handheld devices. | MSN Instant Messenger, Microsoft Live Messenger, Yahoo Messenger, Apple iChat |
| **Conferencing** | |
| Enables user to communicate in a virtual meeting room setting to share work, discussions, planning, using an intranet or Internet environment; can exhibit files, video, and screenshots of content. | Adobe Acrobat Connect, Microsoft Live Meeting or Meeting Space, GoToMeeting, Meeting Bridge, Free Conference, RainDance, WebEx |

## Mouse

The **mouse** is the second-most-commonly used input device. It is manipulated by the user's hand to point, click, and move objects around on the computer screen. A mouse can come in a number of different configurations, including a standard mechanical trackball serial mouse, bus mouse, PS/2 mouse, USB-connected mouse, optical lens mouse, cordless mouse, and optomechanical mouse. Even though "the mouse may be a simple device in concept," it has evolved and increased in complexity and capability over time (Bagaza & Westover, 2016, para. 2). For example, "[g]aming mice take the basic mouse concept and amplify every element to extremes" (Bagaza & Westover, para. 4). Some manufacturers offer specialized features, but there is a common "combination of high-performance parts—laser sensors, light-click buttons, and gold-plated USB connectors—and customization, like adjustable weight, programmable macro commands, and on-the-fly DPI switching. For non-gamers, these features are overkill; for dedicated gamers, they provide a competitive edge" (Bagaza & Westover, para. 4). The **dots per inch (DPI) switch** is an actual switch on a computer mouse that allows you to adjust the mouse's sensitivity to movement, as in faster or slower mouse pointer speeds. Having the ability to do this on the fly or as needed without pausing could enhance the computing or gaming experience.

### Touch Pad

The **touch pad** is a device that senses the pressure of the user's finger along with the movement of the finger on the touch pad to control input positioning. It is an alternative to using a mouse.

### Touch Screen

The **touch screen** is a display used as an input device for interacting with or relating to the display's materials or content. The user can touch or press on the designated display area to respond, execute, or request information or output.

## Processing of Data and Information: Throughput/Processing Components

All of the hardware discussed earlier in this chapter is involved in the **throughput** or **processing** of input data and in the preparation of output data and information. Specific software is used, depending on the application and data involved. One key hardware component, the computer monitor, is a unique example of a visible throughput component—it is the part of the computer that users focus on the most when they are working on a computer. Input data can be visualized and accessed by manipulating the mouse and keyboard input devices, but it is the monitor that receives the user's attention. The monitor is critical for the efficient rendering during this part of the cycle, because it facilitates user access and control of the data and information.

### Monitor

The **monitor** is the visual display that serves as the landscape for all interactions between user and machine. It typically resembles a television screen, and comes in various sizes (usually ranging from 15 to 21 inches) and configurations. Monitors either are based on cathode ray tubes (the conventional monitor with a large section behind the screen) or are thinner, flat-screen liquid crystal display devices. Some computer monitors also have a touch screen that can serve as an input device when the user touches specific areas of the screen.

Monitors vary in their refresh rate (usually measured in megahertz) and dot pitch. Both of these characteristics are important for user comfort. The faster the refresh rate, the cleaner and clearer the image on the screen, because the monitor refreshes the screen contents more frequently. For example, a monitor with a 100 MHz refresh rate refreshes the screen contents 100 times per second. Similarly, the larger the dot pitch factor, the smaller the dots that make up the screen image, which provides a more detailed display on the monitor and also facilitates clarity and ease of viewing.

If equipped with a touch screen, a monitor can also serve as an input device when activated by a stylus or finger pressure. Some users might also consider the monitor to be an output device, because access to input and stored documents is often performed via the screen (e.g., reading a document that is stored on the computer or viewable from the Internet). As we advance to more engaged computing, larger screens and ultra-wide monitors are evolving to provide immersive experiences.

Smartphone displays can be a form of **AMOLED (Active Matrix Organic Light-Emitting Diode)** or **IPS LCD (In-Plane Switching Liquid Crystal Display)**. In the AMOLED type, the individual pixels are lit separately (active matrix); the next-generation super AMOLED type includes touch sensors. The IPS LCD–type uses polarized light passing through a color filter and all of the pixels are backlit. The liquid crystals control the brightness and which pixels are on or off. With the active matrix, you have crisp, vivid colors and darker blacks.

## Dissemination: Output Components

Output devices carry data in a usable form through exit devices in or attached to a computer. Common forms of output include printed documents, audio or video files, physiologic summaries, scan results, and saved files on portable disk drives, such as a CD, DVD, flash drive, or external hard drive. Output devices literally put data and information at the user's fingertips, which can then be used to develop knowledge and even wisdom. The most commonly used output devices include printers, speakers, and portable disk drives.

### Printer

Printers are external components that can be attached to a computer using a printer cord that is secured into the computer's printer port. Printers enable users to print a hard paper copy of documents that are housed on the computer.

The most common printer types are the inkjet and laser printers. Inkjet printers are more economical to use and offer good quality print; they apply ink to paper using a jet-spray mechanism. Laser printers produce publisher-ready quality printing if combined with good-quality paper, but cost more in terms of printing supplies. Both types of printers can print in black and white or in color. Printers can be single function (print only), but typically they are all-in-one machines or multifunction printers that can also scan, fax, and copy. There are printers that can be accessed via the Internet using **Wi-Fi**. There are also three-dimensional (3D) printers that can create a 3D solid object produced layer by layer from a 3D software digital file.

### Speakers

All computers have some sort of speaker setup, usually small speakers embedded in the monitor, in the case, or, if a laptop, close to the keyboard. Often, external speakers are added to a computer system using speaker connectors; these devices provide enhanced sound and a more enjoyable listening experience.

# What Is the Relationship of Computer Science to Knowledge?

Scholars and researchers are beginning to understand the effects that computer systems, architecture, applications, and processes have on the potential for knowledge acquisition and development. Users who have access to contemporary computers equipped with full Internet access have resources at their fingertips that were only dreamed of before the 21st century. Entire library collections are accessible, with many documents available in full printable form. Users are also able to contribute to the development of knowledge through the use of productivity, creativity, and communication software. In addition, using the **World Wide Web (WWW)** interface, users are able to disseminate knowledge on a grand scale with other users. This deluge of information available via computers must be mastered and organized by the user if knowledge is to emerge. Discernment and the ability to critique and filter this information must also be present to facilitate the further development of wisdom.

The development of an understanding of computer science principles as they apply to technology used in nursing can facilitate optimal usage of the technology for knowledge development in the profession. The maxim that "knowledge is power" and that the skillful use of computers lies at the heart of this power is a presumption. Once nurses become comfortable with the various technologies, they can shape them, refine them, and apply them in new and different ways, just as they have always adapted earlier equipment and technologies. Nurses must harness the power of data and information through the use of computer technologies to build knowledge and gain wisdom.

## How Does the Computer Support Collaboration and Information Exchange?

Computers can be linked to other computers through networking software and hardware to promote communication, information exchange, work sharing, and collaboration. Such **networks** can be local or organizationally based, with computers joined together into a local area network; organized on a wider area scope (e.g., a city or district) using a metropolitan area network; or encompassing computers at an even greater distance (e.g., a whole country or continent, or the Internet itself) using a wide area network configuration (Sarkar, 2006). Network interface cards are used to connect a computer and its modem to a network.

Networks within health care can manifest in several different configurations, including client-focused networks, such as in telenursing, e-health, and client support networks; work-related networks, including virtual work and virtual social networks; and learning and research networks, as in communities of practice. These trends are still evolving in most nursing work environments (and most nurses' personal lives), but they are predicted to continue to grow dramatically. We are experiencing one of the greatest upsurges in shared information and our ability to access, exchange, and utilize this information to enhance knowledge.

Virtual social networks are another form of professional network that have expanded phenomenally since the advent of the Internet and other computer software and hardware. Nursing-related virtual social networks provide a cyberspace for nurses to make contacts, share information and ideas, and build a sense of community.

Social communication software is used to provide a dynamic virtual environment, and often virtual social networks provide communicative capabilities through posting tools, such as blogs, forums, and wikis; email for sharing ideas on a smaller scale; collaborative areas for interaction, creating, and building digital artifacts or planning projects; navigation tools for moving through the virtual network landscape; and profiles to provide a space for each member to disclose personal information with others. Nurses who have to engage in shift work often find that virtual social networks can provide a sense of connection with other professionals that is available around the clock. Because time is often a factor in any social interchange, virtual communication offers an alternative for practicing nurses, who can access information and engage in interchanges at any time of day. With active participation, the interchanges and shared information and ideas of the network can culminate in valuable social and cultural capital, available to all members of that network. Often, nursing virtual social networks are created for the purpose of exchanging ideas on practice issues and best practices; to become more knowledgeable about new trends, research, and innovations in health care; or to participate in advocacy, activist, and educational initiatives.

Through the use of portable disk devices, such as flash drives, CDs, and DVDs, as well as Web-based and cloud spaces, people can share information, documents, and communications by exchanging files. Since the advent of the Internet in the mid-1980s, the World Wide Web has evolved to become a viable and user-friendly way for people to collaborate and exchange information, projects, and other knowledge-based files, such as websites, email, social networking applications, and webinar logs. **Box 3-3** provides information on Web 2.0, the latest iteration of the World Wide Web, and beyond.

---

**BOX 3-3 WEB 2.0 AND BEYOND TOOLS**

*Dee McGonigle, Kathleen Mastrian, and Wendy Mahan*

Web 2.0—the name given to the new World Wide Web tools—enables users to collaborate, network socially, and disseminate knowledge with other users on a scale that was once not even comprehensible. These programs promote data and information exchange, feedback, and knowledge development and **dissemination**.

To facilitate a selective review of the Web 2.0 tools available, they have been categorized into three areas here: (1) tools for creating and sharing information, (2) tools for collaborating, and (3) tools for communicating. Examples of tools for creating and sharing information include blogs, podcasts, Flickr, YouTube, Hellodeo, Jing, Screencast-o-matic, Facebook, MySpace, Box, Samepage, Wrike, Snapchat, and MakeBeliefsComix. Examples of tools for collaborating with others include Google Docs, Zoho, wikis, Del.icio.us, and Gliffy. Finally, some tools for communicating with others include Adobe Connect, GoToMeeting, BlueJeans, WebEx Meeting Center, Vyew, Skype, Twitter, and instant messaging.

The application of the creating and sharing information tools has led to an explosion of social networking on the Web. YouTube has promoted the "broadcast yourself" proliferation. Anyone can post a video onto YouTube that is shared with others over the Web. Similarly, Flickr allows users to upload and tag personal photos to share either privately or publicly. Facebook and MySpace both promote socializing on the Web. Facebook is a social utility and MySpace is a place for friends, according to the descriptions found on these websites. Other tools let users create and share recorded messages, diagrams, screen captures, and even custom comic strips.

Collaborating over the Web has become easier. Indeed, it is a way of life for many people. Google Docs and Zoho allow users to create online and share and collaborate in real time. Wikis are server-based software programs that enable users to generate and edit webpage content using any browser. Del.icio.us is a social bookmarking manager that uses tags to identify or describe the bookmarks that can be shared with others.

Communicating with others includes audio- and videoconferencing in real time. Adobe Connect is a comprehensive Web communications solution. Although a fee-based service, it does provide a free trial. Users should read all of the documentation on Adobe's site before downloading, installing, and using this software. Vyew is free, always-on collaboration plus live webinars. Skype allows users to make calls in audio only or with video. Users can download Skype for free but depending on the type of calls made, fees or charges could be assessed. Individuals should read through all of the information before downloading, installing, and using this software. Twitter allows participants to answer the question "What are you doing?" with messages containing 140 or fewer characters. Although Twitter can be used to keep the friends in a person's network updated on daily activities, it can also be used for other purposes, such as asking questions or expressing thoughts. In addition, Twitter can be accessed by cell phones, so users can stay in touch on the go.

Along with all of the advantages and intellectual harvesting capabilities from the use of these tools come serious security issues. Wagner (2007) warned the user to "bear in mind before you jump in that you're giving information to a third-party company to store" (para. 5). He also states that "you should talk to your company's legal and compliance offices to be sure you're obeying the law and regulations with regard to managing company's information" (para. 5). One suggestion that Wagner offers is that if you do not want to involve a third party, "Wikis provide a good alternative for organizations looking to maintain control of their own software. Organizations can install wiki software on their own, internal servers" (para. 6).

This new wave of Web-based tools facilitates the ability to interact, exchange, collaborate, communicate, and share in ways that have only begun to be realized. As the tools and their innovative uses continue to expand, users need to stay vigilant to handle the associated security challenges. These Web 2.0 and beyond tools are providing a new cyber-playground that is limited only by users' own imaginations and intelligence. We encourage you to explore these tools.

## REFERENCE

Wagner, M. (2007). Nine easy Web-based collaborative tools. *Forbes*. Retrieved from http://www.forbes.com/2007/02/26/google-microsoft-bluetie-enttech-cx_mw _0226smallbizresource.html

# Cloud Computing

**Cloud computing** has Web browser–based login-accessible data, software, and hardware that you can access and use. Using the cloud, you could link systems together and reduce costs (Figure 3-4). According to Griffith (2016), "cloud computing means storing and accessing data and programs over the Internet instead of [on] your computer's hard drive. The cloud is just a metaphor for the Internet" (para. 2). IBM (2016) stated that cloud computing, "referred to as simply 'the cloud,' is the delivery of on-demand computing resources—everything from applications to data centers—over the Internet on a pay-for-use basis" (para. 1). IBM described services as elastic resources, either metered or self-service. Elastic resources refer to those that are able to be scaled up or down to meet the consumer's needs. Metered services allow you to pay only for what you use, and self-service refers to having self-service access to all of the IT resources the consumer needs. Woodford (2016) stated that cloud computing is different because it is managed; on-demand; and can be public, private, or a hybrid of both. The **public cloud** is owned and operated by companies offering public access to computing resources. It is believed to be more affordable and economically sound because the user does not need to purchase the hardware, software, or supporting infrastructure, as these are managed and owned by the cloud provider (IBM, 2016). The **private cloud** is operated for a single organization with the infrastructure being managed and/or hosted internally or out-sourced to a third party; it provides added control and avoids multi-tenancy (IBM).

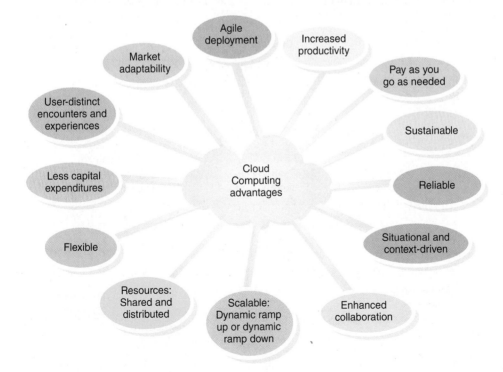

**Figure 3-4** Cloud Computing

As we explore Web-based apps and computing over the Internet, we are cloud computing. Griffith (2016) described some common major examples of cloud computing that you might be using right now: Google Drive, Microsoft Office Online, Microsoft OneDrive, Apple iCloud, Amazon Cloud Drive, Box, Dropbox, and SugarSync. There is also cloud hardware; the primary example of a device that is completely cloud-centric is the Chromebook, a laptop that has just enough local storage and power to run the Chrome OS, which essentially turns the Google Chrome Web browser into an operating system. "With a Chromebook, most everything you do is online: apps, media, and storage are all in the cloud" (Griffith, 2016, para. 16).

**Cloud storage** is data storage provided by networked online servers that are typically outside of the institution whose data are being housed.

There are also additional services based in the cloud that are mainly business related: **software as a service (SaaS), platform as a service (PaaS)**, and **infrastructure as a service (IaaS)** (Figure 3-5). SaaS, such as Salesforce.com refers to cloud-based applications with the following benefits: quickly start using innovative or specific business apps that are scalable to your needs, any connected computer can access the apps and data, and data is not lost if your hard drive crashes because the data is stored in the cloud (Griffith, 2016; IBM, 2016). PaaS provides everything needed to support the cloud application's building and delivery, enabling users to develop and launch custom Web applications rapidly to the cloud (Griffith, 2016; IBM, 2016). IaaS such as Amazon, Microsoft, Google, and Rackspace provide a rentable backbone to companies, enabling the scalable, on-demand infrastructure they need to support their dynamic

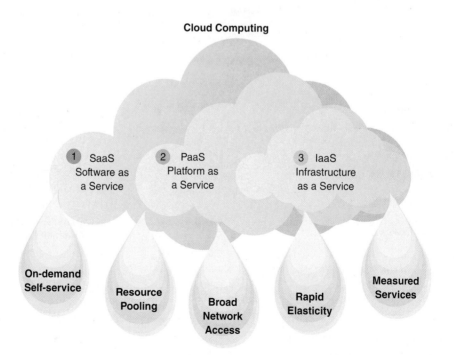

**Figure 3-5** Software as a Service (SaaS), Platform as a Service (PaaS), and Infrastructure as a Service (IaaS)

workloads; the user pays only for what they use and he or she does not have to invest in hardware such as networks, storage, and data center space (Griffith, 2016; IBM, 2016). You can access and receive services from Netflix and Pinterest because they are customers of Amazon's cloud services. According to Griffith (2016), cloud computing is truly big business and could generate 500 billion dollars within the next 5 years.

Cloud computing is Internet computing, and it has the same pitfalls and benefits as using the Internet. Some are not sold on the claims that it is totally reliable, safe, and/or secure. Others believe it is a more environmentally friendly option because it uses fewer resources and less energy, and yet many people can share efficiently managed, centralized cloud-based systems (Woodford, 2016). One of the driving forces behind the initiation of cloud computing was the need for scalable resources that are affordable. As with anything on the Internet, these resources can be shared or privately held. Cloud computing will continue to grow as long as there is demand and it can meet the scalability requirements while maintaining secure, reliable spaces.

In an ideal world, nurses would be able to use and interact with computer technologies effectively to enhance patient care. They would understand computer science and know how to harness its capabilities to benefit the profession and ultimately their patients.

# Looking to the Future

The use of the cloud will continue to expand. The market for **wearable technology**, which is comprised of smaller and faster handheld and portable computer systems, and high-quality voice-activated inventions will further facilitate the use of computers in nursing practice and professional development. The field of computer science will continue to contribute to the evolving art and science of nursing informatics. New trends promise to bring wide-sweeping and (it is hoped) positive changes to the practice of nursing. Computers and other technologies have the potential to support a more client-oriented healthcare system in which clients truly become active participants in their own healthcare planning and decisions. Mobile health technology, telenursing, sophisticated electronic health records, and next-generation technology are predicted to contribute to high-quality nursing care and consultation within healthcare settings, including patients' homes and communities.

Computers are becoming more powerful, yet more compact, which will contribute to the development of several technologic initiatives that are currently still in their infancy, such as **quantum computing**. Some of these initiatives are described here. These predicted innovations are only some of the many computer and technologic applications being developed. As nurses gain proficiency in capitalizing on the creative, time-saving, and interactive capabilities emerging from information technology research, the field of nursing informatics will grow in similar proportions.

## Quantum Computing

**Quantum bits (qubits)** are three-dimensional arrays of atoms in quantum states. A quantum computer is a proposed machine that is not based on the binary system, but instead performs calculations based on the behavior of subatomic particles or qubits. It is estimated that if quantum computing, the act of using a quantum computer, is ever realized, we will be able to execute **millions of instructions per second (MIPS)** due to the qubits existing in more than one state at a time or having the ability to simultaneously execute and process. According to Kennedy (2016), "the era of quantum computers is one step closer" (para. 1) due to the creation of qubits by David Weiss's research team.

## Voice-Activated Communicators

Voice-activated communicators are already on the market, with new iterations being developed by a variety of companies, including Vocera Communications. Vocera (2015) developed the Vocera B3000n Communication Badge, which

> is a lightweight, voice-controlled, wearable device that enables instant two-way or one to many conversations using intuitive and simple commands. The Vocera Badge is widely used by mobile workers who need wearable devices that provide the convenience and expedience of being able to respond to calls without pressing a button (i.e. sterile operating rooms, nuclear power plants, hotel staff, security personnel). (para. 1)

These new technologies will permit nurses to use wireless, hands-free devices to communicate with one another and to record data. This technology is becoming a user-friendly and cost-effective way to increase clinical productivity.

## Game and Simulation Technology

Game and simulation technology is offering realistic, innovative ways to teach content in general, including healthcare informatics concepts and skills. The same technology that powers video games is being used to create dynamic educational interfaces to help students learn about pathophysiology, care guidelines, and a host of other topics. Such applications are also very valuable for client education and health promotion materials. The "serious games" industry is growing now that video game producers are looking beyond mere entertainment to address public and private policy, management, and leadership issues and topics, including those related to health care. For example, the Games for Health Project, initiated by the Robert Wood Johnson Foundation (2015), is working on developing best practices to support innovation in healthcare training, messaging, and illness management. The Serious Games & VE Arcade & Showcase is presented at the annual meetings of the Society for Simulation in Healthcare and is continuing to flourish with numerous products available to demonstrate.

## Virtual Reality

Virtual reality is another technological breakthrough that is and will continue to influence healthcare education and professional development. Virtual reality is a three-dimensional, computer-generated "world" where a person (with the right equipment) can move about and interact as if he or she was actually in the visualized location. The person's senses are immersed in this virtual reality world using special gadgetry, such as head-mounted displays, data gloves, joysticks, and other hand tools. The equipment and special technology provide a sense of presence that is lacking in multimedia and other complex programs. According to Smith (2015), "It's crazy but true: Virtual reality will be a real thing in people's homes by this time next year" (para. 1). There are numerous products available. Virtual Realities (2015) stated that they provide "head mounted displays, head trackers, motion trackers, data gloves, 3D controllers, haptic devices, stereoscopic 3D displays, VR domes and virtual reality software. Virtual Realities' products are used by government, educational, industrial, medical and entertainment markets worldwide" (para. 1). Oculus VR (2015) developed Rift, which is the next generation of virtual reality products, and they are currently distributing the developer kits. HTC (2015) manufactures consumer electronics and developed the Vive headset. The Morpheus headset is used with PlayStation 4.

## Mobile Devices

Mobile devices will be used more by nurses both at the point of care and in planning, documenting, interacting with the interprofessional healthcare team, and research. Nurses also will be using such powerful wearable technologies as nano-based diagnostic sensors in their personal lives, and will be generating their own data streams and receiving data from the wearable and mobile devices their patients use. Silbershatz et al. (2013) stated that Apple iOS and Google Android are "currently dominating mobile computing" (p. 37). Perry (2015) stated that it is "estimated more than 177 million wearable devices will be in use by 2018" (para. 5). Cisco (2014) reported that "by the year 2020, the majority of Generation X and Y professionals believe that smartphones and wearable devices will be the workforce's most important 'connected' device—while the laptop remains the workplace device of choice" (para. 1). Data are truly at our fingertips.

# Summary

The field of computer science is one of the fastest-growing disciplines. Astonishing innovations in computer hardware, software, and architecture have occurred over the past few decades, and there are no indications that this trend will come to a halt anytime soon. Computers have increased in speed, accuracy, and efficiency, yet now cost less and have reduced physical size compared to their forebears. These trends are predicted to continue. Current computer hardware and software serve as vital and valuable tools for both nurses and patients to engage in on-screen and online activities that provide rich access to data and information. Productivity, creativity, and communication software tools also enable nurses to work with computers to further foster knowledge acquisition and development. Wide access to vast stores of information and knowledge shared by others facilitates the emergence of wisdom in users, which can then be applied to nursing in meaningful and creative ways. It is imperative that nurses become discerning, yet skillful users of computer technology to apply the principles of nursing informatics to practice to improve patient care and to contribute to the profession's ever-growing body of knowledge.

# Working Wisdom

Since the beginning of the profession, nurses have applied their ingenuity, resourcefulness, and professional awareness of what works to adapt technology and objects to support nursing care, usually with the intention of promoting efficiency but also in support of client comfort and healing. This resourcefulness could also be applied effectively to the adaptation of information technology within the care environment, to ensure that the technology truly does serve clients and nurses and the rest of the interprofessional team.

Consider this question: "How can you develop competency in using the various computer hardware and software not only to promote efficient, high-quality nursing care and to develop yourself professionally, but also to further the development of the profession's body of knowledge?"

## Application Scenario

Dan P. is a first-year student in graduate studies in nursing. In the past, he has learned to use his family's personal computer to surf the World Wide Web, exchange email with friends, and play some computer games. Now, however, Dan realizes that the computer is a vital tool for his academic success. He has saved up enough money to purchase a laptop computer. He has decided on an Intel processor with 1 TB of storage and 8 GB of RAM. Dan also wishes to choose appropriate software for his system. He is on a limited budget but wants to make the most of his investment.

1. Dan still wants to learn more about computers. *You recommend that he review the following information: Domingo (2016), Knapp (2016), and PCMag Digital Group (2016).*
2. Which of the four categories of software discussed in this chapter would benefit Dan the most in his studies (OS, productivity, creativity, or communication)? *Dan definitely needs an OS—this is critical. He would also directly benefit from productivity software and at least connective email and web browser software from the communication group so he can access the Internet for research, to collaborate with peers, and to communicate with his teachers.*
3. How could Dan afford to install software from all four groups on his new laptop? *If Dan accessed some open source software (e.g., Apache OpenOffice for his productivity software), he could save money to put toward creativity software.*

### THOUGHT-PROVOKING QUESTIONS

1. How can knowledge of computer hardware and software help nurses to participate in information technology adoption decisions in the practice area?
2. How can new computer software help nurses engage in professional development, collaboration, and knowledge dissemination activities at their own pace and leisure?

## References

Alba, D. (2015). Why on earth is IBM still making mainframes? *Wired*. Retrieved from http://www.wired.com/2015/01/z13-mainframe

Anderson, M. (2016). Intel says chips to become slower but more energy efficient. Retrieved from https://thestack.com/iot/2016/02/05/intel-william-holt-moores-law-slower-energy-efficient-chips

Bagaza, L., & Westover, B. (2016). The 10 best computer mice of 2016. *PC Magazine*. Retrieved from http://www.pcmag.com/article2/0,2817,2374831,00.asp

Bandura, A. (2002). Growing primacy of human agency in adaptation and change in the electronic era. *European Psychologist*, 7(1), 2–16.

Cisco. (2014). Working from Mars with an Internet brain implant: Cisco study shows how technology will shape the "Future of Work." Retrieved from http://newsroom.cisco.com/press-release-content?type=webcontent&articleId=1528226

Domingo, J. (2016). The 10 best desktop PCs of 2016. *PC Magazine*. Retrieved from http://www.pcmag.com/article2/0,2817,2372609,00.asp

Evans, D. (2010). Introduction to computing: Explorations in language, logic, and machines. University of Virginia. Retrieved from http://www.computingbook.org

Futuremark. (2016). Best processors May – 2016. Retrieved from http://www.futuremark.com/hardware/cpu

Griffith, E. (2016). What is cloud computing? *PC Magazine*. Retrieved from http://www.pcmag.com/article2/0,2817,2372163,00.asp

HTC. (2015). HTC's VR vision. Finally, the future. Retrieved from http://www.htcvr.com

IBM. (2016). What is cloud computing? Retrieved from https://www.ibm.com/cloud-computing/what-is-cloud-computing

Intel Corporation. (2016). Intel Xeon processor E5 family: Product specifications. Retrieved from http://www.intel.com/content/www/us/en/processors/xeon/xeon-processor-e5-family.html

Kennedy, B. (2016). New, better way to build circuits for the world's first useful quantum computers. *Phys.org*. Retrieved from http://phys.org/news/2016-06-circuits-world-quantum.html#jCp

Knapp, M. (2016). 9 key things to know before you buy a computer. *Gear & Style Cheat Sheet*. Retrieved from http://www.cheatsheet.com/technology/9-tips-for-picking-your-machine-computer-shopping-cheat-sheet.html/?a=viewall

Oculus VR. (2015). Step into the Rift. Retrieved from https://www.oculus.com/en-us/rift

PCMag Digital Group. (2016). Laptops and notebooks. *PC Magazine*. Retrieved from http://www.pcmag.com/reviews/laptop-computers

Perry, L. (2015). Evolving millennial connections using wearables. *Cisco*. Retrieved from http://blogs.cisco.com/tag/wearable-technology

Robert Wood Johnson Foundation. (2015). Games for health. Retrieved from http://gamesforhealth.org/about

Sarkar, N. (2006). *Tools for teaching computer networking and hardware concepts*. Hershey, PA: Idea Group.

Sexton, M. (2016). StarTech unveils USB type-C to HDMI adapter. Retrieved from http://www.tomshardware.com/news/startech-usb-typec-hdmi-adapter,31067.html

Silbershatz, A., Baer Galvin, P., & Gagne, G. (2013). *Operating system concepts* (9th ed.). Hoboken, NJ: John Wiley & Sons.

Smith, D. (2015). 3 virtual reality products will dominate our living rooms by this time next year. *Business Insider*. Retrieved from http://www.businessinsider.com/virtual-reality-is-getting-real-2015-5

Virtual Realities. (2015). Worldwide distributor of virtual reality. Retrieved from https://www.vrealities.com

Vocera. (2015). Vocera badge. Retrieved from http://www.vocera.com/product/vocera-badge

Woodford, C. (2016). Cloud computing. Retrieved from http://www.explainthatstuff.com/cloud-computing-introduction.html

## Objectives

1. Describe cognitive science.

2. Assess how the human mind processes and generates information and knowledge.

3. Explore cognitive informatics.

4. Examine artificial intelligence and its relationship to cognitive science and computer science.

## Key Terms

- » Artificial intelligence
- » Brain
- » Cognitive informatics
- » Cognitive science
- » Computer science
- » Connectionism
- » Decision making
- » Empiricism
- » Epistemology
- » Human Mental Workload (MWL)
- » Intelligence
- » Intuition
- » Knowledge
- » Logic
- » Memory
- » Mind
- » Neuroscience
- » Perception
- » Problem solving
- » Psychology
- » Rationalism
- » Reasoning
- » Wisdom

# CHAPTER 4

# Introduction to Cognitive Science and Cognitive Informatics

Kathleen Mastrian and Dee McGonigle

## Introduction

Cognitive science is the fourth of four basic building blocks used to understand informatics (Figure 4-1). The *Building Blocks of Nursing Informatics* section began by examining nursing science, information science, and computer science, and considering how each relates to and helps one understand the concept of informatics. This chapter explores the building blocks of cognitive science, cognitive informatics (CI), and artificial intelligence (AI).

Throughout the centuries, cognitive science has intrigued philosophers and educators alike. Beginning in Greece, the ancient philosophers sought to comprehend how the mind works and what the nature of knowledge is. This age-old quest to unravel the processes inherent in the working brain has been undertaken by some of the greatest minds in history. However, it was only about 50 years ago that computer operations and actions were linked to cognitive science, meaning theories of the mind, intellect, or brain. This association led to the expansion of cognitive science to examine the complete array of cognitive processes, from lower-level perceptions to higher-level critical thinking, logical analysis, and reasoning.

The focus of this chapter is the impact of cognitive science on nursing informatics (NI). This section provides the reader with an introduction and overview of cognitive science, the nature of knowledge, wisdom, and AI as they apply to the Foundation of Knowledge model and NI. The applications to NI include problem solving, decision support systems, usability issues, user-centered interfaces and systems, and the development and use of terminologies.

## Cognitive Science

The interdisciplinary field of cognitive science studies the mind, intelligence, and behavior from an information-processing perspective. H. Christopher Longuet-Higgins originated the term "cognitive science" in his 1973 commentary on the Lighthill report, which pertained to the state of

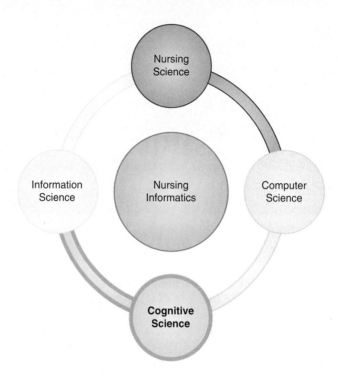

**Figure 4-1** Building Blocks of Nursing Informatics

AI research at that time. The Cognitive Science Society and the *Cognitive Science Journal* date back to 1980 (Cognitive Science Society, 2005). Their interdisciplinary base arises from **psychology**, philosophy, **neuroscience, computer science**, linguistics, biology, and physics; covers **memory**, attention, perception, reasoning, language, mental ability, and computational models of cognitive processes; and explores the nature of the mind, knowledge representation, language, problem solving, decision making, and the social factors influencing the design and use of technology. Simply put, cognitive science is the study of the mind and how information is processed in the mind. As described in the *Stanford Encyclopedia of Philosophy* (2010):

> The central hypothesis of cognitive science is that thinking can best be understood in terms of representational structures in the mind and computational procedures that operate on those structures. While there is much disagreement about the nature of the representations and computations that constitute thinking, the central hypothesis is general enough to encompass the current range of thinking in cognitive science, including connectionist theories which model thinking using artificial neural networks. (para. 9)

**Connectionism** is a component of cognitive science that uses computer modeling through artificial neural networks to explain human intellectual abilities. Neural networks can be thought of as interconnected simple processing devices or simplified models of the brain and nervous system that consist of a considerable number of elements or units (analogs of neurons) linked together in a pattern of connections (analogs of synapses). A neural network that models the entire nervous system would have three types of units: (1) input units (analogs of sensory neurons), which receive information to be processed; (2) hidden units (analogs to all of the other neurons, not sensory or motor), which work in between input and output units; and (3) output units (analogs of motor neurons), where the outcomes or results of the processing are found.

Connectionism (**Figure 4-2**) is rooted in how computation occurs in the brain and nervous system or biologic neural networks. On their own, single neurons have minimal computational capacity. When interconnected with other neurons, however, they have immense computational power. The connectionism system or model learns by modifying the connections linking the neurons. Artificial neural networks are unique computer programs designed to model or simulate their biologic analogs, the neurons of the brain.

The mind is frequently compared to a computer, and experts in computer science strive to understand how the mind processes data and information. In contrast, experts in cognitive science model human thinking using artificial networks provided by computers—an endeavor sometimes referred to as AI. How does the mind process all of the inputs received? Which items and in which ways are things stored or placed into memory, accessed, augmented, changed, reconfigured, and restored? Cognitive science provides the scaffolding for the analysis and modeling of complicated, multifaceted human performance and has a tremendous effect on the issues impacting informatics.

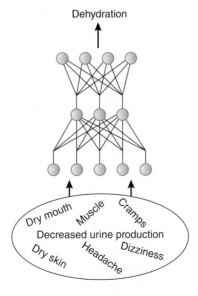

**Figure 4-2** Connectionism

The end user is the focus of this activity because the concern is with enhancing the performance in the workplace; in nursing, the end user could be the actual clinician in the clinical setting, and cognitive science can enhance the integration and implementation of the technologies being designed to facilitate this knowledge worker with the ultimate goal of improving patient care delivery. Technologies change rapidly, and this evolution must be harnessed for the clinician at the bedside. To do this at all levels of nursing practice, one must understand the nature of knowledge, the information and knowledge needed, and the means by which the nurse processes this information and knowledge in the situational context.

## Sources of Knowledge

Just as philosophers have questioned the nature of knowledge, so they have also strived to determine how knowledge arises, because the origins of knowledge can help one understand its nature. How do people come to know what they know about themselves, others, and their world? There are many viewpoints on this issue, both scientific and nonscientific.

According to Holt (2006), "There are two competing traditions concerning the ultimate source of our knowledge: **empiricism** and **rationalism**" (para. 3). Empiricism is based on knowledge being derived from experiences or senses, whereas rationalism contends that "some of our knowledge is derived from reason alone and that reason plays an important role in the acquisition of all of our knowledge" (para. 5). Empiricists do not recognize innate knowledge, whereas rationalists believe that reason is more essential in the acquisition of knowledge than the senses.

Three sources of knowledge have been identified: (1) instinct, (2) reason, and (3) intuition. Instinct is when one reacts without reason, such as when a car is heading toward a pedestrian and he jumps out of the way without thinking. Instinct is found in both humans and animals, whereas reason and intuition are found only in humans. Reason "[c]ollects facts, generalizes, reasons out from cause to effect, from effect to cause, from premises to conclusions, from propositions to proofs" (Sivananda, 2004, para. 4). **Intuition** is a way of acquiring knowledge that cannot be obtained by inference, deduction, observation, reason, analysis, or experience. Intuition was described by Aristotle as "[a] leap of understanding, a grasping of a larger concept unreachable by other intellectual means, yet fundamentally an intellectual process" (Shallcross & Sisk, 1999, para. 4).

Some believe that knowledge is acquired through perception and logic. **Perception** is the process of acquiring knowledge about the environment or situation by obtaining, interpreting, selecting, and organizing sensory information from seeing, hearing, touching, tasting, and smelling. **Logic** is "[a] science that deals with the principles and criteria of validity of inference and demonstration: the science of the formal principles of **reasoning**" (*Merriam-Webster Online Dictionary*, 2007, para. 1). Acquiring knowledge through logic requires reasoned action to make valid inferences.

The sources of knowledge provide a variety of inputs, throughputs, and outputs through which knowledge is processed. No matter how one believes knowledge is acquired, it is important to be able to explain or describe those beliefs, communicate those thoughts, enhance shared understanding, and discover the nature of knowledge.

# Nature of Knowledge

**Epistemology** is the study of the nature and origin of knowledge—that is, what it means to know. Everyone has a conception of what it means to know based on their own perceptions, education, and experiences; knowledge is a part of life that continues to grow with the person. Thus a definition of knowledge is somewhat difficult to agree on because it reflects the viewpoints, beliefs, and understandings of the person or group defining it. Some people believe that knowledge is part of a sequential learning process resembling a pyramid, with data on the bottom, rising to information, then knowledge, and finally wisdom. Others believe that knowledge emerges from interactions and experience with the environment, and still others think that it is religiously or culturally bound. Knowledge acquisition is thought to be an internal process derived through thinking and cognition or an external process from senses, observations, studies, and interactions. Descartes's important premise "called 'the way of ideas' represents the attempt in epistemology to provide a foundation for our knowledge of the external world (as well as our knowledge of the past and of other minds) in the mental experiences of the individual" (*Encyclopedia Britannica*, 2007, para. 4).

For the purpose of this text, knowledge is defined as the awareness and understanding of a set of information and ways that information can be made useful to support a specific task or arrive at a decision. It abounds with others' thoughts and information or consists of information that is synthesized so that relationships are identified and formalized.

# How Knowledge and Wisdom Are Used in Decision Making

The reason for collecting and building data, information, and knowledge is to be able to make informed, judicious, prudent, and intelligent decisions. When one considers the nature of knowledge and its applications, one must also examine the concept of wisdom. **Wisdom** has been defined in numerous ways:

- Knowledge applied in a practical way or translated into actions
- The use of knowledge and experience to heighten common sense and insight to exercise sound judgment in practical matters
- The highest form of common sense resulting from accumulated knowledge or erudition (deep, thorough learning) or enlightenment (education that results in understanding and the dissemination of knowledge)
- The ability to apply valuable and viable knowledge, experience, understanding, and insight while being prudent and sensible
- Focused on our own minds
- The synthesis of our experience, insight, understanding, and knowledge
- The appropriate use of knowledge to solve human problems

In essence, wisdom entails knowing when and how to apply knowledge. The decision-making process revolves around knowledge and wisdom. It is through efforts to understand the nature of knowledge and its evolution to wisdom that one can conceive of, build, and implement informatics tools that enhance and mimic the mind's processes to facilitate **decision making** and job performance.

## Cognitive Informatics

Wang (2003) described CI as an emerging transdisciplinary field of study that bridges the gap in understanding regarding how information is processed in the mind and in the computer. Computing and informatics theories can be applied to help elucidate the information processing of the brain, and cognitive and neurologic sciences can likewise be applied to build better and more efficient computer processing systems. Wang suggested that the common issue among the human knowledge sciences is the drive to develop an understanding of natural intelligence and human problem solving.

Pacific Northwest National Laboratory (PNNL), an organization operated on behalf of the U.S. Department of Energy, suggested the disciplines of neuroscience, linguistics, AI, and psychology constitute this field. PNNL (2008) defined CI as "the multidisciplinary study of cognition and information sciences, which investigates human information processing mechanisms and processes and their engineering applications in computing" (para. 1). CI helps to bridge this gap by systematically exploring the mechanisms of the brain and mind and exploring specifically how information is acquired, represented, remembered, retrieved, generated, and communicated. This dawning of understanding can then be applied and modeled in AI situations resulting in more efficient computing applications.

Wang (2003) explained further:

> *Cognitive informatics attempts to solve problems in two connected areas in a bidirectional and multidisciplinary approach. In one direction, CI uses informatics and computing techniques to investigate cognitive science problems, such as memory, learning, and reasoning; in the other direction, CI uses cognitive theories to investigate the problems in informatics, computing, and software engineering. (p. 120)*

Principles of cognitive informatics and an understanding of how humans interact with computers can be used to build information technology (IT) systems that better meet the needs of users (**Figure 4-3**). If a system is too complex or too taxing for a user, he or she is likely to resist its use. The National Center for Cognitive Informatics and Decision Making in Healthcare (NCCD) was established to respond to "the urgent and long-term cognitive challenges in health IT adoption and meaningful use. NCCD's vision is to become a national resource that provides strategic leadership in patient-centered cognitive support research and applications in health care" (HealthIT.gov, 2013, para. 1). Similarly, Longo (2015) emphasized **Human Mental Workload (MWL)** as a key component in effective system design (**Figure 4-4**). He stated,

> *At a low level of MWL, people may often experience annoyance and frustration when processing information. On the other hand, a high level can also be both problematic and even dangerous, as it leads to confusion, decreases performance in information processing and increases the chances of errors and mistakes. (p. 758)*

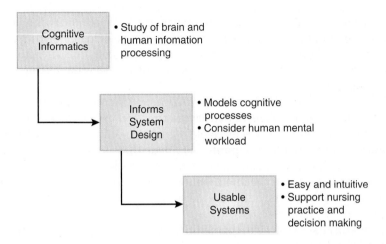

**Figure 4-3** Cognitive Informatics Leads to Usable Systems

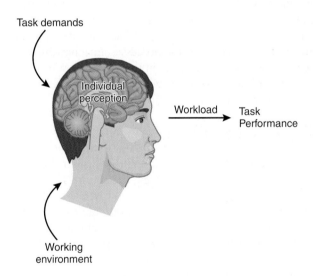

**Figure 4-4** Human Mental Workload

# Cognitive Informatics and Nursing Practice

According to Mastrian (2008), the recognition of the potential application of principles of cognitive science to NI is relatively new. The traditional and widely accepted definition of NI advanced by Graves and Corcoran (1989) is that NI is a combination of nursing science, computer science, and information science used to describe the processes nurses use to manage data, information, and knowledge in nursing practice. Turley (1996) proposed the addition of cognitive science to this mix, as nurse scientists are seen to strive to capture and explain the influence of the human brain on data, information, and knowledge processing and to elucidate how these factors in turn affect nursing decision making. The need to include cognitive sciences is imperative as researchers attempt to model and support nursing decision making in complex computer programs.

In 2003, Wang proposed the term *cognitive informatics* to signify the branch of information and computer sciences that investigates and explains information processing in the human brain. The science of CI grew out of interest in AI, as computer scientists developed computer programs that mimic the information processing and knowledge generation functions of the human brain. CI bridges the gap between artificial and natural intelligence and enhances the understanding of how information is acquired, processed, stored, and retrieved so that these functions can be modeled in computer software.

What does this have to do with nursing? At its very core, nursing practice requires **problem solving** and decision making. Nurses help people manage their responses to illnesses and identify ways that patients can maintain or restore their health. During the nursing process, nurses must first recognize that there is a problem to be solved, identify the nature of the problem, pull information from knowledge stores that is relevant to the problem, decide on a plan of action, implement the plan, and evaluate the effectiveness of the interventions. When a nurse has practiced the science of nursing for some time, he or she tends to do these processes automatically; it is instinctively known what needs to be done to intervene in the problem. What happens, however, if the nurse faces a situation or problem for which he or she has no experience on which to draw? The ever-increasing acuity and complexity of patient situations coupled with the explosion of information in health care has fueled the development of decision support software embedded in the electronic health record. This software models the human and natural decision-making processes of professionals in an artificial program. Such systems can help decision makers to consider the consequences of different courses of action before implementing the action. They also provide stores of information that the user may not be aware of and can use to choose the best course of action and ultimately make a better decision in unfamiliar circumstances.

Decision support programs continue to evolve as research in the fields of cognitive science, AI, and CI is continuously generated and then applied to the development of these systems. Nurses must embrace—not resist—these advances as support and enhancement of the practice of nursing science.

## What Is AI?

The field of AI deals with the conception, development, and implementation of informatics tools based on intelligent technologies. This field captures the complex processes of human thought and intelligence.

Herbert Simon believes that the field of AI could have two functions: "One is to use the power of computers to augment human thinking, just as we use motors to augment human or horse power. . . . The other is to use a computer's artificial intelligence to understand how humans think. In a humanoid way" (Stewart, 1994, para. 13). According to the AAAI (2014), AI is the "scientific understanding of the mechanisms underlying thought and intelligent behavior and their embodiment in machines" (para. 1).

John McCarthy, one of the men credited with founding the field of AI in the 1950s, stated that AI "is the science and engineering of making intelligent machines, especially intelligent computer programs. It is related to the similar task of using computers to understand human intelligence, but AI does not have to confine itself to methods that are biologically observable" (2007, p. 2).

Lamont (2007) interviewed Ray Kurzweil, a visionary who defined AI as "the ability to perform a task that is normally performed by natural intelligence, particularly human natural intelligence. We have in fact artificial intelligence that can perform many tasks that used to require—and could only be done by—human intelligence" (para. 6). The intelligence factor is extremely important in AI and has been defined by McCarthy as "the computational part of the ability to achieve goals in the world. Varying kinds and degrees of intelligence occur in people, many animals, and some machines" (2007, p. 2).

The challenge of this field rests in capturing, mimicking, and creating the complex processes of the mind in informatics tools, including software, hardware, and other machine technologies, with the goal that the tool be able to initiate and generate its own mechanical thought processing. The brain's processing is highly intricate and complicated. This complexity is reflected in Cohn's (2006) comment that "Artificial intelligence is 50 years old this summer, and while computers can beat the world's best chess players, we still can't get them to think like a 4-year-old" (para. 1). AI uses cognitive science and computer science to replicate and generate human intelligence. This field will continue to evolve and produce artificially intelligent tools to enhance nurses' personal and professional lives.

## AI in the Future

As electronic health records become more ubiquitous and we have access to physiologic data streamed in real time, we will have the potential to process large amounts of data using AI tools and we will begin to see data analytics that will enable machine processing that far exceeds the capabilities of the human mind. According to Neill (2013),

> *Perhaps the next great challenge for AI in healthcare is to develop approaches that can be applied to the entire population of patients monitoring huge quantities of data to automatically detect threats to patient safety (including patterns of suboptimal care, as well as outbreaks of hospital acquired illness), and to discover new best practices of patient care. (p. 93)*

# Summary

Cognitive science is the interdisciplinary field that studies the mind, intelligence, and behavior from an information-processing perspective. CI is a field of study that bridges the gap in understanding regarding how information is processed in the mind and in the computer. Computing and informatics theories can be applied to help elucidate the information processing of the brain, and cognitive and neurologic sciences can likewise be applied to build better and more efficient computer processing systems.

AI is the field that deals with the conception, development, and implementation of informatics tools based on intelligent technologies. This field captures the complex processes of human thought and intelligence. AI uses cognitive science and computer science to replicate and generate human intelligence.

The sources of knowledge, nature of knowledge, and rapidly changing technologies must be harnessed by clinicians to enhance their bedside care. Therefore, we must understand the nature of knowledge, the information and knowledge needed, and the means by which nurses process this information and knowledge in their own situational context. The reason for collecting and building data, information, and knowledge is to be able to build wisdom—that is, the ability to apply valuable and viable knowledge, experience, understanding, and insight while being prudent and sensible. Wisdom is focused on our own minds, the synthesis of our experience, insight, understanding, and knowledge. Nurses must use their wisdom and make informed, judicious, prudent, and intelligent decisions while providing care to patients, families, and communities. Cognitive science, CI, and AI will continue to evolve to help build knowledge and wisdom.

## THOUGHT-PROVOKING QUESTIONS

1. How would you describe CI? Reflect on a plan of care that you have developed for a patient. How could CI be used to create tools to help with or support this important work?
2. Think of a clinical setting with which you are familiar and envision how AI tools might be applied in this setting. Are there any current tools in use? Which current or emerging tools would enhance practice in this setting and why?
3. Use your creative mind to think of a tool of the future based on cognitive informatics that would support your practice.

# References

Association for the Advancement of Artificial Intelligence (AAAI). (2014). Homepage. Retrieved from http://www.aaai.org

Cognitive Science Society. (2005). CSJ archive. Retrieved from http://www.cogsci.rpi.edu /CSJarchive/1980v04/index.html

Cohn, D. (2006). AI reaches the golden years. *Wired*. Retrieved from http://archive.wired.com /science/discoveries/news/2006/07/71389

*Encyclopedia Britannica*. (2007). Epistemology. Retrieved from http://www.britannica.com/eb /article-247960/epistemology

Graves, J., & Corcoran, S. (1989). The study of nursing informatics. *Image: Journal of Nursing Scholarship, 21*(4), 227–230.

HealthIT.gov. (2013). National center for cognitive informatics and decision making in healthcare. Retrieved from https://www.healthit.gov/policy-researchers-implementers/national-center-cognitive-informatics-and-decision-making-healthcare

Holt, T. (2006). Sources of knowledge. Retrieved from http://www.theoryofknowledge.info /sourcesofknowledge.html

Lamont, I. (2007). The grill: Ray Kurzweil talks about "augmented reality" and the singularity. *Computer World*. Retrieved from http://www.computerworld.com/action/article.do?comma nd=viewArticleBasic&articleId=306176

Longo, L. (2015). A defeasible reasoning framework for human mental workload representation and assessment. *Behaviour & Information Technology, 34*(8), 758–786. doi:10.1080/0144929X.2015.1015166

Longuet-Higgins, H. C. (1973). Comments on the Lighthill report and the Sutherland reply. *Artificial Intelligence: A Paper Symposium, 35–37.*

Mastrian, K. (2008, February). Invited editorial: Cognitive informatics and nursing practice. *Online Journal of Nursing Informatics, 12*(1). Retrieved from http://ojni.org/12_1/kathy.html

McCarthy, J. (2007). What is artificial intelligence? Retrieved from http://www.formal.stanford .edu/jmc/whatisai.pdf

*Merriam-Webster Online Dictionary.* (2007). Logic. Retrieved from http://www.merriam-webster .com/dictionary/logic

Neill, D. (2013). Using artificial intelligence to improve hospital inpatient care. *IEEE Intelligent Systems, 92–95.*

Pacific Northwest National Laboratory, U.S. Department of Energy. (2008). Cognitive informatics. Retrieved from http://www.pnl.gov/coginformatics

Shallcross, D. J., & Sisk, D. A. (1999). What is intuition? In T. Arnold (Ed.), *Hyponoesis glossary: Intuition.* Retrieved from http://www.hyponoesis.org/Glossary/Definition/Intuition

Sivananda, S. (2004). Four sources of knowledge. *The Divine Life Society.* Retrieved from http://www.dlshq.org/messages/knowledge.htm

*Stanford Encyclopedia of Philosophy.* (2010). Cognitive science. Retrieved from http://plato .stanford.edu/entries/cognitive-science

Stewart, D. (1994). The creator of the first thinking machine on the future of artificial intelligence: Herbert Simon on the mind in the machine. *OMNI Q&A.* Retrieved from http://www.omnimagazine.com/archives/interviews/simon/index.html

Turley, J. (1996). Toward a model for nursing informatics. *Image: Journal of Nursing Scholarship, 28*(4), 309–313.

Wang, Y. (2003). Cognitive informatics: A new transdisciplinary research field. *Brain and Mind, 4*(2), 115–127.

1. Recognize ethical dilemmas in nursing informatics.

2. Examine ethical implications of nursing informatics.

3. Evaluate professional responsibilities for the ethical use of healthcare informatics technology.

4. Explore the ethical model for ethical decision making.

5. Analyze practical ways of applying the ethical model for ethical decision making to manage ethical dilemmas in nursing informatics.

## Key Terms

- » Alternatives
- » Antiprinciplism
- » Applications (Apps)
- » Autonomy
- » Beneficence
- » Bioethics
- » Bioinformatics
- » Care ethics
- » Casuist approach
- » Confidentiality
- » Consequences
- » Courage
- » Decision making

- » Decision support
- » Duty
- » Ethical decision making
- » Ethical dilemma
- » Ethical, social, and legal implications
- » Ethicists
- » Ethics
- » Eudaemonistic
- » Fidelity
- » Good
- » Google Glass

- » Harm
- » Justice
- » Liberty
- » Moral dilemmas
- » Moral rights
- » Morals
- » Negligence
- » Nicomachean
- » Nonmaleficence
- » Principlism
- » Privacy
- » Rights
- » Security

- » Self-control
- » Smartphones
- » Social media
- » Standards
- » Truth
- » Uncertainty
- » Values
- » Veracity
- » Virtue
- » Virtue ethics
- » Wisdom

# CHAPTER 5

# Ethical Applications of Informatics

Dee McGonigle, Kathleen Mastrian, and Nedra Farcus

## Introduction

Those who followed the actual events of Apollo 13, or who were entertained by the movie (Howard, 1995), watched the astronauts strive against all odds to bring their crippled spaceship back to Earth. The speed of their travel was incomprehensible to most viewers, and the task of bringing the spaceship back to Earth seemed nearly impossible. They were experiencing a crisis never imagined by the experts at NASA, and they made up their survival plan moment by moment. What brought them back to Earth safely? Surely, credit must be given to the technology and the spaceship's ability to withstand the trauma it experienced. Most amazing, however, were the traditional nontechnological tools, skills, and supplies that were used in new and different ways to stabilize the spacecraft's environment and keep the astronauts safe while traveling toward their uncertain future.

This sense of constancy in the midst of change serves to stabilize experience in many different life events and contributes to the survival of crisis and change. This rhythmic process is also vital to the healthcare system's stability and survival in the presence of the rapidly changing events of the Knowledge Age. No one can dispute the fact that the Knowledge Age is changing health care in ways that will not be fully recognized and understood for years. The change is paradigmatic, and every expert who addresses this change reminds healthcare professionals of the need to go with the flow of rapid change or be left behind.

As with any paradigm shift, a new way of viewing the world brings with it some of the enduring values of the previous worldview. As health care continues its journey into digital communications, telehealth, and wearable technologies, it brings some familiar tools and skills recognized in the form of **values**, such as **privacy**, **confidentiality**, autonomy, and nonmaleficence. Although these basic values remain unchanged, the **standards** for living out these values will take on new meaning as health professionals confront new and different moral dilemmas brought on by the adoption

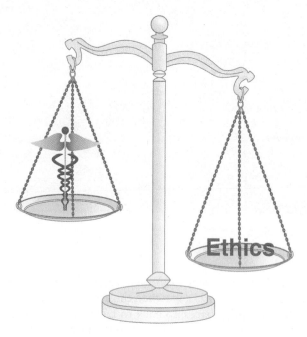

**Figure 5-1** Ethics in Health Care

of technological tools for information management, knowledge development, and evidence-based changes in patient care. Ethical decision-making frameworks will remain constant, but the context for examining these moral issues or ethical dilemmas will become increasingly complex.

This chapter highlights some familiar ethical concepts to consider on the challenging journey into the increasingly complex future of healthcare informatics. Ethics and bioethics are briefly defined, and the evolution of ethical approaches from the Hippocratic ethic era, to principlism, to the current antiprinciplism movement of ethical **decision making** is examined. New and challenging ethical dilemmas are surfacing in the venture into the unfolding era of healthcare informatics (**Figure 5-1**). Also presented in this chapter are findings from some of the more recent literature related to these issues. Readers are challenged to think constantly and carefully about ethics as they become involved in healthcare informatics and to stay abreast of new developments in ethical approaches.

# Ethics

**Ethics** is a process of systematically examining varying viewpoints related to moral questions of right and wrong. **Ethicists** have defined the term in a variety of ways, with each reflecting a basic theoretical philosophic perspective.

Beauchamp and Childress (1994) referred to ethics as a generic term for various ways of understanding and examining the moral life. Ethical approaches to this examination may be normative, presenting standards of right or **good** action; descriptive, reporting what people believe and how they act; or explorative, analyzing the concepts and methods of ethics.

Husted and Husted (1995) emphasized a practice-based ethics, stating "ethics examines the ways men and women can exercise their power in order to bring about human benefit—the ways in which one can act in order to bring about the conditions of happiness" (p. 3).

Velasquez, Andre, Shanks, and Myer (1987) posed the question, "What is ethics?", and answered it with the following two-part response: "First, ethics refers to well-based standards of right and wrong that prescribe what humans ought to do, usually in terms of **rights**, obligations, benefits to society, fairness, or specific virtues" (para. 10), and "Secondly, ethics refers to the study and development of one's ethical standards" (para. 11).

Regardless of the theoretical definition, common characteristics regarding ethics are its dialectical, goal-oriented approach to answering questions that have the potential for multiple acceptable answers.

# Bioethics

**Bioethics** is defined as the study and formulation of healthcare ethics. Bioethics takes on relevant ethical problems experienced by healthcare providers in the provision of care to individuals and groups. Husted and Husted (1995) state the fundamental background of bioethics that forms its essential nature is:

1. The nature and needs of humans as living, thinking beings
2. The purpose and function of the healthcare system in a human society
3. An increased cultural awareness of human beings' essential moral status (p. 7)

Bioethics emerged in the 1970s as health care began to change its focus from a mechanistic approach of treating disease to a more holistic approach of treating people with illnesses. As technology advanced, recognition and acknowledgment of the rights and the needs of individuals and groups receiving this high-tech care also increased.

In today's technologically savvy healthcare environment, patients are being prescribed **applications (apps)** for their **smartphones** instead of medications in some clinical practices. Patients' smartphones are being used to interact with them in new ways and to monitor and assess their health in some cases. With apps and add-ons, for example, a provider can see the patient's ECG immediately, or the patient can monitor his or her ECG and send it to the provider as necessary. Another example would be a sensor attached to the patient's mobile device that could monitor blood glucose levels. We are just beginning to realize the vast potential of these mobile devices—and the threats they sometimes pose. **Google Glass**, for example, can take photos and videos (Stern, 2013) without anyone knowing that this is occurring; in the healthcare environment, such a technological advancement can violate patients' privacy and confidentiality. Wearable technologies provide a data-rich environment for diagnosing, addressing, and monitoring health issues. As we analyze huge patient datasets, concerns arise about privacy, confidentiality, and data sharing (Johns Hopkins, Berman Institute of Bioethics, n.d.). Add these evolving developments to healthcare providers' engagement in social media use with their patients, and it becomes clear that personal and ethical dilemmas abound for nurses in the new über-connected world.

# Ethical Issues and Social Media

As connectivity has improved owing to emerging technologies, a rapid explosion in the phenomenon known as **social media** has occurred. Social media is defined as "a group of Internet-based applications that build on the ideological and technological foundations of Web 2.0 and that allow the creation and exchange of user-generated content" (Spector & Kappel, 2012, p. 1). Just as the electronic health record serves as a real-time event in recording patient–provider contact, so the use of social media represents an instantaneous form of communication. Healthcare providers—particularly nurses—can enhance the patient care delivery system, promote professional collegiality, and provide timely communication and education regarding health-related matters by using this forum (National Council of State Boards of Nursing [NCSBN], 2011, p. 1). In all cases, however, nurses must exercise judicious use of social media to protect patients' rights. Nurses must understand their obligation to their chosen profession, particularly as it relates to personal behavior and the perceptions of their image as portrayed through social media. Above all, nurses must be mindful that once communication is written and posted on the Internet, there is no way to retract what was written; it is a permanent record that can be tracked, even if the post is deleted (Englund, Chappy, Jambunathan, & Gohdes, 2012, p. 242).

Social media platforms include such electronic communication outlets as Facebook, Twitter, LinkedIn, Snapchat, and YouTube. Other widely used means of instantaneous communications include wikis, blogs, tweeting, Skype, and the "hangout" feature on Google+. Even as recently as 5 years ago, some of these means of exchanging information were unknown (Spector & Kappel, 2012, p. 1).

Use of social networking has increased dramatically among all age groups. Zephoria (2016) reported that, in 2016, Facebook had over 1.65 billion active monthly users worldwide as compared to 955 million active monthly users in 2012, and users spend an average of 20 minutes on Facebook per visit. Twitter's influence on health care continues to grow, with Symplur (2016) reporting 1,603,327,260 tweets, including healthcare-related Tweet chats, conferences, and diseases such as breast cancer, diabetes, and irritable bowel syndrome.

The rapid growth of social media has found many healthcare professionals unprepared to face the new challenges or to exploit the opportunities that exist with these forums. The need to maintain confidentiality presents a major obstacle to the healthcare industry's widespread adoption of such technology; thus social networking has not yet been fully embraced by many health professionals (Anderson, 2012, p. 22). Englund and colleagues (2012) noted that undergraduate nursing students may face ambiguous and understudied professional and ethical implications when using social networking venues.

Another confounding factor is the increased use of mobile devices by health professionals as well as the public (Swartz, 2011, p. 345). Smartphones have the capability to take still pictures as well as live recordings; they have found their way into treatment rooms around the globe.

As a consequence of more stringent confidentiality laws and more widespread availability and use of social and mobile media, numerous ethical and legal dilemmas have been posed to nurses. What are not well defined are the expectations of healthcare providers regarding this technology. In some cases, nurses employed in the emergency department (ED) setting have been subjected to video and audio recordings by patients and families when they perform procedures and give care during the ED visit. Nurses would be wise to inquire—before an incident occurs—about the hospital policy regarding audio/video recording by patients and families, as well as the state laws governing two-party consent. Such laws require consent of all parties to any recording or eavesdropping activity (Lyons & Reinisch, 2013, p. 54).

Sometimes the enthusiasm for patient care and learning can lead to ethics violations. In one case, an inadvertent violation of privacy laws occurred when a nurse in a small town blogged about a child in her care whom she referred to as her "little handicapper." The post also noted the child's age and the fact that the child used a wheelchair. A complaint about this breach of confidentiality was reported to the Board of Nursing. A warning was issued to the nurse blogging this information, although a more stringent disciplinary action could have been taken (Spector & Kappel, 2012, p. 2).

In another case cited by Spector and Kappel (2012), a student nurse cared for a 3-year-old leukemia patient whom she wanted to remember after finishing her pediatric clinical experience. She took the child's picture, and in the background of the photo the patient's room number was clearly displayed. The child's picture was posted on the student nurse's Facebook page, along with her statement of how much she cared about this child and how proud she was to be a student nurse. Someone forwarded the picture to the nurse supervisor of the children's hospital. Not only was the student expelled from the program, but the clinical site offer made by the children's hospital to the nursing school was rescinded. In addition, the hospital faced citations for violations of the Health Insurance Portability and Accountability Act (HIPAA) owing to the student nurse's transgression (p. 3).

Nurses sometimes use social network sites or blog about the patients they care for believing that if they omit the patient's name, they are not violating the patient's privacy and confidentiality. "A nurse who posts about caring for an 85-year-old female in her city could cause the patient to be identified by content in the post. This action does not protect the patient" (Henderson & Dahnke, 2015, p. 63). A white paper published by the NCSBN (2011) provides a thorough discussion of the issues associated with nurses' use of social media.

## Ethical Dilemmas and Morals

An **ethical dilemma** arises when moral issues raise questions that cannot be answered with a simple, clearly defined rule, fact, or authoritative view. **Morals** refer to social convention about right and wrong human conduct that is so widely shared that it forms a stable (although usually incomplete) communal consensus (Beauchamp & Childress, 1994). **Moral dilemmas** arise with uncertainty, as is the case when some evidence a person is confronted with indicates an action is morally right and other evidence indicates that this action is morally wrong. **Uncertainty** is stressful and, in the face of inconclusive evidence on both sides of the dilemma, causes the person to question what he or she should do. Sometimes the individual concludes that based on his or her moral beliefs, he or she cannot act. Uncertainty also arises from unanticipated effects or unforeseeable behavioral responses to actions or the lack of action. Adding uncertainty to the situational factors and personal beliefs that must be considered creates a need for an ethical decision-making model to help one choose the best action.

## Ethical Decision Making

**Ethical decision making** refers to the process of making informed choices about ethical dilemmas based on a set of standards differentiating right from wrong. This type of decision making reflects an understanding of the principles and standards of ethical decision making, as well as the philosophic approaches to ethical decision making, and it requires a systematic framework for addressing the complex and often controversial moral questions.

As the high-speed era of digital communications evolves, the rights and the needs of individuals and groups will be of the utmost concern to all healthcare professionals. The changing meaning of communication, for example, will bring with it new concerns among healthcare professionals about protecting patients' rights of confidentiality, privacy, and autonomy. Systematic and flexible ethical decision-making abilities will be essential for all healthcare professionals.

Notably, the concept of nonmaleficence ("do no **harm**") will be broadened to include those individuals and groups whom one may never see in person, but with whom one will enter into a professional relationship of trust and care. Mack (2000)

### RESEARCH BRIEF

Using an online survey of 1,227 randomly selected respondents, Bodkin and Miaoulis (2007) sought to describe the characteristics of information seekers on e-health websites, the types of information they seek, and their perceptions of the quality and ethics of the websites. Of the respondents, 74% had sought health information on the Web, with women accounting for 55.8% of the health information seekers. A total of 50% of the seekers were between 35 and 54 years of age. Nearly two thirds of the users began their searches using a general search engine rather than a health-specific site, unless they were seeking information related to symptoms or diseases. Top reasons for seeking information were related to diseases or symptoms of medical conditions, medication information, health news, health insurance, locating a doctor, and Medicare or Medicaid information. The level of education of information seekers was related to the ratings of website quality, in that more educated seekers found health information websites more understandable, but were more likely to perceive bias in the website information. The researchers also found that the ethical codes for e-health websites seem to be increasing consumers' trust in the safety and quality of information found on the Web, but that most consumers are not comfortable purchasing health products or services online.

The full article appears in Bodkin, C., & Miaoulis, G. (2007). eHealth information quality and ethics issues: An exploratory study of consumer perceptions. *International Journal of Pharmaceutical and Healthcare Marketing*, 1(1), 27–42. Retrieved from ABI/INFORM Global (Document ID: 1515583081).

has discussed the popularity of individuals seeking information online instead of directly from their healthcare providers and the effects this behavior has on patient–provider relationships. He is emphatic in his reminder that "organizations and individuals that provide health information on the Internet have obligations to be trustworthy, provide high-quality content, protect users' privacy, and adhere to standards of best practices for online commerce and online professional services in healthcare" (p. 41).

Makus (2001) suggests that both autonomy and justice are enhanced with universal access to information, but that tensions may be created in patient–provider relationships as a result of this access to outside information. Healthcare workers need to realize that they are no longer the sole providers and gatekeepers of health-related information; ideally, they should embrace information empowerment and suggest websites to patients that contain reliable, accurate, and relevant information (Resnick, 2001).

It is clear that patients' increasing use of the Internet for healthcare information may prompt entirely new types of ethical issues, such as who is responsible if a patient is harmed as a result of following online health advice. Derse and Miller (2008) discuss this issue extensively and conclude that a clear line separates information and practice. Practice occurs when there is direct or personal communication between the provider and the patient, when the advice is tailored to the patient's specific health issue, and when there is a reasonable expectation that the patient will act in reliance on the information.

A summit sponsored by the Internet Healthcare Coalition (www.ihealthcoalition.org) in 2000 developed the E-Health Code of Ethics (eHealth code, n.d.), which includes eight standards for the ethical development of health-related Internet sites: (1) candor, (2) honesty, (3) quality, (4) informed consent, (5) privacy, (6) professionalism, (7) responsible partnering, and (8) accountability. For more information about each of these standards, access the full discussion of the E-Health Code of Ethics (http://www.ihealthcoalition.org/ehealth-code-of-ethics).

It is important to realize that the standards for ethical development of health-related Internet sites are voluntary; there is no overseer perusing these sites and issuing safety alerts for users. Although some sites carry a specific symbol indicating that they have been reviewed and are trustworthy (HONcode and Trust-e), the healthcare provider cannot control which information patients access or how they perceive and act related to the health information they find online. The research brief on the previous page describes one study of consumer perceptions of health information on the Web.

## Theoretical Approaches to Healthcare Ethics

Theoretical approaches to healthcare ethics have evolved in response to societal changes. In a 30-year retrospective article for the *Journal of the American Medical Association*, Pellegrino (1993) traced the evolution of healthcare ethics from the Hippocratic ethic, to principlism, to the current antiprinciplism movement.

The Hippocratic tradition emerged from relatively homogenous societies where beliefs were similar and most societal members shared common values. The emphasis was on **duty**, virtue, and gentlemanly conduct.

**Principlism** arose as societies became more heterogeneous and members began experiencing a diversity of incompatible beliefs and values; it emerged as a foundation for ethical decision making. Principles were expansive enough to be shared by all rational individuals, regardless of their background and individual beliefs. This approach continued into the 1900s and was popularized by two bioethicists, Beauchamp and Childress (1977; 1994), in the last quarter of the 20th century. Principles are considered broad guidelines that provide guidance or direction but leave substantial room for case-specific judgment. From principles, one can develop more detailed rules and policies.

Beauchamp and Childress (1994) proposed four guiding principles: (1) respect for autonomy, (2) nonmaleficence, (3) beneficence, and (4) justice.

- **Autonomy** refers to the individual's freedom from controlling interferences by others and from personal limitations that prevent meaningful choices, such as adequate understanding. Two conditions are essential for autonomy: **liberty,** meaning the independence from controlling influences, and the individual's capacity for intentional action.
- **Nonmaleficence** asserts an obligation not to inflict harm intentionally and forms the framework for the standard of due care to be met by any professional. Obligations of nonmaleficence are obligations of not inflicting harm and not imposing risks of harm. **Negligence**—a departure from the standard of due care toward others—includes intentionally imposing risks that are unreasonable and unintentionally but carelessly imposing risks.
- **Beneficence** refers to actions performed that contribute to the welfare of others. Two principles underlie beneficence: Positive beneficence requires the provision of benefits, and utility requires that benefits and drawbacks be balanced. One must avoid negative beneficence, which occurs when constraints are placed on activities that, even though they might not be unjust, could in some situations cause detriment or harm to others.
- **Justice** refers to fair, equitable, and appropriate treatment in light of what is due or owed to a person. Distributive justice refers to fair, equitable, and appropriate distribution in society determined by justified norms that structure the terms of social cooperation.

Beauchamp and Childress also suggest three types of rules for guiding actions: substantive, authority, and procedural. (Rules are more restrictive in scope than principles and are more specific in content.) Substantive rules are rules of **truth** telling, confidentiality, privacy, and **fidelity,** and those pertaining to the allocation and rationing of health care, omitting treatment, physician-assisted suicide, and informed consent. Authority rules indicate who may and should perform actions. Procedural rules establish procedures to be followed.

The principlism advocated by Beauchamp and Childress has since given way to the **antiprinciplism** movement, which emerged in the 21st century with the expansive technological changes and the tremendous rise in ethical dilemmas accompanying these changes. Opponents of principlism include those who claim that its principles do not represent a theoretical approach as well as those who claim that its principles are too far removed from the concrete particularities of everyday human existence;

are too conceptual, intangible, or abstract; or disregard or do not take into account a person's psychological factors, personality, life history, sexual orientation, or religious, ethnic, and cultural background. Different approaches to making ethical decisions are next briefly explored, providing the reader with an understanding of the varied methods professionals may use to arrive at an ethical decision.

The **casuist approach** to ethical decision making grew out of the call for more concrete methods of examining ethical dilemmas. Casuistry is a case-based ethical reasoning method that analyzes the facts of a case in a sound, logical, and ordered or structured manner. The facts are compared to decisions arising out of consensus in previous paradigmatic or model cases. One casuist proponent, Jonsen (1991), prefers particular and concrete paradigms and analogies over the universal and abstract theories of principlism.

The Husted bioethical decision-making model centers on the healthcare professional's implicit agreement with the patient or client (Husted & Husted, 1995). It is based on six contemporary bioethical standards: (1) autonomy, (2) freedom, (3) veracity, (4) privacy, (5) beneficence, and (6) fidelity.

The **virtue ethics** approach emphasizes the virtuous character of individuals who make the choices. A **virtue** is any characteristic or disposition desired in others or oneself. It is derived from the Greek word *aretai*, meaning "excellence," and refers to what one expects of oneself and others. Virtue ethicists emphasize the ideal situation and attempt to identify and define ideals. Virtue ethics dates back to Plato and Socrates. When asked "whether virtue can be taught or whether virtue can be acquired in some other way, Socrates answers that if virtue is knowledge, then it can be taught. Thus, Socrates assumes that whatever can be known can be taught" (Scott, 2002, para. 9). According to this view, the cause of any moral weakness is not a matter of character flaws but rather a matter of ignorance. In other words, a person acts immorally because the individual does not know what is really good for him or her. A person can, for example, be overpowered by immediate pleasures and forget to consider the long-term **consequences**. Plato emphasized that to lead a moral life and not succumb to immediate pleasures and gratification, one must have a moral vision. He identified four cardinal virtues: (1) **wisdom**, (2) **courage**, (3) **self-control**, and (4) justice.

Aristotle's (350 BC) **Nicomachean** principles also contribute to virtue ethics. According to this philosopher, virtues are connected to will and motive because the intention is what determines if one is or is not acting virtuously. Ethical considerations, according to his **eudaemonistic** principles, address the question, "What is it to be an excellent person?" For Aristotle, this ultimately means acting in a temperate manner according to a rational mean between extreme possibilities.

Virtue ethics has experienced a recent resurgence in popularity (Ascension Health, 2007). Two of the most influential moral and medical authors, Pellegrino and Thomasma (1993), have maintained that virtue theory should be related to other theories within a comprehensive philosophy of the health professions. They argue that moral events are composed of four elements (the agent, the act, the circumstances, and the consequences), and state that a variety of theories must be interrelated to account for different facets of moral judgment.

**Care ethics** is responsiveness to the needs of others that dictates providing care, preventing harm, and maintaining relationships. This viewpoint has been in existence for some time. Engster (2004) stated that "Carol Gilligan's *In a Different Voice* (1982) established care ethics as a major new perspective in contemporary moral and political discourse" (p. 113). The relationship between care and virtue is complex, however. Benjamin and Curtis (1992) base their framework on care ethics; they propose that "critical reflection and inquiry in ethics involves the complex interplay of a variety of human faculties, ranging from empathy and moral imagination on the one hand to analytic precision and careful reasoning on the other" (p. 12). Care ethicists are less stringently guided by rules, but rather focus on the needs of others and the individual's responsibility to meet those needs. As opposed to the aforementioned theories that are centered on the individual's rights, an ethic of care emphasizes the personal part of an interdependent relationship that affects how decisions are made. In this theory, the specific situation and context in which the person is embedded become a part of the decision-making process.

The consensus-based approach to bioethics was proposed by Martin (1999), who claims that American bioethics harbors a variety of ethical methods that emphasize different ethical factors, including principles, circumstances, character, interpersonal needs, and personal meaning. Each method reflects an important aspect of ethical experience, adds to the others, and enriches the ethical imagination. Thus working with these methods provides the challenge and the opportunity necessary for the perceptive and shrewd bioethicist to transform them into something new with value through the process of building ethical consensus. Diverse ethical insights can be integrated to support a particular bioethical decision, and that decision can be understood as a new, ethical whole.

## Applying Ethics to Informatics

With the Knowledge Age has come global closeness, meaning the ability to reach around the globe instantaneously through technology. Language barriers are being broken through technologically based translators that can enhance interaction and exchange of data and information. Informatics practitioners are bridging continents, and international panels, committees, and organizations are beginning to establish standards and rules for the implementation of informatics. This international perspective must be taken into consideration when informatics dilemmas are examined from an ethical standpoint; it promises to influence the development of ethical approaches that begin to accept that healthcare practitioners are working within international networks and must recognize, respect, and regard the diverse political, social, and human factors within informatics ethics.

The various ethical approaches can be used to help healthcare professionals make ethical decisions in all areas of practice. The focus of this text is on informatics. Informatics theory and practice have continued to grow at a rapid rate and are infiltrating every area of professional life. New applications and ways of performing skills are being developed daily. Therefore, education in informatics ethics is extremely important.

Typically, situations are analyzed using past experience and in collaboration with others. Each situation warrants its own deliberation and unique approach, because each individual patient seeking or receiving care has his or her own preferences, quality of life, and healthcare needs in a situational milieu framed by financial, provider, setting, institutional, and social context issues. Clinicians must take into consideration all of these factors when making ethical decisions.

The use of expert systems, **decision support** tools, evidence-based practice, and artificial intelligence in the care of patients creates challenges in terms of who should use these tools, how they are implemented, and how they are tempered with clinical judgment. All clinical situations are not the same, and even though the result of interacting with these systems and tools is enhanced information and knowledge, the clinician must weigh this information in light of each patient's unique clinical circumstances, including that individual's beliefs and wishes. Patients are demanding access to quality care and the information necessary to control their lives. Clinicians need to analyze and synthesize the parameters of each distinctive situation using a specific decision-making framework that helps them make the best decisions. Getting it right the first time has a tremendous impact on expected patient outcomes. The focus should remain on patient outcomes while the informatics tools available are ethically incorporated.

Facing ethical dilemmas on a daily basis and struggling with unique client situations may cause many clinicians to question their own actions and the actions of their colleagues and patients. One must realize that colleagues and patients may reach very different decisions, but that does not mean anyone is wrong. Instead, all parties reach their ethical decision based on their own review of the situational facts and understanding of ethics. As one deals with diversity among patients, colleagues, and administrators, one must constantly strive to use ethical imagination to reach ethically competent decisions.

Balancing the needs of society, his or her employer, and patients could cause the clinician to face ethical challenges on an everyday basis. Society expects judicious use of finite healthcare resources. Employers have their own policies, standards, and practices that can sometimes inhibit the practice of the clinician. Each patient is unique and has life experiences that affect his or her healthcare perspective, choices, motivation, and adherence. Combine all of these factors with the challenges posed by informatics, and it is clear that the evolving healthcare arena calls for an informatics-competent, politically active, consumer-oriented, business-savvy, ethical clinician to rule this ever-changing landscape known as health care.

The goal of any ethical system should be that a rational, justifiable decision is reached. Ethics is always there to help the practitioner decide what is right. Indeed, the measure of an adequate ethical system, theory, or approach is, in part, its ability to be useful in novel contexts. A comprehensive, robust theory of ethics should be up to the task of addressing a broad variety of new applications and challenges at the intersection of informatics and health care.

The information concerning an ethical dilemma must be viewed in the context of the dilemma to be useful. **Bioinformatics** could gather, manipulate, classify, analyze, synthesize, retrieve, and maintain databases related to ethical cases, the effective reasoning applied to various ethical dilemmas, and the resulting ethical decisions. This input would certainly be potent—but the resolution of dilemmas cannot be achieved simply by examining relevant cases from a database. Instead, clinicians must assess each situational context and the patient's specific situation and needs and make their ethical decisions based on all of the information they have at hand.

Ethics is exciting, and competent clinicians need to know about ethical dilemmas and solutions in their professions. Ethicists have often been thought of as experts in the arbitrary, ambiguous, and ungrounded judgments of other people. They know that they make the best decisions they can based on the situation and stakeholders at hand. Just as clinicians try to make the best healthcare decisions with and for their patients, ethically driven practitioners must do the same. Each healthcare provider must critically think through the situation to arrive at the best decision.

To make ethical decisions about informatics technologies and patients' intimate healthcare data and information, the healthcare provider must be competent in informatics. To the extent that information technology is reshaping healthcare practices or promises to improve patient care, healthcare professionals must be trained and competent in the use of these tools. This competency needs to be evaluated through instruments developed by professional groups or societies; such assessment will help with consistency and quality. For the healthcare professional to be an effective patient advocate, he or she must understand how information technology affects the patient and the subsequent delivery of care. Information science and its effects on health care are both interesting and important. It follows that information technology and its **ethical, social, and legal implications** should be incorporated into all levels of professional education.

The need for confidentiality was perhaps first articulated by Hippocrates; thus if anything is different in today's environment, it is simply the ways in which confidentiality can be violated. Perhaps the use of computers for clinical decision support and data mining in research will raise new ethical issues. Ethical dilemmas associated with the integration of informatics must be examined to provide an ethical framework that considers all of the stakeholders. Patients' rights must be protected in the face of a healthcare provider's duty to his or her employer and society at large when initiating care and assigning finite healthcare resources. An ethical framework is necessary to help guide healthcare providers in reference to the ethical treatment of electronic data and information during all stages of collection, storage, manipulation, and dissemination. These new approaches and means come with their own ethical dilemmas. Often they are dilemmas not yet faced owing to the cutting-edge nature of these technologies.

Just as processes and models are used to diagnose and treat patients in practice, so a model in the analysis and synthesis of ethical dilemmas or cases can also be applied. An ethical model for ethical decision making (**Box 5-1**) facilitates the ability to analyze the dilemma and synthesize the information into a plan of action (McGonigle, 2000). The model presented here is based on the letters in the word *ethical*. Each letter guides and prompts the healthcare provider to think critically (think and rethink) through the situation presented. The model is a tool because, in the final analysis, it allows the nurse objectively to ascertain the essence of the dilemma and develop a plan of action.

## BOX 5-1 ETHICAL MODEL FOR ETHICAL DECISION MAKING

- Examine the ethical dilemma (conflicting values exist).
- Thoroughly comprehend the possible alternatives available.
- Hypothesize ethical arguments.
- Investigate, compare, and evaluate the arguments for each alternative.
- Choose the alternative you would recommend.
- Act on your chosen alternative.
- Look at the ethical dilemma and examine the outcomes while reflecting on the ethical decision.

## APPLYING THE ETHICAL MODEL

**Examine the ethical dilemma:**
- Use your problem-solving, decision-making, and critical-thinking skills.
- What is the dilemma you are analyzing? Collect as much information about the dilemma as you can, making sure to gather the relevant facts that clearly identify the dilemma. You should be able to describe the dilemma you are analyzing in detail.
- Ascertain exactly what must be decided.
- Who should be involved in the decision-making process for this specific case?
- Who are the interested players or stakeholders?
- Reflect on the viewpoints of these key players and their value systems.
- What do you think each of these stakeholders would like you to decide as a plan of action for this dilemma?
- How can you generate the greatest good?

**Thoroughly comprehend the possible alternatives available:**
- Use your problem-solving, decision-making, and critical-thinking skills.
- Create a list of the possible alternatives. Be creative when developing your alternatives. Be open minded; there is more than one way to reach a goal. Compel yourself to discern at least three alternatives.
- Clarify the alternatives available and predict the associated consequences—good and bad—of each potential alternative or intervention.
- For each alternative, ask the following questions:
  - Do any of the principles or rules, such as legal, professional, or organizational, automatically nullify this alternative?
  - If this alternative is chosen, what do you predict as the best-case and worst-case scenarios?
  - Do the best-case outcomes outweigh the worst-case outcomes?
  - Could you live with the worst-case scenario?
  - Will anyone be harmed? If so, how will they be harmed?
  - Does the benefit obtained from this alternative overcome the risk of potential harm that it could cause to anyone?

**Hypothesize ethical arguments:**
- Use your problem-solving, decision-making, and critical-thinking skills.
- Determine which of the five approaches apply to this dilemma.
- Identify the moral principles that can be brought into play to support a conclusion as to what ought to be done ethically in this case or similar cases.
- Ascertain whether the approaches generate converging or diverging conclusions about what ought to be done.

**Investigate, compare, and evaluate the arguments for each alternative:**
- Use your problem-solving, decision-making, and critical-thinking skills.
- Appraise the relevant facts and assumptions prudently.
  - Is there ambiguous information that must be evaluated?
  - Are there any unjustifiable factual or illogical assumptions or debatable conceptual issues that must be explored?
- Rate the ethical reasoning and arguments for each alternative in terms of their relative significance.
  - 4 = extreme significance
  - 3 = major significance
  - 2 = significant
  - 1 = minor significance
- Compare and contrast the alternatives available with the values of the key players involved.
- Reflect on these alternatives:
  - Does each alternative consider all of the key players?
  - Does each alternative take into account and reflect an interest in the concerns and welfare of all of the key players?
  - Which alternative will produce the greatest good or the least amount of harm for the greatest number of people?
- Refer to your professional codes of ethical conduct. Do they support your reasoning?

**Choose the alternative you would recommend:**
- Use your problem-solving, decision-making, and critical-thinking skills.
- Make a decision about the best alternative available.
  - Remember the Golden Rule: Does your decision treat others as you would want to be treated?
  - Does your decision take into account and reflect an interest in the concerns and welfare of all of the key players?
  - Does your decision maximize the benefit and minimize the risk for everyone involved?
- Become your own critic; challenge your decision as you think others might. Use the ethical arguments you predict they would use and defend your decision.
  - Would you be secure enough in your ethical decision-making process to see it aired on national television or sent out globally over the Internet?

  - Are you secure enough with this ethical decision that you could have allowed your loved ones to observe your decision-making process, your decision, and its outcomes?

**Act on your chosen alternative:**
- Use your problem-solving, decision-making, and critical-thinking skills.
- Formulate an implementation plan delineating the execution of the decision.
  - This plan should be designed to maximize the benefits and minimize the risks.
  - This plan must take into account all of the resources necessary for implementation, including personnel and money.
- Implement the plan.

**Look at the ethical dilemma and examine the outcomes while reflecting on your ethical decision:**
- Use your problem-solving, decision-making, and critical-thinking skills.
- Monitor the implementation plan and its outcomes. It is extremely important to reflect on specific case decisions and evaluate their outcomes to develop your ethical decision-making ability.
- If new information becomes available, the plan must be reevaluated.
- Monitor and revise the plan as necessary.

The ethical model for ethical decision making was developed by Dr. Dee McGonigle and is the property of Educational Advancement Associates (EAA). The permission for its use in this text has been granted by Mr. Craig R. Goshow, Vice President, EAA.

# Case Analysis Demonstration

The following case study is intended to help readers think through how to apply the ethical model. Review the model and then read through the case. Try to apply the model to this case or follow along as the model is implemented. Readers are challenged to determine their decision in this case and then compare and contrast their response with the decision the authors reached.

> *Allison is a charge nurse on a busy medical–surgical unit. She is expecting the clinical instructor from the local university at 2:00 pm to review and discuss potential patient assignments for the nursing students scheduled for the following day. Just as the university professor arrives, one of the patients on the unit develops a crisis requiring Allison's attention. To expedite the student nurse assignments for the following day, Allison gives her electronic medical record access password to the instructor.*

## Examine the Ethical Dilemma

Allison made a commitment to meet with the university instructor to develop student assignments at 2:00 pm. The patient emergency that developed prevented Allison from living up to that commitment. Allison had an obligation to provide patient care during the emergency and a competing obligation to the professor. She solved the dilemma of competing obligations by providing her electronic medical record access password to the university professor.

By sharing her password, Allison most likely violated hospital policy related to the **security** of healthcare information. She may also have violated the American Nurses Association code of ethics, which states that nurses must judiciously protect information of a confidential nature. Because the university professor was also a nurse and had a legitimate interest in the protected healthcare information, there might not be a code of ethics violation.

## Thoroughly Comprehend the Possible Alternatives Available

The possible **alternatives** available include the following: (1) Allison could have asked the professor to wait until the patient crisis was resolved; (2) Allison could have delegated another staff member to assist the university professor; or (3) Allison could have logged on to the system for the professor.

## Hypothesize Ethical Arguments

The utilitarian approach applies to this situation. An ethical action is one that provides the greatest good for the greatest number; the underlying principles in this perspective are beneficence and nonmaleficence. The rights to be considered are as follows: right of the individual to choose for himself or herself (autonomy); right to truth (**veracity**); right of privacy (the ethical right to privacy avoids conflict and, like all rights, promotes harmony); right not to be injured; and right to what has been promised (fidelity).

Does the action respect the **moral rights** of everyone? The principles to consider are autonomy, veracity, and fidelity.

As for the fairness or justice, how fair is an action? Does it treat everyone in the same way, or does it show favoritism and discrimination? The principles to consider are justice and distributive justice.

Thinking about the common good assumes one's own good is inextricably linked to good of the community; community members are bound by pursuit of common values and goals and ensure that the social policies, social systems, institutions, and environments on which one depends are beneficial to all. Examples of such outcomes are affordable health care, effective public safety, a just legal system, and an unpolluted environment. The principle of distributive justice is considered.

Virtue assumes that one should strive toward certain ideals that provide for the full development of humanity. Virtues are attitudes or character traits that enable one to be and to act in ways that develop the highest potential; examples include honesty, courage, compassion, generosity, fidelity, integrity, fairness, self-control, and prudence. Like habits, virtues become a characteristic of the person. The virtuous person is the ethical person. Ask yourself, what kind of person should I be? What will promote the development of character within myself and my community? The principles considered are fidelity, veracity, beneficence, nonmaleficence, justice, and distributive justice.

In this case, there is a clear violation of an institutional policy designed to protect the privacy and confidentiality of medical records. However, the professor had a legitimate interest in the information and a legitimate right to the information. Allison trusted that the professor would not use the system password to obtain information outside the scope of the legitimate interest. However, Allison cannot be sure that the professor would not access inappropriate information. Further, Allison is responsible for how her access to the electronic system is used. Balancing the rights of everyone—the professor's right to the information, the patients' rights to expect that their information is safeguarded, and the right of the patient in crisis to expect the best possible care—is important and is the crux of the dilemma. Does the patient care obligation outweigh the obligation to the professor? Yes, probably. Allison did the right thing by caring for the patient in crisis. By giving out her system access password, Allison also compromised the rights of the other patients on the unit to expect that their confidentiality and privacy would be safeguarded.

Virtue ethics suggests that individuals use power to bring about human benefit. One must consider the needs of others and the responsibility to meet those needs. Allison must simultaneously provide care, prevent harm, and maintain professional relationships.

Allison may want to effect a long-term change in hospital policy for the common good. It is reasonable to assume that this event was not an isolated incident and that the problem may recur in the future. Can the institutional policy be amended to provide professors with access to the medical records system? As suggested in the HIPAA administrative guidelines, the professor could receive the same staff training regarding appropriate and inappropriate use of access and sign the agreement to safeguard the records. If the institution has tracking software, the professor's access could be monitored to watch for inappropriate use.

Identify the moral principles that can be brought into play to support a conclusion as to what ought to be done ethically in this case or similar cases. The International Council of Nurses (2006) code of ethics states that "The nurse holds in confidence personal information and uses judgment in sharing this information" (p. 4). The code also states, "The nurse uses judgment in relation to individual competence when accepting and delegating responsibilities" (p. 5). Both of these statements apply to the current situation.

Ascertain whether the approaches generate converging or diverging conclusions about what ought to be done. From the analysis, it is clear that the best immediate solution is to delegate assisting the professor with assignments to another nurse on the unit.

## Investigate, Compare, and Evaluate the Arguments for Each Alternative

Review and think through the items listed in Table 5-1.

## Choose the Alternative You Would Recommend

The best immediate solution is to delegate another staff member to assist the professor. The best long-term solution is to change the hospital policy to include access for professors, as described previously.

Table 5-1 Detailed Analysis of Alternative Actions

| Alternative | Good Consequences | Bad Consequences | Do Any Rules Nullify | Expected Outcome | Potential Benefit > Harm |
|---|---|---|---|---|---|
| 1. Wait until crisis was resolved | No policy violation<br><br>Patient rights safeguarded | Not the best use of the professor's time | No | Best: Crisis will require a short time<br><br>Worst: Crisis may take a long time | Patient rights protected<br><br>Collegial relationship jeopardized<br><br>Patient rights may take precedence |
| 2. Delegate to another staff member | No policy violated | Other staff may be equally busy or might not be as familiar with all patients | No | Best: Assignments will be completed<br><br>Worst: May not have benefit of expert advice | Confidentiality of record is assured<br><br>May compromise student learning<br><br>Patient rights may take precedence |
| 3. Log on to the system for the professor | Professor can begin making assignments | May still be a violation of policy regarding system access | Rules regarding access to medical record | Best: Assignments can be completed<br><br>Worst: Abuse of access to information | Potential compromise of records<br><br>Patient in crisis is cared for |

## Act on Your Chosen Alternative

Allison should delegate another staff member to assist the professor in making assignments.

## Look at the Ethical Dilemma and Examine the Outcomes While Reflecting on the Ethical Decision

As already indicated in the alternative analyses, delegation may not be an ideal solution because the staff nurse who is assigned to assist the professor may not possess the same extensive information about all of the patients as the charge nurse. It is, however, the best immediate solution to the dilemma and is certainly safer than compromising the integrity of the hospital's computer system. As noted previously, Allison may want to pursue a long-term solution to a potentially recurring problem by helping the professor gain legitimate access to the computer system with the professor's own password. The system administrator would then have the ability to track who used the system and which types of information were accessed during use.

This case analysis demonstration provides the authors' perspective on this case and the ethical decision made. If your decision did not match this perspective, what was the basis for the difference of opinion? If you worked through the model, you might have reached a different decision based on your individual background and perspective. This does not make the decision right or wrong. A decision should reflect the best decision one can make given review, reflection, and critical thinking about this specific situation.

Six additional cases are provided in the online learner's manual for review. Apply the model to each case study, and discuss these cases with colleagues or classmates.

## New Frontiers in Ethical Issues

The expanding use of new information technologies in health care will bring about new and challenging ethical issues. Consider that patients and healthcare providers no longer have to be in the same place for a quality interaction. How, then, does one deal with licensing issues if the electronic consultation takes place across a state line? Derse and Miller (2008) describe a second-opinion medical consultation on the Internet where the information was provided to the referring physician and not to the patient, thus avoiding the licensing issue. In essence, provider-to-provider consultation does not constitute practicing in a state in which you are not licensed. As new technologies for healthcare delivery are developed, new ethical challenges may arise. It is important for all healthcare providers to be aware of the code of ethics for their specific practices, and to understand the laws governing their practice and private health information.

Consider also the ethical issues created by genomic databases or by sharing of information in a health information exchange to promote population health. Alpert (2008) asks, "Is it wise to put genomic sequence data into electronic medical records that are poorly protected, that cannot adhere well to Fair Information Practice Principles for privacy, and that can potentially be seen by tens of thousands of people/entities, when it is clear that we do not understand the functionality of the genome and likely will not for several years?" (p. 382).

Further, how does one really obtain informed consent for such data collection, when how the data will ultimately be used is not known, but clearly that application will be important to health research uses that go beyond the immediate medical care of the patient? Angst (2009) asks whether the public good outweighs individual interests in such a case because the information contained in these databases is important to developing new understandings and creating new knowledge by matching data in aggregated pools: "Thus, science adds meaning and context to data, but to what extent do we agree to make the data available such that this discovery process can take place, and are the impacts of discovery great enough to justify the risks?" (p. 172). Further, if a voluntary system where patients can opt out of such data collection is adopted, then are healthcare disparities related to incomplete electronic health records created?

In an ideal world, healthcare professionals must not be affected by conflicting loyalties; nothing should interfere with judicious, ethical decision making. As the technologically charged waters of health care are navigated, one must hone a solid foundation of ethical decision making and practice it consistently.

## Summary

As science and technology advance, and policy makers and healthcare providers continue to shape healthcare practices including information management, it is paramount that ethical decisions are made. Healthcare professionals are typically honest, trustworthy, and ethical, and they understand that they are duty bound to focus on the needs and rights of their patients. At the same time, their day-to-day work is conducted in a world of changing healthcare landscapes populated by new technologies, diverse patients, varied healthcare settings, and changing policies set by their employers, insurance companies, and providers. The technologies themselves are not the problem, but the misuse of the technology can cause harm to our patients. If we use them to the patient's advantage while protecting the patient, they can be beneficial tools in accessing our technologically savvy patients to garner the data and information necessary to address their healthcare needs, including patient education, while impacting public health and enhancing our relationship with our patients. Healthcare professionals need to juggle all of these balls simultaneously, and so the ethical considerations must be at the forefront, a task that often results in far too many gray areas or ethical decision-making dilemmas with no clear correct course of action. Patients rely on the ethical competence of their healthcare providers, believing that their situation is unique and will be respected and evaluated based on their own needs, abilities, and limitations. The healthcare professional cannot allow conflicting loyalties to interfere with judicious, ethical decision making. Just as in the opening example of the Apollo mission, it is uncertain where this technologically heightened information era will lead, but if a solid foundation of ethical decision making is relied upon, duties and rights will be judiciously and ethically fulfilled.

### THOUGHT-PROVOKING QUESTIONS

1. Identify moral dilemmas in healthcare informatics that would best be approached with the use of an ethical decision-making framework, such as the use of smartphones to interact with patients as well as to monitor and assess patient health.
2. Discuss the evolving healthcare ethics traditions within their social and historical contexts.
3. Differentiate among the theoretical approaches to healthcare ethics as they relate to the theorists' perspectives of individuals and their relationships.
4. Select one of the healthcare ethics theories and support its use in examining ethical issues in healthcare informatics.
5. Select one of the healthcare ethics theories and argue against its use in examining ethical issues in healthcare informatics.

# References

Alpert, S. (2008). Privacy issues in clinical genomic medicine, or Marcus Welby, M.D., meets the $1000 genome. *Cambridge Quarterly of Healthcare Ethics, 17*(4), 373–384. Retrieved from Health Module (Document ID: 1880623501).

Anderson, K. (2012). Social media a new way to care and communicate. *Australian Nursing Journal, 20*(3), 22–25.

Angst, C. (2009). Protect my privacy or support the common-good? Ethical questions about electronic health information exchanges. *Journal of Business Ethics, 90*(suppl), 169–178. Retrieved from ABI/INFORM Global (Document ID: 2051417481).

Aristotle. (350 BC). *Nichomachean ethics. Book I.* (W. D. Ross, Trans.). Retrieved from http://www .constitution.org/ari/ethic_00.htm

Ascension Health. (2007). Healthcare Ethics: Virtue ethics. Retrieved from http://www .ascensionhealth.org/ethics/public/issues/virtue.asp

Beauchamp, T. L., & Childress, J. F. (1977). *Principles of biomedical ethics.* New York, NY: Oxford University Press.

Beauchamp, T. L., & Childress, J. F. (1994). *Principles of biomedical ethics* (4th ed.). New York, NY: Oxford University Press.

Benjamin, M., & Curtis, J. (1992). *Ethics in nursing* (3rd ed.). New York, NY: Oxford University Press.

Derse, A., & Miller, T. (2008). Net effect: Professional and ethical challenges of medicine online. *Cambridge Quarterly of Healthcare Ethics, 17*(4), 453–464. Retrieved from Health Module (Document ID: 1540615461).

eHealth code. (n.d.). Retrieved from http://www.ihealthcoalition.org/ehealth-code

Englund, H., Chappy, S., Jambunathan, J., & Gohdes, E. (2012, November/December). Ethical reasoning and online social media. *Nurse Educator, 37*, 242–247. http://dx.doi.org/10.1097 /NNE.0b013e31826f2c04

Engster, D. (2004). Care ethics and natural law theory: Toward an institutional political theory of caring. *The Journal of Politics, 66*(1), 113–135.

Henderson, M., & Dahnke, M. (2015). The ethical use of social media in nursing practice. *MEDSURG Nursing, 24*(1), 62–64.

Howard, R. (Director). (1995). *Apollo 13* [Motion picture]. Universal City, CA: MCA Universal Studios.

Husted, G. L., & Husted, J. H. (1995). *Ethical decision-making in nursing* (2nd ed.). New York, NY: Mosby.

International Council of Nurses (ICN). (2006). The ICN code of ethics for nurses. Retrieved from http://www.icn.ch/icncode.pdf

Johns Hopkins, Berman Institute of Bioethics. (n.d.). A blueprint for 21st century nursing ethics. Retrieved from http://www.bioethicsinstitute.org/nursing-ethics-summit-report/literature-review

Jonsen, A. R. (1991). Casuistry as methodology in clinical ethics. *Theoretical Medicine, 12*, 295–307.

Lyons, R., & Reinisch, C. (2013). The legal and ethical implications of social media in the emergency department. *Advanced Emergency Nursing Journal, 35*(1), 53–56. http://dx.doi. org/10.1097/TME.0b013e31827a4926

Mack, J. (2000). Patient empowerment, not economics, is driving e-health: Privacy and ethics issues need attention too! *Frontiers of Health Services Management, 17*(1), 39–43; discussion 49–51. Retrieved from ABI/INFORM Global (Document ID: 59722384).

Makus, R. (2001). Ethics and Internet healthcare: An ontological reflection. *Cambridge Quarterly of Healthcare Ethics, 10*(2), 127–136. Retrieved from Health Module (Document ID: 1409693941).

Martin, P. A. (1999). Bioethics and the whole: Pluralism, consensus, and the transmutation of bioethical methods into gold. *Journal of Law, Medicine & Ethics, 27*(4), 316–327.

McGonigle, D. (2000). The ethical model for ethical decision making. *Inside Case Management, 7*(8), 1–5.

National Council of State Boards of Nursing (NCSBN). (2011). White paper: A nurse's guide to the use of social media. Retrieved from https://www.ncsbn.org/Social_Media.pdf

Pellegrino, E. D. (1993). The metamorphosis of medical ethics: A thirty-year retrospective. *Journal of the American Medical Association, 269*, 1158–1162.

Pellegrino, E., & Thomasma, D. (1993). *The virtues in medical practice.* New York, NY: Oxford University Press.

Resnik, D. (2001). Patient access to medical information in the computer age: Ethical concerns and issues. *Cambridge Quarterly of Healthcare Ethics, 10*(2), 147–154; discussion 154–156. Retrieved from Health Module (Document ID: 1409693961).

Scott, A. (2002). Plato's Meno. Retrieved from http://www.angelfire.com/md2/timewarp/plato.html

Spector, N., & Kappel, D. M. (2012). Guidelines for using electronic and social media: The regulatory perspective. *Online Journal of Nursing, 17*(3). Retrieved from http://www.nursingworld.org/MainMenuCategories/ANAMarketplace/ANAPeriodicals/OJIN/TableofContents/Vol-17-2012/No3-Sept-2012/Guidelines-for-Electronic-and-Social-Media.htm

Stern, J. (2013). Google Glass: What you can and can't do with Google's wearable computer. *ABC News.* Retrieved from http://abcnews.go.com/Technology/google-glass-googles-wearable-gadget/story?id=19091948

Swartz, M. K. (2011, November/December). The potential for social media. *Journal of Pediatric Health Care, 25*, 345.

Symplur. (2016). Why the healthcare Hashtag project? Retrieved from http://www.symplur.com/healthcare-hashtags

Velasquez, M., Andre, C., Shanks, T., & Myer, M. (for the Markkula Center for Applied Ethics). (1987). What is ethics? Retrieved from http://www.scu.edu/SCU/Centers/Ethics/practicing/decision/whatisethics.shtml

Zephoria. (2016). Top 20 valuable Facebook statistics. Retrieved from https://zephoria.com/top-15-valuable-facebook-statistics

# Perspectives on Nursing Informatics

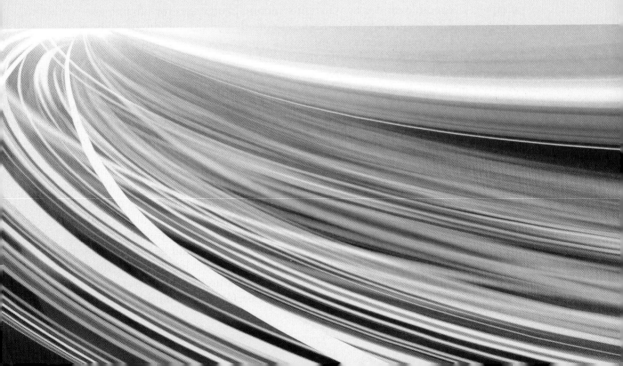

Nursing informatics (NI) is the synthesis of nursing science, information science, computer science, and cognitive science for the purpose of managing and enhancing healthcare data, information, knowledge, and wisdom to improve patient care and the nursing profession. In the *Building Blocks of Nursing Informatics* section, the reader learned about the four sciences of NI, also referred to as the four building blocks, and the ethical application of these sciences to manage patient information. Nursing knowledge workers must be able to understand the evolving specialty of NI to harness and use the tools available for managing the vast amount of healthcare data and information. It is essential that NI capabilities be appreciated, promoted, expanded, and advanced to facilitate the work of the nurse, improve patient care, and enhance the nursing profession.

This section presents the perspectives of nursing experts on NI. The *History and Evolution of Nursing Informatics* chapter begins this exploration by providing the historical development and evolution of NI. This transitions into the *Nursing Informatics as a Specialty* chapter, where the reader learns about NI roles, competencies, and skills. The *Legislative Aspects of Nursing Informatics: HITECH and HIPAA* chapter considers the evolving NI needs of nurses and nurse informaticists based on the current regulations impacting the healthcare arena.

In the *History and Evolution of Nursing Informatics* chapter, interrelationships among major NI concepts are discussed. As data are transformed into information and information into knowledge, increasing complexity and interrelationships ensue. The boundaries between concepts can become blurred, and feedback loops from one concept level to another evolve. Structured languages and human–computer interaction concepts, which are critical elements for NI, are noted in this chapter. Taxonomies and other current structured languages for nursing are listed. Human–computer interaction concepts are briefly defined and discussed because they are critical to the success of informatics solutions. Importantly, the construct of decision making is added to the traditional nursing metaparadigms: nurse, person, health, and environment. Decision making is not only at the crux of nursing practice in all settings and roles, but it is a fundamental concern of NI. The work of nursing is centered on the concepts of NI: data, information, knowledge, and wisdom. Information technology (IT) per se is not the focus; it is the information that the technology conveys that is central. Moreover, NI is no longer the domain of experts in the IT field. More interestingly, one does not need technology to perform informatics. The centerpiece of informatics is the manipulation of data, information, and knowledge, especially related to decision making in any aspect of nursing or in any setting. In a way, nurses are all already informatics nurses. Note that the core concepts and competencies of informatics are particularly well suited to a model of interprofessional education. Ideally, when educational programs are emulating clinical settings, informatics knowledge should be integrated with the processes of interprofessional teams and decision making. Because simulation laboratories are becoming increasingly common fixtures in the delivery of health-related professional education, they provide a perfect opportunity to incorporate the electronic health records applications. The learning laboratory for nursing education will then more closely approximate the IT-enabled clinical settings that are emerging in the real world. A presumption is often made that future graduates will be more computer literate than nurses currently in practice. Although this may be true, computer literacy or comfort does not equate to an understanding of the facilitative and transformative role of information technology. It is essential that the future curricula of basic nursing programs embed the concepts of the role of IT in supporting clinical care delivery. The need for standardizing nursing terminology is also discussed in this chapter as a way to improve the clinical support functions of the electronic health record. The healthcare industry employs the largest number of knowledge workers—a fact that has resulted in the realization that healthcare administrators must begin to change the way they look at their employees. Nurses and physicians are bright, highly skilled, and dedicated to giving the best patient care. Administrators who tap into this wealth of knowledge find that patient care becomes safer and more efficient.

The *Nursing Informatics as a Specialty* chapter discusses NI as a relatively new nursing specialty that combines the building block sciences covered earlier in the text. Combining these sciences results in nurses being able to care for their patients effectively and safely because the information that they need is readily available. Nurses have been actively involved in NI since computers were introduced into health care. With the advent of electronic health records, it became apparent that nursing needed to develop its own language for this evolving field. NI was instrumental in assisting in nursing language development. NI is governed by standards established by the American Nurses Association and is a very diverse field, which results in many nurse informaticist specialists becoming focused on one segment of NI. Although NI is a recognized specialty area of practice, in the future all nurses will be expected to have some knowledge of the field. NI competencies have been developed to ensure that all entry-level nurses are ready to enter a field that is becoming more technologically advanced. The competencies may also be used to determine the educational needs of currently practicing nurses as well as Level 4 nurse informatics specialists. Nurse informatics specialists no longer have to enter the field solely through on-the-job exposure, but can now obtain an advanced degree in NI at many well-established universities throughout the United States. NI has grown tremendously as a specialty since its inception and is predicted to continue growing.

The *Legislative Aspects of Nursing Informatics: HITECH and HIPAA* chapter provides insights into HIPAA rules and an overview of the rules associated with technology implementation as defined by the HITECH Act. Equally important in informatics practice is a thorough understanding of current legislation and regulations that shape 21st century practice. The information provided in this text reflects current rules that were in effect at the time of publication. The reader should follow the rules development and evolution of informatics legislation at the U.S. Department of Health and Human Services website (www.hhs.gov) to obtain the most current information related to health information management.

There is an emerging global focus on information technology to support clinical care and on the potential benefits for clinicians and patients. In the future, nurses will likely have sufficient computing power at their disposal to aggregate and transform additional multidimensional data and information sources (e.g., historical, multisensory, experiential, genetic) into a clinical information system to engage with individuals, families, and groups in ways not yet imagined. Every nurse's practice will make contributions to new nursing knowledge in these dynamically interactive clinical information system environments. With the right tools to support the management of data, complex information processing, and ready access to knowledge, the core concepts and competencies associated with informatics will be embedded in the practice of every nurse, whether administrator, researcher, educator, or practitioner. Information technology is not a panacea, but it provides the profession with unprecedented capacity to generate and disseminate new knowledge more rapidly.

The material within this text is placed within the context of the Foundation of Knowledge model (Figure II-1) to meet the needs of healthcare delivery systems, organizations, patients, and nurses. Through involvement in NI and learning about this evolving specialty, one will be able to use the current theories, architecture, and tools, while beginning to challenge what is known. This questioning and search for what

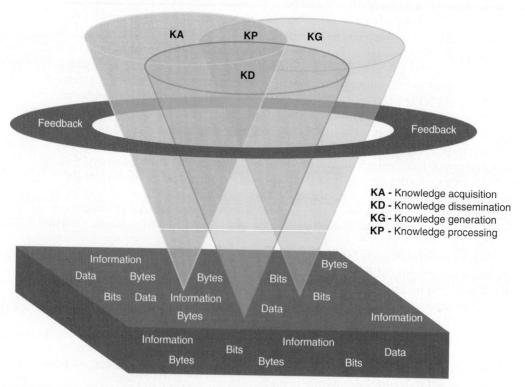

**Figure II-1** Foundation of Knowledge Model
Designed by Alicia Mastrian.

could be will provide the basis for the future landscape of nursing. By using the Foundation of Knowledge model as an organizing framework for this text, the authors have attempted to capture this process.

In this section, the reader learns about NI. Those readers who are beginning their education will consciously focus on input and knowledge acquisition, trying to glean as much information and knowledge as possible. As these readers become more comfortable in their clinical setting and with nursing science, they will begin to take over some of the other knowledge functions. Experienced nurses, also known as "seasoned nurses," question what is known and search for ways to enhance their knowledge and the knowledge of others. What is not available must be created. It is through these leaders, researchers, or clinicians that new knowledge is generated and disseminated and nursing science is advanced. Sometimes, however, to keep up with the explosion of information in nursing and health care, one must continue to rely on the knowledge generated and disseminated by others. In this sense, nurses are committed to lifelong learning and the use of knowledge in the practice of nursing science. How nurses interact within their environment and apply what is learned depends on their placement in the Foundation of Knowledge model.

Readers of this section are challenged to ask how they can (1) apply knowledge gained from the practice setting to benefit patients and enhance their practice, (2) help colleagues and patients understand and use current technology, and (3) use wisdom to help create the theories, tools, and knowledge of the future.

1. Trace the evolution of nursing informatics from concept to specialty practice.

2. Relate nursing informatics metastructures, concepts, and tools to the knowledge work of nursing.

3. Explore the quest for consistent terminology in nursing and describe terminology approaches that accurately capture and codify the contributions of nursing to health care.

4. Explore the concept of nurses as knowledge workers.

5. Explore how nurses can create and derive clinical knowledge from information systems.

## Key Terms

- » Accessibility
- » Cognitive activity
- » Data
- » Data gatherer
- » Enumerative approach
- » Expert systems
- » Industrial Age
- » Information
- » Information Age
- » Information user
- » International Classification of Nursing Practice
- » Knowledge
- » Knowledge builder
- » Knowledge user
- » Knowledge worker
- » Ontological approach
- » Reusability
- » Standardized Nursing Terminology
- » Technologist
- » Terminology
- » Ubiquity
- » Wisdom

# CHAPTER 6

# History and Evolution of Nursing Informatics

Kathleen Mastrian and Dee McGonigle

With contributions by Ramona Nelson, Nancy Staggers, Lynn M. Nagle, and Nicholas Hardiker

## Introduction

The information and knowledge informing the 21st century of healthcare delivery have been growing at an unprecedented pace in recent years. Clinical research in particular has propelled the understanding of the efficacy of various clinical practices, treatment regimens, and interventions. Extended and expanded access to clinical research findings and decision support tools has been significantly influenced by the advent of computerization and the Internet. Indeed, the conduct of research itself has been accelerated by virtue of ubiquitous computing. Working in environments of increasingly complex clinical care and contending with the management of large volumes of data and information, all nurses need to avail themselves of the technological tools that can support quality practice that is optimally safe, informed, and knowledge based. Although the increased deployment of information technologies within healthcare settings presumes that nurses and other health professionals are proficient in the use of computing devices, the processes and potential outcomes associated with informatics are yet to be fully realized or understood. Nurses need to participate in the creation of those possibilities.

Health service organizations, societies, and governments throughout the industrialized world are committed to ensuring that healthcare delivery is safer, knowledge based, cost effective, seamless, and timely. Beyond these deliverables, there are expectations of improved efficiency and quality and of the active engagement of consumers in their care. In particular, given the evolving emphasis on such issues as chronic disease management and aging at home, informatics tools need to include the use of technologies to empower citizens to manage their own health and wellness more effectively.

This chapter explores the history and evolution of nursing informatics and defines and addresses the goal of informatics as it relates to nursing practice. The ways in which nursing informatics supports the creation of a culture of knowledge-based nursing practice that is enabled and advanced through the use of information and communication technologies are described. The chapter also addresses some of the challenges associated with the attainment of this knowledge-based culture, as well as the opportunities for nurses to create and derive knowledge from emerging health information technologies. Finally, the chapter provides a contemplative view of the future for nurses and informatics.

## The Evolution of a Specialty

Nurses have historically gathered and recorded data, albeit in a paper record. For example, nurses gather atomic-level data (e.g., blood pressure, pulse, blood glucose, pallor), aggregate data to derive information (e.g., impending shock), and apply knowledge (e.g., lowering the head of the bed to minimize the potentially deleterious effects of impending shock). Over the years, these data have been recorded into individuals' hard-copy health records, thereby chronicling findings, actions, and outcomes; these data and information were then forever lost unless manually extracted for research purposes. As computers were introduced into health care, and data and information were recorded electronically, a nursing specialty was born.

Florence Nightingale has been credited as one of the first statisticians to collect and use data to change the way she cared for her patients. While serving in the Crimean War, she began to gather data regarding the conditions in which patients were living and the diseases they contracted and from which they died. These data were later used to improve patient conditions at both city and military hospitals (O'Connor & Robertson, 2003). There is no doubt that nursing experiences build knowledge and skill in nursing practice, but paper-based documentation has hindered the ability to share knowledge and to aggregate experiences to build new knowledge.

Nursing informatics pioneers recognized early on that computers had the potential to fundamentally change health care and they became actively involved in shaping how computers were used in health care. For more specific information on nursing informatics pioneers, and to view video recordings of the contributions of each in the nursing informatics history project, please visit this website: https://www.amia.org/working-groups/nursing-informatics/history-project/video-library-1

According to Ozbolt and Saba (2008), one very early pioneer, Harriet Werley, a nurse researcher at Walter Reed Army Research Institute, consulted with IBM in the late 1950s to explore computer use in health care. Ms. Werley recognized the need for a minimum set of data to be collected from every patient, so that comparisons could be made, and thus set the stage for the development of informatics. As computers became more commonplace in the 1970s and 1980s, more nurses became involved with developing approaches to use computers in health care. It is important to note that this was also the time that nurse leaders were writing about the need for and developing terminologies to represent patient data and nursing contributions to health care, were beginning to conduct informatics research, and were advocating for informatics education in nursing curricula (Ozbolt & Saba, 2008).

In 1989, Graves and Cocoran offered what is widely viewed as the seminal definition of nursing informatics (NI). They defined NI as: "a combination of computer science, information science, and nursing science designed to assist in the management and processing of nursing data, information, and knowledge to support the practice of nursing and the delivery of nursing care" (p. 227). In this same article, acknowledging the 1986 work of Blum, Graves and Cocoran provided the definitions and descriptions of the concepts of **data** (discrete entities described objectively without interpretation), **information** (data that are interpreted, organized, or structured), and **knowledge** (information that is synthesized so that relationships are identified and formalized) as these terms apply to the science and practice of NI. They also described what is meant by management and processing. "The management component of informatics is the functional ability to collect, aggregate, organize, move, and re-present information in an economical, efficient way that is useful to the users of the system. . . . In practice, processing is considered as a *transformation* of data or information from one form to another form, usually at a more complex state of organization or meaning. There is a progression of transformation of data into information and of information into knowledge" (p. 227). We will return to a discussion of these concepts later in the chapter. For now, we continue our exploration of the evolution of informatics as a specialty.

In the 1990s, the American Medical Informatics Association was founded with a nursing informatics work group, the American Nurses Association (ANA) recognized nursing informatics as a specialty, ANA published two documents related to informatics practice, and the first informatics certification was established (Ozbolt & Saba, 2008). As nursing informatics pioneers and emerging leaders continued to champion the use of computers in health care, the need for computer-friendly terminologies to represent the work of nursing was increasingly apparent. Several different terminology schemes were developed during this time, and there were also international efforts at developing a standardized nursing terminology to capture and codify the contributions of nursing to health care. At this same time, healthcare organizations were beginning to implement electronic information systems. There was little coordination of these various efforts and approaches. As Ozbolt and Saba (2008) explain, "Faced with the bewildering array of choices and the licensing fees required for the use of NANDA [North American Nursing Diagnosis Association (as it was known until 2002)], NIC [Nursing Interventions Classification], NOC [Nursing Outcomes Classification], and SNOMED [Systematized Nomenclature of Medicine], many health care organizations adopting nursing information systems opted to use their own or vendor-provided, non-standard terms. This approach allowed entry of data via familiar terms, but because the terms were not consistent in definition or usage, investigators could not retrieve meaningful data to analyze for quality improvement or research" (p. 202). We will discuss this issue in more detail later in the chapter.

President Bush's call for electronic health records in 2004 further stimulated the development of nursing informatics, informatics competency identification, and informatics education reform, and spawned several national and international informatics organizations. "While nursing informatics leaders work to transform nursing education and practice, nursing informatics scientists are creating the knowledge and tools that will enable the transformation. As research in nursing terminology and knowledge representation moves from creation to implementation and use, other domains of research reflect the maturation of nursing informatics as a science" (Ozbolt & Saba, 2008 p. 204). In this profound statement, we see the clear connection between nursing science and nursing informatics. That is, knowledge creation in nursing is dependent on knowledge representation in the information management tools that are central to nursing informatics. As the NI pioneers recognized these important connections and synergies, both nursing as a science and nursing informatics as a specialty evolved. Indeed, the evolution is not complete, as you will experience as you read the subsequent chapters in this text.

As the NI specialty was evolving, informatics pioneers and other nurse leaders collaborated on several ANA publications. As mentioned previously, NI was identified by the ANA as a specialty in 1992. In 1994, the first formal document identifying the scope of practice was published, followed by a separate standards of practice document in 1995. In 2001, a combined scope and standards document was published by the ANA, followed by a more robust scope and standards publication in 2008. Finally, in 2015 the ANA released the second edition of *Nursing Informatics: Scope and Standards of Practice.*

## What Is Nursing Informatics?

The ANA's *Nursing Informatics: Scope and Standards of Practice* (2015) offers the following definition of NI:

> *Nursing informatics (NI) is the specialty that integrates nursing science with multiple information and analytical sciences to identify, define, manage, and communicate data, information, knowledge and wisdom in nursing practice. NI supports nurses, consumers, patients, the interprofessional healthcare team, and all other stakeholders in their decision-making in all roles and settings to achieve desired outcomes. This support is accomplished through the use of information structures, information processes, and information technology. (p. 1–2)*

The definition of nursing informatics has undergone several revisions to arrive at this current form. The 1994 ANA definition of informatics indicated that informatics was the integration of nursing science, computer science, and information science, and that nursing informatics supports practice, education, research, and knowledge development (Murphy, 2010). The 2001 version incorporated mention of the support of decision making by patients and providers across all roles and settings and identified information structures, processes, and IT (information technology) as central to informatics (Murphy, 2010). An important change in the 2008 definition of NI is the addition of **wisdom** to the key concepts of the management of data, information, and knowledge (Murphy, 2010). Finally, in the 2015 version, we note that the sciences are no longer limited to nursing science, information science, and computer science. Cognitive science is also a very important part of nursing informatics. Other sciences that may contribute to NI include library science and information management, mathematics, archival science, and the science of terminologies and taxonomies (ANA, 2015).

Let us reflect more carefully on the current definition of NI by deconstructing each of the statements contained in the ANA's (2015) definition (statements from the definition are italicized):

- *Nursing informatics (NI) is the specialty that integrates nursing science with multiple information and analytical sciences to identify, define, manage, and*

*communicate data, information, knowledge and wisdom in nursing practice.*
As we established previously, there are concepts drawn from several sciences
that are integrated to support and contribute to NI. The contributions of these
sciences become apparent in the actions of NI: identify, define, manage, and
communicate. The last part of this statement contains the critical central concepts of NI: the data, information, knowledge, and wisdom that are integral
to our practice. We will explore these central concepts in more detail in the
next section.

- NI *supports nurses, consumers, patients, the interprofessional healthcare team,
  and all other stakeholders in their decision-making in all roles and settings to
  achieve desired outcomes.* This statement refers to the information technology
  (IT) tools that support our practice and help us to collaborate and communicate
  with other healthcare professionals, as well as the evolving trends and tools
  related to patient engagement in managing their own health. All of these contribute to better health outcomes. Examples of such tools are electronic health
  records, bar-code medication administration systems, clinical decision support
  and other expert systems, patient monitoring devices, and telehealth tools. These
  and other NI tools are discussed in subsequent chapters.

- *This support is accomplished through the use of information structures, information processes, and information technology.* This section of the definition
  clearly identifies the need for information technologies to provide structure to
  the data we collect from our patients, and allow for processing of data and
  information to create knowledge and support wisdom in nursing practice.
  Think about the fact that with the advent of clinical information systems (CISs),
  specifically electronic documentation and clinical decision support (CDS)
  applications, every nurse has the capacity to contribute to the advancement of
  nursing knowledge on many levels. Imagine the use of IT solutions to capture
  not only discrete, quantifiable data, but also the nurse's experiential and intuitive personal knowledge not typically documented in paper records. Further
  add to that mix the family history, culture, environmental and social factors,
  past experiences, and perspectives from patients and families, and it becomes
  clear that the possibilities for generating new understandings within populations
  and across the life span and care continuum are endless. Many of these technologies are covered in subsequent chapters.

## The DIKW Paradigm

The conceptual framework underpinning the science and practice of NI centers on
the core concepts of data, information, knowledge, and wisdom, also known as the
DIKW paradigm. As an aside, it is important to note that this paradigm is not exclusive to nursing, and is in fact used by others who work with data and information.
When we assess a patient to determine his or her nursing needs, we gather and then
analyze and interpret data to form a conclusion. This is the essence of nursing science.
Information is composed of data that were processed using knowledge. Knowledge is
the awareness and understanding of a set of information and ways that information
can be made useful to support a specific task or arrive at a decision. When we apply

previous knowledge to data, we convert those data into information, and information into new knowledge—that is, an understanding of which interventions are appropriate in practice. Thus information is data made functional through the application of knowledge. Wisdom is the appropriate application of knowledge to a specific situation. In the practice of nursing science, one expects actions to be ultimately directed by wisdom. Wisdom uses knowledge and experience to heighten common sense and insight to exercise sound judgment in practical matters.

Drawing on the work of Matney, Brewster, Sward, Cloyes, and Staggers (2011), Topaz (2013) provided these expanded definitions and examples of the DIKW paradigm:

- **Data:** The smallest components of the DIKW framework. They are commonly presented as discrete facts; product of observation with little interpretation (Matney et al., 2011). These are the discrete factors describing the patient or his/her environment. Examples include patient's medical diagnosis (e.g. International Statistical Classification of Diseases [ICD-9] diagnosis #428.0: Congestive heart failure, unspecified) or living status (e.g., living alone, living with family, living in a retirement community, etc.). A single piece of data, known as datum, often has little meaning in isolation.

- **Information:** Might be thought of as "data + meaning" (Matney et al., 2011). Information is often constructed by combining different data points into a meaningful picture, given certain context. Information is a continuum of progressively developing and clustered data; it answers questions such as "who," "what," "where," and "when." For example, a combination of patient's ICD-9 diagnosis #428.0 "Congestive heart failure, unspecified" and living status "living alone" has a certain meaning in a context of an older adult.

- **Knowledge:** Information that has been synthesized so that relations and interactions are defined and formalized; it is a build of meaningful information constructed of discrete data points (Matney et al., 2011). Knowledge is often affected by assumptions and central theories of a scientific discipline and is derived by discovering patterns of relationships between different clusters of information. Knowledge answers questions of "why" or "how." For healthcare professionals, the combination of different information clusters, such as the ICD-9 diagnosis #428.0 "Congestive heart failure, unspecified" + living status "living alone" with an additional information that an older man (78 years old) was just discharged from hospital to home with a complicated new medication regimen (e.g., blood thinners) might indicate that this person is at a high risk for drug-related adverse effects (e.g., bleeding).

- **Wisdom:** An appropriate use of knowledge to manage and solve human problems (ANA, 2008; Matney et al., 2011). Wisdom implies a form of ethics, or knowing why certain things or procedures should or should not be implemented in healthcare practice. In nursing, wisdom guides the nurse in recognizing the situation at hand based on patients' values, nurse's experience, and healthcare knowledge. Combining all these components, the nurse decides on a nursing intervention or action. Benner (2000) presents wisdom as a clinical judgment integrating intuition, emotions, and the senses; using the previous examples, wisdom will be displayed when the homecare nurse will consider prioritizing the elderly heart failure patient using blood thinners for an immediate intervention, such as a first nursing visit within the first hours of discharge from hospital to assure appropriate use of medications (para. 2).

Reflect on the examples given by Topaz and create your own application example the DIKW scenario.

In the 2015 *Nursing Informatics: Scope and Standards of Practice*, Ramona Nelson offers a graphic depiction of the DIKW concepts and how these concepts relate to information systems, decision support systems, and expert systems designed to support clinical practice. Her model indicates that as one moves from data to information to knowledge to wisdom, there is increasing complexity (shown as the X-axis) and increasing interactions and relationships (shown as the Y-axis). Information systems are shown at the intersection of data and information, decision support systems are depicted at the intersection of information and knowledge and expert systems, the most complex of the systems, reside at the intersection of knowledge and wisdom (**Figure 6-1**). The development of informatics tools to

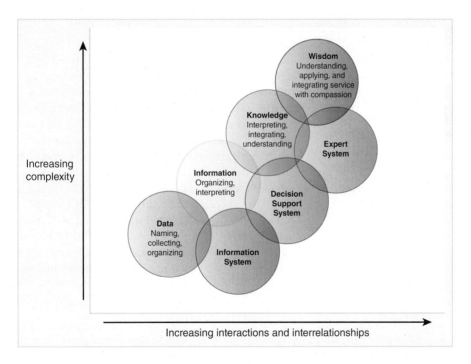

**Figure 6-1** The Relationship of Data, Information, Knowledge, and Wisdom and Automated Systems.

support nursing practice will continue to evolve as we develop more and better understanding of these complex relationships. "The addition of wisdom raises new and important research questions, challenging the profession to develop tools and processes for classifying, measuring, and encoding wisdom as it relates to nursing and informatics education. Research in these directions will help clarify the relationship between wisdom and the intuitive thinking of expert nurses. Such research will be invaluable in building information systems to better support healthcare practitioners in decision-making" (ANA, 2015, p.6).

Central to the development of robust expert systems is the agreement on and use of standard terminologies that accurately codify and capture the nature of nursing in these electronic systems. Consider that physician contributions to the health of a patient have been codified for some time, i.e., ICD-10. What if we were able to code and thus capture nursing contributions in a similar way? This would help to highlight the specific nursing contributions to patient outcomes.

## Capturing and Codifying the Work of Nursing

There are major efforts under way—internationally through the International Council of Nurses' (2013) **International Classification of Nursing Practice** (ICNP) and in many other initiatives among and within countries—in which nurses are attempting to standardize the language of nursing practice (Hannah, White, Nagle, & Pringle, 2009). These efforts are particularly important in the face of the development of EHRs and HIE (health information exchanges) stimulated by the HITECH Act of 2009. The capacity to encourage and enforce consistent nomenclatures that reflect the practice of nurses is now possible. Standardized language gives both the nursing profession and healthcare delivery systems the capability to capture, codify, retrieve, and analyze the impact of nursing care on client outcomes. For example, with the use and documentation of standardized client assessments, including risk measures, interventions based on best practices, and consistently measured outcomes within different care settings and across the continuum of care, there will be an ability to demonstrate more clearly the contributions and impact of nursing care through the analysis of EHR outputs. Additionally, clinical outcomes can be further understood in the context of care environments, particularly implications related to the availability of human and material resources to support care delivery. The standardization of clinical inputs and outputs into EHRs will eventually provide a rich knowledge base from which practice and research can be enhanced, and will inform better administrative and policy decisions (Nagle, White, & Pringle, 2010). Rutherford (2008) echoed these same sentiments:

> A standardized nursing language should be defined so that nursing care can be communicated accurately among nurses and other health care providers. Once standardized, a term can be measured and coded. Measurement of the nursing care through a standardized vocabulary by way of an ED [electronic documentation] will lead to the development of large databases. From these databases, evidence-based standards can be developed to validate the contribution of nurses to patient outcomes. (para. 5)

Thede and Schwiran (2011) identified the benefits of using standardized terminology as (1) better communication among nurse and other healthcare providers, (2) increased visibility of nursing interventions, (3) improved patient care, (4) enhanced data collection to evaluate nursing care outcomes, (5) greater adherence to standards of care, and (6) facilitation of assessment of nursing competency (para. 2).

Think about this. Some EHRs measure height in feet and inches, others in centimeters. Weight may be measured in pounds or kilograms. If we want to compare patient data from multiple EHRs in several different healthcare institutions to develop a model to predict the onset of Type II diabetes, these disparate measures will not translate well. Some EHRs force data collection into coded database fields, and these data are more easily analyzed for trends than that same data recorded as free text. Clinicians used to recording data (charting) as text may resist the use of the coded data fields typically presented as dropdown menus in the EHR. As Skrocki (2013) pointed out, "Data interoperability is hindered when clinicians utilize free text documentation. Although text data can be searched with a specific word or word phases, it does not allow for optimal data sharing. When an organization transfers data to another organization, standardized codified data allows for better data interpretation" (p. 77).

Although significant progress has been made in this standardization work, it is still evolving. Box 6-1 discusses standardizing terminologies in nursing; it was contributed by Nicholas Hardiker (2011), a leader in the development of standardized languages that support clinical applications of information and communication technology.

## BOX 6-1 THE NEED FOR STANDARDIZED TERMINOLOGIES TO SUPPORT NURSING PRACTICE

*Nicholas Hardiker*

Agreement on the consistent use of a term, such as "impaired physical mobility," allows that term to be used for a number of purposes: to provide continuity of care from care provider to care provider, to ensure care quality by facilitating comparisons between care providers, or to identify trends through data aggregation. Since the early 1970s, there has been a concerted effort to promote consistency in nursing terminology. This work continues today, driven by the following increasing demands placed on health-related information and knowledge:

- **Accessibility:** It should be easy to access the information and knowledge needed to deliver care or manage a health service.
- **Ubiquity:** With changing models of healthcare delivery, information and knowledge should be available anywhere.
- Longevity: Information should be usable beyond the immediate clinical encounter.
- **Reusability:** Information should be useful for a range of purposes.

Without consistent terminology, nursing runs the risk of becoming invisible; it will remain difficult to quantify nursing, the unique contribution and impact of nursing will go unrecognized, and the nursing component of electronic health record systems will remain at best rudimentary. Not least, without consistent terminology, the nursing knowledge base will suffer in terms of development and in terms of access, thereby delaying the integration of evidence-based health care into nursing practice.

External pressures merely compound this problem. For example, in the United States, the Health Information Technology for Economic and Clinical Health (HITECH) Act, signed in January 2009, provides a financial incentive for the use of electronic health records; similar steps are being taken in other regions. The HITECH Act mandates that EHRs are used in a meaningful way; achieving this goal will be problematic without consistent terminology. Finally, the current and future landscape of information and communication technologies (e.g., connection anywhere, borderless communication, Web-based applications, collaborative working, disintermediation and reintermediation, consumerization, ubiquitous advanced digital content [van Eecke, da Fonseca Pinto, & Egyedi, 2007]) and their inevitable infiltration into health care will only serve to reinforce the need for consistent nursing terminology while providing an additional sense of urgency.

This box explains what is meant by a standardized nursing terminology and lists several examples. It describes in detail the different approaches taken in the development of two example terminologies. It presents, in the form of an international technical standard, a means of ensuring consistency among the plethora of contemporary standardized nursing terminologies, with a view toward harmonization and possible convergence. Finally, it provides a rationale for the shared development of models of terminology use—models that embody both clinical and pragmatic knowledge to ensure that contemporary nursing record systems reflect the best available evidence and fit comfortably with routine practice.

## STANDARDIZED NURSING TERMINOLOGIES

A term at its simplest level is a word or phrase used to describe something concrete (e.g., *leg*) or abstract (e.g., *plan*). A nursing **terminology** is a body of the terms used in nursing. Many nursing terminologies exist, both formal and informal. Nursing terminologies allow nurses to consistently capture, represent, access, and communicate nursing data, information, and knowledge. A **standardized nursing terminology** is a nursing terminology that is in some way approved by an appropriate authority (de jure standardization) or by general consent (de facto standardization).

In North America, one such authority is the ANA (2007), which operates a process of de jure standardization through its Committee for Nursing Practice Information Infrastructure (CNPII). The ANA-approved list of nursing languages is presented in **Box 6-2**.

CNPII has also recognized two data element sets: the Nursing Minimum Data Set (NMDS) and the Nursing Management Minimum Data Set (NMMDS). Work on a standardized data element set for nursing, which in the United States began in the 1980s with the NMDS (Werley & Lang, 1988), provided an additional catalyst for the development of many of the aforementioned nursing terminologies that could provide values (e.g., chronic pain) for particular data elements in the NMDS (e.g., nursing diagnosis). The data element sets provide a framework for the uniform collection and management of nursing data; the use of a standardized nursing terminology to represent those data serves further to enhance consistency.

## APPROACHES TO NURSING TERMINOLOGY

From relatively humble beginnings, nursing terminologies have evolved significantly over the past several decades in line with best practices in terminology work. The **enumerative approach** consists of simple lists of words or phrases represented in a list or a simple hierarchy. In the nursing diagnosis terminology system of the North American Nursing Diagnosis Association (NANDA), a nursing diagnosis has an associated name or label and a textual definition (NANDA International, 2008). Each nursing diagnosis may have a set of defining characteristics and related or risk factors. These additional features do not constitute part of the core terminology but instead are intended to be used as an aid to diagnosis. What an enumerative approach to standardizing terminology may lack in terms of hierarchical sophistication, it makes up for in terms of simplicity and potential ease of implementation and use.

In contrast, the **ontological approach** is compositional in nature and provides a partial representation of the entities within a domain and the relationships that hold between them. The evolution of this approach to terminology standardization has been facilitated by advances in knowledge representation (e.g., the refinement of the description logic that underpins many contemporary ontologies) and in their accompanying technologies (e.g., automated reasoners that can check consistency and identify equivalence) as well as the subsumption (i.e., subclass–superclass) relationships within those ontologies.

ICNP version 2 is an example of an ontology. ICNP is described as a unified nursing language system. It seeks to provide a resource that can be used to develop local terminologies and to facilitate cross-mapping between terminologies to compare and combine data from different sources; the existence of a number of overlapping but inconsistent standardized nursing terminologies is problematic in terms of data comparison and aggregation. The core of ICNP is represented in the Web ontology language (OWL), a recommendation of the World Wide Web Consortium (W3C), and a de facto standard language for representing ontologies (McGuiness & van Harmelen, 2004). Because it is underpinned by description logic, OWL permits the use of automated reasoners that can check consistency, identify equivalence, and support classification within the ICNP ontology.

The results of contemporary terminology work are encouraging. Nevertheless, further work is needed to harmonize standardized nursing terminologies and to scale up and mainstream the development and implementation of models of terminology use.

In an ideal world, one would see standardized nursing terminologies and the structures and systems that support their implementation and use merely as means to an end—that is, as tools to support good nursing practice and good patient care. Standardized nursing terminologies are important, but they do not obviate the need to think and work creatively, to do right by the people in our care, and to continue to advance nursing.

## REFERENCES

American Nurses Association (ANA). (2007). Nursing practice information infrastructure. Retrieved from http://www.nursingworld.org/MainMenuCategories/Policy-Advocacy /Positions-and-Resolutions/ANAPositionStatements/Position-Statements-Alphabetically /Privacyand Confidentiality.html

McGuiness, D. L., & van Harmelen, F. (Eds.). (2004). OWL Web ontology language overview. World Wide Web Consortium. Retrieved from http://www.w3.org/TR/owl-features

NANDA International. (2008). *Nursing diagnoses: Definitions and classification 2009– 2011 edition*. Indianapolis, IN: Wiley-Blackwell.

van Eecke, P., da Fonseca Pinto, P., & Egyedi, T., for the European Commission. (2007). EU study on the specific policy needs for ICT standardisation [Final report]. Retrieved from http://ec.europa.eu/idabc/en/document/7040/254.html

Werley, H. H., & Lang, N. M. (Eds.). (1988). *Identification of the Nursing Minimum Data Set*. New York, NY: Springer.

## BOX 6-2 ANA-RECOGNIZED TERMINOLOGIES THAT SUPPORT NURSING PRACTICE (AUGUST 2012)

1. NANDA: Nursing Diagnoses, Definitions, and Classification, 1992; website: www.nanda.org
2. Nursing Interventions Classification System (NIC), 1992; website: nursing .uiowa.edu/cncce/nursing-interventions-classification-overview
3. Clinical Care Classification (CCC), 1992; formerly Home Health Care Classification (HHCC); website: www.sabacare.com
4. Omaha System, 1992; website: www.omahasystem.org
5. Nursing Outcomes Classification (NOC), 1997; Sue Moorehead, PhD, RN, Center Director; website: nursing.uiowa.edu/cncce/nursing-outcomes-classification-overview
6. Nursing Management Minimum Data Set (NMMDS), 1998; website: www.nursing.umn.edu/sites/nursing.umn.edu/files/nmds-monograph.pdf
7. PeriOperative Nursing Data Set (PNDS), 1999; website: www.aorn.org
8. SNOMED CT, 1999; website: www.ihtsdo.org/snomed-ct
9. Nursing Minimum Data Set (NMDS), 1999; website: www.nursing.umn .edu/sites/nursing.umn.edu/files/usa-nmds.pdf
10. International Classification for Nursing Practice (ICNP), 2000; website: www.icn.ch/icnp.htm
11. ABC Codes, 2000; website: www.abccodes.com
12. Logical Observation Identifiers Names and Codes (LOINC), 2002; website: www.loinc.org

At least two decades of work has been directed toward articulating standardized data elements that reflect nursing practice. The nursing profession has been steadily moving toward consensus on the adoption of data standards. In fact, several "consensus conferences" have been hosted in recent years by the University of Minnesota, with the goal of developing "a national action plan and harmonize existing and new efforts of multiple individuals and organizations to expedite integration of standardized nursing data within EHRs and ensure their availability in clinical data repositories for secondary use" (Westra et al., 2015 para. 3). Consider that as clinical information systems are widely implemented, as standards for nursing documentation and reporting are adopted, and as healthcare IT solutions continue to evolve, the synthesis of findings from a variety of methods and worldviews becomes much more feasible. As we move toward a standard terminology to capture the work of nursing, we also will have the ability to mine electronic record data to tease out best practices and promote care improvements. Information technology is not a panacea for all of the challenges found in health care, but it will provide the nursing profession with an unprecedented capacity to generate and disseminate new knowledge at rapid speed, thus supporting the knowledge work of nursing.

## The Nurse as a Knowledge Worker

As we have already established, all nurses use data and information. This information is then converted to knowledge. The nurse then acts on this knowledge by initiating a plan of care, updating an existing one, or maintaining status quo. Does this use of knowledge make the nurse a **knowledge worker**?

The term *knowledge worker* was first coined by Peter Drucker in his 1959 book, *Landmarks of Tomorrow* (Drucker, 1994). Knowledge work is defined as nonrepetitive, nonroutine work that entails a significant amount of **cognitive activity** (Sorrells-Jones & Weaver, 1999a). Drucker (1994) describes a knowledge worker as one who has advanced formal education and is able to apply theoretical and analytical knowledge. According to Drucker, the knowledge worker must be a continuous learner and a specialist in a field. McCormick (2009) estimates that a knowledge worker spends at least 50% of his or her work time searching for and evaluating information.

According to Androwich (2010), it is important to understand that there is a dual role for accessing and using information (content) in health care. In the first instance, when the nurse is caring for an individual patient, evidence-based information (content) and patient data need to be available at the point of care to inform the present patient encounter. In the second instance, patient data that are entered by the nurse in the process of documentation need to be entered in such a manner that they are able to be aggregated to inform future patient encounters.

The world is transitioning from the **Industrial Age** to the **Information Age** (Snyder-Halpern, Corcoran-Perry, & Narayan, 2001; Sorrells-Jones & Weaver, 1999a). In the early 1900s, the workforce consisted predominantly of farmers. After World War I, the workforce began to become predominantly industrial. This transition occurred when many farmers and domestic help moved to the cities to take jobs at factories. Today, the industrial worker is slowly being replaced by the **technologist** (Drucker, 1994); the technologist is adept at using both mind and hand. Many industrial workers are finding it increasingly more difficult to obtain jobs because they do not have the educational base or mindset required of knowledge workers (Drucker, 1994). The technologist is no longer trained on the job, as industrial workers traditionally were, which can cause significant problems for the industrial worker who does not have the education required to transition to a knowledge worker position (Drucker, 1994; Sorrells-Jones & Weaver, 1999a).

Knowledge workers are innovators, and the work they produce is the foundation for organizational sustainability and growth. Knowledge workers are specialized, have advanced education, and typically have a high degree of autonomy and control over their own work environments (Davenport, Thomas, & Cantrell, 2002; Sorrells-Jones & Weaver, 1999a). Such individuals are most efficient when they are working in a multidisciplinary team. These teams are typically composed of members with complementary knowledge bases. The team members possess problem-solving and decision-making skills and advanced interpersonal skills. All members of the team are considered equal and are there to contribute their expertise. Leadership shifts and changes as the team tackles different parts of the project, with the topic expert taking the lead. A well-functioning team can consistently outperform an individual (Sorrells-Jones & Weaver, 1999b). Many of these teams become focused and passionate about the project on which they are working.

A key impediment to team effectiveness is a lack of understanding among team members and a lack of respect for one another's knowledge and experience (Sorrells-Jones & Weaver, 1999a). Another barrier to efficiency within the multidisciplinary team is the individual knowledge worker who does not want to give up his or her own identity even though he or she may be swayed by other professional opinions. Professionals have a more difficult time adjusting to working in a team than do nonprofessionals. Professionals fail very few times in their lives, which often results in their not being able to learn from their failures (Sorrells-Jones & Weaver, 1999b). Knowledge workers also tend to be resistant to change, and as a result they dig in their heels and refuse to adapt to changes that management has implemented to improve the work process or workflow (Davenport et al., 2002).

Companies that employ knowledge workers have been forced to change their management structures to better support these employees. Management no longer commands, but rather seeks to inspire workers to produce the best product (Drucker, 1992). Companies that rely on knowledge workers have come to the realization that the machines are unproductive without the knowledge of those workers. Loyalty is no longer purchased with a paycheck but is earned by giving knowledge workers the ability to use their knowledge effectively and innovatively (Drucker, 1992). In turn, the physical environment and workplace arrangements have been adjusted to maximize the workflow of the knowledge workers (Davenport et al., 2002). Many of these changes have occurred in the business world but have been slow to be adopted in health care.

Right now, health care is in the process of transitioning from the Industrial Age to the Information Age. This transition has proved challenging because of the success of healthcare institutions that have enjoyed using current management methods. Its history of success will make it difficult for the healthcare industry to abandon the old so as to learn the new. A new philosophy recognizing that employees are mature, self-reliant, independent-thinking adults who function as partners in carrying out the work of the organization is needed. The organization needs to view (knowledge worker) employees as an asset and supply the resources, tools, information, and power they need to self-manage their work. Innovation needs to be supported, especially when it meets the customers' needs, desires, and wishes (Weaver & Sorrells-Jones, 1999).

Nursing entails a significant amount of knowledge and nonknowledge work. Knowledge work includes such duties as interpreting trends in laboratories and symptoms. Nonknowledge work includes such tasks as calling the laboratory to check on laboratory results or making beds. Nurses, on a daily basis, rely on their extensive clinical information and specialized knowledge to implement and evaluate the processes and outcomes related to patient care (Snyder-Halpern et al., 2001).

Snyder-Halpern and colleagues (2001) have identified four tasks associated with human information processing: (1) data gathering, (2) information use, (3) creative application of knowledge to clinical practice, and (4) generation of new knowledge. These four tasks are associated with four roles that nursing takes on as a knowledge worker: **data gatherer, information user, knowledge user,** and **knowledge builder,** respectively.

Nurses are data gatherers by nature. They collect and record objective clinical data on a daily basis. These items include such things as patient history information, vital signs, and patient assessment data. Nurses as data gatherers transition to information users when they begin to interpret the data that they have collected and recorded. Nurses as information users then structure the clinical data into information that can be used to guide patient care decisions (Snyder-Halpern et al., 2001). An example of this is when the nurse notices that the patient's blood pressure is elevated. Information users transition to knowledge users when they begin to notice trends in a patient's clinical data and determine whether the clinical data fall within or outside of the normal data range. Nurses transition from knowledge users to knowledge builders when they examine clinical data and trends across groups of patients. These trends are interpreted and compared to current scientific data to determine whether these data would improve the nursing knowledge domain. An example of the transition of a nurse as knowledge user to a nurse as knowledge builder is an observation of medication compliance rates over a specified time period for patients diagnosed with chronic high blood pressure, with the nurse then comparing these rates to evidence-based literature to determine if this information improves the nursing knowledge base (Snyder-Halpern et al., 2001).

Snyder-Halpern and colleagues (2001) found that as nurses assumed each of these roles, they required different types of decision support processes to support their knowledge needs. The data gatherer requires a system that captures and stores data accurately and reliably and allows the data to be readily accessed. Most current healthcare decision support systems (DSSs) support the nurse in this role. The information user role requires a system that can transform clinical data into a format that allows for easy recognition of patterns and trends. These systems recognize the trend and display it for the nurse, who in turn uses this information to adjust the plan of care for the patient. The information user role is generally well supported by current

DSSs. The knowledge user role is the least supported role, and many systems are currently looking at ways to support nurses in this role. One advantage of these DSSs is their ability to bring knowledge to nurses so that they do not have to retrieve the information themselves, which allows them to adjust a patient's plan of care in a more efficient and timely manner. The knowledge builder role is typically seen in conjunction with the nurse researcher role and quality management roles. These roles typically look at aggregated data that have been captured over time and from numerous patients, with these data then being compared to clinical variables and interventions; this analysis results in the development of new domain knowledge (Snyder-Halpern et al., 2001).

Most of the available DSS tools for nursing practice, although promising, are simplistic and in early development. Typically, DSS includes such tools as (1) computerized alerts and reminders (e.g., medication due, patient has an allergy, potassium level abnormal), (2) clinical guidelines (e.g., best practice for prevention of skin breakdown), (3) online information retrieval (e.g., CINAHL, drug information), (4) clinical order sets and protocols, and (5) online access to organizational policies and procedures. In the future, these tools may be expanded to include applications with embedded case-based reasoning.

In the context of nursing practice supported by CISs, nurses will eventually have access to evidence and knowledge derived from large aggregates of clinical data, including nursing interventions and resultant outcomes. Experiential evidence provides practice guidelines and directives to ensure concurrence with optimal clinical decisions and actions. To illustrate, consider this example: A nurse assesses a patient who has experienced a stroke for signs of skin breakdown, photographs and documents early ulcerations, and submits the photos and documentation to CIS. The nurse receives an option to review the best practices for care of the patient and to submit a request for a consult to a wound management specialist. The ongoing clinical findings, treatment, and response are logged and aggregated with similar cases, thereby contributing to the knowledge base related to nursing and care of the integumentary system.

The informational elements of CISs can also be designed to include specifics about individuals' multicultural practices and beliefs. Consider the situation where a client voices concerns about her prescribed dietary treatment and expresses a preference for a female care provider. With a query to the CIS for the client's history and sociocultural background, the nurse obtains explanations for these requests that derive from the patient's religious and cultural background and makes a notation to highlight and carry this information forward in the electronic record for any future admissions. Future systems may also be designed to provide access to standards of ethical practice and online access to experts in the field of moral reasoning to guide clinical interactions and decision making.

Through each and every instance of interacting with the CIS, nurses add to these repositories of knowledge by chronicling their daily clinical challenges and queries. The continued expansion and aggregation of knowledge about clients and populations; their personal, cultural, physical, and clinical presentations; and individuals' experiences and the guidance received from others enhance the delivery of personalized, knowledge-based care.

Graves and Corcoran (1989) have suggested that nursing knowledge is "simultaneously the laws and relationships that exist between the elements that describe the phenomena of concern in nursing (factual knowledge) and the laws or rules that the nurse uses to combine the facts to make clinical nursing decisions" (p. 230). In their view, not only does knowledge support decision making, but it also leads to new discoveries. Thus one might think about the future creation of nursing knowledge as being the discovery of new laws and relationships that can continue to advance nursing practice.

New technologies have made the capture of multifaceted data and information possible through the use of such technologies as digital imaging (e.g., photography to support wound management). Now included as part of the clinical record, such images add a new dimension to the assessment, monitoring, and treatment of illness and the maintenance of wellness. Beyond the use of computer keyboards, input devices are being integrated with CISs and used to gather data and information for the following clinical and administrative purposes:

- Biometrics (e.g., facial recognition, security)
- Voice and video recordings (e.g., client interviews and observations, diagnostic procedures, ultrasounds)
- Voice-to-text files (e.g., voice recognition for documentation)
- Medical devices, (e.g., infusion pumps, ventilators, hemodynamic monitors)
- Bar-code and radio-frequency identification (RFID) technologies (e.g., medication administration)
- Telehomecare monitoring (e.g., for use in diabetes and other chronic disease management)

These are but a few of the emerging capabilities that allow for numerous data inputs to be transposed, combined, analyzed, and displayed to provide information and views of clinical situations currently not possible in a world dominated by hard-copy documentation. Through the application of information and communication technologies to support the capture and processing (i.e., interpretation, organization, and structuring) of all relevant clinical data, relationships can be identified and formalized into new knowledge. This transformational process is at the core of generating new nursing knowledge at a rate never experienced before; in the context of current research paradigms, the same relationships would likely take years to uncover.

As CISs advance, nurses will eventually become generators of new knowledge by virtue of designs that embed machine learning and case-based reasoning methods within their core functionality. This functionality will become possible only with national and international adoption of standardized nursing language, as previously described. Imagine the power of having access to systems that aggregate the same data elements and information garnered from multiple clinical situations and provide a probability estimate of the likely outcome for individuals of a certain age, with a specific diagnosis and comorbid conditions, medication profile, symptoms, and interventions. How much more rapidly would an understanding of the efficacy of clinical interventions be elucidated? Historically, some knowledge might have taken years of research to discover (e.g., that long-standing practices are sometimes more harmful than beneficial). A case in point is the long-standing practice of instilling endotracheal tubes with normal saline before suctioning (O'Neal, Grap, Thompson, & Dudley, 2001). Based on the evidence gathered through several studies, the potentially deleterious effects of this practice have become widely recognized. Conceivably, a meta-analysis approach to clinical studies will be expedited by convergence of large clinical data repositories across care settings, thereby making available to practitioners the collective contributions of health professionals and longitudinal outcomes for individuals, families, and populations.

Nurses need to be engaged in the design of CIS tools that support access to and the generation of nursing knowledge. As we have emphasized, the adoption of clinical data standards is of particular importance to the future design of CIS tools. We are also beginning to see the development and use of **expert systems** that implement knowledge automatically without human intervention. For example, an insulin pump that senses the patient's blood glucose level and administers insulin based on those data is a form of expert system. The expert system differs from decision support tools in that the decision support tools require the human to act on the information provided, whereas the expert system intervenes automatically based on an algorithm that directs the intervention. Consider that as CISs are widely implemented, as standards for nursing documentation and reporting are adopted, and as healthcare IT solutions continue to evolve, the synthesis of findings from a variety of methods and worldviews becomes much more feasible.

### BOX 6-3 CASE STUDY: CASTING TO THE FUTURE

In the year 2025, nursing practice enabled by technology has created a professional culture of reflection, critical inquiry, and interprofessional collaboration. Nurses use technology at the point of care in all clinical settings (e.g., primary care, acute care, community, and long-term care) to inform their clinical decisions and effect the best possible outcomes for their clients. Information is gathered and retrieved via human–technology biometric interfaces including voice, visual, sensory, gustatory, and auditory interfaces, which continuously monitor physiologic parameters for potentially harmful imbalances. Longitudinal records are maintained for all citizens from their initial prenatal assessment to death; all lifelong records are aggregated into the knowledge bases of expert systems. These systems provide the basis of the artificial intelligence being embedded in emerging technologies. Smart technologies and invisible computing are ubiquitous in all sectors where care is delivered. Clients and families are empowered to review and contribute actively to their record of health and wellness. Invasive diagnostic techniques are obsolete, nanotechnology therapeutics are the norm, and robotics supplement or replace much of the traditional work of all health professions. Nurses provide expertise to citizens to help them effectively manage their health and wellness life plans, and navigate access to appropriate information and services.

# The Future

The future landscape is yet to be fully understood, as technology continues to evolve with a rapidity and unfolding that is rich with promise and potential peril. **Box 6-3** helps us to imagine what future practice might entail. It is anticipated that computing power will be capable of aggregating and transforming additional multidimensional data and information sources (e.g., historical, multisensory, experiential, and genetic sources) into CIS. With the availability of such rich repositories, further opportunities will open up to enhance the training of health professionals, advance the design and application of CDSs, deliver care that is informed by the most current evidence, and engage with individuals and families in ways yet unimagined.

The basic education of all health professions will evolve over the next decade to incorporate core informatics competencies. In general, the clinical care environments will be connected, and information will be integrated across disciplines to the benefit of care providers and citizens alike. The future of health care will be highly dependent on the use of CISs and CDSs to achieve the global aspiration of safer, quality care for all citizens.

The ideal is a nursing practice that has wholly integrated informatics and nursing education and that is driven by the use of information and knowledge from a myriad of sources, creating practitioners whose way of being is grounded in informatics. Nursing research is dynamic and an enterprise in which all nurses are engaged by virtue of their use of technologies to gather and analyze findings that inform specific clinical situations. In every practice setting, the contributions of nurses to health and well-being of citizens will be highly respected and parallel, if not exceed, the preeminence granted physicians.

# Summary

In this chapter, we have traced the development of informatics as a specialty, defined nursing informatics, and explored the DIKW paradigm central to informatics. We also explored the need for and the development of standardized terminologies to capture and codify the work of nursing and how informatics supports the knowledge work of nursing. This chapter advanced the view that every nurse's practice will make contributions to new nursing knowledge in dynamically interactive CIS environments. The core concepts associated with informatics will become embedded in the practice of every nurse, whether administrator, researcher, educator, or practitioner. Informatics will be prominent in the knowledge work of nurses, yet it will be a subtlety because of its eventual fulsome integration with clinical care processes. Clinical care will be substantially supported by the capacity and promise of technology today and tomorrow.

Most importantly, readers need to contemplate a future without being limited by the world of practice as it is known today. Information technology is not a panacea for all of the challenges found in health care, but it will provide the nursing profession with an unprecedented capacity to generate and disseminate new knowledge at rapid speed. Realizing these possibilities necessitates that all nurses understand and leverage the informatician within and contribute to the future.

**THOUGHT-PROVOKING QUESTIONS**

1. How is the concept of wisdom in NI like or unlike professional nursing judgment? Can any aspect of nursing wisdom be automated?
2. How can a single agreed-upon model of terminology use (with linkages to a single terminology) help to integrate knowledge into routine clinical practice?
3. Can you create examples of how expert systems (not decision support systems but true expert systems) can be used to support nursing practice?
4. How would you incorporate the data-to-wisdom continuum into a job description for nurse?
5. What are the possibilities to accelerate the generation and uptake of new nursing knowledge?

# References

American Nurses Association (ANA). (2008). *Nursing informatics: Scope and standards of practice*. Springfield, MD: Nursesbooks.org.

American Nurses Association (ANA). (2015). *Nursing informatics: Scope and standards of practice* (2nd ed.). Silver Spring, MD: Nursesbooks.org.

Androwich, I. (2010, June). Paper presented at Delaware Valley Nursing Informatics Annual Meeting, Malvern, PA.

Benner, P. (2000). The wisdom of our practice. *The American Journal of Nursing, 100*(10), 99–101, 103, 105.

Blum, B. (1986). *Clinical information systems*. New York, NY: Springer-Verlag.

Davenport, T. H., Thomas, R., & Cantrell, S. (2002). The mysterious art and science of knowledge worker performance. *MIT Sloan Management Review, 44*(1), 23–30.

Drucker, P. F. (1992). The new society of organizations. *Harvard Business Review, 70*(5), 95–104.

Drucker, P. F. (1994). The age of social transformation. *Atlantic Monthly, 274*(5), 52–80.

Graves, J., & Corcoran, S. (1989). The study of nursing informatics. *Image, 21*(4), 227–230.

Hannah, K. J., White, P., Nagle, L. M., & Pringle, D. M. (2009). Standardizing nursing information in Canada for inclusion in electronic health records: C-HOBIC. *Journal of the American Medical Informatics Association, 16*(4), 524–530.

Hardiker, N. (2011). Developing standardized terminologies to support nursing practice. In D. McGonigle & K. Mastrian (Eds.), *Nursing informatics and the foundation of knowledge* (2nd ed., pp. 111–120). Sudbury, MA: Jones & Bartlett Learning.

Matney, S., Brewster, P., Sward, K., Cloyes, K., & Staggers, N. (2011). Philosophical approaches to the data–information–knowledge–wisdom framework. *Advances in Nursing Science, 34*(1), 6–18.

McCormick, J. (2009, May 14). Preparing for the future of knowledge work: A day in the life of the knowledge worker. *Infomanagment Direct Online*. Retrieved from http://www.information-management.com/infodirect/2009_121/knowledge_worker_information_management_ecm_content_management-10015405-1.html

Murphy, J. (2010). Nursing informatics: The intersection of nursing, computer, and information sciences. *Nursing Economic$, 28*(3), 204–207.

Nagle, L. M., White, P., & Pringle, D. (2010). Realizing the benefits of standardized measures of clinical outcomes. *Electronic Healthcare, 9*(2), e3–e9.

O'Connor, J. J., & Robertson, E. F. (2003). Florence Nightingale. Retrieved from http://www-history.mcs.st-andrews.ac.uk/history/Printonly/Nightingale.html

O'Neal, P. V., Grap, M. J., Thompson, C., & Dudley, W. (2001). Level of dyspnea experienced in mechanically ventilated adults with and without saline instillation prior to endotracheal suctioning. *Intensive Critical Care Nursing, 17*(6), 356–363.

Ozbolt, J., & Saba, V. (2008). A brief history of nursing informatics in the United States of America. *Nursing Outlook, 56(5),* 199–205.

Rutherford, M. (2008). Standardized nursing language: What does it mean for nursing practice? *OJIN: The Online Journal of Issues in Nursing, 13*(1). doi:10.3912/OJIN.Vol13No01PPT05

Skrocki, M. (2013). Standardization needs for effective interoperability. *Transactions of the International Conference on Health Information Technology Advancement.* Paper 32, 76–83. Retrieved from http://scholarworks.wmich.edu/ichita_transactions/32

Snyder-Halpern, R., Corcoran-Perry, S., & Narayan, S. (2001). Developing clinical practice environments supporting the knowledge work of nurses. *Computers in Nursing, 19*(1), 17–26.

Sorrells-Jones, J., & Weaver, D. (1999a). Knowledge workers and knowledge-intense organizations, Part 1: A promising framework for nursing and healthcare. *Journal of Nursing Administration, 29*(7/8), 12–18.

Sorrells-Jones, J., & Weaver, D. (1999b). Knowledge workers and knowledge-intense organizations, Part 3: Implications for preparing healthcare professionals. *Journal of Nursing Administration, 29*(10), 14–21.

Thede, L., Schwiran, P. (2011). Informatics: The standardized nursing terminologies: A national survey of nurses' experiences and sttitudes—Survey I*. *OJIN: The Online Journal of Issues in Nursing, 16*(2). doi: 10.3912/OJIN.Vol16No02InfoCol01

Topaz, M. (2013). Invited editorial: The hitchhiker's guide to nursing informatics theory: Using the Data-Knowledge-Information-Wisdom framework to guide informatics research. *Online Journal of Nursing Informatics (OJNI), 17*(3). Retrieved from http://ojni.org/issues/?p=2852

Weaver, D., & Sorrells-Jones, J. (1999). Knowledge workers and knowledge-intense organizations, Part 2: Designing and managing for productivity. *Journal of Nursing Administration, 29*(9), 19–25.

Westra, B., Latimer, G., Matney, S., Park, J., Sensmeier, J., Simpson, R., . . . Delaney, C. (2015). A national action plan for sharable and comparable nursing data to support practice and translational research for transforming health care. *Journal of the American Medical Informatics Assocociation, 22*(3), 600–607. doi:10.1093/jamia/ocu011

1. Describe the nursing informatics specialty.
2. Explore the scope and standards of nursing informatics practice.
3. Assess the evolving roles and competencies of nursing informatics practice.
4. Appreciate the future of nursing informatics in our rich, technology-laden healthcare environments.

## Key Terms

- » Advocate/policy developer
- » Certification
- » Consultant
- » Data
- » Decision support/outcomes manager
- » Educator
- » Entrepreneur
- » Informatics
- » Informatics innovator
- » Informatics nurse specialist
- » Information
- » Knowledge
- » Knowledge worker
- » Medical informatics
- » Nursing informatics competencies
- » Product developer
- » Project manager
- » Researcher
- » TIGER initiative

# CHAPTER 7

# Nursing Informatics as a Specialty

Dee McGonigle, Kathleen Mastrian, Julie A. Kenney, and Ida Androwich

## Introduction

In the previous chapter, you reviewed the history and evolution of nursing informatics, and the ways that all nurses use informatics for practice. In this chapter, we will focus on nursing **informatics** as a specialty. Nursing informatics (NI) is an established, yet ever-evolving, specialty. Those choosing NI as a career find it full of numerous and varied opportunities. Previously, most nurse informaticists entered the field by showing an understanding and enthusiasm for working with computers. Now, however, nurses have many educational opportunities available to become formally trained in the field of NI to become an informatics nurse specialist (INS). We will explore the scope and standards of NI; NI roles, education, and specialization; rewards of working in the field; and organizations and professional journals of the INS.

## Nursing Contributions to Healthcare Informatics

Nursing has been involved in the purchase, design, and implementation of information systems (ISs) since the 1970s (Saba & McCormick, 2006). One of the first health IS vendors studied how nurses managed patient care and realized that nursing activity was the core of patient activity and needed to be the foundation of the health or clinical IS. Nursing informaticists have been instrumental in developing, critiquing, and promoting standard nursing terminologies to be used in the health IS. Nursing is involved heavily in the design of educational materials for practicing nurses, student nurses, other healthcare workers, and patients. Computers have revolutionized the way individuals access information and have revolutionized educational and social networking processes.

## Scope and Standards

NI is important to nursing and health care because it focuses on representing nursing **data, information,** and **knowledge.** As identified in the earlier edition of the *Nursing Informatics: Scope and Standards of Practice*, NI meets the following needs for health informatics (American Nurses Association [ANA], 2008; Brennan, 1994):

- Provides a nursing perspective
- Showcases nursing values and beliefs
- Provides a foundation for nurses in NI
- Produces unique knowledge
- Distinguishes groups of practitioners
- Emphasizes the interest for nursing
- Provides needed nursing language and word context

In 2008, the ANA published a revised scope and standards of nursing informatics practice. This publication included the most recent INS standards of practice and the INS standards of professional performance, and addressed the who, what, when, where, how, why, and functional roles of INS practice. There were three overarching standards of practice (ANA, 2008, p. 33):

1. Incorporate theories, principles, and concepts from appropriate sciences into informatics practice.
2. Integrate ergonomics and human–computer interaction (HCI) principles into informatics solution design, development, selection, implementation, and evaluation.
3. Systematically determine the social, legal, and ethical impact of an informatics solution within nursing and health care.

The standards of practice and professional performance for an INS are listed in Box 7-1.

In 2015, the second edition of the ANA's *Nursing Informatics: Scope and Standards of Practice* was released. The ANA described the functional areas of nursing informatics as follows (p. 19):

- Administration, leadership, and management
- Systems analysis and design
- Compliance and integrity management
- Consultation
- Coordination, facilitation, and integration
- Development of systems, products, and resources
- Educational and professional development
- Genetics and genomics
- Information management/operational architecture
- Policy development and advocacy
- Quality and performance improvement
- Research and evaluation
- Safety, security, and environmental health

---

**BOX 7-1 INFORMATICS NURSE SPECIALIST STANDARDS OF PRACTICE AND PERFORMANCE**

**STANDARDS OF PROFESSIONAL PRACTICE FOR NURSING INFORMATICS**

Standard 1: Assessment
Standard 2: Diagnosis, Problems, and Issues Identification
Standard 3: Outcomes Identification
Standard 4: Planning
Standard 5: Implementation
Standard 5A: Coordination of Activities
Standard 5B: Health Teaching and Health Promotion
Standard 5C: Consultation
Standard 6: Evaluation

**STANDARDS OF PROFESSIONAL PERFORMANCE FOR NURSING INFORMATICS**

Standard 7: Ethics
Standard 8: Education
Standard 9: Evidence-Based Practice and Research
Standard 10: Quality of Practice
Standard 11: Communication
Standard 12: Leadership
Standard 13: Collaboration
Standard 14: Professional Practice Evaluation
Standard 15: Resource Utilization
Standard 16: Environmental Health

Data from American Nurses Association (ANA). (2015). *Nursing informatics: Scope and standards of practice* (2nd ed.). Silver Spring, MD: Nursesbooks.org.

---

As INSs assume their roles, it is evident that typical roles cover more than one functional area and that our "informatics solutions are more closely integrated with the delivery of care" (ANA, 2015, p. 36). The ANA also denoted telehealth as an integrated functional area that is a dynamic health information technology. As nursing, information, computer, and cognitive sciences continue to evolve, so will NI functions. With the rapid advancements we have already seen in the previous decade, we know that the INSs of the future will be assuming roles and working in areas that we have not imagined yet.

# Nursing Informatics Roles

NI has become a viable and essential nursing specialty with the introduction of computers and the EHR to health care. Many nurses entered the NI field because of their natural curiosity and their dedication to being lifelong learners. Others who entered this field might have done so by accident: Perhaps they were comfortable working with computers and their coworkers used them as a resource for computer-related questions. The introduction of the EHR has forced all clinicians to learn to use this new technology and incorporate it into their already busy days. According to one estimate, nurses spend as little as 10–15% of their days with their patients and as much as 28–50% of their day documenting (Healthcare Information and Management Systems Society [HIMSS] Nursing Informatics Awareness Task Force, 2007; Munyisia, Yu, & Hailey, 2014). Assisting nurses to incorporate this new technology into their daily workflow is one of many challenges that the INS may tackle. Even though INSs appear to work behind the scenes, INSs impact the health and clinical outcomes of patients.

The INS may take on numerous roles; refer to **Figure 7-1**. For example, one position that INSs fill quite well is the role of the **project manager**, as a result of their ability to simultaneously manage multiple complex situations. Because of the breadth of the NI field, however, many INSs find that they need to further specialize. The following list includes some typical INS positions. It is far from comprehensive, because this field changes rapidly, as does technology (ANA, 2015; Thede, 2003).

- *Project Manager.* In the project manager role, the INS is responsible for the planning and implementation of informatics projects. The INS uses communication, change management, process analysis, risk assessment, scope definition, and team building. This role acts as the liaison among clinicians, management, IS, stakeholders, vendors, and all other interested parties.
- *Consultant.* The INS who takes on the **consultant** role provides expert advice, opinions, and recommendations based on his or her area of expertise. Flexibility, good communication skills, excellent interpersonal skills, and extensive clinical and informatics knowledge are highly desirable skill sets needed by the NI consultant.
- *Educator.* The success or failure of an informatics solution can be directly related to the education and training that were provided for end users. The INS who chooses the **educator** role develops and implements educational materials and sessions and provides education about the system to new or current employees during a system implementation or an upgrade.
- *Researcher.* The **researcher** role entails conducting research (especially data mining) to create new informatics and clinical knowledge. Research may range from basic informatics research to developing clinical decision support tools for nurses.
- *Product Developer.* An INS in the **product developer** role participates in the design, production, and marketing of new informatics solutions. An understanding of business and nursing is essential in this role.
- *Decision Support/Outcomes Manager.* Nurses assuming the role of **decision support/outcomes manager** use tools to maintain data integrity and reliability.

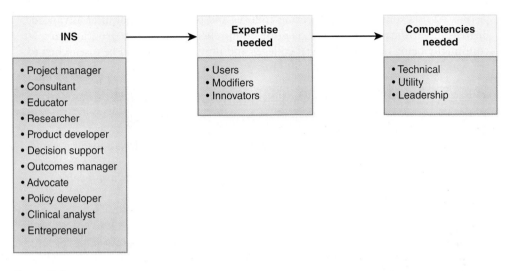

**Figure 7-1** NI Roles

Contributing to the development of a nursing knowledge base is an integral component of this role.

- *Advocate/Policy Developer.* INSs are key to advocating for the patients and healthcare systems and developing the infrastructure of health policy. Policy development on a local, national, and international level is an integral part of the **advocate/policy developer** role.
- *Clinical Analyst/System Specialist.* INSs may work at varying levels and serve as a link between nursing and information services in healthcare organizations.
- *Entrepreneur.* Those nurses involved in the **entrepreneur** role combine their passion, skills, and knowledge to develop marketable business ideas by analyzing nursing information needs and developing and marketing solutions.

## Specialty Education and Certification

Many nurses who entered into NI did so without any formal education in this field. In many cases, these nurses served as the unit resource for computer or program questions. Often, they acquired their skills through on-the-job training or by attending classes. Although this pathway to the NI field is still available today, more formal ways of acquiring these skills exist. The informatics nurse has a bachelor of science degree in nursing and additional knowledge and expertise in the informatics field (ANA, 2015). The INS holds an advanced degree or a post-master's certificate and is prepared to assume roles requiring this advanced knowledge. INSs may attend informatics conferences and obtain contact hours or continuing education units.

Box 7-2 lists some of the pioneering colleges and universities that offer advanced degrees or certificates in NI. This is not a comprehensive list; new programs are continually being developed. Local colleges and universities should be researched to see which may have informatics programs.

## BOX 7-2 FORMAL NURSING INFORMATICS EDUCATIONAL PROGRAMS

### GRADUATE DEGREE PROGRAMS

Chamberlin College of Nursing: www.chamberlain.edu/admissions/graduate/Master-of-Science-in-Nursing/informatics-track

Duke University: http://nursing.duke.edu/academics/programs/msn/health-informatics-major

Excelsior College: www.excelsior.edu/nursing-masters-informatics-faq

Loyola University Chicago: www.luc.edu/hsm

New York University: http://nursing.nyu.edu/academics/masters

Northeastern University: www.healthinformatics.neu.edu

University of Alabama at Birmingham: www.uab.edu/nursing/home/msn/nursing-informatics-major

University of Colorado at Denver: www.ucdenver.edu/academics/colleges/nursing/programs-admissions/masters-programs/ms-program/specialties/healthcareinformatics/Pages/default.aspx

University of Iowa: http://informatics.grad.uiowa.edu/health-informatics/curriculum

University of Kansas: http://nursing.kumc.edu/academics/master-of-science/nursing-informatics.html

University of Maryland: www.nursing.umaryland.edu/academics/grad/specialties/ni

University of North Carolina at Chapel Hill: http://nursing.unc.edu/academics/graduate-practice-programs/master_of_science_in_nursing/health-care-systems-msn/

University of Pittsburgh: www.nursing.pitt.edu/degree-programs/master-science-nursing-msn/msn-program-majors/nursing-informatics/nursing

University of Utah: http://nursing.utah.edu/programs/msnursinginformatics.php

University of Washington: www.son.washington.edu/portals/cipct

Vanderbilt University: www.nursing.vanderbilt.edu/msn/ni.html

### CERTIFICATE PROGRAMS

Chamberlain College of Nursing: www.chamberlain.edu/admissions/graduate/graduate-certificate-programs

Indiana University: nursing.iupui.edu/continuing/informatics.shtml

Loyola University Chicago: www.luc.edu/media/lucedu/nursing/pdfs/Informatics%20Certificate.pdf

Northeastern University: www.ccis.northeastern.edu/program/health-informatics-grad-certificate/

Penn State University: www.worldcampus.psu.edu/degrees-and-certificates/nursing-informatics-certificate/overview

University of Iowa: informatics.grad.uiowa.edu/health-informatics/curriculum

Nurses who choose to specialize in NI have two **certification** options available to them. The first is obtained through the American Nurses Credentialing Center (ANCC). The ANCC's examination is specific for the informatics nurse. The applicant must be a licensed registered nurse with at least 2 years of recent experience and have a baccalaureate degree in nursing. The applicant must have completed 30 contact hours of continuing education in informatics. The applicant must meet one of the following criteria: (1) 2,000 hours practicing as an informatics nurse, (2) 1,000 hours practicing as an informatics nurse and 12 semester hours of graduate academic credit toward an NI degree, or (3) completion of an NI degree that included at least 200 supervised practicum hours. For further information on this certification examination, visit www.nursecredentialing.org/Certification/NurseSpecialties/Informatics. This website includes the aforementioned criteria and provides further information about test eligibility, fees, examination content, examination locations, study materials, and practice tests.

The second certification examination is sponsored by the Healthcare Information and Management Systems Society (HIMSS). Candidates who successfully pass this examination are designated as certified professionals in healthcare information and management systems. The HIMSS examination is open to any candidate who is involved in healthcare informatics. Candidates must hold positions in the following fields: administration/management, clinical IS, e-health, IS, or management engineering. Candidates may include any of the following: chief executive officers, chief information officers, chief operating officers, senior executives, senior managers, IS technical staff, physicians, nurses, consultants, attorneys, financial advisors, technology vendors, academicians, management engineers, and students. Candidates must meet the following criteria to be eligible to sit for the examination: a baccalaureate degree plus 5 years of associated information and management systems experience, with 3 of those years being in health care; or a graduate degree plus 3 years of associated information and management systems experience, with 2 of those years being in health care. The information discussed in this text and additional information about the examination can be found by visiting http://www.himss.org/ASP/certification_cphims.asp.

## Nursing Informatics Competencies

One challenge that has been identified in the literature and continues to plague health care is the vast differences in computer literacy and information management skills that healthcare workers possess (Gassert, 2008; McNeil, Elfrink, Beyea, Pierce, & Bickford, 2006; Topkaya & Kaya, 2014). Gassert (2008) felt that new graduates were not adequately literate. Barton (2005) believed that new nurses should have the following critical skills: use e-mail, operate Windows applications, search databases, and know how to work with the institution-specific nursing software used for charting and medication administration. These skills should not be limited to just new nurses, but instead should be required of all nurses and healthcare workers.

Staggers, Gassert, and Curran (2001) advocated that nursing students and practicing nurses should be educated on core NI competencies. Although information technology and informatics concepts certainly need to be incorporated into nursing school curricula, progress in this area has been slow. In the 1980s, a nursing group of the International Medical Informatics Association convened to develop the first level of nursing competencies. While developing these competencies, the nursing group found that nurses fell in to one of the following three categories: (1) user, (2) developer, or (3) expert. These categories have since been expanded.

Staggers and colleagues (2001) decided that the NI competencies developed in the 1980s were inadequate and needed to be updated. These authors reviewed 35 NI competency articles and 14 job descriptions, which resulted in 1,159 items that were sorted into three broad categories: (1) computer skills, (2) informatics knowledge, and (3) informatics skills. These items were then placed in a database, where redundant items were removed. When this process was completed, 313 items remained.

When these items were then further subdivided, Staggers and colleagues, along with the American Medical Informatics Association (AMIA) work group, realized that these competencies were not universal to all nurses; thus, before it could be determined if the competency was an NI competency, nursing skill levels needed to be defined. The group determined that practicing nurses could be classified into four categories: (1) beginning nurse, (2) experienced nurse, (3) **informatics nurse specialist**, and (4) **informatics innovator**. Each of these skill levels needed to be defined before Staggers and colleagues (2001) could determine which level was the most appropriate for that skill set. Table 7-1 provides the definition criteria for each skill level. Once the levels were defined, the group determined that 305 items were NI competencies and placed them into appropriate categories.

Staggers, Gassert, and Curran (2002) conducted the seminal work in this area, a Delphi study to validate the placement of the competencies into the correct skill level. Of the 305 original competencies identified, 281 achieved an 80% approval rating for both importance as a competency and placement in the correct practice level. The authors stressed that this is a comprehensive list; thus, for a nurse to enter a particular skill level, he or she need not have mastered every item listed for that skill level. For a list of competencies by skill level, see Table 7-2.

In 2004, a group of nurses came together after attending a national informatics conference to ensure that nursing was equally recognized in the national informatics movement. This so-called Technology Informatics Guiding Education Reform (TIGER) team determined that using informatics was a core competency for all healthcare workers. They also determined that many nurses lack information technology skills, which limits their ability to access evidence-based information that could otherwise be incorporated into their daily practice. This group is currently working on a plan to include informatics courses in all levels of nursing education; when that effort is complete, they will examine how to get the information out to practicing nurses who are not currently enrolled in an academic program (HIMSS, 2016). Many of the items identified by the TIGER team as lacking in both nursing students and practicing nurses are items that Staggers et al. (2002) determined to be NI competencies. To learn more about the **TIGER initiative**, visit http://www.himss.org/professionaldevelopment/tiger-initiative.

Through the work of Hunter et al. (2011; 2013; 2015) and McGonigle et al. (2014; 2015), the competencies for nursing informatics practice Levels 1 through 4 have been further refined with two self-assessment tools developed. Hunter and colleagues focused on the Level 1 and Level 2 competencies and developed the self-assessment of

TABLE 7-1 Definitions of Four Levels of Practicing Nurses

### Beginning Nurse

- Has basic computer technology skills and information management skills
- Uses institution's information systems and the contained information to manage patients

### Experienced Nurse

- Proficient in a specialty
- Highly skilled in using computer technology skills and information management skills to support his or her specialty area of practice
- Pulls trends out of data and makes judgments based on this information
- Uses current systems, but will collaborate with informatics nurse specialist regarding concerns or suggestions provided by staff

### Informatics Nurse Specialist

- RN with advanced education who possesses additional knowledge and skills specific to computer technology and information management
- Focuses on nursing's information needs, which include education, administration, research, and clinical practice
- Application and integration of the core informatics sciences: information, computer, and nursing science
- Uses critical thinking, process skills, data management skills, systems life cycle development, and computer skills

### Informatics Innovator

- Conducts informatics research and generates informatics theory
- Vision of what is possible
- Keen sense of timing to make things happen
- Creative in developing solutions
- Leads the advancement of informatics practice and research
- Sophisticated level of skills and understanding in computer technology and information management
- Cognizant of the interdependence of systems, disciplines, and outcomes and is able to finesse situations to obtain the best outcome

Reproduced from Staggers, N., Gassert, C., & Curran, C. (2001). Informatics competencies for nurses at four levels of practice. *Journal of Nursing Education, 40*(7), 303–316. With permission of SLACK Incorporated.

competencies TANIC tool, Tiger-based Assessment of Nursing Informatics Competencies. McGonigle and colleagues focused on the competencies related to the advanced levels 3 and 4, developing the self-assessment of competencies NICA L3/L4 tool, Nursing Informatics Competency Assessment Level 3/Level 4 (ANA, 2015, p. 43).

Table 7-2  Nursing Informatics Compentencies by Skill Level

Based on research conducted by Hunter, McGonigle, and Hebda (2013), the online self-assessment instrument, TIGER-based Assessment of Nursing Informatics Competencies (TANIC) was developed. This instrument assesses the Level I: Beginning Nurse and Level 2: Experienced Nurse competencies.

### Level 1: Beginning Nurse

- Start the computer and log on securely to access select applications/software

- Access and send email

- Collect and enter patient data into the information system

### Level 2: Experienced Nurse

- Identify the risks and limitations of surfing the Internet to locate evidence-based practice information

- Gather data to draw and synthesize conclusions

- Explain how to sustain the integrity of information resources

Based on the research conducted by McGonigle, Hunter, Hebda, and Hill (2014), the online self-assessment instrument, Nursing Informatics Competency Assessment – Level 3/Level 4 (NICA L3/L4) was developed. This instrument assesses the Level 3: Informatics Nurse Specialist and Level 4: Informatics Innovator competencies.

### Level 3: Informatics Nurse Specialist

- Fluent in nursing informatics and nursing terminologies

- Applies aspects of human technology interface to screen, device, and software design

- Teach nurses how to locate, access, retrieve, and evaluate information

### Level 4: Informatics Innovator

- Analyze systems

- Transform software programs to support data analysis and aggregation

- Lead research efforts to determine and address application needs

### References

Hill, T., McGonigle, D., Hunter, K., Sipes, C. & Hebda, T. (2014). An instrument for assessing advanced nursing informatics competencies. *Journal of Nursing Education and Practice, 4*(7), 104–112.

Hunter, K., McGonigle, D. & Hebda, T. (2011, December). Operationalizing TIGER NI competencies for online assessment of perceived competency. *TIGER Initiative Foundation Newsletter*. Retrieved from http://www.thetigerinitiative.org [must subscribe to access]

Hunter, K., McGonigle, D., & Hebda, T. (2013). TIGER-based measurement of nursing informatics competencies: The development and implementation of an online tool for self-assessment. *Journal of Nursing Education and Practice, 3*(12), 70–80. doi: 10.5430/jnep.v3n12p70

Hunter, K., McGonigle, D., Hebda, T., Sipes, C., Hill, T., & Lamblin, J. (2015). TIGER-based assessment of nursing informatics competencies (TANIC). In A. Rocha, S. Correia, S. Costanza, & L. Reis (Eds.). *New contributions in information systems and technologies: Volume 1 (advances in intelligent systems and computing)* (pp. 171–177). Basel, Switzerland: Springer. DOI: 10.1007/978-3-319-16486-1_7

McGonigle, D., Hunter, K., Hebda, T., & Hill, T. (2014). *Self-assessment of Level 3 and Level 4 NI competencies tool development.* Retrieved from http://www.himss.org/file/1307246/download?token=cNOya_Lm

McGonigle, D., Hunter, K., Hebda, T., Sipes, C., Hill, T., & Lamblin, J. (2015). Nursing informatics competencies assessment Level 3 and Level 4 (NICA L3/L4). In A. Rocha, S. Correia, S. Costanza, & L. Reis (Eds.). *New contributions in information systems and technologies: Volume 1 (advances in intelligent systems and computing)* (pp. 209–214). Basel, Switzerland: Springer. DOI: 10.1007/978-3-319-16486-1_21

It is critical that nurses and INSs can demonstrate competence. As there were many definitions of the term *competency*, the authors of these tools first had to define the term competency. Hunter et al. (2013) concluded that

> *Competency, then, is a concept applicable to multiple situations. At its most basic, competency denotes having the knowledge, skills, and ability to perform or do a specific task, act, or job. Depending on the context, competency can refer to adequate or expert performance. For this research, competency was used to mean adequate knowledge, skills, and ability. Nursing-informatics competency was defined as adequate knowledge, skills, and ability to perform specific informatics tasks.* (p. 71)

The teams began instrument development by synthesizing both seminal and current literature to construct instrument items; they reviewed, formatted, and initiated instrument testing with a Delphi study and then piloted the resulting instrument with experts. Cronbach's alpha values were calculated. The TANIC Cronbach was 0.944 for clinical information management, 0.948 for computer skills, and 0.980 for information literacy. The NICA L3/L4 reliability estimates were as follows: computer skills, 0.909; informatics knowledge, 0.982; and informatics skills, 0.992. The Cronbach's reliability estimates for each tool showed strong internal consistency reliability.

The TANIC self-assessment instrument has four parts, including questions about demographics and the self-assessment, consisting of 85 items covering basic computer literacy, clinical information management, and information literacy. The NICA L3/L4 self-assessment instrument also has four parts: questions about demographics and the 178 item self-assessment, consisting of computer skills, informatics knowledge, and informatics skills.

These tools and those that will follow are extremely important because they help each of us identify our own level of comfort with technology and our self-confidence in our ability to perform these skills/tasks. Nurse educators in all practice settings and school-based programs must help their nurses or nursing students recognize deficits in their current knowledge and skills. The nurse educators can facilitate the professional development of their nurses or nursing students through the identification of courses or skill-based labs that will help them turn their deficits into strengths.

# Rewards of NI Practice

NI is a nursing specialty that does not focus on direct patient care but instead focuses on enhancing patient care and safety and improving the workflow and work processes of nurses and other healthcare workers. The INS is instrumental in designing the electronic healthcare records that healthcare workers use on a daily basis. This nurse is also responsible for designing tools that allow healthcare workers to access patient information more efficiently than they have been able to do so in the past. Watching these changes take place brings great satisfaction to the INS.

Change is a factor that an INS deals with on a daily basis. This dynamic nature of the position is probably its most difficult aspect, because people deal with change differently. Understanding change theory and processes and appreciating how change affects people assist the INS in developing strategies to encourage healthcare workers to accept changes and become proficient in informatics solutions that have been implemented. Seeing the change adopted with a minimal amount of discord is very rewarding to the INS.

The INS also participates in informatics organizations that allow INSs to network and share experiences with one another. Such interactions allow INSs to bring these new solutions back to their respective organizations and improve informatics trouble spots. Attending professional conferences allows the INS to stay abreast of changes in the industry. Continuing education may help the INS to improve a process or workflow within the hospital or to change the way a system upgrade is rolled out.

# NI Organizations and Journals

One of the first informatics organizations founded was HIMSS. HIMSS, which celebrated its 55th year in 2016, was launched in 1961 and now has offices throughout the United States and Europe. HIMSS currently represents more than 20,000 individuals and 300 corporations. This organization supports both local and national chapters. It has many associated work groups, one of which is an NI work group. HIMSS is well known for its development of industry-wide policies and its educational and professional development initiatives, all of which are directed toward the goal of ensuring safe patient care. Membership in HIMSS offers many advantages for nurses, such as access to numerous weekly and monthly publications, and two scholarly journals, the *Journal of Healthcare Information Management* and the *Online Journal of Nursing Informatics*. HIMSS offers many educational programs, including virtual expos, which allow participants to experience the expo without having to travel. These educational opportunities allow participants to network with colleagues and peers, which is a valuable asset in this field. HIMSS also periodically conducts NI workforce surveys. It is interesting to review the most current survey results and compare them to your setting and role.

The American Medical Informatics Association (AMIA) was founded in 1990 when three health informatics associations merged. AMIA currently has more than 3,000 members who reside in 42 countries. This organization focuses on the development and application of biomedical and healthcare informatics. Members include physicians, nurses, dentists, pharmacists, health information technology professionals, and biomedical engineers. AMIA offers many benefits to its members, such as weekly and monthly publications and a scholarly journal, *JAMIA—The Journal of the*

*American Medical Informatics Association*. Members may join a working group that is specific to their specialty, including an NI work group. AMIA offers multiple educational opportunities and many opportunities for networking with colleagues.

The American Nursing Informatics Association (ANIA) was established in 1992 to provide an opportunity for southern California informatics nurses to meet. It has since grown to a national organization whose members include healthcare professionals who work with clinical IS, educational applications, data collection/research applications, administrative/DSS, and those who have an interest in the field of NI. In 2009, ANIA merged with the Capital Area Roundtable on Informatics in Nursing (CARING). Membership benefits include the following:

- Access to a network of more than 3,200 informatics professionals in 50 states and 30 countries
- Active email list
- Quarterly newsletter indexed in CINAHL and Thomson
- Job bank with employee-paid postings
- Reduced rate at the ANIA Annual Conference
- Reduced rate for *CIN: Computers, Informatics, Nursing*
- ANIA Online Library of on-demand and webinar education activities
- Membership in the Alliance for Nursing Informatics
- Web-based meetings
- In-person meetings and conferences held nationally and worldwide

The Alliance for Nursing Informatics (ANI) is a coalition of NI groups that represents more than 3,000 nurses and 20 distinct NI groups in the United States. Its membership represents local, national, and international NI members and groups. These individual groups have developed organizational structures and have established programs and publications. ANI functions as the link between NI organizations and the general nursing and healthcare communities and serves as the united voice of NI.

These groups have been instrumental in establishing the informatics community. **Box 7-3** lists some of these organizations and their publications, but many other informatics groups exist.

# The Future of Nursing Informatics

NI is still in its infancy, as is the technology that the INS uses on a daily basis. NI will continue to influence development of the EHR; in turn, the EHR will continue to improve and will one day accurately capture the care nurses give to their patients. This is a formidable challenge because much of the care provided by nurses is intangible in nature. In the future, the EHR will provide data to the INS that can then be used to improve nursing workflow and to determine whether current practices are the most efficient and beneficial to the patient.

Nursing and health care are on a roller-coaster ride that will undoubtedly prove very interesting. New technology is being introduced at a breakneck speed, and nursing and health care must be ready to ride this roller coaster. Programs need to be developed to keep nurses and healthcare workers abreast of the new technological changes as they occur, and educating new and current nurses presents a significant challenge to the INS. Therefore, the INS's future looks very promising and rewarding.

**BOX 7-3 NURSING INFORMATICS WEBSITES AND CORRESPONDING JOURNALS**

**Alliance for Nursing Informatics**
Website: www.allianceni.org

**American Health Information Management Association**
Website: www.ahima.org
Journal: *Journal of AHIMA & Perspectives in Health Information Management* (online)

**American Medical Informatics Association**
Website: www.amia.org
Journal: *JAMIA—Journal of the American Medical Informatics Association*
NI website: www.amia.org/programs/working-groups/nursing-informatics

**American Nursing Informatics Association**
(includes Capital Area Roundtable on Informatics in Nursing [CARING])
    Website: www.ania.org
Resources link: www.ania.org/Resources.htm
Journal: *CIN: Computers, Informatics, Nursing*

**Health Information and Management Systems Society**
Website: www.himss.org
Chapter websites: www.himss.org/ASP/chaptersHome.asp
Journal: *The Journal of Healthcare Information Management*
NI website: www.himss.org/asp/topics_nursingInformatics.asp

**International Medical Informatics Association**
Website: www.imia.org
Journal: *International Journal of Medical Informatics*
NI website: www.imia.org/ni

**Online Journal of Nursing Informatics**
Website: www.himss.org/ojni

According to the ANA (2015), five trends will influence the future of nursing informatics:

1. Changing practice roles in nursing
2. Increasing informatics competence requirements for all nurses
3. Rapidly evolving technology
4. Regulatory changes and quality standards that include healthcare consumers as partners in healthcare models
5. Care delivery models and innovation (p. 52)

As the future becomes yesterday, people are waking up to the fact that we need the healthcare team prepared with informatics competencies. All healthcare providers should receive education on informatics because they need basic informatics skills, such as the ability to use search engines to find information about a specific topic. Consequently, all healthcare providers need to be able to attend classes to improve their computer skills and knowledge. Those entering the nursing field need a general knowledge of computer capabilities. Many new trends—such as Web 2.0, increased attention to evidence-based practice, and a better understanding of genomics—will impact care delivery in the 21st century, and NI nurses need to be prepared to lead these efforts to improve care and help nurses have a voice in the informatics skills they need, as well as in the advances and tools they use, including the EHR (Bakken, Stone, & Larson, 2008; Lavin, Harper, & Barr, 2015).

Change plays a significant part in health care today, and those interested in NI must embrace change. They must also be good at enticing others to embrace change. Nevertheless, NI candidates must realize that change is often accompanied by resistance. For their part, INSs must be ready to leave the bedside, because nurses entering into this field will no longer be giving hands-on care. NI is a very challenging but very rewarding field. In an ideal world, all healthcare agencies will employ at least one INS, and all nurses will embrace the **knowledge worker** title.

## Summary

Nursing informatics is a specialty that integrates nursing science, computer science, and information science to manage and communicate data, information, knowledge, and wisdom in nursing practice. Our definition: the synthesis of nursing science, information science, computer science, and cognitive science for the purpose of managing, disseminating, and enhancing healthcare data, information, knowledge, and wisdom to improve collaboration and decision making, provide high-quality patient care, and advance the profession of nursing. Informatics practices support nurses as they seek to care for their patients effectively and safely, by making the information that they need more readily available. Nurses have been actively involved in this field since computers were introduced to health care. With the advent of the EHR, it became apparent that nursing needed to develop its own terminology related to the new technology and its applications; NI has been instrumental in this process.

Today, the healthcare industry employs the largest number of knowledge workers in the world. Nurses, as knowledge workers in technology-laden healthcare facilities, must continuously improve their informatics competencies. The INS is instrumental in leading the advancement of informatics concepts and tools in all settings and across all specialties. NI is a specialty governed by standards that have been established by the ANA. Because NI is a very diverse field, many INSs eventually specialize in one segment of the field. While NI is an established specialty, the core NI principles are utilized by all nurses. **Nursing informatics competencies** have been developed to encompass all levels of practice and ensure that entry-level nurses are ready to enter the more technologically advanced field of nursing, as well as establish advanced competencies for the INS's specialty practice. These competencies may be used to determine the educational needs of current staff members.

The growth of the NI field has resulted in the formation of numerous NI organizations or subgroups of the **medical informatics** organizations. Nurses no longer have to enter the field by chance but can obtain an advanced degree in NI at many well-established universities. In addition, INSs may continue their learning by attending the numerous conferences offered.

NI has grown tremendously as a specialty since its inception and has the expectation of continued growth. The NI specialty not only engages nurses and patients, but also engages data to improve patient outcomes, enhance patient care, and advance the science of nursing. It will be interesting to see where NI and INSs take health care in the future.

## THOUGHT-PROVOKING QUESTIONS

1. A hospital is seeking to update its EHR. It has been suggested that an INS be hired. This position does not involve direct patient care and the administration is struggling with how to justify the position. How can this position be justified?
2. It is important that all nurses be informatics competent at all levels. In particular, at which levels should the INS be able to exhibit competency? Provide several examples of the knowledge and skills that an INS might demonstrate.
3. How does nursing move from measuring the tasks completed to measuring the final outcome of the patient? How can the INS help us reach this goal?

# References

Alliance for Nursing Informatics. (2013). Homepage. Retrieved from http://www.allianceni.org

American Medical Informatics Association. (2013). Homepage. Retrieved from http://www.amia.org

American Nurses Association (ANA). (2008). *Nursing informatics: Scope and standard of practice*. Silver Spring, MD: Nursesbooks.org.

American Nurses Association (ANA). (2015). *Nursing informatics: Scope and standard of practice* (2nd ed.). Silver Spring, MD: Nursesbooks.org.

Androwich, I. (2010, June). Paper presented at Delaware Valley Nursing Informatics Annual Meeting, Malvern, PA.

Bakken, S., Stone, P., & Larson, E. (2008). A nursing informatics research agenda for 2008–2018: Contextual influences and key components. *Nursing Outlook, 56*(5), 206–214.

Barton, A. J. (2005). Cultivating informatics competencies in a community of practice. *Nursing Administration Quarterly, 29*(4), 323–328.

Brennan, P. F. (1994). On the relevance of discipline to informatics. *Journal of the American Medical Informatics Association, 1*(2), 200–201.

Davenport, T. H., Thomas, R., & Cantrell, S. (2002). The mysterious art and science of knowledge worker performance. *MIT Sloan Management Review, 44*(1), 23–30.

Drucker, P. F. (1992). The new society of organizations. *Harvard Business Review, 70*(5), 95–104.

Drucker, P. F. (1994). The age of social transformation. *Atlantic Monthly, 274*(5), 52–80.

Gassert, C. (2008). Technology and informatics competencies. *Nursing Clinics of North America, 43*(4), 507–521. doi: 10.1016/j.cnur.2008.06.005

Health Information and Management Systems Society (HIMSS). (2006). *HIMSS dictionary of healthcare information technology terms, acronyms and organizations*. Chicago, IL: Author.

Health Information and Management Systems Society (HIMSS). (2013). Homepage. Retrieved from http://www.himss.org

Health Information and Management Systems Society (HIMSS). (2016). The TIGER initiative. Retrieved from http://www.himss.org/professionaldevelopment/tiger-initiative

HIMSS Nursing Informatics Awareness Task Force. (2007). An emerging giant: Nursing informatics. *Nursing Management, 13*(10), 38–42.

Hunter, K., McGonigle, D. & Hebda, T. (2011, December). Operationalizing TIGER NI competencies for online assessment of perceived competency. *TIGER Initiative Foundation Newsletter*. Retrieved from http://www.thetigerinitiative.org

Hunter, K., McGonigle, D., & Hebda, T. (2013). TIGER-based measurement of nursing informatics competencies: The development and implementation of an online tool for self-assessment. *Journal of Nursing Education and Practice (JNEP), 3*(12), 70–80. doi: 10.5430/jnep.v3n12p70

Hunter, K., McGonigle, D., Hebda, T., Sipes, C., Hill, T., & Lamblin, J. (2015). TIGER-Based assessment of nursing informatics competencies (TANIC). In A. Rocha, S. Correia, S. Costanza,

& L. Reis (Eds.), *New contributions in information systems and technologies: Volume 1 (Advances in intelligent systems and computing)* (pp. 171–177). Basel, Switzerland: Springer. DOI: 10.1007/978-3-319-16486-1_7

Lavin, M., Harper, E., & Barr, N. (2015). Health information technology, patient safety, and professional nursing care documentation in acute care settings. *OJIN The Online Journal of Issues in Nursing, 20*(2). doi: 10.3912/OJIN.Vol20No02PPT04

McCormick, J. (2009, May 14). Preparing for the future of knowledge work: A day in the life of the knowledge worker. *Infomanagment Direct Online*. Retrieved from http://www.information-management.com/infodirect/2009_121/knowledge_worker_information_management_ecm_content_management-10015405-1.html

McGonigle, D., Hunter, K., Hebda, T., & Hill, T. (2014). *Self-assessment of Level 3 and Level 4 NI competencies tool development.* Retrieved from http://www.himss.org/file/1307246/download?token=cNOya_Lm

McGonigle, D., Hunter, K., Hebda, T., Sipes, C., Hill, T., & Lamblin, J. (2015). Nursing informatics competencies assessment Level 3 and Level 4 (NICA L3/L4). In A. Rocha, S. Correia, S. Costanza, & L. Reis (Eds.), *New contributions in information systems and technologies: Volume 1 (Advances in intelligent systems and computing)* (pp. 209–214). Basel, Switzerland: Springer. DOI: 10.1007/978-3-319-16486-1_21

McNeil, B. J., Elfrink, V., Beyea, S. C., Pierce, S., & Bickford, C. J. (2006). Computer literacy study: Report of qualitative findings. *Professional Nursing, 22*(1), 52–59.

*Merriam-Webster Online.* (2011). Worker. Retrieved from http://mw1.merriam-webster.com/dictionary/worker

Munyisia, E., Yu, P., & Hailey, D. (2014). The effect of an electronic health record system on nursing staff time in a nursing home: A longitudinal study. *Australasian Medical Journal, 7*(7), 285–293. http//dx.doi.org/10.4066/AMJ.2014.2072

O'Connor, J. J., & Robertson, E. F. (2003). *Florence Nightingale.* Retrieved from http://www-history.mcs.st-andrews.ac.uk/history/Printonly/Nightingale.html

Saba, V. K., & McCormick, K. A. (Eds.). (2006). *Essentials of nursing informatics* (4th ed.). New York, NY: McGraw-Hill.

Snyder-Halpern, R., Corcoran-Perry, S., & Narayan, S. (2001). Developing clinical practice environments supporting the knowledge work of nurses. *Computers in Nursing, 19*(1), 17–26.

Sorrells-Jones, J., & Weaver, D. (1999a). Knowledge workers and knowledge-intense organizations, Part 1: A promising framework for nursing and healthcare. *Journal of Nursing Administration, 29*(7/8), 12–18.

Sorrells-Jones, J., & Weaver, D. (1999b). Knowledge workers and knowledge-intense organizations, Part 3: Implications for preparing healthcare professionals. *Journal of Nursing Administration, 29*(10), 14–21.

Staggers, N., Gassert, C., & Curran, C. (2001). Informatics competencies for nurses at four levels of practice. *Journal of Nursing Education, 40*(7), 303–316.

Staggers, N., Gassert, C., & Curran, C. (2002). A Delphi study to determine informatics competencies for nurses at four levels of practice. *Nursing Research, 51*(6), 383–390.

Thede, L. Q. (2003). *Informatics and nursing: Opportunities and challenges* (2nd ed.). Philadelphia, PA: Lippincott Williams & Wilkins.

Topkaya, S. & Kaya, N. (2014). Nurses' computer literacy and attitudes towards the use of computers in health care. Retrieved from http://nursing-informatics.com/niassess/Topkaya_2014.pdf

Weaver, D., & Sorrells-Jones, J. (1999). Knowledge workers and knowledge-intense organizations, Part 2: Designing and managing for productivity. *Journal of Nursing Administration, 29*(9), 19–25.

Wickramasinghe, N., & Ginzberg, M. J. (2001). Integrating knowledge workers and the organization: Role of IT. *International Journal of Health Care Quality Assurance, 14*(6), 245–253.

1. Explore the Health Insurance Portability and Accountability Act (HIPAA) of 1996.

2. Describe the purposes of the Health Information Technology for Economic and Clinical Health (HITECH) Act of 2009.

3. Explore how the HITECH Act is enhancing the security and privacy protections of HIPAA.

4. Determine how the HITECH Act and its impact on HIPAA apply to nursing practice.

5. Identify informatics technologies likely to be legislated in the future.

## Key Terms

- » Access
- » Agency for Healthcare Research and Quality
- » American National Standards Institute
- » American Recovery and Reinvestment Act
- » Centers for Medicare and Medicaid Services
- » Certified EHR technology
- » Civil monetary penalties
- » Compliance
- » Confidentiality
- » Consequences
- » Electronic health records
- » Enterprise integration
- » Entities
- » Gramm-Leach-Bliley Act
- » Health disparities
- » Health information technology
- » Health Insurance Portability and Accountability Act
- » Health Level Seven
- » Healthcare-associated infections
- » International Standards Organization
- » Meaningful use
- » National Institute of Standards and Technology
- » Office of Civil Rights
- » Office of the National Coordinator for Health Information Technology
- » Open Systems Interconnection
- » Patient-centered care
- » Policies
- » Privacy
- » Protected health information
- » Qualified electronic health record
- » Rights
- » Sarbanes-Oxley Act
- » Security
- » Standards
- » Standards-developing organizations
- » Treatment/payment/operations

# CHAPTER 8

# Legislative Aspects of Nursing Informatics: HITECH and HIPAA

Kathleen M. Gialanella, Kathleen Mastrian, and Dee McGonigle

## Introduction

Two key pieces of legislation have shaped the nursing informatics landscape: the Health Insurance Portability and Accountability Act (HIPAA) of 1996 and the Health Information Technology for Economic and Clinical Health Act (HITECH) of 2009. This chapter presents an overview of the HITECH Act, including the Medicare and Medicaid health information technology (HIT) provisions of the law. Nurses need to be familiar with the goals and purposes of this law, know how it enhances the security and privacy protections of the **Health Insurance Portability and Accountability Act** (HIPAA) of 1996, and appreciate how it otherwise affects nursing practice in the emerging electronic health records age. The concepts of "meaningful use" and "certified EHR technology" also are explored in this chapter, as well as potential future legislation regulating medical devices and apps and the movement toward payment based on quality. **Figure 8-1** provides a snapshot of the legislation affecting the informatics landscape.

## HIPAA Came First

HIPAA was signed into law by President Bill Clinton in 1996. Hellerstein (1999) summarized the intent of the act as follows: to curtail healthcare fraud and abuse, enforce standards for health information, guarantee the security and privacy of health information, and ensure health insurance portability for employed persons. **Consequences** were put into place for institutions and individuals who violate the requirements of this act. For this text, we concentrate on the health information security and privacy aspects of HIPAA, which are outlined as follows:

> *The privacy provisions of the federal law, the Health Insurance*
> *Portability and Accountability Act of 1996 (HIPAA), apply to*
> *health information created or maintained by healthcare providers*

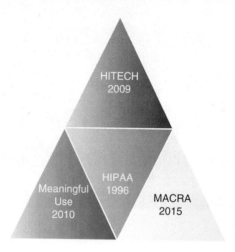

**Figure 8-1** Health Informatics Regulations

*who engage in certain electronic transactions, health plans, and healthcare clearinghouses. The U.S. Department of Health and Human Services (USDHHS) issued the regulation, "Standards for Privacy of Individually Identifiable Health Information," applicable to* **entities** *covered by HIPAA. The Office for Civil Rights (OCR) is the Departmental component responsible for implementing and enforcing the privacy regulation. (U.S. Department of Health and Human Services, 2015, para. 5–6)*

The need and means to guarantee the security and privacy of health information was the focus of numerous debates. Comprehensive standards for the implementation of this portion of the Act eventually were finalized, but the process to adopt final standards took years. In August 1998, the USDHHS released a set of proposed rules addressing health information management. Proposed rules specific to health information privacy and security were released in November 1999. The purpose of the proposed rules was to balance patients' rights to privacy and providers' needs for access to information (Hellerstein, 2000).

Hellerstein (2000) summarized the proposed privacy rules. The rules do the following:

- Define protected health information as "information relating to one's physical or mental health, the provision of one's health care, or the payment for that health care, that has been maintained or transmitted electronically and that can be reasonably identified with the individual it applies to" (Hellerstein, 2000, p. 2). **Figure 8-2** depicts the types of information protected under HIPAA.
- Propose that authorization by patients for release of information is not necessary when the release of information is directly related to treatment and payment for treatment. Specific patient authorization is not required for research, medical or police emergencies, legal proceedings, and collection of data for public health concerns. All other releases of health information require a specific form for each release and only information pertinent to the issue at

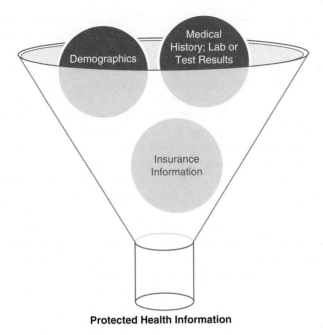

**Protected Health Information**

**Figure 8-2** What Is Protected Health Information?

hand is allowed to be released. All releases of information must be formally documented and accessible to the patient on request.

- Establish patient ownership of the healthcare record and allow for patient-initiated corrections and amendments.
- Mandate administrative requirements for the protection of healthcare information. All healthcare organizations are required to have a privacy official and an office to receive privacy violation complaints. A specific training program for employees that includes a certification of completion and a signed statement by all employees that they will uphold privacy procedures must be developed and implemented. All employees must re-sign the agreement to uphold privacy every 3 years. Sanctions for violations of policy must be clearly defined and applied.
- Mandate that all outside entities that conduct business with healthcare organizations (e.g., attorneys, consultants, auditors) must meet the same standards as the organization for information protection and security.
- Allow protected health information to be released without authorization for research studies. Patients may not access their information in blinded research studies because this access may affect the reliability of the study outcomes.
- Propose that protected health information may be deidentified before release in such a manner that the identity of the patient is protected. The healthcare organization may code the deidentification so that the information can be reidentified once it has been returned.
- Apply only to health information maintained or transmitted by electronic means.

As concerns mounted and deadlines loomed, the healthcare arena prepared to comply with the requirements of the law. The administrative simplification portion of this law was intended to decrease the financial and administrative burdens by standardizing the electronic transmission of certain administrative and financial transactions. This section also addressed the security and privacy of healthcare data and information for the covered entities of healthcare providers who transmit any health information in electronic form in connection with a covered transaction, health plans, and healthcare clearinghouses (Centers for Medicare & Medicaid Services, 2014).

The privacy requirements, which went into effect on April 14, 2003, limited the release of protected health information without the patient's knowledge and consent. Covered entities must comply with the requirements. Notably, they must dedicate a privacy officer, adopt and implement privacy procedures, educate their personnel, and secure their electronic patient records. Most individuals are familiar with the need to notify patients of their privacy rights, having signed forms on interacting with healthcare providers.

According to the USDHHS (2002), the privacy rule provides certain rights to patients: the right to request restrictions to access of the health record; the right to request an alternative method of communication with a provider; the right to receive a paper copy of the notice of privacy practices; the right to file a complaint if the patient believes his or her privacy rights were violated; the right to inspect and copy one's health record; the right to request an amendment to the health record; and the right to see an account of disclosures of one's health record. This places the burden of maintaining privacy and accuracy on the healthcare system, rather than the patient.

On October 16, 2003, the electronic transaction and code set standards became effective. At the time, they did not require electronic transmission, but rather mandated that if transactions were conducted electronically, they must comply with the required federal standards for electronically filed healthcare claims. "The Secretary has made the Centers for Medicare & Medicaid Services (CMS) responsible for enforcing the electronic transactions and code sets provisions of the law" ("Guidance on Compliance with HIPAA Transactions and Code Sets," 2003, para. 3).

The security requirements went into effect on April 21, 2005, and required the covered entities to put safeguards that protect the confidentiality, integrity, and availability of protected health information when stored and transmitted electronically into place.

The safeguards that were addressed were administrative, physical, and technical. The administrative safeguards refer to the documented formal policies and procedures that are used to manage and execute the security measures. They govern the protection of healthcare data and information and the conduct of the personnel. The physical safeguards refer to the policies and procedures that must be in place to limit physical access to electronic information systems. Technical safeguards are the policies and procedures used to control access to healthcare data and information. Safeguards need to be in place to control access whether the data and information are at rest, residing on a machine or storage medium, being processed, or in transmission, such as being backed up to storage or disseminated across a network.

## Overview of the HITECH Act

The federal Health Information Technology for Economic and Clinical Health Act of 2009 (HITECH Act; Leyva & Leyva, 2011), enacted February 17, 2009, is part of the

**American Recovery and Reinvestment Act** (ARRA). The ARRA, also known as the "Stimulus" law, was enacted to stimulate various sectors of the U.S. economy during the most severe recession this country had experienced since the Great Depression of the late 1920s and early 1930s. The **health information technology** (HIT) industry was one area where lawmakers saw an opportunity to stimulate the economy and improve the delivery of health care at the same time. This explains why the title of the HITECH Act contains the phrase "for Economic and Clinical Health."

The ARRA is a lengthy piece of legislation that is organized into two major sections: Division A and Division B. Each division contains several titles. Title XIII of Division A of the ARRA is the HITECH Act. It addresses the development, adoption, and implementation of HIT **policies** and **standards** and provides enhanced **privacy** and **security** protections for patient information—an area of the law that is of paramount concern in nursing informatics. Title IV of Division B of the ARRA is considered part of the HITECH Act. It addressed Medicare and Medicaid HIT and provided significant financial incentives to healthcare professionals and hospitals that adopted and engaged in the **"meaningful use"** of **electronic health records** (EHRs) technology.

At the time the HITECH Act was enacted, it was estimated that less than 8% of U.S. hospitals used a basic EHR system in at least one of their clinical units, and less than 2% of U.S. hospitals had an EHR system in all of their clinical settings (Ashish, 2009). Not surprisingly, the cost of an EHR system has been a major barrier to widespread adoption of this technology in most healthcare facilities. The HITECH Act sought to change that situation by providing each person in the United States with an EHR. In addition, a nationwide HIT infrastructure would be developed so that access to a person's EHR will be readily available to every healthcare provider who treats the patient, no matter where the patient may be located at the time treatment is rendered. According to the Office of the National Coordinator for Health Information Technology (2015), three out of four hospitals now have at least a basic EHR with clinician notes, and for larger acute care hospitals, nearly 97% have EHR technology certified by USDHHS.

## Definitions

The HITECH Act includes some important definitions that anyone involved in nursing informatics should know:

- **"Certified EHR Technology"**: An EHR that meets specific governmental standards for the type of record involved, whether it is an ambulatory EHR used by office-based healthcare practitioners or an inpatient EHR used by hospitals. The specific standards that are to be met for any such EHRs are set forth in federal regulations.
- **"Enterprise Integration"**: The electronic linkage of healthcare providers, health plans, the government, and other interested parties to enable the electronic exchange and use of health information among all the components in the health care infrastructure.
- **"Healthcare Provider"**: Hospitals, skilled nursing facilities, nursing homes, long-term care facilities, home health agencies, hemodialysis centers, clinics, community mental health centers, ambulatory surgery centers, group practices, pharmacies and pharmacists, laboratories, physicians, and therapists, among others.

- "Health Information Technology" (HIT): "Hardware, software, integrated technologies or related licenses, intellectual property, upgrades, or packaged solutions sold as services that are designed for or support the use by healthcare entities or patients for the electronic creation, maintenance, access, or exchange of health information."
- "**Qualified Electronic Health Record**": "An electronic record of health-related information on an individual." A "qualified" EHR contains a patient's demographic and clinical health information, including the medical history and a list of health problems, and is capable of providing support for clinical decisions and entry of physician orders. It must also have the capacity "to capture and query information relevant to health care quality" and "exchange electronic health information with, and integrate such information from other sources" (Readthestimulus.org, 2009, pp. 32–35).

## Purposes

The HITECH Act established the **Office of the National Coordinator for Health Information Technology** (ONC) within the USDHHS. The ONC is headed by the national coordinator, who is responsible for overseeing the development of a nationwide HIT infrastructure that supports the use and exchange of information to achieve the following goals:

1. Improve healthcare quality by enhancing coordination of services between and among the various healthcare providers a patient may have, fostering more appropriate healthcare decisions at the time and place of delivery of services, and preventing medical errors and advancing the delivery of **patient-centered care**
2. Reduce the cost of health care by addressing inefficiencies, such as duplication of services within the healthcare delivery system, and by reducing the number of medical errors
3. Improve people's health by promoting prevention, early detection, and management of chronic diseases
4. Protect public health by fostering early detection and rapid response to infectious diseases, bioterrorism, and other situations that could have a widespread impact on the health status of many individuals
5. Facilitate clinical research
6. Reduce health disparities
7. Better secure patient health information

Improving healthcare quality has been an ongoing challenge in the United States. According to the **Agency for Healthcare Research and Quality** (AHRQ), quality health care is care that is "safe, timely, patient centered, efficient, and equitable" (AHRQ, 2009, p. 1). AHRQ, an agency within USDHHS, has been releasing a national healthcare quality report (NHQR) every year since 2003. Access the most recent report at www.ahrq.gov/research/findings/nhqrdr/index.html. The NHQR emphasized the need for HIT to support the goal of improving quality of care.

*Providers need reliable information about their performance to guide improvement activities. Realistically, HIT infrastructure is needed to ensure that relevant data are collected regularly, systematically, and unobtrusively while protecting patient privacy and confidentiality . . . . Systems need to generate information that can be understood by end users and that are interoperable across different institutions' data platforms... Quality improvement typically requires examining patterns of care across panels of patients rather than one patient at a time . . . Ideally, performance measures should be calculated automatically from health records in a format that can be easily shared and compared across all providers involved with a patient's care. (AHRQ, 2009, p. 13)*

The prevalence of **healthcare-associated infections** serves as an excellent example of how use of EHR technology and a nationwide HIT infrastructure can play a significant role in addressing healthcare quality issues. According to the NHQR, "wound infections are a common occurrence following surgery, but hospitals can reduce the risk of these health care–associated infections by making sure patients receive an appropriate antibiotic within an hour before their procedures" (AHRQ, 2009, p. 110). The **Centers for Medicare and Medicaid Services** (CMS) already has the capacity to track Medicare patients who receive this prophylactic treatment and the rate of post-surgical wound infections for those patients who do and do not receive the treatment. Imagine being able to track this issue for all surgical patients and developing evidence-based care plans to ensure that all patients within the infrastructure receive the same quality of care. This is just one of many examples in which the end result of EHR adoption is better patient outcomes.

EHR technology also will make it easier for all providers involved in a patient's care to readily access that patient's complete and current healthcare record, thereby allowing providers to make well-informed, efficient, and effective decisions about a patient's care at the time those decisions need to be made. This is of tremendous benefit to the patient and promotes a higher level of patient-centered care. It also allows effective coordination of care between and among all providers involved in the patient's care, including doctors, nurses, therapists, nutritionists, hospitals, nursing homes, rehabilitation facilities, home health agencies, laboratories, and other diagnostic centers, thereby assuring the continuum of patient care.

Such an integrated system would have clear benefits for patients and providers alike. For example, imagine how much easier it would be for a patient with a rare form of cancer to obtain a second oncologist's opinion before beginning a course of treatment. The patient's complete record, including the results of numerous diagnostic tests conducted at multiple sites, such as blood tests, biopsies, radiographs, and scans, would be readily available to the second oncologist. Imagine how much easier it would be for a patient with end-stage renal disease, who is receiving outpatient hemodialysis several times a week, to receive appropriate treatment if he or she is suddenly hospitalized or would like to take a vacation out of state. Imagine how much easier it would be for nurses to complete a medication reconciliation for a newly admitted patient. The possibilities are endless, and the savings realized from enhancing quality, avoiding duplication of services, and streamlining delivery of patient care are obvious.

Reducing healthcare errors has been another ongoing challenge in the United States. Healthcare providers strive to meet the standard of care and avoid harm to patients. Patients have a right to receive appropriate care, but that does not always happen. Ten years ago, the Institute of Medicine's Committee on the Quality of Health Care in America undertook a comprehensive literature review and summarized the results of more than 40 studies about healthcare errors in its seminal report, *To Err Is Human: Building a Safer Health System* (Institute of Medicine, 2000). That report concluded that approximately 44,000–98,000 people in the United States die each year as a result of healthcare errors. Many thousands more who do not die are seriously injured from such errors. In addition to the human pain and suffering associated with healthcare errors, the monetary costs of these errors are substantial. Although some progress in reducing healthcare errors has been made since the release of *To Err Is Human*, substantial work remains to be done. It is anticipated that a nationwide HIT infrastructure will contribute to a reduction in healthcare errors by providing mechanisms to assist with the prevention of errors and to provide timely warnings of the possibility of a repetitive error that may affect many patients.

Containing and reducing healthcare costs in the United States, where more than $2 trillion is spent on health care each year (Keehan, Sisko, & Truffler, 2008), is another daunting challenge. Using EHR technology and a nationwide HIT infrastructure to improve quality and reduce errors within the healthcare delivery system is one way to address this challenge. Imagine the billions of dollars that could be saved just by reducing the estimated 1.7 million cases of healthcare-associated infections contracted by patients in U.S. hospitals each year (AHRQ, 2009, p. 108).

Promoting prevention, early detection, and management of chronic diseases is another purpose of the HITECH Act. The delivery of health care in the United States traditionally has been based on a disease model rather than a wellness model. Having an EHR for each individual could help with the necessary transition as providers and their patients become more aware of the variables that positively or negatively impact health. The ability to identify appropriate choices to promote wellness and either prevent illness and injury or detect and manage chronic diseases sooner will be enhanced.

Chronic diseases are of major concern to this country, not only because of the impact they have on individuals, but also because of the tremendous cost associated with providing treatment for patients with these conditions. Adult-onset diabetes, for example, has reached epidemic proportions. A national HIT infrastructure will help providers better identify those patients who are at risk for developing this disease and provide treatment strategies to avoid it. For those patients who develop type 2 diabetes, their providers will be able to diagnose the condition much sooner and manage it more effectively because of the vast resources that a national HIT infrastructure can provide.

Improving public health is another purpose of the HITECH Act. The recent Zika virus challenge is illustrative of how a national HIT infrastructure can protect public health by fostering early detection and rapid response to infectious diseases, bioterrorism, and other situations that could have a widespread impact on the health status of many individuals and groups.

The impact that a national HIT infrastructure will have on clinical research is self-evident. Once the infrastructure becomes operational, the amount of data that will become readily available for clinical research will increase exponentially compared to what is available today. The ability of researchers to conduct studies and provide clinicians with the most current evidence-based practice will be of tremendous benefit to patients everywhere.

Reducing **health disparities** is another purpose of the HITECH Act. According to the AHRQ (2013), "Health care disparities are differences or gaps in the care experienced by one population compared with another population" (p. 1). Detailed information about healthcare disparities can be found at the website for the Office of Minority Health and Health Disparities at www.cdc.gov/omhd. The AHRQ routinely examines the issue of disparities in health care and reports its findings to the public. The National Healthcare Disparities Report of 2012 confirms that some Americans continue to receive inferior care because of such factors as race, ethnicity, and socioeconomic status (AHRQ, 2013). This report found disparities in the following areas:

- Across all dimensions of healthcare quality: Effectiveness, patient safety, timeliness, and patient centeredness
- Across all dimensions of access to care: Facilitators and barriers to care and health care utilization
- Across many levels and types of care: Preventive care, treatment of acute conditions, and management of chronic diseases
- Across many clinical conditions: Cancer, diabetes, end-stage renal disease, heart disease, HIV disease, mental health and substance abuse, and respiratory diseases
- Across many care settings: Primary care, home health care, hospice care, emergency department, hospitals, and nursing homes
- Within many subpopulations: Women, children, older adults, residents of rural areas, and individuals with disabilities and other special healthcare needs (AHRQ, 2013, pp. H1–H4)

All patients, regardless of race, ethnicity, or socioeconomic status, should receive care that is effective, safe, and timely. When the national HIT infrastructure contemplated by the HITECH Act is fully implemented, such disparities are bound to decrease. The ability to monitor for disparities and promote the delivery of appropriate care to all patients will be enhanced. Clinicians will be prompted to base their treatments on appropriate factors and avoid biased care.

Perhaps the most important task facing the national coordinator during the development and implementation of a nationwide HIT infrastructure is ensuring the security of the patient health information within that system. The ability to secure and protect confidential patient information has always been of paramount importance to clinicians, who view this consideration as an ethical and legal obligation of practice. Patients value their privacy and they have a right to expect that their confidential health information will be properly safeguarded. Nurses have been complying with the regulatory requirements of HIPAA for years, and the HITECH Act has enhanced the security and privacy protections each patient has a right to expect under HIPAA. The specific changes are discussed in greater detail later in this chapter.

# How a National HIT Infrastructure Is Being Developed

Developing a national HIT infrastructure is an enormous and extremely complex undertaking that requires extensive financial, technologic, and human resources. The HITECH Act established the ONC, as noted earlier, and the USDHHS appointed a national coordinator, who is responsible for the development of the infrastructure.

The HITECH Act also established two committees within the ONC: the HIT Policy Committee and the HIT Standards Committee.

The Policy Committee is responsible for making recommendations to the coordinator about how to implement the requirements of the HITECH Act, such as the technologies to use in the infrastructure. The Policy Committee has a total of 20 members, one of whom must be a member from a labor organization and two of whom must be healthcare providers. At least one of the healthcare providers must be a physician. There is no specific requirement that a nurse be on the Policy Committee. A complete list of the Policy Committee members is available at www.healthit.hhs.gov.

The Standards Committee is responsible for recommending standards by which health information is to be electronically exchanged. The HITECH Act does not designate the number of members to be on the committee; however, its members include healthcare providers, ancillary healthcare workers, consumers of health care, and others. Again, there is no specific requirement that a nurse be on the Standards Committee, and a complete list of the Standards Committee members is available at www.healthit.gov.

The HITECH Act also made provisions to include meaningful public input in the development of a national HIT infrastructure. Both the Policy Committee and the Standards Committee hold public meetings, and anyone interested in this process can participate. A schedule of meetings, committee agendas, and the transcripts of past meeting are posted at www.healthit.gov.

The national coordinator has several duties. He or she decides whether to endorse the recommendations of the Policy and Standards Committees and acts as a liaison among the committees and various federal agencies involved in the process of developing a national HIT infrastructure. He or she consults with these other agencies, including the National Institute of Standards and Technology, and along with those agencies updates the Federal HIT Strategic Plan (U.S. Department of Commerce, 2011). The initial Federal HIT Strategic Plan was published in June 2008, before the enactment of the HITECH Act, and the plan has been updated frequently to reflect evolving IT strategies. The most current plan can be accessed at www.healthit.gov/policy-researchers-implementers/health-it-strategic-planning.

The HITECH Act also provides significant monetary incentives for providers who engaged in meaningful use of HIT. "Meaningful use" was defined as "using electronic health records (EHRs) in a meaningful manner, which includes, but is not limited to electronically capturing health information in a coded format, using that information to track key clinical conditions, communicating that information to help coordinate care, and initiating the reporting of clinical quality measures and public health information" (CMS, 2010, para. 3).

Monetary incentives are available to clinicians and facilities that implement EHR systems that meet the specific standards. Providers that fail to adopt such systems within a specified time frame may be subject to significant governmental penalties.

## How the HITECH Act Changed HIPAA

### HIPAA Privacy and Security Rules

Nurses have been complying with HIPAA for years. HIPAA was enacted by the federal government for several purposes, including better portability of health insurance as a worker moved from one job to another; deterrence of fraud, abuse, and waste within the healthcare delivery system; and simplification of the administrative functions associated with the delivery of health care, such as reimbursement claims sent to Medicare and Medicaid. Simplification of administrative functions entailed the adoption of electronic transactions that included sensitive healthcare information. To protect the privacy and security of health information, two sets of federal regulations were implemented. The Privacy Rule became effective in 2003, and the Security Rule became effective in 2005. Many practitioners that refer to HIPAA are not referring to the comprehensive federal statute enacted in 1996, but rather to the Privacy Rule and the Security Rule—that is, the federal regulations that were adopted years after HIPAA became law.

Under the Privacy Rule, patients have a right to expect privacy protections that limit the use and disclosure of their health information. Under the Security Rule, providers are obligated to safeguard their patients' health information from improper use or disclosure, maintain the integrity of the information, and ensure its availability. Both rules apply to **protected health information** (PHI), defined as any physical or mental health information created, received, or stored by a "covered entity" that can be used to identify an individual patient, regardless of the form of the health information (i.e., it can be electronic, handwritten, or verbal) (Legal Information Institute [LII], 2013). Covered entities include hospitals and other healthcare providers that transmit any health information electronically, as well as health insurance companies and healthcare clearinghouses (LII, 2013).

Clinicians have become very knowledgeable about the requirements of the Privacy and Security Rules. They are familiar with their obligations to protect patient information and the **rights** afforded to their patients under these regulations. Patients are entitled to a notice of privacy practices from their healthcare provider. Inpatients are entitled to opt out of the facility's directory, thereby protecting disclosure of information that they are even a patient in the facility. Under certain circumstances, patients must authorize disclosure of their PHI before it can be released by the provider. Patients can request and obtain access to their own healthcare records and may request that corrections and additions be made to their records. Providers must consider a patient's request to amend a healthcare record, but they are not required to make such an amendment if the request is unwarranted. Unauthorized access or use or any loss of healthcare information must be disclosed to any patient affected by the breach. Patients may request an accounting of anyone who accessed their healthcare information, and the provider is required to provide that information in a timely manner. Finally, patients have a right to complain if they perceive that the privacy or security of their healthcare information has been compromised in some way. Such complaints can be made directly to the provider or to the **Office of Civil Rights** (OCR).

The OCR, which is part of the USDHHS, is responsible for enforcing HIPAA. It provides significant information and guidance to clinicians who must comply with the Privacy and Security Rules. It has been tracking complaints and investigating violations since 2003. Guidance and information about the complaint process and the violations that the OCR has handled are available on its website at www.healthit .gov/providers-professionals/model-notices-privacy-practices. As an example, one such violation involved a nurse practitioner who had privileges within a healthcare system. She accessed her ex-husband's medical records without his authorization by using the system-wide EHRs. A complaint was filed and the OCR investigated the matter. The OCR resolved the complaint with the healthcare system. As part of this resolution, the healthcare system curtailed the nurse practitioner's access to its EHRs and it required her to undergo remedial training. In addition, it reported the nurse practitioner to her professional board (USDHHS, Office of Civil Rights, n.d.)

Many businesses are moving to enact a "bring your own device" (BYOD) policy for employees. This policy, which helps to streamline the lives of employees by maintaining personal and business information on one device, can also result in cost savings for the organization overall. BYOD is an issue, however, when dealing with PHI. Healthcare organizations typically do not encourage use of personal devices for professional matters, and in many instances they actually have policies in place forbidding employees from using personal devices in the workplace. According to HIT Consultant (2013), approximately 50% of healthcare organizations report that personal mobile devices can be used to access the Internet within their facilities but these devices are not given access to the organization's network. Typically, only devices that are issued by the organization, secured, and routinely audited are able to access to the network. Nurses must exercise caution when bringing their personal devices into the healthcare organization to ensure that they are not violating any specifics of the BYOD policy.

**Compliance** with the Privacy and Security Rules is mandatory for all covered entities, and the HITECH Act extends compliance with these requirements directly to other entities that are business associates of a covered entity. Requirements include designation of privacy and information security officials to protect health information and appropriate handling of any complaints. Sanctions must be imposed if a violation of HIPAA occurs. The Privacy and Security Rules also mandate that certain physical and technical safeguards be implemented for PHI, and they require entities to conduct periodic training of all staff to ensure compliance with these safeguards. Most entities adhere to industry standards and provide their personnel with yearly training. In addition, entities are to conduct regular audits to ensure compliance, and any breaches in the privacy or security of PHI must be remedied immediately. It is important to avoid a security incident as such incidents trigger certain notification requirements and may be associated with monetary penalties.

## The HITECH Act Enhanced HIPAA Protections

The HITECH Act has had a significant impact on HIPAA's Privacy and Security Rules in the following ways:

- USDHHS is to provide annual guidance about how to secure health information.
- Notification requirements in the event of a breach in the security of health information have been enhanced.
- HIPAA requirements now apply directly to any business associates of a covered entity.
- The rules that pertain to providing an accounting to patients who want to know who accessed their health information have changed.
- Enforcement of HIPAA has been strengthened.

These measures are being implemented to provide further assurance that health information will be protected as the country transitions to a nationwide HIT infrastructure. Several other organizations are also involved in the privacy and security aspects of the HIT infrastructure development (Box 8-1).

## BOX 8-1 OTHER ORGANIZATIONS ASSISTING HIPAA

*Dee McGonigle, Kathleen Mastrian, and Nedra Farcus*

Several other organizations have been involved in HIPAA implementation. The **American National Standards Institute** (ANSI) X12N and **Health Level Seven** (HL7) standards organizations worked together to develop an electronic standard for claims attachments to recommend to USDHHS (Spencer & Bushman, 2006, para. 2). ANSI (n.d.) was founded in 1918 and has served as the coordinator of the U.S. voluntary standards and conformity assessment system (para. 1). ANSI provides a forum where the private and public sectors can cooperatively work together toward the development of voluntary national consensus standards and the related compliance programs (para. 2). HL7 (n.d.) is one of several ANSI-accredited **standards-developing organizations (SDOs)** operating in the healthcare arena (para. 1). It states that its mission is to provide standards for interoperability that improve care delivery, optimize workflow, reduce ambiguity, and enhance knowledge transfer among all stakeholders, including healthcare providers, government agencies, the vendor community, fellow SDOs, and patients (para. 5).

HL7 was initially associated with HIPAA in 1996 through the creation of a claims attachments special interest group charged with standardizing the supplemental information needed to support healthcare insurance and other e-commerce transactions. The initial deliverable of this group was six claim attachments. This special interest group is currently known as the Attachment Special Interest Group. As the attachment projects continue, they are slated to include skilled nursing facilities, home health care, preauthorization, and referrals.

The "Level Seven" in HL7's name refers to the highest level of the **International Standards Organization's** (ISO's) communications model for **Open Systems Interconnection** (OSI) application level. The application level addresses definition of the data to be exchanged, the timing of the interchange, and the communication of certain errors to the application. The seventh level supports such functions as security checks, participant identification, availability checks, exchange mechanism negotiations and, most importantly, data exchange structuring (HL7, n.d., para. 5).

The OSI was an attempt to standardize networking by the ISO. HL7 addresses the distinct requirements of the systems in use in hospitals and other facilities, is more concerned with application than the other levels, and considers user authentication and privacy (Webopedia, 2008). The lower levels of OSI address hardware, software, and data reformatting.

HL7's mission is supported through two separate groups, the Extensible Markup Language (XML) special interest group and the structured documents technical committee. The XML special interest group makes recommendations on use of XML standards for all of HL7's platform- and vendor-independent healthcare specifications (HL7, n.d., para. 21). XML began as a simplified subset of the standard generalized markup language; its major purpose is to facilitate the exchange of structured data across different information systems, especially via the Internet. It is considered an extensible language because it permits users to define their own elements, thereby supporting customization to enable purpose-specific development. The structured documents technical committee supports the

HL7 mission through development of structured document standards for health care (para. 21). HL7 also organizes, maintains, and sustains a repository for the vocabulary terms used in its messages to provide a shared, well-defined, and unambiguous knowledge base of the meaning of the data transferred.

ISO (2008a) is a network of the national standards institutes of 157 countries. It includes one member per country, and a central secretariat in Geneva, Switzerland, coordinates the system (para. 1). ISO is a nongovernmental organization; its members are not delegations of national governments (unlike the case in the United Nations system). Nevertheless, ISO occupies a special position between the public and private sectors. On the one hand, many of its member institutes are part of the governmental structure of their countries or are mandated by their government. On the other hand, other members have their roots uniquely in the private sector, having been set up by national partnerships of industry associations (ISO, 2008a, para. 2).

This placement enables ISO to become a bridging organization where members can reach agreement on solutions that meet both the requirements of business and the broader needs of society, consumers, and users. These international agreements become standards that use the prefix ISO followed by the number of the standard. An example is the health informatics, health cards, numbering system, and registration procedure for issuer identifiers, ISO 20302:2006; it is designed to confirm, via a numbering system and registration procedure, the identities of both the healthcare application provider and the health card holder so that information may be exchanged by using cards issued for healthcare service (ISO, 2008b, para. 12). ISO provides standards for interoperability that improve care delivery, optimize workflow, reduce ambiguity, and enhance knowledge transfer among all of its stakeholders, including healthcare providers, government agencies, the vendor community, fellow SDOs, and patients. The standards are used on a voluntary basis because ISO has no power to force their enactment.

All of the organizations described here have guidelines, standards, and rules to help healthcare entities collect, store, manipulate, dispose of, and exchange secure PHI. Many SDOs work to help develop standards. HIPAA guarantees the security and privacy of health information and curtails healthcare fraud and abuse while enforcing standards for health information.

## UNITED STATES AND BEYOND

Health care was not the only focus of U.S. legislative acts. One often sees "GLBA" and "SOX" when searching for information on HIPAA. The **Gramm-Leach-Bliley Act** (GLBA) is federal legislation in the United States to control how financial institutions handle the private information they collect from individuals. The **Sarbanes-Oxley Act** (SOX) is legislation put in place to protect shareholders and the public from deceptive accounting practices in organizations.

Privacy and data regulations are also being established around the world. See a map of the world depicting the laws of various countries at this website: www.dlapiperdataprotection.com/#handbook/world-map-section. It is quite evident that privacy and security have become global concerns.

Avoiding security incidents has become a paramount concern for healthcare organizations and providers. Providers must protect their information and prevent unauthorized persons from accessing, using, disclosing, changing, or destroying a patient's health information, or otherwise interfering with the operations of a health information system, such as an EHR. To facilitate a provider's ability to do this, the HITECH Act requires USDHHS to provide annual guidance to secure health information. PHI can be secured or unsecured. PHI is considered unsecured if the provider does not follow the guidance provided by USDHHS for implementing technologies and methodologies that make PHI "unusable, unreadable, or indecipherable to unauthorized individuals" (USDHHS, 2009). PHI can be secured through encryption, shredding and other forms of complete destruction, or electronic media sanitation. Figure 8-3 depicts some common causes of PHI vulnerabilities.

The distinction between secured and unsecured PHI is important because providers that experience a breach in the privacy or security of their PHI must adhere to certain notification requirements depending on the type of PHI affected by the breach. The HITECH Act enhanced the breach notification requirements of HIPAA. If the PHI is unsecured, the provider must take certain steps to notify those individuals who have been affected. Providers can avoid these onerous breach notification requirements if the PHI is secured in accordance with the specifications of USDHHS.

A breach is considered discovered as soon as an employee other than the individual who committed the breach knows or should have known of the breach, such as unauthorized access or even an unsuccessful attempt to access information. For example, if a nurse knows that a colleague has accessed or attempted to access the record of a patient for whom the colleague is not providing care (e.g., the nurse practitioner who accessed her ex-husband's EHR, as discussed previously), the nurse's employer is deemed to have discovered the breach as soon as the nurse learned of it. The discovery of a breach triggers the beginning of the time frame during which the provider must fulfill the notification requirements. A provider must fulfill these

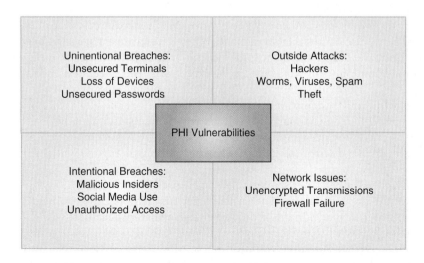

**Figure 8-3** Vulnerability of Private Health Information

requirements within a reasonable period of time; under no circumstances may a provider take more than 60 days from discovery of the breach. It is easy to understand why providers require their employees to report knowledge of such breaches immediately to the privacy or information security officer. A provider's failure to adhere to the breach notification requirements could result in OCR sanctions, including monetary penalties.

Whenever a breach involves unsecured PHI, covered entities are responsible for alerting each affected individual by mail, or by e-mail if preferred by the individual. If there is insufficient contact information for 10 or more patients, the provider is required to place conspicuous postings on the home page of its website or in major print or broadcast media (without identifying patients). A toll-free telephone number must be provided so that affected individuals can call for information about the breach. For breaches involving unsecured PHI of more than 500 individuals, a prominent media outlet must also be notified. Notice must be given to USDHHS as well, and USDHHS will post the information on its public website (USDHHS, 2009). It is easy to see why providers would want to avoid these requirements by making sure their PHI is secured. Having to post such notices undermines the trust that exists between healthcare providers and the patients and communities they serve.

The HITECH Act has improved the privacy and security of patient health information by applying the requirements of HIPAA directly to the business associates of covered entities. In the past, it was up to the covered entity to enter into contracts with its business associates to ensure compliance with HIPAA. Now business associates are responsible for their own compliance. An example of such a business associate is a HIT company hired by a hospital to implement or upgrade an EHR system. The technology company has access to the hospital's EHR system and must comply with the HIPAA Privacy and Security Rules, just as covered entities must comply with these rules. This includes being subject to enforcement by the OCR for any violations.

Existing accounting rules are enhanced under the HITECH Act, giving patients the right to **access** their EHR and receive an accounting of all disclosures. Before the HITECH Act, HIPAA regulations provided an exception to the accounting requirements. Providers and other covered entities were not required to include in the accounting any disclosures that were made to facilitate **treatment/payment/operations**—treatment of patients, the payment for services, or the operations of the entity—a provision commonly known as the "TPO exception." This exception ended in January 2011 for providers that recently implemented new EHR systems. For those providers with EHR systems that were implemented before the HITECH Act, the TPO exception ended in January 2014. It is easy to understand why this exception has ended. As all providers implement comprehensive EHR systems, it will be very easy to generate an electronic record with an accounting of anyone who accessed a patient's record.

Finally, the HITECH Act strengthens the enforcement of HIPAA. USDHHS can conduct audits, which will be even easier to accomplish once a nationwide HIT infrastructure is in place. In addition, stiffer **civil monetary penalties** (CMP) for violations of HIPAA became effective as soon as the HITECH Act became law in February 2009. CMPs are divided into three tiers. A Tier 1 CMP, in which the covered entity had no reason to know of a violation, is $100 per incident, up to a cap of

$25,000 per year. A Tier 2 CMP, in which the covered entity had reasonable cause to know of a violation, is $1,000 per incident, up to a cap of $100,000 per year. A Tier 3 CMP, in which the covered entity engaged in willful neglect that resulted in a breach, is $10,000 per incident, up to a cap of $250,000 per year. In addition, the HITECH Act gives authority to impose an additional CMP of $50,000 to $1.5 million if the covered entity does not properly correct a violation. Criminal penalties also can be imposed when warranted. It is imperative that providers avoid these penalties.

Before enactment of the HITECH Act, the federal government alone enforced HIPAA. Now, state attorneys general can play a significant role in the enforcement and prosecution of HIPAA violations. Once the HITECH Act became law, state attorneys general were authorized to pursue civil claims for HIPAA violations and collect up to $25,000 plus attorneys' fees. As of 2012, individuals who are damaged by such violations became eligible to share in any monetary awards obtained by these state officials.

# Implications for Nursing Practice

## Being Involved and Staying Informed

The development and implementation of a nationwide EHR system holds great promise for nursing practice and nursing informatics. The profession of nursing will benefit from the many enhancements such an infrastructure has to offer, including the ability to improve the delivery of nursing care and the quality of that care, the ability to make more efficient and timely nursing care decisions for patients, the ability to avoid errors that may harm patients, and the ability to promote health and wellness for the patients whom nurses serve. On a broader scale, nurse researchers will have the ability to more readily access data that can be used to continue to foster evidence-based practice. The possibilities seem endless. For those who devote their professional careers to nursing informatics or plan to do so, the opportunities abound. Much work remains to be done as this country transitions to a nationwide HIT infrastructure, and moves beyond meaningful use requirements.

All nurses need to be engaged in this process, whether they treat patients, are managers within healthcare organizations, teach, develop computer programs, or help create institutional or governmental policies. Nurses, as the end users of developing technologies, cannot afford to be left behind in these exciting times. Their voices must be heard, whether it is within the facility where they work as changes to the EHR system are contemplated, or whether it is in the public policy arena. How often are nurses the last to know that a new EHR system has been adopted by their hospital? How many times have nurses been trained to use a system that would have benefited from their input before it was implemented or even purchased? Nurses often are not invited to the table when entities make decisions about informatics, so they should not be afraid to ask to be included, whether it is to be heard within the workplace or within the governmental agencies that are overseeing the changes that are taking place.

Even nurses who do not get involved in this process need to stay current with the rapid changes that are taking place. Information about federal initiatives is available from the ONC and the OCR. Both offices are housed within USDHHS and are excellent resources for additional information about the HITECH Act and HIPAA. Regulations to implement the HITECH Act and enhance the HIPAA protections required by it are being proposed and adopted at a rapid pace. See www.healthit.gov to access the most current information.

## Protecting Yourself

Nurses who strive to protect the privacy and security of patient information are protecting themselves from ethical lapses and violations of law. The American Nurses Association's (ANA's) Code of Ethics for Nurses with Interpretive Statements mandates that nurses protect a patient's rights to privacy and **confidentiality.**

Associated with the right to privacy, the nurse has a duty to maintain confidentiality of all patient information. Nurses who engage with social media need to be especially cognizant of the potential for breaching the confidentiality of patient information. Box 8-2 provides more information related to nurses' use of social media. Refer also to

---

### BOX 8-2 USE OF SOCIAL NETWORKS BY NURSES

*Glenn Johnson and Jeff Swain*

New opportunities to share information via social networks have grabbed the headlines. Since their inception in 2004, the growth in popularity of social networking tools, such as Facebook (www.facebook.com) and Twitter (www.twitter.com), has been phenomenal. What makes these sites so attractive? Web-based applications, such as Facebook, allow users to connect and share information in ways that were not previously possible. Users develop online profiles that contain information they select to share with others. Using simple online utilities, users can easily connect and share their profiles, communicating with friends over the Internet. Virtual groups of users with similar profiles may be created, connecting users with others who have similar interests. Twitter, a micro-blogging platform, allows users to create interpersonal networks for socializing, support, and information sharing. The power of such tools as Twitter lies in their being lightweight, their limiting of updates to 140 or fewer characters, and their convenience—users can update their status from any device that has an Internet connection or text messaging capabilities.

The popularity of social and mobile networking applications is one indication of how new Web-based technologies are changing communication preferences. The Web is no longer a destination place, but instead has become a vehicle of communication where individuals use application software ("apps"), which are installed or downloaded, to connect with others. Individuals act as their own portal and can connect from anywhere with their various communities. This makes it difficult to separate out various communities and social networks. Where once it was relatively easy to separate work relationships from friends and family, networked communities tend to overlap, blurring the boundaries between them. The phenomenon of overlapping networks means that the unintended audience is almost always greater than the intended one. A status update that may be construed as harmless and funny to one's friends could be taken an entirely different way by family or colleagues. This is not to say networked communities are harmful or bad. Indeed, the benefits of such communities far exceed their negatives. However, the immediacy and the permanence of the updates shared mean that the user must think about the impact beyond the intended audience in ways never before required (Johnson & Swain, 2011).

Nurses and other healthcare workers who use social media must be aware that the overlapping of networks may unintentionally create privacy and confidentiality breaches. Even when patients are not identified by name, general sharing of information or venting about a difficult day may constitute a privacy breach. The National Council of State Boards of Nursing (NCSBN, 2011) has collaborated with the ANA to develop specific guidelines for the use of social media by nurses. See www.ncsbn.org/Social_Media.pdf to read a white paper discussing common misconceptions about social media, consequences for breaching confidentiality using social media, guidelines for appropriate use of social media, and case scenarios with discussion.

## REFERENCES

Johnson, G., & Swain, J. (2011). Professional development and collaboration tools. In D. McGonigle & K. Mastrian (Eds.), *Nursing informatics and the foundation of knowledge* (2nd ed., pp. 185–195). Burlington, MA: Jones & Bartlett Learning.

National Council of State Boards of Nursing. (2011). White paper: A nurse's guide to the use of social media. Retrieved from https://www.ncsbn.org/Social_Media.pdf

the ethical use of social media discussed in Chapter 5. The patient's well-being could be jeopardized and the fundamental trust between patient and nurse destroyed by unnecessary access to data or by the inappropriate disclosure of identifiable patient information. The rights, well-being, and safety of the individual patient should be the primary factors in arriving at any professional judgment concerning the disposition of confidential information received from or about the patient, whether oral, written, or electronic. The standard of nursing practice and the nurse's responsibility to provide quality care require that relevant data be shared with only those members of the healthcare team who have a need to know that information. Only information pertinent to a patient's treatment and welfare should be disclosed, and only to those directly involved with the patient's care. When using electronic communications, special effort should be made to maintain data security (ANA, 2010, p. 6).

The similarities between these ethical obligations and the legal requirements of HIPAA and other federal and state privacy and confidentiality laws are readily apparent to nurses. By complying with their ethical code, nurses were complying with the Privacy and Security Rules before they were required to do so. Since the adoption of the HIPAA Privacy and Security Rules, and now with the passage of the HITECH

Act, it is more important than ever for nurses to understand their obligations in this area and avoid the pitfalls of violations.

In addition to the sanctions imposed by the OCR, violations can lead to disciplinary actions by employers and professional licensing boards, as well as litigation. Such actions can have a serious negative impact on the nurse's reputation and financial well-being. If a nurse is terminated for invading a patient's privacy or breaching the confidentiality of a patient's information, some state laws require reporting the information to prospective employers of the nurse; other laws require reporting to the State Board of Nursing. State Boards of Nursing have the authority to publicly discipline a nurse who has engaged in professional misconduct by invading a patient's privacy, which includes inappropriately accessing a patient's EHR, and breaching confidentiality of patient information, such as allowing or tolerating unauthorized access to a patient's EHR. These types of situations can also cause patients to file complaints with the OCR and lawsuits against the offenders. Nurses must be ever mindful of their obligations to report a breach in the privacy or security of PHI to their employers, even if it entails reporting a colleague.

Finally, some view the EHR as a convenient method for employers to monitor the performance of its nurses. Clearly, an EHR system provides a wealth of information that can be, and often is required to be, monitored. Audits are required to make sure that no breaches in the system's security occur. Audits are not necessarily required to determine, for example, which nurses are failing to complete the hospital's documentation requirements in a timely fashion, which nurses are improperly altering (attempting to correct) the record, or which nurses are dispensing more pain medication than the average. Nurses have been challenged by employers who allege failure to document, improper or false documentation, and suspected diversion of narcotics. These types of situations are unsettling and may be on the rise as more providers adopt or augment EHR systems. Thus it behooves every nurse who works with such a system to obtain proper training and to know the policies and procedures that pertain to its use.

Social media can and should be used in an appropriate manner by professionals to educate and promote health behaviors in the clients they serve, communicate with clients if they choose this method of communication, and network with other professionals by sharing information (deidentified) and knowledge. As Gagnon and Sabus (2015) suggest, "the reach of social media for health and wellness presents exciting opportunities for the health care professional with a well-executed social media presence. Social media give health care providers a far-reaching platform on which to contribute high-quality online content and amplify positive and accurate health care information and messages. It also provides a forum for correcting misinformation and addressing misconceptions" (p. 410). They advocated for healthcare professionals to practice digital professionalism, and for social media use to be one of the professional competencies for health professional education. Bazan (2015) suggested that social media can be used to consult with other healthcare providers, such as in a professional Facebook group using direct private messaging between the two providers, but cautioned that posting to the main social site cannot contain any hint of PHI. He also shared information about a progressive practice that communicates with patients via private messaging on Facebook. Remember that everything you do electronically leaves a digital footprint! Proceed with caution and be certain that your digital interactions comply completely with professional ethics, laws, and organizational policies.

## Future Regulations

CMS recently released new legislation, the Medicare Access and CHIP Reauthorization Act of 2015 (MACRA; USDHHS, 2016). Although this legislation primarily affects provider payments, all members of the healthcare team will have a hand in ensuring quality care. The final implementation guidelines have yet to be released, but this new legislation is expected to replace the former CMS meaningful use guidelines. For more information on this program, refer to the chapter on *Workflow and Meaningful Use*.

The U.S. Food and Drug Administration (FDA), a division of USDHHS, is responsible for regulating medical devices to ensure public safety. In 2015, the FDA released a guidance document for manufacturers, developers, and FDA staff related to mobile medical applications. At the current time, the most common types of these applications, or apps, are not regulated by the FDA because they are not defined as medical devices. An app is defined as a medical device and may be subject to regulation by the FDA if "the intended use of a mobile app is for the diagnosis of a disease or other conditions, or the cure, mitigation, treatment, or prevention of disease, or if it is intended to affect the structure or function of the body of man" (FDA, 2015, p. 8). The guidance document also provides a list of examples of apps that are not currently viewed as medical devices, such as apps that help users organize personal medical data, track fitness, or self-manage a disease. If, however, the mobile app is an accessory to a regulated medical device, then it is also considered a medical device and is subject to FDA oversight. We need to be aware that as these mobile apps become more sophisticated in the future, they may indeed be subject to more stringent oversight by the FDA to ensure consumer safety.

## Summary

The HITECH Act and the HIPAA Privacy and Security Rules are intended to enhance the rights of individuals. These laws provide patients with greater access and control over their PHI. They can control its uses, dissemination, and disclosures. Covered entities must establish not only a required level of security for PHI, but also sanctions for employees who violate the organization's privacy policies and administrative processes for responding to patient requests regarding their information. Therefore, they must be able to track the PHI, note access from the perspective of which information was accessed and by whom, and identify any disclosures. Finally, readers should recognize that there is global awareness of the need for privacy protections for personal information or PHI. Over the next few years, international efforts will accelerate, enhancing international data exchange.

## THOUGHT-PROVOKING QUESTIONS

1. One of the largest problems with healthcare information security has always been inappropriate use by authorized users. How do HIPAA and the HITECH Act help to curb this problem?
2. How do you envision Health Level Seven, HIPAA, and the HITECH Act evolving in the next decade?
3. If you were the privacy officer in your organization, how would you address the following?
   a. Tracking each point of access of the patient's database, including who entered the data.
   b. Encouraging employees to report privacy and security breaches.
   c. The healthcare professionals are using smartphones, iPads, and other mobile devices. How do you address privacy when data can literally walk out of your setting?
   d. You observe one of the healthcare professionals using his smartphone to take pictures of a patient. He sees you and says, in front of the patient, "I am not capturing her face!" How do you respond to this situation?

# References

Agency for Healthcare Research and Quality (AHRQ). (2009). *National healthcare quality report (NHQR) 2009: Crossing the quality chasm: A new healthcare system for the 21st century.* Washington, DC: National Academies Press.

Agency for Healthcare Research and Quality (AHRQ). (2013). *2012 national healthcare disparities report.* Retrieved from https://archive.ahrq.gov/research/findings/nhqrdr/nhdr12

American National Standards Institute (ANSI). (n.d.). ANSI: A historical overview. Retrieved from http://ansi.org/about_ansi/introduction/history.aspx?menuid=1

American Nurses Association (ANA). (2010). *Code of ethics for nurses with interpretive statements.* Retrieved from http://www.nursingworld.org/codeofethics

Ashish, J. (2009). Use of electronic health records in U.S. hospitals. *New England Journal of Medicine, 360*(16), 1628–1638.

Bazan, J. (2015). HIPAA in the age of social media. *Optometry Times, 7*(2), 16–18.

Centers for Medicare and Medicaid Services (CMS). (2010). Meaningful use. Retrieved from https://www.cms.gov/EHRIncentivePrograms/30_Meaningful_Use.asp

Centers for Medicare and Medicaid Services (CMS). (2014). Introduction to administrative simplification. Retrieved from https://www.cms.gov/eHealth/downloads/eHealthU_IntroAdminSimp.pdf

Egger, E. (2000). HIPAA offers hospitals the good, the bad, and the ugly. *Health Care Strategic Management, 18*(4), 1, 21–23.

Food and Drug Administration (FDA). (2015). *Mobile medical applications. Guidance for industry and food and drug administration staff.* Retrieved from http://www.fda.gov/downloads/MedicalDevices/DeviceRegulationandGuidance/GuidanceDocuments/UCM263366.pdf

Gagnon, K., & Sabus, C. (2015). Professionalism in a Digital Age: Opportunities and considerations for using social media in health care. *Physical Therapy, 95*(3), 406–414. doi:10.2522/ptj.20130227

Guidance on compliance with HIPAA transactions and code sets. (2003). Retrieved from https://www.ihs.gov/hipaa/documents/guidance-final.pdf

Health Level Seven (HL7). (n.d.). What is HL7? Retrieved from http://www.hl7.org

Hellerstein, D. (1999). HIPAA's impact on healthcare. *Health Management Technology, 20*(3), 10.

Hellerstein, D. (2000). HIPAA and health information privacy rules: Almost there. Health Management Technology, 21(4), 26.

HIT Consultant. (2013). 3 Do's and don'ts of effective HIPAA compliance for BYOD & mHealth. Retrieved from http://hitconsultant.net/2013/06/11/3-dos-and-donts-of-effective-hipaa-compliance-for-byod-mhealth

Institute of Medicine. (2000). *To err is human: Building a safer health system*. Washington, DC: National Academies Press.

International Standards Organization (ISO). (2008a). About ISO. Retrieved from http://www.iso.org/iso/about.htm

International Standards Organization (ISO). (2008b). Health informatics. Retrieved from http://www.iso.org/iso/iso_catalogue/catalogue_tc/catalogue_detail.htm?csnumber=35376

Keehan, S., Sisko, A.Q., & Truffler, C. (2008). Health spending projections through 2017: The baby-boom generation is coming to Medicare. *Health Affairs, 27*(2), 145–155.

Legal Information Institute (LII). (2013). 45 CFR 160.103—Definitions. Retrieved from https://www.law.cornell.edu/cfr/text/45/160.103

Leyva, C., & Leyva, D. (2011). HITECH Act. Retrieved from http://www.hipaasurvivalguide.com/hitech-act-text.php

Office of the National Coordinator for Health Information Technology. (2015, June). Non-federal acute care hospital electronic health record adoption, Health IT Quick-Stat #47. Retrieved from http://dashboard.healthit.gov/quickstats/pages/FIG-Hospital-EHR-Adoption.php

Privacy Commissioner. (2007). Health information privacy code. Retrieved from http://www.privacy.org.nz/health-information-privacy-code

Readthestimulus.org. (2009). Committee print, January 16, 2009. Retrieved from http://govinfo.sla.org/2009/02/08/readthestimulusorg

Savage, M. (2006). Security news: Perfect HIPAA security impossible, experts say. *TechTarget*. Retrieved from http://searchsecurity.techtarget.com/originalContent/0,289142,sid14_gci1268986,00.html

Spencer, J., & Bushman, M. (2006). HIPAAdvisory: The next HIPAA frontier: Claims attachments. Retrieved from http://www.worldprivacyforum.org/wp-content/uploads/2006/02/WPF_HHS_NPRM_HIPAAclaims_fs.pdf

U.S. Department of Commerce. (2011). National Institute of Standards and Technology (NIST). Retrieved from http://www.nist.gov/index.html

U.S. Department of Health and Human Services (HHS). (2002). Federal Register, Part V, Department of Health and Human Services: Standards for privacy of individually identifiable health information; Final rule. Retrieved from https://aspe.hhs.gov/report/standards-privacy-individually-identifiable-health-information-final-privacy-rule-preamble

U.S. Department of Health and Human Services (HHS). (2009). Federal Register: 45 CFR Parts 160 and 164: Breach Notification for Unsecured Protected Health Information; Interim.

U.S. Department of Health and Human Services (HHS). (2015). The privacy act. Retrieved from http://www.hhs.gov/foia/privacy

U.S. Department of Health and Human Services (HHS). (2016). Administration takes first step to implement legislation modernizing how Medicare pays physicians for quality. Retrieved from http://www.hhs.gov/about/news/2016/04/27/administration-takes-first-step-implement-legislation-modernizing-how-medicare-pays-physicians.html

U.S. Department of Health and Human Services (HHS), Office of Civil Rights (OCR). (n.d.). Health information privacy: All case examples. Retrieved from http://www.hhs.gov/ocr/privacy/hipaa/enforcement/examples/allcases.html#case1

Webopedia. (2008). The 7 layers of the OSI model. Retrieved from http://www.webopedia.com/quick_ref/OSI_Layers.asp

# Nursing Informatics Administrative Applications: Precare and Care Support

Nursing informatics (NI) and information technology (IT) have invaded nursing, and some nurses are happy with the capabilities afforded by this specialty. Others, however, remain convinced that the changes wrought by IT are nothing more than a nuisance. In the past, nursing administrators have found the implementation of technology tools to be an expensive venture with minimal rewards. This disappointment is likely related to their lack of knowledge about NI, which caused nursing administrators to listen to vendors or other colleagues; in essence, it was decision making based on limited and biased information. There were at least two reasons for the experience of limited rewards. First, nurses were rarely included in the testing and implementation of products designed for nurses and nursing tasks. Second, the new products they purchased had to interface with old, legacy systems that were not at all compatible or seemed compatible until the glitches arose. These glitches caused frustration for clinicians and administrators alike. They purchased tools that should have made the nurses happy, but instead all they did was grumble.

The good news is that approaches have changed as a result of the difficult lessons learned from the early forays into technology tools. Nursing personnel are involved both at the agency level and at the vendor level, in the decision-making process and development of new systems and products charged with enhancing the practice of nursing. Older legacy systems are being replaced with newer systems that have more capacity to interface with other systems. Nurses and administrators have become more astute in the realm of NI, but there is still a long way to go. The *Systems Development Life Cycle: Nursing Informatics and Organizational Decision Making* chapter introduces the system development life cycle, which is used to make important and appropriate organizational decisions for technology adoption.

Administrators need information systems that facilitate their administrative role, and they particularly need systems that provide financial, risk management, quality assurance, human resources, payroll, patient registration, acuity, communication, and scheduling functions. The administrator must be open to learning about all of the tools available. One of the most important tasks that an administrator can oversee and engage in is data mining, or the extraction of data and information from big data, sizeable datasets that have been collected and warehoused. Data mining helps to identify patterns in aggregate data, gain insights, and ultimately discover and generate knowledge applicable to nursing science. To take advantage of these benefits, nursing administrators must become astute informaticists—knowledge workers who harness the information and knowledge at their fingertips to facilitate the practice of their clinicians, improve patient care, and advance the science of nursing.

Clinical information systems (CIS) have traditionally been designed for use by one unit or department within an institution. However, because clinicians working in other areas of the organization need access to this information, these data and information are generally used by more than one area. The new initiatives arising with the integration of the electronic health record place institutions in the position of striving to manage their CIS through the electronic health record. Currently, there are many CISs, including nursing, laboratory, pharmacy, monitoring, and order entry, plus additional ancillary systems to meet the individual institutions' needs. The *Administrative Information Systems* chapter provides an overview of administrative information systems and helps the reader to understand the powerful data aggregation and data mining tools afforded by these systems.

*The Human–Technology Interface* chapter discusses the need to improve quality and safety outcomes significantly in the United States. Through the use of IT, the designs for human–technology interfaces can be radically improved so that the technology better fits both human and task requirements. A number of useful tools are currently available for the analysis, design, and evaluation phases of development life cycles and should be used routinely by informatics professionals to ensure that technology better fits both task and user requirements. In this chapter, the authors stress that the focus on interface improvement using these tools has dramatically improved patient safety in a specific area of health care: anesthesiology. With increased attention from informatics professionals and engineers, the same kinds of improvements are being made in other areas. This human–technology interface is a crucial area if the theories, architectures, and tools provided by the building block sciences are to be implemented.

Each organization must determine who can access and use its information systems and provide robust tools for securing information in a networked environment. The *Electronic Security* chapter addresses the important safeguards for protecting information. As new technologies designed to improve interprofessional collaboration and enhance patient care are adopted, barriers to implementation and resistance by practitioners to change are frequently encountered. The *Workflow and Beyond Meaningful Use* chapter provides insights into clinical workflow analysis and provides advice on improving efficiency and effectiveness while reviewing what we have learned as we tried to achieve meaningful use of caring technologies.

Pause to reflect on the Foundation of Knowledge model (Figure III-1) and its relationship to both personal and organizational knowledge management. Consider that organizational decision making must be driven by appropriate information and knowledge developed in the organization and applied with wisdom. Equally important to adopting technology within an organization is the consideration of the knowledge base and knowledge capabilities of the individuals within that organization. Administrators must use the system development life cycle wisely and carefully consider organizational workflow as they adopt NI technology for meaningful use.

The reader of this section is challenged to ask the following questions: (1) How can I apply the knowledge gained from my practice setting to benefit my patients and enhance my practice?; (2) How can I help my colleagues and patients understand and use the current technology that is available?; and (3) How can I use my wisdom to create the theories, tools, and knowledge of the future?

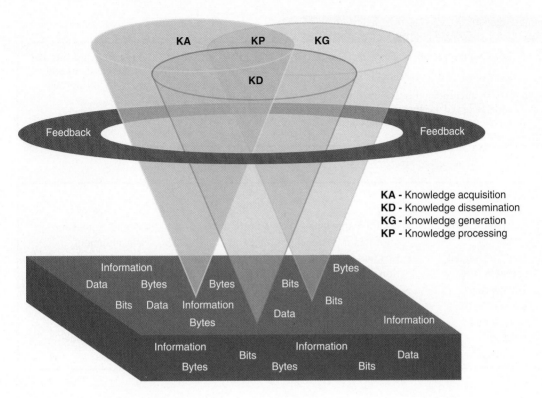

**Figure III-1** Foundation of Knowledge Model
Designed by Alicia Mastrian

## Objectives

1. Describe the systems development life cycle (SDLC).

2. Explore selected approaches to SDLC.

3. Assess interoperability and its importance in addressing and meeting the challenges of implementing the HITECH Act in health care.

4. Reflect on the past to move forward into the future to determine how new systems will be developed, integrated, and made interoperable in health care.

## Key Terms

- » Chief information officer
- » Computer-aided software engineering
- » Dynamic system development method
- » End users
- » Health management information system
- » Hospital information system
- » Information technology
- » Integration
- » Interoperability
- » Iteration
- » Milestones
- » MoSCoW
- » Object-oriented systems development
- » Open source software
- » Prototype
- » Rapid application development
- » Rapid prototyping
- » Repository
- » Systems development life cycle
- » TELOS strategy
- » Waterfall model

# CHAPTER 9

# Systems Development Life Cycle: Nursing Informatics and Organizational Decision Making

Dee McGonigle and Kathleen Mastrian

## Introduction

The following case scenario demonstrates the need to have all of the stakeholders involved from the beginning to the end of the **systems development life cycle** (SDLC). Creating the right team to manage the development is key. Various methodologies have been developed to guide this process. This chapter reviews the following approaches to SDLC: waterfall, rapid prototyping or rapid application development (RAD), object-oriented system development (OOSD), and dynamic system development method (DSDM). When reading about each approach, think about the case scenario and how important it is to understand the specific situational needs and the various methodologies for bringing a system to life. As in this case, it is generally necessary or beneficial to use a hybrid approach that blends two or more models for a robust development process.

As the case demonstrates, the process of developing systems or SDLC is an ongoing development with a life cycle. The first step in developing a system is to understand the problems or business needs. It is followed by understanding the solution or how to address those needs; developing a plan; implementing the plan; evaluating the implementation; and, finally, maintenance, review, and destruction. If the system needs major upgrading outside of the scope of the maintenance phase, if it needs to be replaced because of technological advances, or if the business needs change, a new project is launched, the old system is destroyed, and the life cycle begins anew.

SDLC is a way to deliver efficient and effective information systems (ISs) that fit with the strategic business plan of an organization. The business plan stems from the mission of the organization. In the world of health care, its development includes a needs assessment for the entire organization, which should include outreach linkages (as seen in the case scenario) and partnerships and merged or shared functions. The organization's participating physicians and other ancillary professionals and their offices are included in thorough needs assessments. When developing a strategic plan, the design must take into account the existence of the organization within the larger healthcare delivery system and assess the various factors outside of the organization itself, including technological, legislative, and environmental issues that impact the organization. The plan must identify the needs of the organization as a whole and propose solutions to meet those needs or a way to address the issues.

SDLC can occur within an organization, be outsourced, or be a blend of the two approaches. With outsourcing, the team hires an outside organization to carry out all or some of the development. Developing systems that truly meet business needs is not an easy task and is quite complex. Therefore, it is common to run over budget and miss milestones. When reading this chapter, reflect on the case scenario and in general the challenges teams face when developing systems.

## CASE SCENARIO

Envision two large healthcare facilities that merge resources to better serve their community. This merger is called the Wellness Alliance, and its mission is to establish and manage community health programming that addresses the health needs of the rural, underserved populations in the area. The Wellness Alliance would like to establish pilot clinical sites in five rural areas to promote access and provide health care to these underserved consumers. Each clinical site will have a full-time program manager and three part-time employees (a secretary, a nurse, and a doctor). Each program manager will report to the wellness program coordinator, a newly created position within the Wellness Alliance.

Because you are a community health nurse with extensive experience, you have been appointed as the wellness program coordinator. Your directive is to establish these clinical sites within 3 months and report back in 6 months as to the following: (1) community health programs offered, (2) level of community involvement in outreach health programs and clinical site–based programming, (3) consumer visits made to the clinical site, and (4) personnel performance.

You are excited and challenged, but soon reality sets in: You know that you have five different sites with five different program managers. You need some way to gather the vital information from each of them in a similar manner so that the data are meaningful and useful to you as you develop your reports and evaluate the strengths and weaknesses of the pilot project. You know that you need a system that will handle all of the pilot project's information needs.

Your first stop is the chief information officer of the health system, a nurse informaticist. You

know her from the **health management information system** mini-seminar that she led. After explaining your needs, you share with her the constraint that this system must be in place in 3 months when the sites are up and running before you make your report. When she begins to ask questions, you realize that you do not know the answers. All you know is that you must be able to report on which community health programs were offered, track the level of community involvement in outreach health programs and clinical site–based programming, monitor consumer visits made to the clinical site, and monitor the performance of site personnel. You know that you want accessible, real-time tracking, but as far as programming and clinical site–related activities are concerned, you do not have a precise description of either the process or procedures that will be involved in implementing the pilot, or the means by which they will gather and enter data.

The chief information officer requires that you and each program manager remain involved in the development process. She assigns an **information technology** (IT) analyst to work with you and your team in the development of a system that will meet your current needs. After the first meeting, your head is spinning: The IT analyst has challenged your team not only to work out the process for your immediate needs, but also to envision what your needs will be in the future. At the next meeting, you tell the analyst that your team does not feel comfortable trying to map everything out at this point. He states that there are several ways to go about building the system and software by using the SDLC. Noticing the blank look on everyone's faces, he explains that the SDLC is a series of actions used to develop an

IS. The SDLC is similar to the nursing process, in which the nurse must assess, diagnose, plan, implement, evaluate, and revise. If the plan developed in this way does not meet the patient's need or if a new problem arises, the nurse either revises and updates the plan or starts anew. Likewise, you will plan, analyze, design, implement, operate, support, and secure the proposed community health system.

The SDLC is an iterative process—a conceptual model that is used in project management describing the phases involved in building or developing an IS. It moves from assessing feasibility or project initiation, to design analysis, to system specification, to programming, to testing, to implementation, to maintenance, and to destruction—literally from beginning to end. As the IT analyst describes this process, once again he sees puzzled looks. He quickly states that even the destruction of the system is planned—that is, how it will be retired, broken down, and replaced with a new system. Even during upgrades, destruction tactics can be invoked to secure the data and even decide if servers are to be disposed of or repurposed. The security people will tell you that this is their phase, where they make sure that any sensitive information is properly handled and decide whether the data are to be securely and safely archived or destroyed.

After reviewing all of the possible methods and helping you to conduct your feasibility and business study, the analyst chooses the DSDM. This SDLC model was chosen because it works well when the time span is short and the requirements are fluctuating and mainly unknown at the outset. The IT analyst explains that this model works well on tight schedules and is a highly iterative and incremental approach that stresses continuous user input and involvement. As part of this highly iterative process, the team will revisit and loop through the same development activities numerous times; this repetitive examination provides ever-increasing levels of detail, thereby improving accuracy. The analyst explains that you will use a mockup of the **hospital information system** (HIS) and design for what is known; you will then create your own mini-system that will interface with the HIS. Because time is short, the analysis, design, and development phases will occur simultaneously while you are formulating and revising your specific requirements through the iterative process so that they can be integrated into the system.

The functional model **iteration** phase will be completed in 2 weeks based on the information that you have given to the analyst. At that time, the prototype will be reviewed by the team. The IT analyst tells you to expect at least two or more iterations of the prototype based on your input. You should end with software that provides some key capabilities. Design and testing will occur in the design and build iteration phase and continue until the system is ready for implementation, the final phase. This DSDM should work well because any previous phase can be revisited and reworked through its iterative process.

One month into the SDLC process, the IT analyst tells the team that he will be leaving his position at Wellness Alliance. He introduces his replacement. She is new to Wellness Alliance and is eager to work with the team. The initial IT analyst will be there 1 more week to help the new analyst with the transition. When he explains that you are working through DSDM, she looks a bit panicky and states that she has never used this approach. She has used the waterfall, prototyping, iterative enhancement, spiral, and object-oriented methodologies—but never the DSDM. From what she heard, DSDM is new and often runs amok because of the lack of understanding as to how to implement it appropriately. After 1 week on the project, the new IT analyst believes that this approach was not the best choice. As the leader of this SDLC, she is growing concerned about having a product ready at the point when the clinical sites open. She might combine another method to create a hybrid approach with which she would be more comfortable; she is thinking out loud and has everyone very nervous.

The IT analyst reviews the equipment that has arrived for the sites and is excited to learn that the computers were ordered from Apple. They will be powerful and versatile enough for your needs.

Two months after the opening of the clinical sites, you, as the wellness program coordinator are still tweaking the system with the help of the IT analyst. It is hard to believe how quickly the team was able to get a robust system in place. As you think back on the process, it seems so long ago that you reviewed the HIS for deficiencies and screen shots. You reexamined your requirements and watched them come to life through five prototype iterations and constant security updates. You trained your personnel on its use, tested its performance, and made final adjustments before implementation. Your own stand-alone system that met your needs was installed and fully operational on the Friday before you opened the clinic doors on Monday, 1 day ahead of schedule. You are continuing to evaluate and modify the system, but that is how the SDLC works: It is never finished, but rather constantly evolving.

# Waterfall Model

The **waterfall model** is one of the oldest methods and literally depicts a waterfall effect—that is, the output from each previous phase flows into or becomes the initial input for the next phase. This model is a sequential development process in that there is one pass through each component activity from conception or feasibility through implementation in a linear order. The deliverables for each phase result from the inputs and any additional information that is gathered. There is minimal or no iterative development where one takes advantage of what was learned during the development of earlier deliverables. Many projects are broken down into six phases (**Figure 9-1**), especially small- to medium-size projects.

## Feasibility

As the term implies, the feasibility study is used to determine whether the project should be initiated and supported. This study should generate a project plan and estimated budget for the SDLC phases. Often, the **TELOS strategy**—technological and systems, economic, legal, operational, and schedule feasibility—is followed. Technological and systems feasibility addresses the issues of technological capabilities, including the expertise and infrastructure to complete the project. Economic feasibility is the cost–benefit analysis, weighing the benefits versus the costs to determine whether the project is fiscally possible and worth undertaking. Formal assessments should include return on investment. Legal feasibility assesses the legal ramifications

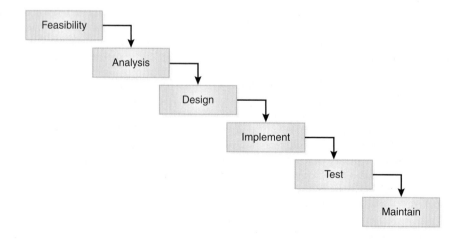

**Figure 9-1** Waterfall Phases

of the project, including current contractual obligations, legislation, regulatory bodies, and liabilities that could affect the project. Operational feasibility determines how effective the project will be in meeting the needs and expectations of the organization and actually achieving the goals of the project or addressing and solving the business problem. Schedule feasibility assesses the viability of the time frame, making sure it is a reasonable estimation of the time and resources necessary for the project to be developed in time to attain the benefits and meet constraints. TELOS helps to provide a clear picture of the feasibility of the project.

## Analysis

During the analysis phase, the requirements for the system are teased out from a detailed study of the business needs of the organization. As part of this analysis, work flows and business practices are examined. It may be necessary to consider options for changing the business process.

## Design

The design phase focuses on high- and low-level design and interface and data design. At the high-level phase, the team establishes which programs are needed and ascertains how they will interact. At the low-level phase, team members explore how the individual programs will actually work. The interface design determines what the look and feel will be or what the interfaces will look like. During data design, the team critically thinks about and verifies which data are required or essential.

The analysis and design phases are vital in the development cycle, and great care is taken during these phases to ensure that the software's overall configuration is defined properly. Mockups or prototypes of screenshots, reports, and processes may be generated to clarify the requirements and get the team or stakeholders on the same page, limiting the occurrence of glitches that might result in costly software development revisions later in the project.

## Implement

During this phase, the designs are brought to life through programming code. The right programming language, such as C++, Pascal, Java, and so forth, is chosen based on the application requirements.

## Test

The testing is generally broken down into five layers: (1) the individual programming modules, (2) **integration**, (3) volume, (4) the system as a whole, and (5) beta testing. Typically, the programs are developed in a modular fashion, and these individual modules are then subjected to detailed testing. The separate modules are subsequently synthesized, and the interfaces between the modules are tested. The system is evaluated with respect to its platform and the expected amount or volume of data. It is then tested as a complete system by the team. Finally, to determine if the system performs appropriately for the user, it is beta tested. During beta testing, users put the new system through its paces to make sure that it does what they need it to do to perform their jobs.

## Maintain

Once the system has been finalized from the testing phase, it must be maintained. This could include user support through actual software changes necessitated through use or time.

According to Isaias and Issa (2015), "one common trait covers all the variations of this model: It is a sequential model. Each of its stages must be entirely concluded before the next can begin" (p. 23). The main lack of iterative development is seen as a major weakness, according to Purcell (2007). No projects are static, and typically changes occur during the SDLC. As requirements change, there is no way to address them formally using the waterfall method after project requirements are developed. The waterfall model should be used for simple projects when the requirements are well known and stable from the outset.

# Rapid Prototyping or Rapid Application Development

As technology advances and faster development is expected, **rapid prototyping**, also known as **rapid application development** (RAD), provides a fast way to add functionality through prototyping and user testing. It is easier for users to examine an actual **prototype** rather than documentation. A rapid requirements-gathering phase relies on workshops and focus groups to build a prototype application using real data. This prototype is then beta tested with users, and their feedback is used to perfect or add functionality and capabilities to the system (**Figure 9-2**).

According to Alexandrou (2016), "RAD (rapid application development) proposes that products can be developed faster and of higher quality" (para. 1). The RAD approach uses informal communication, repurposes components, and typically follows a fast-paced schedule. Object-oriented programming using such languages as C++ and Java promotes software repurposing and reuse.

The major advantage is the speed with which the system can be deployed; a working, usable system can be built within 3 months. The use of prototyping allows the developers to skip steps in the SDLC process in favor of getting a mockup in front of the user. At times, the system may be deemed acceptable if it meets a predefined minimum set of requirements rather than all of the identified requirements.

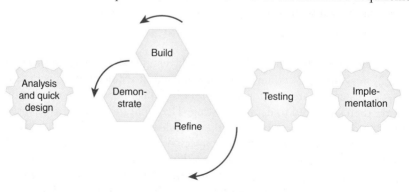

**Figure 9-2** Rapid Application Development (RAD) or Rapid Prototyping

This rapid deployment also limits the project's exposure to change elements. Unfortunately, the fast pace can be its biggest disadvantage in some cases. Once one is locked into a tight development schedule, the process may be too fast for adequate testing to be put in place and completed. The most dangerous lack of testing is in the realm of security.

The RAD approach is chosen because it builds systems quickly through user-driven prototyping and adherence to quick, strict delivery **milestones**. This approach continues to be refined and honed, and other contemporary manifestations of RAD continue to emerge in the agile software development realm.

# Object-Oriented Systems Development

The **object-oriented systems development** model blends SDLC logic with object-oriented modeling and programming power (Stair & Reynolds, 2016). Object-oriented modeling makes an effort to represent real-world objects by modeling the real-world entities or things (e.g., clinic, patient, account, nursing or healthcare professional) into abstract computer software objects. Once the system is object oriented, all of the interactions or exchanges take place between or among the objects. The objects are derived from classes, and each object is comprised of data and the actions that can be enacted on that data. Class hierarchy allows objects to inherit characteristics or attributes from parent classes, which fosters object reuse, resulting in less coding. The object-oriented programming languages, such as C++ and Java, promote software repurposing and reuse. Therefore, the class hierarchy must be clearly and appropriately designed to reap the benefits of this SDLC approach, which uses object-oriented programming to support the interactions of objects.

For example, in the case scenario, a system could be developed for the Wellness Alliance to manage the community health programming for the clinic system being set up for outreach. There could be a class of programs, and *well-baby care* could be an object in the class of programs; *programs* is a relationship between Wellness Alliance and well-baby care. The program class has attributes, such as *clinic site*, *location address*, or *attendees* or *patients*. The relationship itself may be considered an object having attributes, such as *pediatric programs*. The class hierarchy from which all of the system objects are created with resultant object interactions must be clearly defined.

The OOSD model is a highly iterative approach. The process begins by investigating where object-oriented solutions can address business problems or needs, determining user requirements, designing the system, programming or modifying object modeling (class hierarchy and objects), implementing, user testing, modifying, and reimplementing the system, and ends with the new system being reviewed regularly at established intervals and modifications being made as needed throughout its life.

# Dynamic System Development Method

The **dynamic system development method** is a highly iterative and incremental approach with a high level of user input and involvement. The iterative process requires repetitive examination that enhances detail and improves accuracy. The DSDM has three phases: (1) preproject, (2) project life cycle (feasibility and business studies, functional model iteration, design and build iteration, and implementation), and (3) postproject.

In the preproject phase, buy-in or commitment is established and funding is secured. This helps to identify the stakeholders (administration and **end users**) and gain support for the project. In the second phase, the project's life cycle begins. This phase includes five steps: (1) feasibility, (2) business studies, (3) functional model iteration, (4) design and build iteration, and (5) implementation (**Figure 9-3**).

In steps 1 and 2, the feasibility and business studies are completed. The team ascertains if this project meets the required business needs while identifying the potential risks during the feasibility study. In step 1, the deliverables are a feasibility report, project plan, and a risk log. Once the project is deemed feasible, step 2, the business study, is begun. The business study extends the feasibility report by examining the processes, stakeholders, and their needs. It is important to align the stakeholders with the project and secure their buy-in because it is necessary to have user input and involvement throughout the entire DSDM process. Therefore, bringing them in at the beginning of the project is imperative.

Using the **MoSCoW** approach, the team works with the stakeholders to develop a prioritized requirements list and a development plan. MoSCoW stands for "Must have, Should have, Could have, and Would have." The "must have" requirements are needed to meet the business needs and are critical to the success of the project. "Should have" requirements are those that would be great to have if possible, but the success of the project does not depend on them being addressed. The "could

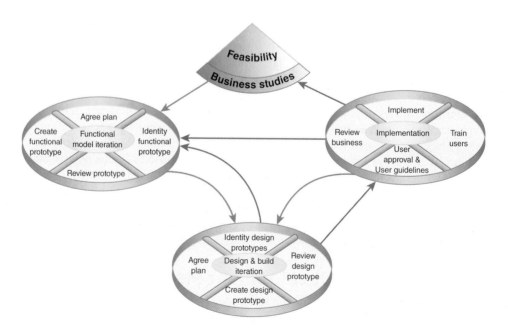

**Figure 9-3** Dynamic System Development Method (DSDM)
Copyright 2014 Agile Business Consortium Limited. Reproduced by kind permission.

have" requirements are those that would be nice to have met, and the "would have" requirements can be put off until later; these may be undertaken during future developmental iterations. Timeboxing is generally used to develop the project plan. In timeboxing, the project is divided into sections, each having its own fixed budget and dates or milestones for deliverables. The MoSCoW approach is then used to prioritize the requirements within each section; the requirements are the only variables because the schedule and budget are set. If a project is running out of time or money, the team can easily omit the requirements that have been identified as the lowest priority to meet their schedule and budget obligations. This does not mean that the final deliverable, the actual system, would be flawed or incomplete. Instead, because the team has already determined the "must have" or "should have" items, it still meets the business needs. According to Haughey (2010), the 80/20 rule, or Pareto principle, can be applied to nearly everything. The Pareto principle states that 80% of the project comes from 20% of the system requirements; therefore, the 20% of requirements must be the crucial requirements or those with the highest priority. One also must consider the pancake principle: The first pancake is not as good as the rest, and one should know that the first development will not be perfect. This is why it is extremely important to clearly identify the "must have" and "should have" requirements.

In the third step of the project life cycle phase, known as functional model iteration, the deliverables are a functional model and prototype ready for user testing. Once the requirements are identified, the next step is to translate them into a functional model with a functioning prototype that can be evaluated by users. This could take several iterations to develop the desired functionality and incorporate the users' input. At this stage, the team should examine the quality of the product and revise the list requirements and risk log. The requirements are adjusted, the ones that have been realized are deleted, and the remaining requirements are prioritized. The risk log is revised based on the risk analysis completed during and after prototype development.

The design and build iteration step focuses on integrating functional components and identifying the nonfunctional requirements that need to be in the tested system. Testing is crucial; the team will develop a system that the end users can safely use on a daily basis. The team will garner user feedback and generate user documentation. These efforts provide this step's deliverable, a tested system with documentation for the next and final phase of the development process.

In the final step of the project life cycle phase, known as implementation, deliverables are the system (ready to use), documentation, and trained users. The requirements list should be satisfied, along with the users' needs. Training users and implementing the approved system is the first part of this phase, and the final part consists of a full review. It is important to review the impact of the system on the business processes and to determine if it addressed the goals or requirements established at the beginning of the project. This final review determines if the project is completed or if further development is necessary. If further development is needed, preceding phases are revisited. If the project is complete and satisfies the users, then it moves into maintenance and ongoing development.

The final phase is labeled "postproject." In this phase, the team verifies that the system is functioning properly. Once verified, the maintenance schedule is begun. Because the DSDM is iterative, this postproject phase is seen as ongoing development and any of the deliverables can be refined. This is what makes the DSDM such an iterative development process.

DSDM is one of an increasing number of agile methodologies being introduced, such as Scrum and Extreme Programming. These new approaches address the organizational, managerial, and interpersonal communication issues that often bog down SDLC projects. Empowerment of teams and user involvement enhance the iterative and programming strengths provided in these SDLC models.

## Computer-Aided Software Engineering Tools

When reviewing SDLC, the **computer-aided software engineering** (CASE) tools that will be used must be described.

CASE tools promote adherence to the SDLC process since they automate several required tasks; this provides standardization and thoroughness to the total systems development method (Stair & Reynolds, 2016). These tools help to reduce cost and development time while enriching the quality of the product. CASE tools contain a **repository** with information about the system: models, data definitions, and references linking models together. They are valuable in their ability to make sure the models follow diagramming rules and are consistent and complete.

The various types of tools can be referred to as upper-CASE tools or lower-CASE tools. The upper-CASE tools support the analysis and design phases, whereas the lower-CASE tools support implementation. The tools can also be general or specific in nature, with the specific tools being designed for a particular methodology.

Two examples of CASE tools are Visible Analyst and Rational Rose. According to Andoh-Baidoo, Kunene, and Walker (2009), Visible Analyst "supports structured and object-oriented design (UML)," whereas Rational Rose "supports solely object-oriented design (UML)" (p. 372). Both tools can "build and reverse database schemas for SQL and Oracle" and "support code generation for pre-.NET versions of Visual Basic" (p. 372). Visible Analyst can also support shell code generation for pre-.NET versions of C and COBOL, whereas Rational Rose can support complete code for C++ and Java. In addition, Andoh-Baidoo et al. found that Rational Rose "[p]rovides good integration with Java, and incorporates common packages into class diagrams and decompositions through classes" (p. 372).

CASE tools have many advantages, including decreasing development time and producing more flexible systems. On the down side, they can be difficult to tailor or customize and use with existing systems.

## Open Source Software and Free/Open Source Software

Another area that must be discussed with SDLC is **open source software** (OSS). An examination of job descriptions or advertisements for candidates shows that many ISs and IT professionals need a thorough understanding of SDLC and OSS development tools (e.g., PHP, MySQL, and HTML). With OSS, any programmer can implement, modify, apply, reconstruct, and restructure the rich libraries of source codes available from proven, well-tested products.

As Karopka, Schmuhl, and Demski (2014) noted,

*Free/Libre Open Source Software (FLOSS) has been successfully adopted across a wide range of different areas and has opened new ways of value creation. Today there are hundreds of examples of successful FLOSS projects and products. . . . Especially in times of financial crisis and austerity the adoption of FLOSS principles opens interesting alternatives and options to tremendously lower total cost of ownership (TCO) and open the way for a continuous user-driven improvement process. (para. 6)*

To transform health care, it is necessary for clinicians to use information systems that can share patient data (Goulde & Brown, 2006; NORC, 2014). This all sounds terrific and many people wonder why it has not happened yet, but the challenges are many. How does one establish the networks necessary to share data between and among all healthcare facilities easily and securely? "Healthcare IT is beginning to adopt open source software to address these challenges" (Goulde & Brown, p. 4). Early attempts at OSS ventures in the healthcare realm failed because of a lack of support or buy-in for sustained effort, technologic lags, authority and credibility, and other such issues. "Spurred by a greater sense of urgency to adopt IT, health industry leaders are showing renewed interest in open source solutions" (Goulde & Brown, p. 5).

Karopka et al., (2014) concluded that

*North America has the longest tradition in applying FLOSS-HC delivery. It is home of many mature, stable and widely disseminated FLOSS applications. Some of them are even used on a global scale. The deployment of FLOSS systems in healthcare delivery is comparatively low in Europe. (para. 48)*

Health care is realizing the benefits of FLOSS. According to Goulde and Brown (2006), "other benefits of open source software—low cost, flexibility, opportunities to innovate—are important but independence from vendors is the most relevant for health care" (p. 10).

## Interoperability

**Interoperability**, the ability to share information across organizations, will remain paramount under the HITECH Act. The ability to share patient data is extremely important, both within an organization and across organizational boundaries (Figure 9-4).

According to the Health Information and Management Systems Society (HIMSS; Murphy, 2015), "an acceptable 2015 [interoperability standards] Advisory and more complete 2016 Advisory will not be achievable without the inclusion of health IT security standards" (para. 4). Few healthcare systems take advantage of the full potential of the current state of the art in computer science and health informatics (HIMSS, 2010). The consequences of this situation include a drain on financial resources from the economy, the inability to truly mitigate the occurrence of medical errors, and a lack of national preparedness to respond to natural and manmade epidemics and disasters. HIMSS has created the Integration and Interoperability Steering Committee

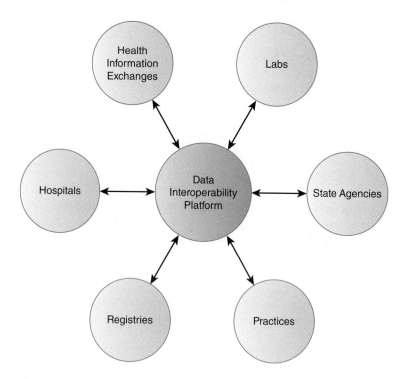

**Figure 9-4** Interoperability

to guide the industry on allocating resources to develop and implement standards and technology needed to achieve interoperability (para. 2).

As we enter into SDLCs, we must be aware of how this type of development will affect both our own healthcare organization and the healthcare delivery system as a whole. In an ideal world, we would all work together to create systems that are integrated within our own organization while having the interoperability to cross organizational boundaries and unite the healthcare delivery system to realize the common goal of improving the quality of care provided to consumers.

## Summary

At times during the SDLC, new information affects the outputs from earlier phases; the development effort may be reexamined or halted until these modifications can be reconciled with the current design and scope of the project. At other times, teams are overwhelmed with new ideas from the iterative SDLC process that result in new capabilities or features that exceed the initial scope of the project. Astute team leaders will preserve these ideas or initiatives so they can be considered at a later time. The team should develop a list of recommendations to improve the current software when the project is complete. This iterative and dynamic exchange makes the SDLC robust.

As technology and research continue to advance, new SDLC models are being pioneered and revised to enhance development techniques. The interpretation and implementation of any model selected reflect the knowledge and skill of the team applying the model. The success of the project is often directly related to the quality of the organizational decision making throughout the project—that is, how well the plan was followed and documented. United efforts to create systems that are integrated and interoperable will define the future of health care.

### THOUGHT-PROVOKING QUESTIONS

1. Reflect on the SDLC in relation to the quality of the organizational decision making throughout the project. What are some of the major stumbling blocks faced by healthcare organizations?
2. Why is it important for all nurses and healthcare professionals to understand the basics of how information systems are selected and implemented?

# References

Alexandrou, M. (2016). Rapid application development (RAD) methodology. *Infolific*. Retrieved from http://www.infolific.com/technology/methodologies/rapid-application-development

Andoh-Baidoo, F., Kunene, K., & Walker, R. (2009). An evaluation of CASE tools as pedagogical aids in software development courses. *2009 SWDSI Proceedings*. Retrieved from http://www.swdsi.org/swdsi2009/Papers/9K10.pdf

Goulde, M., & Brown, E. (2006). Open source software: A primer for health care leaders. *Protocode*. Retrieved from http://www.protecode.com/an-open-source-world-a-primer-on-licenses-obligations-and-your-company

Haughey, D. (2010). Pareto analysis step by step. *Project Smart*. Retrieved from http://www.projectsmart.co.uk/pareto-analysis-step-by-step.html

Health Information and Management Systems Society (HIMSS). (2010). Interoperability & standards. Retrieved from http://www.himss.org/library/interoperability-standards?navItemNumber=13323

Isaias, P. & Issa, T. (2015). *High level models and methodologies for information systems*. New York, NY: Springer.

Karopka, T., Schmuhl, H., & Demski, H. (2014). Free/Libre open source software in health care: A review. *Healthcare Informatics Research, 20*(1), 11–22. PMCID: PMC3950260

Murphy, K. (2007). HIMSS has ideas for 2015 interoperability standards advisory. *HealthIT Interoperability*. Retrieved from http://healthitinteroperability.com/news/himss-has-ideas-for-2015-interoperability-standards-advisory

NORC. (2014). Data sharing to enable clinical transformation at the community level: IT takes a village. Retrieved from http://www.healthit.gov/sites/default/files/beacondatasharingbrief062014.pdf

Purcell, J. (2007). Comparison of software development lifecycle methodologies. *SANS Institute*. Retrieved from https://software-security.sans.org/resources/paper/cissp/comparison-software-development-lifecycle-methodologies

Stair, R., & Reynolds, G. (2016). *Principles of information systems* (12th ed.). Boston, MA: Cengage Learning.

## Objectives

1. Explore agency-based health information systems.
2. Evaluate how administrators use core business systems in their practice.
3. Assess the function and information output from selected information systems used in healthcare organizations.

## Key Terms

- » Acuity systems
- » Admission, discharge, and transfer systems
- » American National Standards Institute (ANSI)
- » Attribute
- » Care plan
- » Case management information systems
- » Clinical documentation systems
- » Clinical information systems
- » Collaboration
- » Columns
- » Communication systems
- » Computerized physician (provider) order entry systems

- » Core business systems
- » Data dictionary
- » Data file
- » Data mart
- » Data mining
- » Data warehouse
- » Database
- » Database management system
- » Decision support
- » Drill-down
- » Electronic health record
- » Entity
- » Entity–relationship diagram
- » Fields
- » Financial systems
- » Information systems
- » Information technology

- » International Organization for Standardization (ISO)
- » Interoperability
- » Key field
- » Knowledge exchange
- » Laboratory information systems
- » Managed care information systems
- » Order entry systems
- » Patient care information system
- » Patient care support system
- » Patient centered
- » Pharmacy information systems
- » Picture and archiving

- » communication system
- » Primary key
- » Query
- » Radiology information system
- » Records
- » Relational database management system (RDMS)
- » Repository
- » Rows
- » Scheduling systems
- » Stakeholders
- » Standardized plan of care
- » Structured Query Language (SQL)
- » Table
- » Tiering
- » Triage
- » Tuples

# CHAPTER 10

# Administrative Information Systems

Marianela Zytkowski, Susan Paschke, Kathleen Mastrian, and Dee McGonigle

## Introduction

To compete in the ever-changing healthcare arena, organizations require quick and immediate access to a variety of types of information, data, and bodies of knowledge for daily clinical, operational, financial, and human resource activities. Information is continuously shared between units and departments within healthcare organizations and is also required or requested from other healthcare organizations, regulatory and government agencies, educational and philanthropic institutions, and consumers. Organizations need interoperable systems that are accessible for data storage and retrieval.

The healthcare context is distinct from other organizations that use information systems.

Fichman, Kohli, and Krishnan (2011) identify six important elements of health care that influence the development and implementation of information systems:

- The stakes are life and death.
- Healthcare information is highly personal.
- Health care is highly influenced by regulation and competition.
- Health care is professionally driven and hierarchical.
- Health care is multidisciplinary.
- Healthcare information system implementation is complex, with important implications for learning and adaptation (pp. 420–423).

Healthcare organizations integrate a variety of clinical and administrative types of **information systems** (ISs). These systems collect, process, and distribute patient-centered data to aid in managing and providing care. Together, they create a comprehensive record of the patient's medical history and support organizational processes. Each of these systems is unique in the way it functions and provides information to clinicians and administrators. An understanding of how each of these types of systems works within healthcare organizations is fundamental in the study of informatics. This chapter will focus on the administrative organizational systems.

# Types of Healthcare Organization Information Systems

## Case Management Information Systems

**Case management information systems** identify resources, patterns, and variances in care to prevent costly complications related to chronic conditions and to enhance the overall outcomes for patients with chronic illness. These systems span past episodes of treatment and search for trends among the records. Once a trend is identified, case management systems provide **decision support** promoting preventive care. Care plans are a common tool found in case management systems. A **care plan** is a set of care guidelines that outline the course of treatment and the recommended interventions that should be implemented to achieve optimal results. By using a **standardized plan of care**, these systems present clinicians with treatment protocols to maximize patient outcomes and support best practices. Information technology in health care is positioned to support the development of interdisciplinary care plans. In the health informatics pathway, Standard 5 deals with documentation: "Health informatics professionals will understand the content and diverse uses of health information. They will accurately document and communicate appropriate information using legal and regulatory processes" (National Consortium for Health Science Education, 2012, para. 11).

Case management information systems are especially beneficial for patient populations with a high cost of care and complex health needs, such as the elderly or patients with chronic disease conditions. Avoiding complications requires identifying the right resources for care and implementing preventive treatments across all medical visits. Ultimately, this preventive care decreases the costs of care for patients with chronic illnesses and supports a better quality of life. Such systems increase the value of individual care while controlling the costs and risks associated with long-term health care.

Case management systems are increasingly being integrated with electronic health records (EHRs). Information collected by these systems is processed in a way that helps to reduce risks, ensure quality, and decrease costs. A presentation of results of the 2012 Health Information Technology Survey, conducted by the Case Management Society of America (CMSA, 2014), revealed several key trends in information technology, including the increased use of social media and wireless communications, the use of IT to support care transitions and prevent readmissions, expanded use of patient engagement technologies (text messaging, email, portals, smartphone apps), and work toward the integration of case management software into the EHR.

# Communication Systems

**Communication systems** promote interaction among healthcare providers and between providers and patients. Such systems have historically been kept separate from other types of health information systems and from one another. Healthcare professionals overwhelmingly recognize the value of these systems, however, so they are now more commonly integrated into the design of other types of systems as a newly developing standard within the industry. Examples of communication systems include call light systems, wireless telephones, pagers, email, and instant messaging, which have traditionally been forms of communication targeted at clinicians. Other communication systems target patients and their families. Some patients are now able to access their electronic chart from home via an Internet connection. They can update their own medical record to inform their physician of changes to their health or personal practices that impact their physical condition. Inpatients in hospital settings also receive communication directly to their room. Patients and their families may, for example, review individualized messages with scheduled tests and procedures for the day and confirm menu choices for their meals. These types of systems may also communicate educational messages, such as smoking cessation advice.

As health care begins to introduce more of this technology into practice, the value of having communication tools integrated with other types of systems is being widely recognized. Integrating communication systems with clinical applications provides a real-time approach that facilitates interactions among the entire healthcare team, patients, and their families to enhance care. These systems enhance the flow of communication within an organization and promote an exchange of information to care better for patients. The next generation of communication systems will be integrated with other types of healthcare systems and guaranteed to work together smoothly. The Research Brief discusses the economic impact of communication inefficiencies in U.S. hospitals. As hospitals and physician practices strive to become more patient centered, communication technologies will be an integral part of this goal. Many of us have experienced the anxiety of waiting for news about a loved one during a surgical procedure. Newer communication techniques, such as surgical tracking boards that communicate about the process, help to ease these anxieties. Gordon and colleagues (2015) report high patient and family satisfaction with a HIPAA-compliant surgical instant messaging system to communicate real-time surgical progress with patient-designated recipients. They stated that

> [w]hile this study focused on the discipline of surgery, we can easily imagine the benefits of this type of communications application outside of the surgical model that we have studied. The results of any laboratory, pathology, or radiography studies can be instantaneously shared with concerned family members all over the globe. In the critical care setting, doctors can communicate with a patient's extended support group more efficiently and in a less stress-inducing environment than the typical crowded consultation room outside of the intensive care unit. News of the arrival of a newborn baby boy or girl can be sent to eager aunts, uncles, and grandparents back home. The opportunities for enhancing communication pertaining to medical issues are seemingly limitless. (p. 6)

What are some other ways that new communication technologies could be used to increase patient and family satisfaction with health care in your practice?

# Core Business Systems

**Core business systems** enhance administrative tasks within healthcare organizations. Unlike **clinical information systems** (CISs), whose aim is to provide direct patient care, these systems support the management of health care within an organization. Core business systems provide the framework for reimbursement, support of best practices, quality control, and resource allocation. There are four common core business systems: (1) admission, discharge, and transfer (ADT) systems; (2) financial systems; (3) acuity systems; and (4) scheduling systems.

**Admission, discharge, and transfer systems** provide the backbone structure for the other types of clinical and business systems (Hassett & Thede, 2003). These systems were among the first to be automated in health care. Admitting, billing, and bed management departments most commonly use ADT systems. These systems hold key information on which all other systems rely. For example, ADT systems maintain the patient's name; medical record number; visit or account number; and demographic information, such as age, gender, home address, and contact information. Such systems are considered the central source for collecting this type of patient information and communicating it to other types of healthcare information systems.

---

### RESEARCH BRIEF

Researchers attempted to quantify the costs of poor communication, termed "communication inefficiencies," in hospitals. This qualitative study was conducted in seven acute care hospitals of varying sizes via structured interviews with key informants at each facility. The interview questions focused on four broad categories: (1) communication bottlenecks, (2) negative outcomes as a result of those bottlenecks, (3) subjective perceptions of the potential effectiveness of communication improvements on the negative outcomes, and (4) ideas for specific communication improvements. The researchers independently coded the interview data and then compared results to extract themes.

All of the interviewees indicated that communication was an issue. Inefficiencies revolved around time spent tracking people down to communicate with them, with various estimates provided: 3 hours per nursing shift wasted tracking people down, 20% of productive time wasted on communication bottlenecks, and a reported average of five to six telephone calls to locate a physician. Several respondents pointed to costly medical errors that were the direct result of communication issues. Communication lapses also resulted in inefficient use of clinician resources and increased length of stay for patients.

The researchers developed a conceptual model of communication quality with four primary dimensions: (1) efficiency of resource use, (2) effectiveness of resource use, (3) quality of work life, and (4) service quality. They concluded that the total cost of communication inefficiencies in U.S. hospitals is more than $12 billion annually and estimated that a 500-bed hospital could lose as much as $4 million annually because of such problems. They urge the adoption of information technologies to redesign workflow processes and promote better communication.

The full article appears in Agarwal, R., Sands, D., Schneider, J., & Smaltz, D. (2010). Quantifying the economic impact of communication inefficiencies in U.S. hospitals. *Journal of Healthcare Management*, 55(4), 265–281.

**Financial systems** manage the expenses and revenue for providing health care. The finance, auditing, and accounting departments within an organization most commonly use financial systems. These systems determine the direction for maintenance and growth for a given facility. They often interface to share information with materials management, staffing, and billing systems to balance the financial impact of these resources within an organization. Financial systems report fiscal outcomes, which can then be tracked and related to the organizational goals of an institution. These systems are key components in the decision-making process as healthcare institutions prepare their fiscal budgets. They often play a pivotal role in determining the strategic direction for an organization.

**Acuity systems** monitor the range of patient types within a healthcare organization using specific indicators. They track these indicators based on the current patient population within a facility. By monitoring the patient acuity, these systems provide feedback about how intensive the care requirement is for an individual patient or group of patients. Identifying and classifying a patient's acuity can promote better organizational management of the expenses and resources necessary to provide care. Acuity systems help predict the ability and capacity of an organization to care for its current population. They also forecast future trends to allow an organization to successfully strategize on how to meet upcoming market demands.

**Scheduling systems** coordinate staff, services, equipment, and allocation of patient beds. They are frequently integrated with the other types of core business systems. By closely monitoring staff and physical resources, these systems provide data to the financial systems. For example, resource-scheduling systems may provide information about operating room use or availability of intensive care unit beds and regular nursing unit beds. These systems also provide great assistance to financial systems when they are used to track medical equipment within a facility. Procedures and care are planned when the tools and resources are available. Scheduling systems help to track resources within a facility while managing the frequency and distribution of those resources.

## Order Entry Systems

**Order entry systems** are one of the most important systems in use today. They automate the way that orders have traditionally been initiated for patients—that is, clinicians place orders using these systems instead of creating traditional handwritten transcriptions onto paper. Order entry systems provide major safeguards by ensuring that physician orders are legible and complete, thereby providing a level of patient safety that was historically missing with paper-based orders. **Computerized physician (provider) order entry systems** provide decision support and automated alert functionality that was unavailable with paper-based orders.

The seminal report by the Institute of Medicine estimated that medical errors cost the United States approximately $37.6 billion each year; nearly $17 billion of those costs are associated with preventable errors (Kohn, Corrigan, Donaldson, & Institute of Medicine, 2000). Consequently, the federal Agency for Healthcare Research and Quality Patient Safety Network (2015) continued to recommend eliminating reliance on handwriting for ordering medications. Because of the global concern for patient safety as a result of incorrect and misinterpreted orders, healthcare organizations are incorporating order entry systems into their operations as a standard tool for practice. Such systems allow for clear and legible orders, thereby both promoting patient safety and streamlining care. Although much of the health information technology literature suggests that physicians are resistant to adopting health information technology, a recent study by Elder, Wiltshire, Rooks, BeLue, and Gary (2010) found that physicians who use **information technology** were more satisfied overall with their careers. The *Informatics Tools to Promote Patient Safety and Quality Outcomes* chapter provides more information about the use of computerized physician order entry systems in clinical care.

## Patient Care Support Systems

Most specialty disciplines within health care have an associated **patient care information system**. These patient-centered systems focus on collecting data and disseminating information related to direct care. Several of these systems have become mainstream types of systems used in health care. The four systems most commonly encountered in health care include (1) clinical documentation systems, (2) pharmacy information systems, (3) laboratory information systems, and (4) radiology information systems.

**Clinical documentation systems**, also known as "clinical information systems," are the most commonly used type of **patient care support system** within healthcare organizations. CISs are designed to collect patient data in real time. They enhance care by putting data at the clinician's fingertips and enabling decision making where it needs to occur—that is, at the bedside. For that reason, these systems often are easily accessible at the point of care for caregivers interacting with the patient. CISs are **patient centered**, meaning they contain the observations, interventions, and outcomes noted by the care team. Team members enter information, such as the plan of care, hemodynamic data, laboratory results, clinical notes, allergies, and medications. All members of the treatment team use clinical documentation systems; for example, pharmacists, allied health workers, nurses, physicians, support staff, and many others access the clinical record for the patient using these systems. Frequently these types of systems are also referred to as the electronic patient record or **electronic health record**. *The Electronic Health Record and Clinical Informatics* chapter provides a comprehensive overview of CISs and the electronic health record.

**Pharmacy information systems** also have become mainstream patient care support systems. They typically allow pharmacists to order, manage, and dispense medications for a facility. They also commonly incorporate information regarding allergies and height and weight to ensure effective medication management. Pharmacy information systems streamline the order entry, dispensing, verification, and authorization process for medication administration. They often interface with clinical documentation and order entry systems so that clinicians can order and document the administration of medications and prescriptions to patients while having the benefits of decision support alerting and interaction checking.

**Laboratory information systems** were perhaps some of the first clinical information systems ever used in health care. Because of their long history of use within medicine, laboratory systems have been models for the design and implementation of other types of patient care support systems. Laboratory information systems report on blood, body fluid, and tissue samples, along with biological specimens collected at the bedside and received in a central laboratory. They provide clinicians with reference ranges for tests indicating high, low, or normal values to make care decisions. Often, the laboratory system provides result information in the EHR and directs clinicians toward the next course of action within a treatment regimen.

The final type of patient care support system commonly found within health care is the **radiology information system** (RIS) found in radiology departments. These systems schedule, result, and store information related to diagnostic radiology procedures. One feature found in most radiology systems is a **picture archiving and communication system** (PACS). The PACS may be a stand-alone system, kept separate from the main radiology system, or it can be integrated with the RIS and CIS. These systems collect, store, and distribute medical images, such as computed tomography scans, magnetic resonance images, and X-rays. PACS replace traditional hard-copy films with digital media that are easy to store, retrieve, and present to clinicians. The benefit of RIS and PACS is their ability to assist in diagnosing and storing vital patient care support data. Imaging studies can be available in minutes as opposed to 2–6 hours for images in a film-based system. The digital workstations provide enhanced imaging capabilities and on-screen measurement tools to improve diagnostic accuracy. Finally, the archive system stores images in a database that is readily accessible, so that images can be easily retrieved and compared to subsequent testing or shared instantly with consultants.

The mobility of patients both geographically and within a single healthcare delivery system challenges information systems because data must be captured wherever and whenever the patient receives care. In the past, **managed care information systems** were implemented to address these issues. Consequently, data can be obtained at any and all of the areas where a patient interacts with the healthcare system. Patient-tracking mechanisms continue to be honed, but the financial impact of health care also has changed these systems to some extent. The information systems currently in use enable nurses and physicians to make clinical decisions while being mindful of their financial ramifications. In the future, vast improvements in information systems and systems that support health information exchange are likely to continue to emerge.

One such trend is the incentive to develop accountable care organizations encouraged by the Patient Protection and Affordable Care Act of 2010. According to the Centers for Medicare and Medicaid Services (2015), "Accountable Care Organizations (ACOs) are groups of doctors, hospitals, and other health care providers, who come together voluntarily to give coordinated high quality care to their Medicare patients. The goal of coordinated care is to ensure that patients, especially the chronically ill, get the right care at the right time, while avoiding unnecessary duplication of services and preventing medical errors" (para. 1–2). Members of an ACO share data and information to better coordinate care and they also share in any health care cost savings generated when the coordination of care reduces unnecessary and duplicated costs.

# Interoperability

A key component to coordinated care is the **interoperability** of healthcare information systems. In 2015, the Office of the National Coordinator for Health IT (ONC) released an interoperability roadmap to promote ease of access and use of electronic healthcare data. Interoperability is defined as "the ability of a system to exchange electronic health information with and use electronic health information from other systems without special effort on the part of the user" (Healthcare Information and Management Systems Society [HIMSS], 2015, para. 2). The final goal of the national roadmap emphasis on interoperability is driven by the need to "achieve nationwide interoperability to enable a learning health system, with the person at the center of a system that can continuously improve care, public health, and science through real-time data access" (ONC, 2015, p. vii). As we develop more sophisticated electronic systems, we are realizing the huge potential benefits of exchanging secure and precise healthcare data. However, in the current landscape, several things need to happen to realize this goal. Chief among them is a worldwide commitment to interoperability. HIMSS (2013) identified three types of health information technology interoperability—foundational, structural, and semantic—each with increasing complexity. Foundational interoperability is basic data reception from one system to another without interpretation. Structural interoperability is more complex and depends on consistency of clinical terminology and meaning of the data. Semantic interoperability depends on data that is consistent and codified allowing for information system interpretation and analysis of the data. Semantic interoperability is considered the highest and most complex form of interoperability. Semantic interoperability is necessary for seamless health information exchange.

Suppose you have a joint replacement patient who is being discharged from the acute care facility to a rehabilitation center. You create a discharge summary for the patient in a PDF format and send it via a secure electronic exchange to the new facility. The staff at the rehabilitation center is able to read and understand the report and a staff assistant can scan a copy of the discharge summary into the electronic record for the rehabilitation facility. This is an example of functional interoperability. If each facility uses Health Level Seven standards for data exchange and collects certain minimum data, then it might be possible for certain data fields from one facility to populate automatically into an appropriate data field in the new facility. This is an example of structural interoperability. To achieve true semantic interoperability, systems must use the same standardized terminologies or disparate terminologies must be mapped, and the two systems must be able to "talk" to each other to exchange data seamlessly and to populate the data into to the appropriate fields in the new system. True semantic interoperability enables machine-to-machine data exchange.

> *Consistently representing electronic health information across different stakeholders and systems is the bedrock of successful interoperability. In a learning health system, while user interfaces can and should be different depending on the user, the format in which electronic health information is shared between health IT systems must be consistent and machine readable, so that the meaning and integrity of information is retained as a variety of users interact with it. (ONC, 2015, p. 28)*

For more detailed information on interoperability, download and read the ONC's Interoperability Roadmap: https://www.healthit.gov/sites/default/files/hie-interoperability/nationwide-interoperability-roadmap-final-version-1.0.pdf

# Aggregating Patient and Organizational Data

Many healthcare organizations now aggregate data in a **data warehouse** (DW) for the purpose of mining the data to discover new relationships and to build organizational knowledge. Rojas (2015) stated that

> *Hospitals and medical centers have more to gain from big data analytics than perhaps any other industry. But as data sets continue to grow, healthcare facilities are discovering that success in data analytics has more to do with storage methods than with analysis software or techniques. Traditional data silos are hindering the progress of big data in the healthcare industry, and as terabytes turn into petabytes, the most successful hospitals are the ones that are coming up with new solutions for storage and access challenges. (para. 1)*

When disparate information systems within an organization are unable to interface with any other information systems (either within or outside of the organization), the result is poor communication, billing errors, and issues with continuity of care. By developing a single comprehensive database, healthcare systems are able to facilitate interprofessional communications, yet maintain compliance with privacy regulations. **Figure 10-1** depicts moving from siloed to integrated data.

Based on the size of the organization, data **triage** and **tiering** might be necessary. These decision-making processes related to data storage are based on predictions related to how quickly data might need to be accessed.

Consider the case of Intermountain, a chain of 22 hospitals in Salt Lake City. With 4.7 petabytes of data under its management, cloud storage becomes cost prohibitive. The network estimates the size of the hospital chain's data will grow by 25–30% each year until it reaches 15 petabytes in 5 years. With such massive data needs, Intermountain found ways to cut costs and streamline efficiency. One way was through data tiering, which is the creation of data storage tiers that can be accessed at the appropriate speeds. Tiering is currently done manually through triaging, but several different organizations are exploring autotiering, which automatically stores data according to availability needs (Rojas, 2015, para. 9–10).

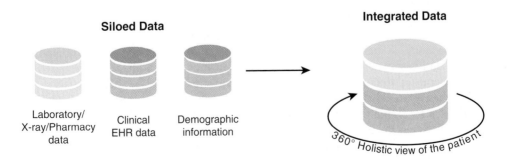

**Figure 10-1** Moving from Data Silos to Integrated Data
Data from Smart Data Collective. (2015). 2 critical obstacles facing retailers for data driven marketing. Retrieved from http://www.smartdatacollective.com/lbedgood/349875/two-critical-obstacles
-facing-retailers-data-driven-marketing

The most basic element of a database system is the data. Data refers to raw facts that can consist of unorganized text, graphics, sound, or video. Information is data that have been processed—it has meaning; information is organized in a way that people find meaningful and useful. Even useful information can be lost if one is mired in unorganized information. Computers can come to the rescue by helping to create order out of chaos. Computer science and information science are designed to help cut down the amount of information to a more manageable size and organize it so that users can cope with it more efficiently through the use of databases and database programs technology. Learning about basic databases and database management programs is paramount so that users can apply data and information management principles in health care.

A **database** is a structured or organized collection of data that is typically the main component of an information system. Databases and database management software allow the user to input, sort, arrange, structure, organize, and store data and turn those data into useful information. An individual can set up a personal database to organize recipes, music, names and addresses, notes, bills, and other data. In health care, databases and information systems make key information available to healthcare providers and ancillary personnel to promote the provision of quality patient care. **Box 10-1** provides a detailed description of a database.

---

### BOX 10-1 OVERVIEW OF DATABASE CONSTRUCTION

Databases consist of **fields** (**columns**) and **records** (**rows**). Within each record, one of the fields is identified as the **primary key** or **key field**. This primary key contains a code, name, number, or other information that acts as a unique identifier for that record. In the healthcare system, for example, a patient is assigned a patient number or ID that is unique for that patient. As you compile related records, you create **data files** or **tables**. A data file is a collection of related records. Therefore, databases consist of one or more related data files or tables.

An **entity** represents a table, and each field within the table becomes an **attribute** of that entity. The database developer must critically think about the attributes for each specific entity. For example, the entity "disease" might have the attributes of "chronic disease," "acute disease," or "communicable disease." The name of the entity, "disease," implies that the entity is about diseases. The fields or attributes are "chronic," "acute," or "communicable."

The **entity–relationship diagram** specifies the relationship among the entities in the database. Sometimes the implied relationships are readily apparent based on the entities' definitions; however, all relationships should be specified as to how they relate to one another. Typically, three relationships are possible: (1) one to one, (2) one to many, and (3) many to many. A one-to-one relationship exists between the entities of the table about a patient and the table about the patient's birth. A one-to-many relationship could exist when one entity is repeatedly used by another entity. Such a one-to-many relationship could then be a table query for age that could be used numerous times for one patient entity. The many-to-many relationship reflects entities that are all used repeatedly by other

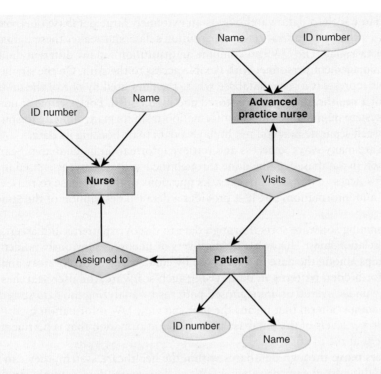

**Figure 10-2** Example of an Entity Relationship Diagram (ERD)

entities. This is easily explained by the entities of patient and nurse. The patient could have several nurses caring for him or her, and the nurse could have many patients assigned to him or her (see **Figure 10-2**).

The relational model is a database model that describes data in which all data elements are placed in relation in two-dimensional tables; the relations or tables are analogous to files. A **relational database management system (RDMS)** is a system that manages data using this kind of relational model. A relational database could link a patient's table to a treatment table (e.g., by a common field, such as the patient ID number). To keep track of the tables that constitute a database, the **database management system** uses software called a **data dictionary**. The data dictionary contains a listing of the tables and their details, including field names, validation settings, and data types. The data type refers to the type of information, such as a name, a date, or a time.

The database management system is an important program because before it was available, many health systems and businesses had dozens of database files with incompatible formats. Because patient data come from a variety of sources, these separated, isolated data files required duplicate entry of the same information, thereby increasing the risk of data entry error. The design of the relational databases eliminates data duplication. Some examples of popular database management system software include Microsoft's Access or Visual FoxPro, Corel's Paradox, Oracle's Oracle Database 10g, and IBM's DB2.

On a large scale, a data warehouse is an extremely large database or **repository** that stores all of an organization's or institution's data and makes these data available for **data mining**. The DW can combine an institution's many different databases to provide management personnel with flexible access to the data. On the smaller scale, a **data mart** represents a large database where the data used by one of the units or a division of a healthcare system are stored and maintained. For example, a university hospital system might store clinical information from its many affiliate hospitals in a DW, and each separate hospital might have a data mart housing its data.

There are many ways to access and retrieve information in databases. Searching information in databases can be done through the use of a **query**, as is used in Microsoft's Access database. A query asks questions of the database to retrieve specific data and information. **Box 10-2** provides a detailed description of the **Structured Query Language (SQL)**.

Data mining software sorts thorough data to discover patterns and ascertain or establish relationships. This software discovers or uncovers previously unidentified relationships among the data in a database by conducting an exploratory analysis looking for hidden patterns in data. Using such software, the user searches for previously undiscovered or undiagnosed patterns by analyzing the data stored in a DW. **Drill-down** is a term that means the user can view DW information by drilling down to lower levels of the database to focus on information that is pertinent to his or her needs at the moment.

As users move through databases within the healthcare system, they can access anything from enterprise-wide DWs to data marts. For example, an infection-control nurse might notice a pattern of methicillin-resistant *Staphylococcus aureus* infections in the local data mart (a single hospital within a larger system). The nurse might want to find out if the outbreak is local (data mart) or more widespread in the system (DW). The nurse might also query the database to determine if certain patient attributes (e.g., age or medical diagnosis) are associated with the incidence of infection.

These kinds of data mining capabilities are also quite useful for healthcare practitioners who wish to conduct clinical research studies. For example, one might query a database to tease out attributes (patient characteristics) associated with asthma-related hospitalizations. For a more detailed description and review of data mining, refer to the *Data Mining as a Research Tool* chapter.

According to Mishra, Sharma, and Pandey (2013), there is a new set of challenges and opportunities for managing data, data mining, and establishing algorithms in the cloud. Data mining in the cloud is emerging and evolving. This frontier is becoming a potent way to take advantage of the power of cloud computing and combine it with SQL. The world as we know it is changing: "Clouds" are leading us to develop revolutionary data mining technologies. There are five typical clinical applications for databases: (1) hospitals, (2) clinical research, (3) clinical trials, (4) ambulatory care, and (5) public health. Some healthcare systems are connecting their hospitals together by choosing a single CIS to capture data on a system-wide basis. In such healthcare organizations, multiple application programs share a pool of related data. Think about how potent such databases might potentially be in managing organizations and providing insights into new relationships that may ultimately transform the way work is done.

## BOX 10-2 SQL

SQL was originally called SEQUEL, or Structured English Query Language. SQL, still pronounced "sequel," now stands for Structured Query Language; it is a database querying language, rather than a programming language. It is a standard language for accessing and manipulating databases. SQL is "used with relational databases; it allows users to define the structure and organization of stored data, verify and maintain data integrity, control access to the data, and define relationships among the stored data items" (University of California at San Diego, 2010, para. 8). In this way, it simplifies the process of retrieving information from a database in a functional or usable form while facilitating the reorganization of data within the databases.

The relational database management system is the foundation or basis for SQL. An RDMS stores data in "database objects called tables" (W3Schools.com, 2010, para. 6). A table is a collection of related data that consists of columns and rows; as noted earlier, columns are also referred to as fields, and rows are also referred to as records or **tuples**. Databases can have many tables, and each table is identified by a name (see the Database Example: School of Nursing Faculty).

SQL statements handle most of the actions users need to perform on a database. SQL is an **International Organization for Standardization (ISO)** standard and **American National Standards Institute (ANSI)** standard, but many different versions of the SQL language exist (Indiana University, 2010). To remain compliant with the ISO and ANSI standards, SQL must handle or support the major commands of SELECT, UPDATE, DELETE, INSERT, and WHERE in a similar manner (W3Schools.com, 2010). The SELECT command allows you to extract data from a database. UPDATE updates the data, DELETE deletes the data, and INSERT inserts new data. WHERE is used to specify selection criteria, thereby restricting the results of the SQL query. Thus SQL allows you to create databases and manipulate them by storing, retrieving, updating, and deleting data.

### Database Example: School of Nursing Faculty

#### Table Named "Faculty"

| P_ID | Last Name | First Name | Department Affiliation | Office Phone Number | Office Location | UserID |
|------|-----------|------------|------------------------|---------------------|-----------------|--------|
| 1 | Eggleers | Renee | Informatics | 444-111-1104 | 104A | Eggleersr100 |
| 2 | Feistyz | Judi | Gerontology | 444-111-2202 | 202b | Feistyzj562 |
| 3 | Martinez | Bethann | Neurology | 444-111-3336 | 336C | Martinezb789 |
| 4 | Smythe | Ralph | Informatica | 444-111-1110 | 110A | Smyther355 |

The database example provided here reflects the faculty listing for a school of nursing. The table that contains the data is identified by the name "Faculty." The faculty members are each categorized by the following fields (columns): Last Name, First Name, Department Affiliation, Office Phone Number, Office Location, and UserID. Each individual faculty member's information is a record (tuple or row).

Using the SQL command SELECT, all of the records in the "Faculty" table can be selected:

SELECT*FROM Faculty

This command would SELECT all (*) of the records FROM the table known as FACULTY. The asterisk (*) is used to select all of the columns.

# Department Collaboration and Exchange of Knowledge and Information

The implementation of systems within health care is the responsibility of many people and departments. All systems require a partnership of collaboration and knowledge sharing to implement and maintain successful standards of care. **Collaboration** is the sharing of ideas and experiences for the purposes of mutual understanding and learning. **Knowledge exchange** is the product of collaboration when sharing an understanding of information promotes learning from past experiences to make better future decisions.

Depending on the type of project, collaboration may occur at many different levels within an organization. At an administrative level, collaboration among key stakeholders is critical to the success of any project. **Stakeholders** have the most responsibility for completing the project. They have the greatest influence in the overall design of the system, and ultimately they are the people who are most impacted by a system implementation. Together with the organizational executive team, stakeholders collaborate on the overall budget and time frame for a system implementation.

Collaboration may also occur among the various departments impacted by the system. These groups frequently include representatives from information technology, clinical specialty areas, support services, and software vendors. Once a team is assembled, it defines the objectives and goals of the system. The team members work strategically to align their goals with the goals of the organization where the system is to be used. The focus for these groups is on planning, resource management, transitioning, and ongoing support of the system. Their collaboration determines the way in which the project is managed, the deliverables for the project, the individuals held accountable for the project, the time frame for the project, opportunities for process improvement using the system, and the means by which resources are allocated to support the system.

From collaboration comes the exchange of information and ideas through knowledge sharing. Specialists exchange knowledge within their respective areas of expertise to ensure that the system works for an entire organization. From one another, they learn requirements that make the system successful. This exchange of ideas is what makes healthcare information systems so valuable. A multidisciplinary approach ensures that systems work in the complex environment of healthcare organizations that have diverse and complex patient populations.

## Summary

The integration of technology within healthcare organizations offers limitless possibilities. As new types of systems emerge, clinicians will become smarter and more adept at incorporating these tools into their daily practice. Success will be achieved when health care incorporates technology systems in a way that they are not viewed as separate tools to support healthcare practices, but rather as necessary instruments to provide health care. Patients, too, will become savvier at using healthcare information systems as a means of communication and managing their personal and preventive care. In the future, these two mindsets will become expectations for health care and not simply a high-tech benefit, as they are often viewed today.

Ultimately, it is not the type of systems adopted that is important, but rather the method in which they are put into practice. In an ideal world, robust and transparent information technologies will support clinical and administrative functions and promote safe, quality, and cost-effective care.

### THOUGHT-PROVOKING QUESTIONS

1. Which type of technology exists today that could be converted into new types of information systems to be used in health care?
2. How could collaboration and knowledge sharing at a single organization be used to help individuals preparing for information technology at a different facility?
3. Explore the administrative information systems and their applications in your healthcare organization.
   a. What are the main systems used?
   b. How is data shared among systems?
   c. What examples of functional, structural, and semantic interoperability can you identify?

# References

Agency for Healthcare Research and Quality (AHRQ) Patient Safety Network. (2015). Patient safety primers: Medication errors. Retrieved from http://psnet.ahrq.gov/primer .aspx?primerID=23

Case Management Society of America (CMSA). (2014, September 12). Health IT survey. Retrieved from http://www.cmsa.org/Individual/NewsEvents/2010HealthITSurvey /tabid/539/Default.aspx

Centers for Medicare and Medicaid Services (CMS). (2015). Accountable care organizations. Retrieved from https://www.cms.gov/Medicare/Medicare-Fee-for-Service-Payment/ACO /index.html

Elder, K., Wiltshire, J., Rooks, R., BeLue, R., & Gary, L. (2010, Summer). Health information technology and physician career satisfaction. *Perspectives in Health Information Management*, 1–18. Retrieved from ProQuest Nursing & Allied Health Source (Document ID: 2118694921).

Fichman, R. G., Kohli, R., & Krishnan, R. (2011). Editorial overview: The role of information systems in healthcare; current research and future trends. *Information Systems Research*, 22(3), 419–428. doi:10.1287/isre.1110.0382

Gordon, C. R., Rezzadeh, K. S., Li, A., Vardanian, A., Zelken, J., Shores, J. T., . . . Jarrahy, R. (2015). Digital mobile technology facilitates HIPAA-sensitive perioperative messaging, improves physician-patient communication, and streamlines patient care. *Patient Safety In Surgery*, 9(1), 1–7. doi:10.1186/s13037-015-0070-9

Hassett, M., & Thede, L. (2003). Information in practice: Clinical information systems. In B. Cunningham (Ed.), *Informatics and nursing opportunities and challenges* (2nd ed., rev., pp. 222–239). Philadelphia, PA: Lippincott Williams & Wilkins.

Healthcare Information and Management Systems Society (HIMSS). (2013). Definition of interoperability. Retrieved from http://www.himss.org/library/interoperability-standards /what-is-interoperability

Healthcare Information and Management Systems Society (HIMSS). (2015). ONC releases final interoperability roadmap. Retrieved from http://www.himss.org/news /onc-releases-final-interoperability-roadmap?ItemNumber=44779

Indiana University. (2010). University information technology services knowledge base: What is SQL? Retrieved from http://kb.iu.edu/data/ahux.html

Kohn, L. T., Corrigan, J., Donaldson, M. S., & Institute of Medicine (U.S.). Committee on Quality of Health Care in America. (2000). *To err is human: Building a safer health system.* Washington, DC: National Academy Press.

Mishra, N., Sharma, S. & Pandey, A. (2013). High performance cloud data mining algorithm and data mining in clouds. *IOSR Journal of Computer Engineering*, 8(4), 54–61. Retrieved from http://www.iosrjournals.org/iosr-jce/papers/Vol8-Issue4/I0845461 .pdf

National Consortium for Health Science Education. (2012). Health informatics pathway standards and accountability criteria. Retrieved from http://www.healthscienceconsortium .org/wp-content/uploads/2015/07/Health-Informatics-Standards.pdf

Office of the National Coordinator for Health Information Technology (ONC). (2015). Connecting health and care for the nation: A shared nationwide interoperability roadmap. Final version 1.0. Retrieved from https://www.healthit.gov/sites/default/files/hie -interoperability/nationwide-interoperability-roadmap-final-version-1.0.pdf

Rojas, N. (2015). Healthcare industry finds new solutions to big data storage challenges. *Data Science Central*. Retrieved from http://www.datasciencecentral.com/profiles/blogs/healthcare-industry-finds-new-solutions-to-big-data-storage

University of California at San Diego. (2010). Data warehouse terms. Retrieved from http://blink.ucsd.edu/technology/help-desk/queries/warehouse/terms.html#s

W3Schools.com. (2010). Introduction to SQL. Retrieved from http://www.w3schools.com/SQL/sql_intro.asp

## Key Terms

- » Cognitive task analysis
- » Cognitive walkthrough
- » Cognitive work analysis
- » Earcons
- » Ergonomics
- » Field study
- » Gulf of evaluation
- » Gulf of execution
- » Heuristic evaluation
- » Human–computer interaction
- » Human factors
- » Human–technology interaction
- » Human–technology interface
- » Mapping
- » Situational awareness
- » Task analysis
- » Usability
- » Workarounds

# CHAPTER 11

# The Human–Technology Interface

Dee McGonigle, Kathleen Mastrian, and Judith A. Effken

## Introduction

One of this chapter's authors stayed in a new hotel on the outskirts of London. When she entered her room, she encountered three wall-mounted light switches in a row, but with no indication of which lights they operated. In fact, the mapping of switches to lights was so peculiar that she was more often than not surprised by the light that came on when she pressed a particular switch. One might conclude that the author had a serious problem, but she prefers to attribute her difficulty to poor design.

When these kinds of technology design issues surface in health care, they are more than just an annoyance. Poorly designed technology can lead to errors, lower productivity, or even the removal of the system (Alexander & Staggers, 2009). Unfortunately, as more and more kinds of increasingly complex health information technology applications are integrated, the problem becomes even worse (Johnson, 2006). However, nurses are very creative and, if at all possible, will design workarounds that allow them to circumvent troublesome technology. However, workarounds are only a Band-Aid; they are not a long-term solution.

In his classic book *The Psychology of Everyday Things*, Norman (1988) argued that life would be a lot simpler if people who built the things that others encounter (such as light switches) paid more attention to how they would be used. At least one everyday thing meets Norman's criteria for good design: the scythe. Even people who have never encountered one will pick up a scythe in the manner needed to use it because the design makes only one way feasible. The scythe's design fits perfectly with its intended use and a human user. Would it not be great if all technology were so well fit to human use? In fact, this is not such a far-fetched idea. Scientists and engineers are making excellent strides in understanding human–technology interface problems and proposing solutions to them.

As you read through this chapter, reflect on the everyday items you use. What makes them easy or difficult to use? Is it evident that the developer

207

thought about how they would be used to facilitate their design and function? Next, turn your attention to the technologies you use. Is it evident that the developer thought about how the technology would be used to facilitate its design and function? Think about your smartphone. How easy is it to hold your smartphone? Is it intuitive and easy to access and use? What improvements would you make? Does the electronic health record (EHR) system you use support your workflow and patient needs? Do you use workarounds to avoid items that you feel should not be there or are not needed at the time of entry? Do you think that the developer understood you, as the user, or did not realize how their technology tool would be used? By the end of this chapter, you should be able to critically examine the human–technology interfaces currently available in health care and describe models, strategies, and exemplars for improving interfaces during the analysis, design, and evaluation phases of the development life cycle.

## The Human–Technology Interface

What is the **human–technology interface**? Broadly speaking, anytime a human uses technology, some type of hardware or software enables and supports the interaction. It is this hardware and software that defines the interface. The array of light switches described previously was actually an interface (although not a great one) between the lighting technology in the room and the human user.

In today's healthcare settings, one encounters a wide variety of human–technology interfaces. Those who work in hospitals may use bar-coded identification cards to log their arrival time into a human resources management system. Using the same cards, they might log into their patients' EHR, access their patient's drugs from a drug administration system, and even administer the drugs using bar-coding technology. Other examples of human–technology interfaces one might encounter include a defibrillator, a patient-controlled analgesia (PCA) pump, any number of physiologic monitoring systems, electronic thermometers, and telephones and pagers. According to Rice and Tahir (2014),

> [R]ecent studies have found that rapid implementation of new medical technology—electronic health records, patient monitoring devices, surgical robots and other tools—can lead to adverse patient events when it is not thoughtfully integrated into workflow. The right processes require understanding the devices and the users. Testing in controlled environments often does not adequately consider the "human factor," or how people interact with technology in high-pressure, real-life situations. (p. 12)

The human interfaces for each of these technologies are different and can even differ among different brands or versions of the same device. For example, to enter data into an EHR, one might use a keyboard, a light pen, a touch screen, or voice. Healthcare technologies may present information via computer screen, printer, or smartphone. Patient data might be displayed in the form of text, images (e.g., the results of a brain scan), or even sound (an echocardiogram); in addition, the information may be arrayed or presented differently, based on roles and preferences. Some human–technology interfaces mimic face-to-face human encounters. For example, faculty members are increasingly using videoconferencing technology to communicate with their students. Similarly, telehealth allows nurses to use telecommunication and videoconferencing software to communicate more effectively and more frequently with patients at home by using the technology to monitor patients' vital signs, supervise their wound care, or demonstrate a procedure. According to Gephart and Effken (2013), "The National eHealth Collaborative Technical Expert Panel recommends fully integrating patient-generated data (e.g., home monitoring of daily weights, blood glucose, or blood pressure readings) into the clinical workflow of healthcare providers" (para. 3). Telehealth technology has fostered other virtual interfaces, such as system-wide intensive care units in which intensivists and specially trained nurses monitor critically ill patients in intensive care units, some of whom may be in rural locations. Sometimes telehealth interfaces allow patients to interact with a virtual clinician (actually a computer program) that asks questions, provides social support, and tailors education to identify patient needs based on the answers to screening questions. These human–technology interfaces have been remarkably successful; sometimes patients even prefer them to live clinicians.

Human–technology interfaces may present information using text, numbers, images, icons, or sound. Auditory, visual, or even tactile alarms may alert users to important information. Users may interact with (or control) the technology via keyboards, digital pens, voice activation, or even touch.

A small, but growing, number of clinical and educational interfaces rely heavily on tactile input. For example, many students learn to access an intravenous site using virtual technology. Other, more sophisticated virtual reality applications help physicians learn to do endoscopies or practice complex surgical procedures in a safe environment. Still others allow drug researchers to design new medications by combining virtual molecules (here, the tactile response is quite different for molecules that can be joined from those that cannot). In each of these training environments, accurately depicting tactile sensations is critical. For example, feeling the kind and amount of pressure required to penetrate the desired tissues, but not others, is essential to a realistic and effective learning experience.

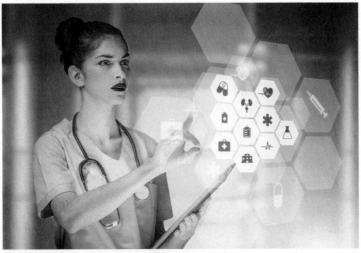

The growing use of large databases for research has led to the design of novel human–technology interfaces that help researchers visualize and understand patterns in the data that generate new knowledge or lead to new questions. Many of these interfaces now incorporate multidimensional visualizations, in addition to scatter plots, histograms, or cluster representations (Vincent, Hastings-Tolsma, & Effken, 2010). Some designers, such as Quinn (the founder of the Design Rhythmics Sonification Research Laboratory at the University of New Hampshire) and Meeker (2000), use variations in sound to help researchers hear the patterns in large datasets. In Quinn and Meeker's (2000) "climate symphony," different musical instruments, tones, pitches, and phrases are mapped onto variables, such as the amounts and relative concentrations of minerals, to help researchers detect patterns in ice core data covering more

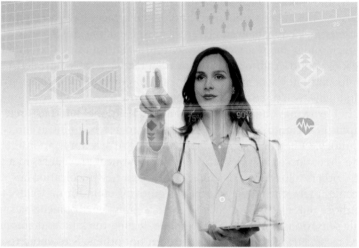

© Innocenti/Cultura/Getty

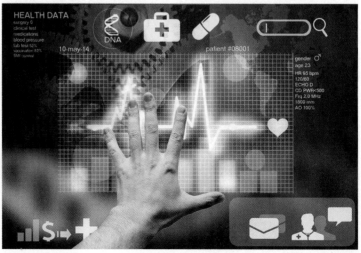

© Carlos Amarillo/Shutterstock

than 110,000 years. Climate patterns take centuries to emerge and can be difficult to detect. The music allows the entire 110,000 years to be condensed into just a few minutes, making detection of patterns and changes much easier.

The human–technology interface is ubiquitous in health care and takes many forms. A look at the quality of these interfaces follows. Be warned: It is not always a pretty picture.

# The Human–Technology Interface Problem

In *The Human Factor*, Vicente (2004) cited the many safety problems in health care identified by the Institute of Medicine's (1999) report and noted how the technology (defined broadly) used often does not fit well with human characteristics. As a case in point, Vicente described his own studies of nurses' PCA pump errors. Nurses made the errors, in large part, because of the complexity of the user interface, which required as many as 27 steps to program the device. Vicente and his colleagues developed a PCA in which programming required no more than 12 steps. Nurses who used it in laboratory experiments made fewer errors, programmed drug delivery faster, and reported lower cognitive workloads compared to the commercial device. Further evidence that human–technology interfaces do not work as well as they might is evident in the following events.

Doyle (2005) reported that when a bar-coding medication system interfered with their workflow, nurses devised **workarounds,** such as removing the armband from the patient and attaching it to the bed, because the bar-code reader failed to interpret bar codes when the bracelet curved tightly around a small arm. Koppel et al. (2005) reported that a widely used computer-based provider order entry (CPOE) system meant to decrease medication errors actually facilitated 22 types of errors because the information needed to order medications was fragmented across as many as 20 screens, available medication dosages differed from those the physicians expected, and allergy alerts were triggered only after an order was written.

Han et al. (2005) reported increased mortality among children admitted to Children's Hospital in Pittsburgh after CPOE implementation. Three reasons were cited for this unexpected outcome. First, CPOE changed the workflow in the emergency room. Before CPOE, orders were written for critical time-sensitive treatment based on radio communication with the incoming transport team before the child arrived. After CPOE implementation, orders could not be written until the patient arrived and was registered in the system (a policy that was later changed). Second, entering an order required as many as 10 clicks and took as long as 2 minutes; moreover, computer screens sometimes froze or response time was slow. Third, when the team changed its workflow to accommodate CPOE, face-to-face contact among team members diminished. Despite the problems with study methods identified by some of the informatics community, there certainly were serious human–technology interface problems.

In 2005, a *Washington Post* article reported that Cedars-Sinai Medical Center in Los Angeles had shut down a $34 million system after 3 months because of the medical staff's rebellion. Reasons for the rebellion included the additional time it took to complete the structured information forms, failure of the system to recognize misspellings (as nurses had previously done), and intrusive and interruptive auto-mated alerts (Connolly, 2005). Even though physicians actually responded appro-priately to the alerts, modifying or canceling 35% of the orders that triggered them, designers had not found the right balance of helpful-to-interruptive alerts. The system simply did not fit the clinicians' workflow.

Such unintended consequences (Ash, Berg, & Coiera, 2004) or unpredictable outcomes (Aarts, Doorewaard, & Berg, 2004) of healthcare information systems may be attributed, in part, to a flawed implementation process, but there were clearly also **human–technology interaction** issues. That is, the technology was not well matched to the users and the context of care. In the pediatric case, a system developed for medi-cal–surgical units was implemented in a critical care unit.

Human–technology interface problems are the major cause of as many as 87% of all patient monitoring incidents (Walsh & Beatty, 2002). It is not always that the tech-nology itself is faulty. In fact, the technology may perform flawlessly, but the interface design may lead the human user to make errors (Vicente, 2004).

Rice and Tahir (2014) reported on two errors that remind us we still have a long way to go to ensure patient safety: In 2011, a pop-up box on a digital blood glucose reader was misread and the patient was given too much insulin, sending her into a diabetic coma; in 2013, a patient did not receive his psychiatric medicine for almost 3 weeks because the pharmacy's computer system was set to automatically discon-tinue orders for certain drugs, and there was no alert built in to notify the team providing care to this patient that the drug was suspended. The real issue is that the healthcare personnel–technology interfaces continue to cause these adverse events and near-misses. It is important to remember that it is not only a technology or human interface issue. Many of these problems occur when new technology is introduced or existing technology is modified. In addition, we must examine how the technology tools are tested, how the human users are prepared for their use, and how the tools are integrated into the care delivery process (Rice & Tahir, 2014).

## Improving the Human–Technology Interface

Much can be learned from the related fields of cognitive engineering, **human factors**, and **ergonomics** (**Figures 11-1 and 11-2**) about how to make interfaces more compat-ible with their human users and the context of care. Each of these areas of study is multidisciplinary and integrates knowledge from multiple disciplines (e.g., computer science, engineering, cognitive engineering, psychology, and sociology).

These areas are also concerned with health issues arising from computer and other technology use. Longo and Reese (2014) reminded us that

> *Nearly 20 years ago, the American Optometric Association termed computer vision syndrome (CVS) as the complex of eye and vision problems related to near work experienced while using a computer. CVS symptoms reflect the current broad diagnosis of asthenopia (ICD-9, 368.13) [2017 ICD-10-CM H53.149] also referred to as eyestrain. Symptoms include: fatigue, blurred distal or proximal vision, headache, dry or irritated eyes, neck and/or back-aches, blurred near vision and diplopia (double vision). (p. 8)*

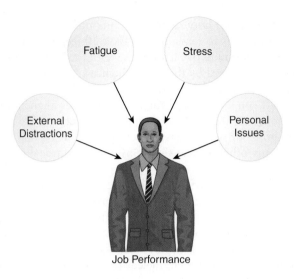

**Figure 11-1** Human Factors and Ergonomics

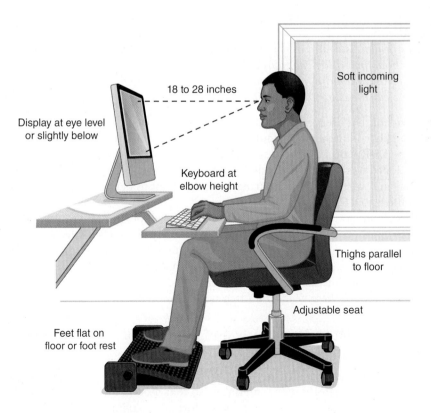

**Figure 11-2** Human Factors and Ergonomics, Continued

Longo and Reese described how to prevent computer vision syndrome. One of the best ways to help your eyes is to remember to look 20 feet away from your screen every 20 minutes for a minimum of 20 seconds. With the increased smartphone use, we are seeing neck issues caused by the tilt of the head (with the chin on the chest) while looking down at the smartphone or other handheld device. You should hold your phone up so that you are keeping your neck and eyes aligned properly with the device's screen for more comfortable viewing and interactions. We must all be aware of our posture and how our work areas are set up when using our computers, smartphones, tablets, and any other devices that consume a great deal of our time during our work or personal hours.

Effken (2016) proposed the ecological approach to interface design to help us realize a more meaningful EHR. This approach borrowed from a small field of psychology, ecological psychology, which "emerged after the 3-Mile Island nuclear fiasco to allow complex processes (like nuclear power plants) to be more easily and safely controlled by operators. Ecological displays subsequently have enhanced the control of airplanes, bottling plants—and even nuclear power plants. In the 1990s, the approach began to be extended to the complexities of healthcare" (Effken, para. 2). Ecological displays help the user identify deviations from normal physical or physiological processes. According to Effken,

> Given the current pressure to achieve meaningful use of the EHR and the availability of new, more flexible technology, this seems like an ideal time for informaticists (and nurse informaticists, in particular) to consider seriously how the ecological approach might be applied to make the meaning of the EHR's data more transparent to clinician and patient users, as well as to make clear the value proposition of various treatments. (para. 8)

It is evident that users and clinicians need the technology and interfaces necessary to quickly comprehend the multiple discrete data that are contained in distinct parts of the EHR. "Because these are exactly the kind of complex problems that they were developed to solve, the analysis and design approaches derived from ecological psychology are worth examining further as we attempt to derive a more meaningful EHR" (Effken, 2016, para. 8).

Over the years, three axioms have evolved for developing effective **human–computer interactions** (Staggers, 2003): (1) Users must be an early and continuous focus during interface design; (2) the design process should be iterative, allowing for evaluation and correction of identified problems; and (3) formal evaluation should take place using rigorous experimental or qualitative methods. These axioms still apply today and, even after all of these years, are often not followed.

## Axiom 1: Users Must Be an Early and Continuous Focus During Interface Design

Rubin (1994) used the term *user-centered design* to describe the process of designing products (e.g., human–technology interfaces) so that users can carry out the tasks needed to achieve their goals with "minimal effort and maximal efficiency" (p. 10).

Thus, in user-centered design, the end user is emphasized. This is still a focus of human–technology interface design today.

Vicente (2004) argued that technology should fit human requirements at five levels of analysis (physical, psychological, team, organizational, and political). Physical characteristics of the technology (e.g., size, shape, or location) should conform to the user's size, grasp, and available space. Information should be presented in ways that are consistent with known human psychological capabilities (e.g., the number of items that can be remembered is seven plus or minus two). In addition, systems should conform to the communication, workflow, and authority structures of work teams; to organizational factors, such as culture and staffing levels; and even to political factors, such as budget constraints, laws, or regulations.

A number of analysis tools and techniques have been developed to help designers better understand the task and user environment for which they are designing. Discussed next are task analysis, cognitive task analysis, and cognitive work analysis (CWA).

**Task analysis** examines how a task must be accomplished. Generally, analysts describe the task in terms of inputs needed for the task, outputs (what is achieved by the task), and any constraints on actors' choices on carrying out the task. Analysts then lay out the sequence of temporally ordered actions that must be carried out to complete the task in flowcharts (Vicente, 1999). A worker's tasks must be analyzed. Task analysis is very useful in defining what users must do and which functions might be distributed between the user and technology (U.S. Department of Health and Human Services, 2013). **Cognitive task analysis** usually starts by identifying, through interviews or questionnaires, the particular task and its typicality and frequency. Analysts then may review the written materials that describe the job or are used for training and determine, through structured interviews or by observing experts perform the task, which knowledge is involved and how that knowledge might be represented. Cognitive task analysis can be used to develop training programs. Zupanc and colleagues (2015) reported on the use of cognitive task analysis techniques to develop a framework from which a colonoscopy training program could be designed. "Task analysis methods (observation, a think-aloud protocol and cued-recall) and subsequent expert review were employed to identify the competency components exhibited by practicing endoscopists with the aim of providing a basis for future instructional design" (Zupanc et al., p. 10). The resulting colonoscopy competency framework consisted of "twenty-seven competency components grouped into six categories: clinical knowledge; colonoscope handling; situation awareness; heuristics and strategies; clinical reasoning; and intra and inter-personal" (Zupanc et al., p. 10).

**Cognitive work analysis** was developed specifically for the analysis of complex, high-technology work domains, such as nuclear power plants, intensive care units, and emergency departments, where workers need considerable flexibility in responding to external demands (Burns & Hajdukiewicz, 2004; Vicente, 1999). A complete CWA includes five types of analysis: (1) work domain, (2) control tasks, (3) strategies, (4) social–organizational, and (5) worker competencies. The work domain analysis describes the functions of the system and identifies the information that users need to accomplish their task goals. The control task analysis investigates the control structures through which the user interacts with or controls the system. It also identifies which variables and relations among variables discovered in the work domain analysis are relevant for particular situations so that context-sensitive interfaces can present the right information (e.g., prompts or alerts) at the right time. The strategies analysis looks at how work is actually done by users to facilitate the design of appropriate human–computer dialogues. The social–organizational analysis identifies the responsibilities of various users (e.g., doctors, nurses, clerks, or therapists) so that the system can support collaboration, communication, and a viable organizational structure. Finally, the worker competencies analysis identifies design constraints related to the users themselves (Effken, 2002).

Specialized tools are available for the first three types of CWA (Vicente, 1999). Analysts typically borrow tools (e.g., ethnography) from the social sciences for the two remaining types. Hajdukiewicz, Vicente, Doyle, Milgram, and Burns (2001) used CWA to model an operating room environment. Effken (2002) and Effken et al. (2001) used CWA to analyze the information needs for an oxygenation management display for an ICU. Other examples of the application of CWA in health care are described by Burns and Hajdukiewicz (2004) in their chapter on medical systems (pp. 201–238). Ashoon et al. (2014) used team CWA to reveal the interactions of the healthcare team in the context of work models in a birthing unit. They felt that team CWA enhances CWA in complex environments, such as health care, that require effective teamwork because it reveals additional constraints relevant to the workings of the team. The information gleaned about the teamwork could be used for systems design applications.

## Axiom 2: The Design Process Should Be Iterative, Allowing for Evaluation and Correction of Identified Problems

Today, both principles and techniques for developing human–technology interfaces that people can use with minimal stress and maximal efficiency are available. An excellent place to start is with Norman's (1988, pp. 188–189) principles:

1. Use both knowledge in the world and knowledge in the head. In other words, pay attention not only to the environment or to the user, but to both, and to how they relate. By using both, the problem actually may be simplified.
2. Simplify the structure of tasks. For example, reduce the number of steps or even computer screens needed to accomplish the goal.
3. Make things visible: Bridge the **gulf of execution** and the **gulf of evaluation**. Users need to be able to see how to use the technology to accomplish a goal (e.g., which buttons does one press and in which order to program this PCA?); if they do, then designers have bridged the gulf of execution. They also need to be able to see the effects of their actions on the technology (e.g., if a nurse practitioner prescribes a drug to treat a certain condition, the actual patient response may not be perfectly clear). This bridges the gulf of evaluation.
4. Get the mappings right. Here, the term **mapping** is used to describe how environmental facts (e.g., the order of light switches or variables in a physiologic monitoring display) are accurately depicted by the information presentation.

5. Exploit the power of constraints, both natural and artificial. Because of where the eyes are located in the head, humans have to turn their heads to see what is happening behind them; however, that is not true of all animals. As the location of one's eyes constrains what one can see, so also do physical elements, social factors, and even organizational policy constrain the way tasks are accomplished. By taking these constraints into account when designing technology, it can be made easier for humans use.

6. Design for error. Mistakes happen. Technology should eliminate predictable errors and be sufficiently flexible to allow humans to identify and recover from unpredictable errors.

7. When all else fails, standardize. To get a feel for this principle, think how difficult it is to change from a Macintosh to a Windows environment or from the iPhone operating system to Android.

Kirlik and Maruyama (2004) described a real-world human–technology interface that follows Norman's principles. In their classic analogy, the authors observed how a busy expert short-order cook strategically managed to grill many hamburgers at the same time, but each to the customer's desired level of doneness. The cook put those burgers that were to be well-done on the back and far right portion of the grill, those to be medium well-done in the center of the grill, and those to be rare at the front of the grill, but farther to the left. The cook moved all burgers to the left as grilling proceeded and turned them over during their travel across the grill. Everything the cook needed to know was available in this simple interface. As a human–technology interface, the grill layout was elegant. The interface used knowledge housed both in the environment and in the expert cook's head; also, things were clearly visible, both in the position of the burgers and in the way they were moved. The process was clearly and effectively standardized, with built-in constraints. What might it take to create such an intuitive human–technology interface in health care?

Several useful books have been written about effective interface design (e.g., Burns & Hajdukiewicz, 2004; Cooper, 1995; Mandel, 1997; McKay, 2013; Wigdor & Wixon, 2011). In addition, a growing body of research is exploring new ways to present clinical data that might facilitate clinicians' problem identification and accurate treatment (Agency for Healthcare Research and Quality, 2010). Just as in other industries, health care is learning that big data can provide big insights if it can be visualized, accessed, and meaningful (Intel IT Center, 2013). Often, designers use graphical objects to show how variables relate. The first to do so were likely Cole and Stewart (1993), who used changes in the lengths of the sides and area of a four-sided object to show the relationship of respiratory rate to tidal volume. Other researchers have demonstrated that histograms and polygon displays are better than numeric displays for detecting changes in patients' physiologic variables (Gurushanthaiah, Weinger, & Englund, 1995). When Horn, Popow, and Unterasinger (2001) presented physiologic data via a single circular object with 12 sectors (where each sector represented a different variable), nurses reported that it was easy to recognize abnormal conditions, but difficult to comprehend the patient's overall status. This kind of graphical object approach has been most widely used in anesthesiology, where a number of researchers have shown improved clinician **situational awareness** or problem detection time by mapping physiologic variables onto display objects that have meaningful shapes, such as using a bellows-like object to represent ventilation (Agutter et al., 2003; Blike, Surgenor, Whallen, & Jensen, 2000; Michels, Gravenstein, & Westenskow, 1997; Zhang et al., 2002).

Effken (2006) compared a prototype display that represented physiologic data in a structured pictorial format with two bar graph displays. The first bar graph display and the prototype both presented data in the order that experts were observed to use them. The second bar graph display presented the data in the way that nurses collected them. In an experiment in which resident physicians and novice nurses used simulated drugs to treat observed oxygenation management problems using each display, residents' performance was improved with the displays ordered as experts used them, but nurses' performance was not improved. Instead, nurses performed better when the variables were ordered as they were used to collecting them, demonstrating the importance of understanding user roles and the tasks they need to accomplish.

Data also need to be represented in ways other than visually. Gaver (1993) proposed that because ordinary sounds map onto familiar events, they could be used as icons to facilitate easier technology navigation and use and to provide continuous background information about how a system is functioning. In health care, auditory displays have been used to provide clinicians with information about patients' vital signs (e.g., in pulse oximetry), such as by altering volume or tone when a significant change occurs (Sanderson, 2006).

Admittedly, auditory displays are probably more useful for quieter areas of the hospital, such as the operating room. Perhaps that is why researchers have most frequently applied the approach in anesthesiology. For example, Loeb and Fitch (2002) reported that anesthesiologists detected critical events more quickly when auditory information about heart rate, blood pressure, and respiratory parameters was added to a visual display. Auditory tones also have been combined as **earcons** to represent relationships among data elements, such as the relationship of systolic to diastolic blood pressure (Watson & Gill, 2004).

## Axiom 3: Formal Evaluation Should Take Place Using Rigorous Experimental or Qualitative Methods

Perhaps one of the highest accolades that any interface can achieve is to say that it is transparent. An interface becomes transparent when it is so easy to use that users no longer think about it, but only about the task at hand. For example, a transparent clinical interface would enable clinicians to focus on patient decisions rather than on how to access or combine patient data from multiple sources. In **Figure 11-3**, instead of the nurse interacting with the computer, the nurse and the patient interact through the technology interface. The more transparent the interface, the easier the interaction should be.

**Usability** is a term that denotes the ease with which people can use an interface to achieve a particular goal. Usability of a new human–technology interface needs to be evaluated early and often throughout its development. Typical usability indicators include ease of use, ease of learning, satisfaction with using, efficiency of use, error tolerance, and fit of the system to the task (Staggers, 2003). Some of the more commonly used approaches to usability evaluation are discussed next.

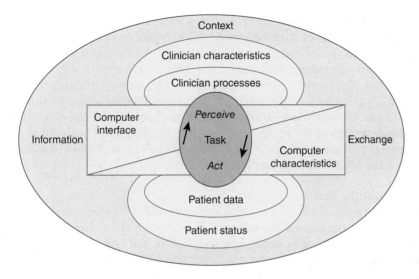

**Figure 11-3** Nurse–Patient Interaction Framework in Which the Technology Supports the Interaction

Modified from Staggers, N., & Parks, P. L. (1993). Description and initial applications of the Staggers & Parks nurse–computer interaction framework. *Computers in Nursing, 11,* 282–290. Reprinted by permission of AMIA.

## Surveys of Potential or Actual Users

Chernecky, Macklin, and Waller (2006) assessed cancer patients' preferences for website design. Participants were asked their preferences for a number of design characteristics, such as display color, menu buttons, text, photo size, icon metaphor, and layout, by selecting on a computer screen their preferences for each item from two or three options.

## Focus Groups

Typically used at the very start of the design process, focus groups can help the designer better understand users' responses to potential interface designs and to content that might be included in the interface.

## Cognitive Walkthrough

In a **cognitive walkthrough,** evaluators assess a paper mockup, working prototype, or completed interface by observing the steps users are likely to take to use the interface to accomplish typical tasks. This analysis helps designers determine how understandable and easy to learn the interface is likely to be for these users and the typical tasks (Wharton, Rieman, Lewis, & Polson, 1994).

## Heuristic Evaluation

A **heuristic evaluation** has become the most popular of what are called "discount usability evaluation" methods. The objective of a heuristic evaluation is to detect problems early in the design process, when they can be most easily and economically corrected. The methods are termed "discount" because they typically are easy to do, involve fewer than 10 experts (often experts in relevant fields such as human–computer technology or cognitive engineering), and are much less expensive than other methods. They are called "heuristic" because evaluators assess the degree to which the design complies with recognized usability rules of thumb or principles (the heuristics), such as those proposed by Nielsen (1994) and available on his website (www.useit.com/papers/heuristic/heuristic_list.html).

For example, McDaniel and colleagues (2002) conducted a usability test of an interactive computer-based program to encourage smoking cessation by low-income women. As part of the initial evaluation, healthcare professionals familiar with the intended users reviewed the design and layout of the program. The usability test revealed several problems with the decision rules used to tailor content to users that were corrected before implementation.

## Formal Usability Test

Formal usability tests typically use either experimental or observational studies of actual users using the interface to accomplish real-world tasks. A number of researchers use these methods. For example, Staggers, Kobus, and Brown (2007) conducted a usability study of a prototype electronic medication administration record. Participants were asked to add, modify, or discontinue medications using the system. The time they needed to complete the task, their accuracy in the task, and their satisfaction with the prototype were assessed (the last criterion through a questionnaire). Although satisfaction was high, the evaluation also revealed design flaws that could be corrected before implementation.

## Field Study

In a **field study**, end users evaluate a prototype in the actual work setting just before its general release. For example, Thompson, Lozano, and Christakis (2007) evaluated the use of touch-screen computer kiosks containing child health–promoting information in several low-income, urban community settings through an online questionnaire that could be completed after the kiosk was used. Most users found the kiosk easy to use and the information it provided easy to understand. Researchers also gained a better understanding of the characteristics of the likely users (e.g., 26% had never used the Internet and 48% had less than a high school education) and the information most often accessed (television and media use, and smoke exposure).

Dykes and her colleagues (2006) used a field test to investigate the feasibility of using digital pen and paper technology to record vital signs as a way to bridge an organization from a paper to an electronic health record. In general, satisfaction with the tool increased with use, and the devices conformed well to nurses' workflow. However, 8% of the vital sign entries were recorded inaccurately because of inaccurate handwriting recognition, entries outside the recording box, or inaccurate data entry (the data entered were not valid values). The number of modifications needed in the tool and the time that would be required to make those changes ruled out using the digital pen and paper as a bridging technology.

Ideally, every healthcare setting would have a usability laboratory of its own to test new software and technology in its own setting before actual implementation. However, this can be expensive, especially for small organizations. Kushniruk and Borycki (2006) developed a low-cost rapid usability engineering method for creating a portable usability laboratory consisting of video cameras and other technology that one can take out of the laboratory into hospitals and other locations to test the technology on site using as close to a real world environment as possible. This is a much more cost-effective and efficient solution and makes it possible to test all technologies before their implementation.

## A Framework for Evaluation

Ammenwerth, Iller, and Mahler (2006) proposed a fit between individuals, tasks, and technology (FITT) model that suggests that each of these factors be considered in designing and evaluating human–technology interfaces. It is not enough to consider only the user and technology characteristics; the tasks that the technology supports must be considered as well. The FITT model builds on DeLone and McLean's (1992) information success model, Davis's (1993) technology acceptance model, and Goodhue and Thompson's (1995) task technology fit model. A notable strength of the FITT model is that it encourages the evaluator to examine the fit between the various pairs of components: user and technology, task and technology, and user and task.

Johnson and Turley (2006) compared how doctors and nurses describe patient information and found that doctors emphasized diagnosis, treatment, and management, whereas the nurses emphasized functional issues. Although both physicians and nurses share some patient information, how they thought about patients differed. For that reason, an EHR needs to present information (even the same information) to the two groups in different ways.

Hyun, Johnson, Stetson, and Bakken (2009) used a combination of two models (technology acceptance model and task–technology fit model) to design and evaluate an electronic documentation system for nurses. To facilitate the design, they employed multiple methods, including brainstorming of experts, to identify design requirements. To evaluate how well the prototype design fit both task and user, nurses were asked to carry out specific tasks using the prototype in a laboratory setting, and then complete a questionnaire on ease of use, usefulness, and fit of the technology with their documentation tasks. Because the researchers engaged nurses at each step of the design process, the result was a more useful and usable system.

## Future of the Human–Technology Interface

Increased attention to improving the human–technology interface through human factors approaches has already led to significant improvements in one area of health care: anesthesiology. Anesthesia machines that once had hoses that would fit into any delivery port now have hoses that can only be plugged into the proper port. Anesthesiologists have also been actively working with engineers to improve the computer interface through which they monitor their patients' status and are among the leaders in investigating the use of audio techniques as an alternative way to help anesthesiologists maintain their situational awareness. As a result of these efforts, anesthesia-related deaths dropped from 2 in 20,000 to 1 in 200,000 in less than 10 years (Vicente, 2004). It is hoped that continued emphasis on human factors (Vicente, 2004) and user-centered design (Rubin, 1994) by informatics professionals and human–computer interactions experts will have equally successful effects on other parts of the healthcare system. The increased amount of informatics research in this area is encouraging, but there is a long way to go.

A systematic review of clinical technology design evaluation studies (Alexander & Staggers, 2009) found 50 nursing studies. Of those, nearly half (24) evaluated effectiveness, fewer (16) evaluated satisfaction, and still fewer (10) evaluated efficiency. The evaluations were not systematic—that is, there was no attempt to evaluate the same system in different environments or with different users. Most evaluations were done in a laboratory, rather than in the setting where the system would be used. The authors argued for a broader range of studies that use an expanded set of outcome measures. For example, instead of looking at user satisfaction, evaluators should dig deeper into the design factors that led to the satisfaction or dissatisfaction. In addition, performance measures, such as diagnostic accuracy, errors, and correct treatment, should be used.

Rackspace, Brauer, and Barth (2013) reported on a social study of the human cloud formed in part by data collected from wearable technologies; they focused on assessing attitudes and "exploring how cloud computing is enabling this new generation of smart devices" (p. 2). Today, smartphones, glasses, clothing, watches, cameras, and monitors for health or patient tracking, to name but a few devices, are available to this purpose.

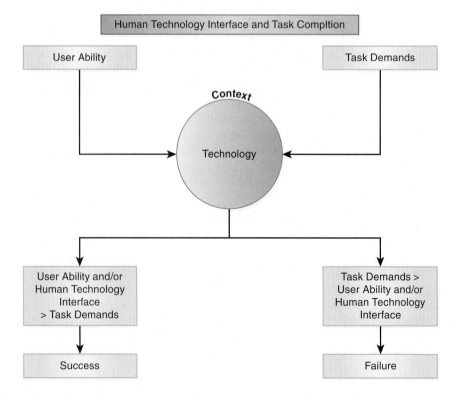

**Figure 11-4** Human Technology Interface and Task Completion

The additional technologies that are entering our lives on a daily basis can enhance or challenge our ability to complete both our activities of daily living and our professional tasks. As our home monitoring and patient technologies increase, the user's (patient's or nurse's) ability to use the technology is paramount. No matter who is using the technology, the human–technology interface addresses the user's ability and the technology's functionality to complete the task demands (see Figure 11-4).

As our technologies continue to evolve, we are creating more design issues. The proliferation of smart devices and wearable technology brings new concerns related to human–technology interfaces. According to Madden (2013), wearable technologies are adding another wrinkle into the design process—namely, human behavior. How will someone use this technology? How will individuals behave with it on their person? How will they wear it? How and when will they enable and use it? Will others be able to detect the technologies (that is, will someone be able to wear Google Glass and take pictures or videos of other people's actions), and will users be able to seamlessly move among all of the capabilities of his or her wearable technologies? The human–technology interface must address these issues. There is a long way to go.

## Summary

There are at least three messages the reader should take away from the discussion in this chapter. First, if there is to be significant improvement in quality and safety outcomes in the United States through the use of information technology, the designs for human–technology interfaces must be radically improved so that the technology better fits human and task requirements. However, that improvement will be possible only if clinicians identify and report problems, rather than simply creating workarounds. That means that each clinician has a responsibility to participate in the design process and to report designs that do not work.

Second, a number of useful tools are currently available for the analysis, design, and evaluation phases of development life cycles. They should be used routinely by informatics professionals to ensure that technology better fits both task and user requirements.

Third, focusing on interface improvement using these tools has had a huge impact on patient safety in the area of anesthesiology and medication administration. With increased attention from informatics professionals and engineers, the same kind of

### THOUGHT-PROVOKING QUESTIONS

1. You are a member of a team that has been asked to evaluate a prototype smartphone-based application for calculating drug dosages. Based on what you know about usability testing, which kind of test (or tests) might you do and why?
2. Is there a human–technology interface that you have encountered that you think needs improvement? If you were to design a replacement, which analysis techniques would you choose? Why?
3. Which type of functionality and interoperability would you want from your smartphone, watch, clothing, glasses, camera, and monitor? Provide a detailed response.

improvement should be possible in other areas regardless of the technologies actually employed there. In the ideal world, one can envision that every human–technology interface will be designed to enhance users' workflow, will be as easy to use as banking ATMs, and will be fully tested before its implementation in a setting that mirrors the setting where it will be used.

# References

Aarts, J., Doorewaard, H., & Berg, M. (2004). Understanding implementation: The case of a computerized physician order entry system in a large Dutch university medical center. *Journal of the American Medical Association, 11*, 207–216.

Agency for Healthcare Research and Quality (AHRQ). (2010). Improving data collection across the health care system. Retrieved from http://www.ahrq.gov/research/findings/final-reports/iomracereport/reldata5.html

Agutter, J., Drews, F., Syroid, N., Westneskow, D., Albert, R., Strayer, D., . . . Weinger, M. (2003). Evaluation of graphic cardiovascular display in a high-fidelity simulator. *Anesthesia and Analgesia, 97*, 1403–1413.

Alexander, G., & Staggers, N. (2009). A systematic review of the designs of clinical technology findings and recommendations for future research. *Advances in Nursing Science, 32*(3), 252–279.

Ammenwerth, E., Iller, C., & Mahler, C. (2006). IT-adoption and the interaction of task, technology and individuals: A fit framework and a case study. *BMC Medical Informatics and Decision Making, 6*, 3.

Ash, J. S., Berg, M., & Coiera, E. (2004). Some unintended consequences of information technology in health care: The nature of patient care information system-related errors. *Journal of the American Medical Informatics Association, 11*, 104–112.

Ashoon, M., Burns, C., d'Entremont, B., & Momtahan, K. (2014). Using team cognitive work analysis to reveal healthcare team interactions in a birthing unit. *Ergonomics, 57*(7), 973–986.

Blike, G. T., Surgenor, S. D., Whallen, K., & Jensen, J. (2000). Specific elements of a new hemodynamics display improves the performance of anesthesiologists. *Journal of Clinical Monitoring & Computing, 16*, 485–491.

Burns, C. M., & Hajdukiewicz, J. R. (2004). *Ecological interface design.* Boca Raton, FL: CRC Press.

Chernecky, C., Macklin, D., & Waller, J. (2006). Internet design preferences of patients with cancer. *Oncology Nursing Forum, 33*, 787–792.

Cole, W. G., & Stewart, J. G. (1993). Metaphor graphics to support integrated decision making with respiratory data. *International Journal of Clinical Monitoring and Computing, 10*, 91–100.

Connolly, C. (2005, March 21). Cedars-Sinai doctors cling to pen and paper. *Washington Post*, p. A01.

Cooper, A. (1995). *About face: Essentials of window interface design.* New York, NY: Hungry Minds, Inc.

Davis, F. D. (1993). User acceptance of information technology: System characteristics, user perceptions and behavioral impacts. *International Journal of Man–Machine Studies, 38*, 475–487.

DeLone, W. H., & McLean, E. (1992). Information systems success: The question for the dependent variable. *Information Systems Research, 3*(1), 60–95.

Doyle, M. (2005). *Impact of the Bar Code Medication Administration (BCMA) system on medication administration errors.* Unpublished doctoral dissertation, University of Arizona, Tucson, AZ.

Dykes, P. C., Benoit, A., Chang, F., Gallagher, J., Li, Q., Spurr, C., . . . Prater, M. (2006). The feasibility of digital pen and paper technology for vital sign data capture in acute care settings. In *AMIA 2006 Symposium Proceedings* (pp. 229–233). Washington, DC: American Medical Informatics Association.

Effken, J., Loeb, R., Johnson, K., Johnson, S., & Reyna, V. (2001). Using cognitive work analysis to design clinical displays. In V. L. Patel, R. Rogers, & R. Haux (Eds.), *Proceedings of MedInfo-2001* (pp. 27–31). London, UK: IOS Press.

Effken, J. (2016, February). Proposed: An ecological interface design approach to a more meaningful EHR. *Online Journal of Nursing Informatics (OJNI), 19*(3). Retrieved from http://www.himss.org/proposed-ecological-interface-design-approach-more-meaningful-ehr

Effken, J. A. (2002). Different lenses, improved outcomes: A new approach to the analysis and design of healthcare information systems. *International Journal of Medical Informatics, 65,* 59–74.

Effken, J. A. (2006). Improving clinical decision making through ecological interfaces. *Ecological Psychology, 18*(4), 283–318.

Gaver, W. W. (1993). What in the world do we hear? An ecological approach to auditory event perception. *Ecological Psychology, 5,* 1–30.

Gephart, S., & Effken, J. (2013). Using health information technology to engage patients in their care. *Online Journal of Nursing Informatics (OJNI), 17*(3). Retrieved from http://ojni.org/issues/?p=2848

Goodhue, D. L., & Thompson, R. L. (1995). Task–technology fit and individual performance. *MIS Quarterly, 19*(2), 213–236.

Gurushanthaiah, K. I., Weinger, M. B., & Englund, C. E. (1995). Visual display format affects the ability of anesthesiologists to detect acute physiologic changes: A laboratory study employing a clinical display simulator. *Anesthesiology, 83,* 1184–1193.

Hajdukiewicz, J. R., Vicente, K. J., Doyle, D. J., Milgram, P., & Burns, C. M. (2001). Modeling a medical environment: An ontology for integrated medical informatics design. *International Journal of Medical Informatics, 62,* 79–99.

Han, Y. Y., Carcillo, J. A., Venkataraman, S. T., Clark, R. S. B., Watson, R. S., Nguyen, T., . . . Orr, R. (2005). Unexpected increased mortality after implementation of a commercially sold computerized physician order entry system. *Pediatrics, 116,* 1506–1512.

Horn, W., Popow, C., & Unterasinger, L. (2001). Support for fast comprehension of ICU data: Visualization using metaphor graphics. *Methods in Informatics Medicine, 40,* 421–424.

Hyun, S., Johnson, S. B., Stetson, P. D., & Bakken, S. (2009). Development and evaluation of nursing user interface screens using multiple methods. *Journal of Biomedical Informatics, 42*(6), 1004–1012.

Institute of Medicine. (1999). *To err is human: Building a safer health system.* Washington, DC: Author.

Intel IT Center. (2013). Big data visualization: Turning big data into big insights. Retrieved from http://www.intel.com/content/dam/www/public/us/en/documents/white-papers/big-data-visualization-turning-big-data-into-big-insights.pdf

Johnson, C. M., & Turley, J. P. (2006). The significance of cognitive modeling in building healthcare interfaces. *International Journal of Medical Informatics, 75*(2), 163–172.

Johnson, C. W. (2006). Why did that happen? Exploring the proliferation of barely usable software in healthcare systems. *Quality & Safety in Healthcare, 15*(suppl 1), 176–181.

Kirlik, A., & Maruyama, S. (2004). Human–technology interaction and music perception and performance: Toward the robust design of sociotechnical systems. *Proceedings of the IEEE, 92*(4), 616–631.

Koppel, R., Metlay, J. P., Cohen, A., Abaluck, B., Localio, A. R., Kimmel, S. E., & Stron, B. (2005). Role of computerized physician order entry systems in facilitating medication errors. *Journal of the American Medical Association, 293*(10), 1197–1203.

Kushniruk, A. W., & Borycki, E. M. (2006). Low-cost rapid usability engineering: Designing and customizing usable healthcare information systems. *Healthcare Quarterly (Toronto, Ont.), 9*(40), 98–100, 102.

Loeb, R. G., & Fitch, W. T. (2002). A laboratory evaluation of an auditory display designed to enhance intraoperative monitoring. *Anesthesia and Analgesia, 94*, 362–368.

Longo, B., & Reese, C. (2014). Human–technology interface: Computers & vision health. *Nevada RNformation, 23*(1), 8–19.

Madden, S. (2013). With wearable tech like Google Glass, human behavior is now a design problem. *Gigaom.* Retrieved from http://gigaom.com/2013/06/15/with-wearable-tech-like -google-glass-human-behavior-is-now-a-design-problem

Mandel, T. (1997). *The elements of user interface design.* New York, NY: John Wiley & Sons.

McDaniel, A., Hutchinson, S., Casper, G. R., Ford, R. T., Stratton, R., & Rembush, M. (2002). Usability testing and outcomes of an interactive computer program to promote smoking cessation in low income women. In *Proceedings AMIA 2002* (pp. 509–513). Washington, DC: American Medical Informatics Association.

McKay, E. (2013). *UI is communication: How to design intuitive, user-centered interfaces by focusing on effective communication.* New York, NY: Elsevier.

Michels, P., Gravenstein, D., & Westenskow, D. R. (1997). An integrated graphic data display improves detection and identification of critical events during anesthesia. *Journal of Clinical Monitoring & Computing, 13*, 249–259.

Nielsen, J. (1994). Heuristic evaluation. In J. Nielsen & R. L. Mack (Eds.), *Usability inspection methods* (pp. 25–62). New York, NY: John Wiley & Sons.

Norman, D. A. (1988). *The psychology of everyday things.* New York, NY: Basic Books.

Quinn, M., & Meeker, L. (2000). Research set to music: The climate symphony and other sonifications of ice core, radar, DNA, seismic and solar wind data. Retrieved from http:// www.drsrl.com/climate_paper.html

Rackspace, Brauer, C. & Barth, J. (2013). The human cloud: Wearable technology from novelty to productivity. A social study into the impact of wearable technology. Retrieved from http:// www.rackspace.co.uk/sites/default/files/whitepapers/The_Human_Cloud_-_June_2013.pdf

Rice, S. & Tahir, D. (2014). The human factor. *Modern Healthcare, 44*(33), 12–15.

Rubin, J. (1994). *Handbook of usability testing: How to plan, design, and conduct effective tests.* New York, NY: Wiley & Sons.

Sanderson, P. (2006). The multimodal world of medical monitoring displays. *Applied Ergonomics, 37*, 501–512.

Staggers, N. (2003). Human factors: Imperative concepts for information systems in critical care. *AACN Clinical Issues, 14*(3), 310–319.

Staggers, N., Kobus, D., & Brown, C. (2007). Nurses' evaluations of a novel design for an electronic medication administration record. *CIN: Computers, Informatics, Nursing, 25*(2), 67–75.

Thompson, D. A., Lozano, P., & Christakis, D. A. (2007). Parent use of touchscreen computer kiosks for child health promotion in community settings. *Pediatrics, 119*(3), 427–434.

U.S. Department of Health and Human Services. (2013). Usability.gov: Task analysis. Retrieved from http://www.usability.gov/how-to-and-tools/methods/task-analysis.html

Vicente, K. (2004). *The human factor.* New York, NY: Routledge.

Vicente, K. J. (1999). *Cognitive work analysis: Toward safe, productive, and healthy computer-based work.* Mahwah, NJ: Lawrence Erlbaum Associates.

Vincent, D., Hastings-Tolsma, M., & Effken, J. (2010). Data visualization and large nursing datasets. *Online Journal of Nursing Informatics, 14*(2). Retrieved from http://ojni.org/14_2 /Vincent.pdf

Walsh, T., & Beatty, P. C. W. (2002). Human factor error and patient monitoring. *Physiological Measurement, 23,* R111–R132.

Watson, G., & Gill, T. (2004). Earcon for intermittent information in monitoring environments. In *Proceedings of the 2004 Conference of the Computer–Human Interaction Special Interest Group of the Human Factors and Ergonomics Society of Australia* (OzCHI2004), Wollonggong, New South Wales, November 22–24, 1994.

Wharton, C., Rieman, J., Lewis, C., & Polson, P. (1994). The cognitive walkthrough: A practitioner's guide. In J. Nielsen & R. L. Mack (Eds.), *Usability inspection methods* (pp. 105–139). New York, NY: John Wiley & Sons.

Wigdor, D., & Wixon, D. (2011). *Brave NUI world: Designing natural user interfaces for touch and gesture.* New York, NY: Elsevier.

Zhang, Y., Drews, F. A., Westenskow, D. R., Foresti, S., Agutter, J., Burmedez, J. C., . . . Loeb, R. (2002). Effects of integrated graphical displays on situation awareness in anaesthesiology. *Cognition, Technology & Work, 4,* 82–90.

Zupanc, C., Burgess-Limerick, R., Hill, A., Riek, S., Wallis, G., Plooy, A., . . . Hewett, D. (2015). A competency framework for colonoscopy training derived from cognitive task analysis techniques and expert review. *BMC Medical Education, 15,* 1–11.

## Key Terms

- » Antivirus software
- » Authentication
- » Baiting
- » Biometrics
- » Brute force attack
- » Confidentiality
- » Electronic protected health information (EPHI)
- » Firewall
- » Flash drives
- » Hackers
- » Integrity
- » Intrusion detection devices
- » Intrusion detection system
- » Jump drives
- » Malicious code
- » Malicious insiders
- » Malware
- » Mask
- » Negligent insider
- » Network
- » Network accessibility
- » Network availability
- » Network security
- » Password
- » Phishing
- » Proxy server
- » Radio frequency identification (RFID)
- » Ransomware
- » Scareware
- » Secure information
- » Security breaches
- » Shoulder surfing
- » Social engineering
- » Spear phishing
- » Spyware
- » Thumb drives
- » Trojan horses
- » Viruses
- » Worms
- » Zero day attack

# CHAPTER 12

# Electronic Security

Lisa Reeves Bertin, Kathleen Mastrian, and Dee McGonigle

## Introduction

In addition to complying with federal HIPAA and HITECH guidelines regarding the privacy of patient information, healthcare systems need to be vigilant in the way that they secure information and manage network security. Mowry and Oakes (n.d.) discuss the vulnerability of electronic health records to data breaches. They suggest that as many as 77 persons could view a patient's record during a hospital stay. It is critical for information technology (IT) policies and procedures to ensure appropriate access by clinicians and to protect private information from inappropriate access. However, authentication procedures can be cumbersome and time consuming, thus reducing clinician performance efficiency.

Physicians spend on average 7 minutes per patient encounter, with nearly 2 minutes of that time being devoted to managing logins and application navigation. Likewise, an average major healthcare provider must deal with more than 150 applications—most requiring different user names and passwords—making it difficult for caregivers to navigate and receive contextual information. Healthcare organizations must strike the right balance, in terms of simplifying access to core clinical datasets while maximizing the time providers can interact with patients without jeopardizing data integrity and security (Mowry & Oakes, n.d., para. 7).

This chapter explores use of information and processes for securing information in a health system computer network.

## Securing Network Information

Typically, a healthcare organization has computers linked together to facilitate communication and operations within and outside the facility. This is commonly referred to as a **network**. The linking of computers together and to the outside world creates the possibility of a breach of network security and exposes the information to unauthorized use. With the advent of smart devices, managing all of these risks has become a nightmare for some institutions' security processes. In the past, stationary devices or computers resided within healthcare facilities. Today, smart devices travel in and out of healthcare organizations with patients, family members, and other visitors, as well as employees—both staff and healthcare providers alike. According to Sullivan (2012), "Even as they promise better health and easier care delivery, wireless medical devices (MDs) carry significant security risks. And the situation is only getting trickier as more and more MDs come with commercial operating systems that are both Internet-connected and susceptible to attack" (para. 1).

The three main areas of secure network information are (1) **confidentiality,** (2) availability, and (3) **integrity.** An organization must follow a well-defined policy to ensure that private health information remains appropriately confidential. The confidentiality policy should clearly define which data are confidential and how those data should be handled. Employees also need to understand the procedures for releasing confidential information outside the organization or to others within the organization and know which procedures to follow if confidential information is accidentally or intentionally released without authorization. In addition, the organization's confidentiality policy should contain consideration for elements as basic as the placement of monitors so that information cannot be read by passersby. **Shoulder surfing,** or watching over someone's back as that person is working, is still a major way that confidentiality is compromised.

Availability refers to network information being accessible when needed. This area of the policy tends to be much more technical in nature. An accessibility policy covers issues associated with protecting the key hardware elements of the computer network and the procedures to follow in case of a major electric outage or Internet outage. Food and drinks spilled onto keyboards of computer units, dropping or jarring hardware, and electrical surges or static charges are all examples of ways that the hardware elements of a computer network may be damaged. In the case of an electrical outage or a weather-related disaster, the network administrator must have clear plans for data backup, storage, and retrieval. There must also be clear procedures and alternative methods of ensuring that care delivery remains largely uninterrupted.

Another way organizations protect the availability of their networks is to institute an acceptable use policy. Elements covered in such policy could include which types of activities are acceptable on the corporate network. For example, are employees permitted to download music at work? Restricting downloads is a very common way for organizations to prevent viruses and other malicious code from entering their networks. The policy should also clearly define which activities are not acceptable and identify the consequences for violations.

The last area of information security is integrity. Employees need to have confidence that the information they are reading is true. To accomplish this, organizations need clear policies to clarify how data are actually inputted, determine who has the authorization to change such data, and track how and when data are changed. All three of these areas use authorization and authentication to enforce the corporate policies. Access to networks can easily be grouped into areas of authorization (e.g., users can be grouped by job title). For example, anyone with the job title of "floor supervisor" might be authorized to change the hours worked by an employee, whereas an employee with the title of "patient care assistant" cannot make such changes.

## Authentication of Users

**Authentication** of employees is also used by organizations in their security policies. The most common ways to authenticate rely on something the user knows, something the user has, or something the user is (**Figure 12-1**).

Something a user knows is a **password**. Most organizations today enforce a strong password policy, because free software available on the Internet can break a password from the dictionary very quickly. Strong password policies include using combinations of letters, numbers, and special characters, such as plus signs and ampersands. Some organizations are suggesting the use of passphrases to increase the strength of a password. See **Box 12-1** for an overview of best practices to create strong passwords. Policies typically include the enforcement of changing passwords every 30 or 60 days.

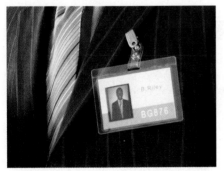

A © Photos.com

**Weak password:**
BobandSue

**Strong password:**
M2f4#eegh/

B

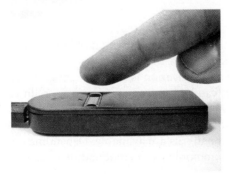

C © Gary James Calder/Shutterstock

**Figure 12-1** Ways to Authenticate Users
A. An ID badge, B. Examples of weak and strong passwords, C. A finger on a biometric scanner.

## BOX 12-1 BEST PRACTICES FOR CREATING AND MANAGING PASSWORDS

### DO

- Review the specific system guidelines for users—most will have information on password parameters and allowable characters.
- Use a combination of letters, numbers, special characters (!, $, %, &, *) and upper- and lowercase.
- Longer passwords are harder to crack. Consider at least 8 characters if the system allows.
- Choose a password that is based on a phrase: Use portions or abbreviations of the words in the phrase, or use substitutions (e.g., $ for S, 4 for "for") to create the password. Example phrase: "Lucy in the Sky with Diamonds" was released in 1967; example password: LUit$wdia67.
- Think carefully about the password and create something that is easy for you to remember.
- Change your password frequently, and do so immediately if you believe your system or email has been hacked.
- Consider using a password manager program to help you create strong passwords and store them securely.

### DO NOT:

- Share your password with anyone.
- Post your passwords in plain sight.
- Use dictionary words or any personal characteristics (your name, phone number, or birthday).
- Use a string of numbers.
- Use the same password for multiple sites.

Data from Pennsylvania State Information Technology Services. (2015). Password best practices. Retrieved from http://its.psu.edu/legacy/be-safe/password-best-practices.html

Passwords should never be written down in an obvious place, such as a sticky note attached to the monitor or under the keyboard.

The second area of authentication is something the user has, such as an identification (ID) card. ID cards can be magnetic, similar to a credit card, or have a **radio frequency identification (RFID)** chip embedded into the card.

The last area of authentication is **biometrics**. Devices that recognize thumb prints, retina patterns, or facial patterns are available. Depending on the level of security needed, organizations commonly use a combination of these types of authentication.

## Threats to Security

The largest benefit of a computer network is the ability to share information. However, organizations need to protect that information and ensure that only authorized individuals have access to the network and the data appropriate to their role. Threats to data security in healthcare organizations are becoming increasingly prevalent. A nationwide survey by the Computing Technology Industry Association (CompTIA) found that human error was responsible for more than half of **security breaches**. Human error was categorized as failure to follow policies and procedures, general carelessness, lack of experience with websites and applications, and being unaware of new threats (Greenberg, 2015). According to Degaspari (2010), "Given the volume of electronic patient data involved, it's perhaps not surprising that breaches are occurring. According to the Department of Health and Human Services' Office of Civil Rights (OCR), 146 data breaches affecting 500 or more individuals occurred between December 22, 2009, and July 28, 2010. The types of breaches encompass theft, loss, hacking, and improper disposal; and include both electronic data and paper records" (para. 4). The Fifth Annual Benchmark Study on Privacy & Security of Healthcare Data (Ponemon Institute, 2015) reported that "[m]ore than 90 percent of healthcare organizations represented in this study had a data breach, and 40 percent had more than five data breaches over the past two years" (para. 3). Interestingly, the most common type of data breach was related to a criminal attack on the healthcare organization (up 125% in the last 5 years). Key terms related to criminal attacks are **brute force attack** (software used to guess network passwords) and **zero day attack** (searching for and exploiting software vulnerabilities). Of the intentional data breaches (as opposed to unintentional), "45 percent of healthcare organizations say the root cause of the data breach was a criminal attack and 12 percent say it was due to a malicious insider" (Ponemon Institute, para. 4). That leaves nearly 43% of data breaches in the unintentional category. The Healthcare Information and Management Systems Society (HIMSS) 2015 survey reported the **negligent insider** as the most common source of a security breach. Examples of unintentional/negligent breaches include lost or stolen devices, or walking away from a workstation without logging off. If you use a device in your work and it is lost or stolen, or you violate policy by walking away from a workstation without logging off, this may be considered negligence and you may be subject to discipline or even lose your job. An interesting example of an unintentional data breach was reported on the OCR website: A company leased photocopier equipment and returned it without erasing the healthcare data stored on the copier hard drive, resulting in a settlement of over $1.2 million (U.S. Department of Health and Human Services, n.d.). Healthcare organizations need to be proactive in anticipating the potential for and preventing security breaches.

The first line of defense is strictly physical. A locked office door, an operating system that locks down after 5 minutes of inactivity, and regular security training programs are extremely effective in this regard. Proper workspace security discipline is a critical aspect of maintaining security. Employees need to be properly trained to be aware of computer monitor visibility, shoulder surfing, and policy regarding the removal of computer hardware. A major issue facing organizations is removable storage devices (Figure 12-2). CD/DVD burners, **jump drives, flash drives**, and **thumb drives** (which use USB port access) are all potential security risks. These devices can be slipped into a pocket and, therefore, are easily removed from the organization. One

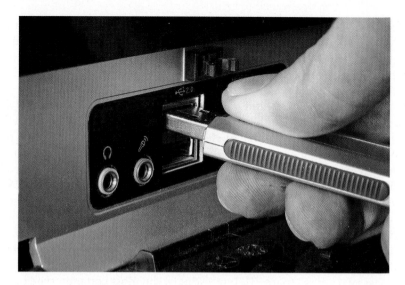

**Figure 12-2** A Removable Storage Device
© Alex Kotlov/Shutterstock

way to address this physical security risk is to limit the authorization to write files to a device. Organizations are also turning off the CD/DVD burners and USB ports on company desktops.

The most common security threats a corporate network faces are **hackers, malicious code** (**spyware**, adware, **ransomware, viruses, worms, Trojan horses**), and **malicious insiders**. Acceptable use policies help to address these problems. For example, employees may be restricted from downloading files from the Internet. Downloaded files, including email attachments, are the most common way viruses and other malicious codes enter a computer network. Network security policies typically prohibit employees from using personal CDs/DVDs and USB drives, thereby preventing the transfer of malicious code from a personal computer to the network.

Let's look more closely at some of these common network security threats. We typically think of hackers as outsiders who attempt to break into a network by exploiting software and network vulnerabilities, and indeed these black hat (malicious) hackers (crackers) do exist. However, more organizations are looking to employ ethical hackers (white hat hackers), those who are skilled at looking for and closing network security vulnerabilities (Caldwell, 2011).

Spyware and adware are normally controlled in a corporate network by limiting the functions of the browsers used to surf the Internet. For example, the browser privacy options can control how cookies are used. A cookie is a very small file written to the hard drive of a computer whose user is surfing the Internet. This file contains information about the user. For example, many shopping sites write cookies to the user's hard drive containing the user's name and preferences. When that user returns to the site, the site will greet her by name and list products in which she is possibly interested. Weather websites send cookies to users' hard drives with their

ZIP code so that when each user returns to that site, the local weather forecast is immediately displayed. On the negative side, cookies can follow the user's travels on the Internet. Marketing companies use spying cookies to track popular websites that could provide a return on advertising expenditures. Spying cookies related to marketing typically do not track keystrokes in an attempt to steal user IDs and passwords; instead, they simply track which websites are popular, and these data are used to develop advertising and marketing strategies. Nurse informaticists exploring new healthcare technologies on the Internet may find that ads for these technologies begin to pop up the next few times they are on the Internet. Spyware that does steal user IDs and passwords contains malicious code that is normally hidden in a seemingly innocent file download. This threat to security explains why healthcare organizations typically do not allow employees to download files. The rule of thumb to protect the network and one's own computer system is to only download files from a reputable site that provides complete contact information. Be aware that malicious code is sometimes hidden in an email link or in a file sent by a trusted contact whose email has been hacked. If you are not expecting a file from an email contact, or if you receive an email with only a link in it—resist the urge to download or click!

A relatively new threat to healthcare organizations is ransomware—malicious code that blocks the organization from using their computer systems until a ransom is paid to the hacker. Consider this recent case of ransomware intrusion:

> In February 2016 a hospital in Los Angeles made headlines for giving in to the ransom demand of hackers who used encryption to cripple its internal computer network, including electronic patient records, for three weeks, causing it to lose patients and money. After the hackers initially demanded $3.4 million, the hospital paid them $17,000. In explaining his decision, Allen Stefanek, president of Hollywood Presbyterian Medical Center, said, "The quickest and most efficient way to restore our systems and administrative functions was to pay the ransom." The money was transferred through Bitcoin, a cryptocurrency that permits anonymity. (Goldsborough, 2016, para. 2–3)

In addition to strict policies related to network security, organizations may also use such devices as firewalls (covered in the next section) and **intrusion detection devices** to protect from hackers. Protect yourself at home by ensuring that you have an updated version of antivirus software, be wary of unusual emails, and develop strong passwords and change them frequently. If your email is hacked, report it to the proper authorities as soon as possible, warn your contacts that you have been hacked, change your password, and check to see that your antivirus software is up to date.

Another huge threat to corporate security is **social engineering,** or the manipulation of a relationship based on one's position (or pretend position) in an organization. For example, someone attempting to access a network might pretend to be an employee from the corporate IT office, who simply asks for an employee's user ID and password. The outsider can then gain access to the corporate network. Once this access has been obtained, all corporate information is at risk. A second

## BOX 12-2 IDENTIFYING PHISHING SCAMS

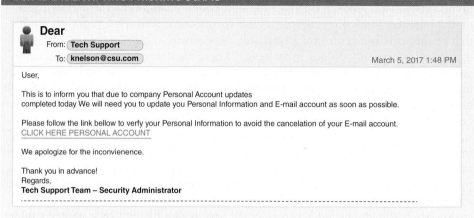

**Dear**

From: Tech Support
To: knelson@csu.com

March 5, 2017 1:48 PM

User,

This is to inform you that due to company Personal Account updates
completed today We will need you to update you Personal Information and E-mail account as soon as possible.

Please follow the link bellow to verfy your Personal Information to avoid the cancelation of your E-mail account.
CLICK HERE PERSONAL ACCOUNT

We apologize for the inconvenience.

Thank you in advance!
Regards,
**Tech Support Team – Security Administrator**

Example of a Phishing Scam Email

Check suspicious emails for grammar and spelling errors, generic greetings (User, Dear, Dearest, etc.), requests for immediate action, or requests for personal information (passwords, bank account numbers). Some phishing emails may appear to come from your bank or other trusted organization. Think carefully about why a seemingly legitimate organization might be asking for information they should already have, or ask yourself why they might need to know what they are asking for. Be aware of your organization's procedures for reporting phishing scams, and do so immediately.

Data from Pennsylvania State University Office of Information Security. (2016). Stop phishing scams. Retrieved from http://phishing.psu.edu/what-is-phishing

example of social engineering is a hacker impersonating a federal government agent. After talking an employee into revealing network information, the hacker has an open door to enter the corporate network. A related type of social engineering is **phishing**. Phishing is an attempt to steal information by manipulating the recipient of an email or phone call to provide passwords or other private information. Box 12-2 contains an example of a phishing email and tips for identifying phishing scams.

Additional types of social engineering schemes include **spear phishing**, which is a more specifically targeted scheme where the attacker takes advantage of contact information provided in an organization's directory and tailors the scam email to a specific person; **baiting**, where a malware-infected USB flash drive is left in a public area, thus tricking the finder into loading it to identify its owner; and **scareware**, where the scam email reports that the user has been hacked and tricks them into giving the hacker remote access to the computer to "fix" it (TechTarget, n.d.).

Another example of an important security threat to a corporate network is the malicious insider. This person can be a disgruntled or recently fired employee whose rights of access to the corporate network have not yet been removed. In the case of a recently fired employee, his or her network access should be suspended immediately upon notice of termination. To avoid the potentially hazardous issues created by malicious insiders, healthcare organizations need some type of policy and specific procedures to monitor employee activity to ensure that employees carry out only those duties that are part of their normal job. Separation of privileges is a common security tool; no one employee should be able to complete a task that could cause a critical event without the knowledge of another employee. For example, the employee who processes the checks and prints them should not be the same person who signs those checks. Similarly, the employee who alters pay rates and hours worked should be required to submit a weekly report to a supervisor before the changes take effect. Software that can track and monitor employee activity is also available. This software can log which files an employee accesses, whether changes were made to files, and whether the files were copied. Depending on the number of employees, organizations may also employ a full-time electronic auditor who does nothing but monitor activity logs. More than half of healthcare organizations have hired full-time employees to provide network security (HIMSS, 2015). Additional strategies for securing networks suggested in this most recent HIMSS survey were mock cyberdefense exercises, sharing information between and among healthcare organizations, monitoring vendor intelligence feeds, and subscribing to security alerts and tips from US_CERT (United States Computer Emergency Readiness Team).

## Security Tools

A wide range of tools are available to an organization to protect the organizational network and information. These tools can be either a software solution, such as **antivirus software,** or a hardware tool, such as a proxy server. Such tools are effective only if they are used along with employee awareness training. The 2015 HIMSS Cybersecurity Survey results indicate that an average of 11 different software tools were used by respondents to provide network security, with antivirus technology, firewalls, and data encryption as the most common tools.

For example, email scanning is a commonly used software tool. All incoming email messages are scanned to ensure they do not contain a virus or some other malicious code. This software can find only viruses that are currently known, so it is important that the virus software be set to search for and download updates automatically. Organizations can further protect themselves by training employees to never open an email attachment unless they are expecting the attachment and know the sender. Even IT managers have fallen victim to email viruses that sent infected emails to everyone in their address book. Employees should be taught to protect their organization from new viruses that may not yet be included in their scanning software by never opening an email attachment unless the sender is known and the attachment is expected. Email scanning software and antivirus software should never be turned off, and updates should be installed at least weekly—or, ideally, daily. Software is also available to scan instant messages and to delete automatically any spam email.

Many antivirus and adware software packages are available for fees ranging from free to more than $25 per month (for personal use) to several thousands of dollars per month (to secure an organization's network). The main factors to consider when purchasing antivirus software are its effectiveness (i.e., the number of viruses it has missed), the ease of installation and use, the effectiveness of the updates, and the help and user support available. Numerous websites compare and contrast the most recent antivirus software packages. Be aware, however, that some of these sites also sell antivirus software, so they may present biased information.

Firewalls are another tool used by organizations to protect their corporate networks when they are attached to the Internet. A **firewall** can be either hardware, software, or a combination of both that examines all incoming messages or traffic to the network. The firewall can be set up to allow only messages from known senders into the corporate network. It can also be set up to look at outgoing information from the corporate network. If the message contains some type of corporate secret, the firewall may prevent the message from leaving. In essence, firewalls serve as electronic security guards at the gate of the corporate network.

Proxy servers also protect the organizational network. Proxy servers prevent users from directly accessing the Internet. Instead, users must first request passage from the proxy server. The server looks at the request and makes sure the request is from a legitimate user and that the destination of the request is permissible. For example, organizations can block requests to view a website with the word "sex" in the title or the actual uniform resource locator of a known pornography site. The proxy server can also lend the requesting user a **mask** to use while he or she is surfing the Web. In this way, the corporation protects the identity of its employees. The **proxy server** keeps track of which employees are using which masks and directs the traffic appropriately.

With hacking becoming more common, healthcare organizations must have some type of protection to avoid this invasion. An **intrusion detection system** (both hardware and software) allows an organization to monitor who is using the network and which files that user has accessed. Detection systems can be set up to monitor a single computer or an entire network. Corporations must diligently monitor for unauthorized access of their networks. Anytime someone uses a secured network, a digital footprint of all of the user's travels is left, and this path can be easily tracked by electronic auditing software.

## Offsite Use of Portable Devices

Offsite uses of portable devices, such as laptops, tablets, home computing systems, smartphones, smart devices, and portable data storage devices, can help to streamline the delivery of health care. For example, home health nurses may need to access **electronic protected health information (EPHI)** via a wireless laptop connection during a home visit, or a physician might use a smartphone to get specific patient information related to a prescription refill in response to a patient request. These mobile devices are invaluable to healthcare efficiency and responsiveness to patient need in such cases. At the very least, however, agencies should require data encryption when EPHI is being transmitted over unsecured networks or transported on a mobile device as a way of protecting sensitive information. Hotspots provided by companies, such as coffee shops or restaurants, and by airports are not secured networks. Virtual private networks (VPNs) must be used to ensure that all data transmitted on unsecured networks are encrypted. The user must log into the VPN to reach the organization's network.

Only data essential for the job should be maintained on the mobile device; other nonclinical information, such as Social Security numbers, should never be carried outside the secure network. Some institutions make use of thin clients, which are basic interface portals that do not keep **secure information** stored on them. Essentially, users must log in to the network to get the data they need. Use of thin clients may be problematic in patient care situations where the user cannot access the network easily. For example, some rural areas of the United States do not have wireless or cellular data coverage. In these instances, private health information may need to be stored in a clinician's laptop or tablet. This is comparable to home health nurses carrying paper charts in their cars to make home visits, and it entails the same responsibilities accompanying such use of private information outside the institution's walls.

What happens if one of these devices is lost or stolen? The agency is ultimately responsible for the integrity of the data contained on these devices and is required by HIPAA regulations (U.S. Department of Health and Human Services, 2006) to have policies in place covering such items as appropriate remote use, removal of devices from their usual physical location, and protection of these devices from loss or theft. Simple rules, such as covering laptops left in a car and locking car doors during transport of mobile devices containing EPHI, can help to deter theft. If a device is lost or stolen, the agency must have clear procedures in place to help ensure that sensitive data are not released or used inappropriately. Software packages that provide for physical tracking of the static and mobile computer inventory including laptops, smartphones, and tablets are being used more widely and can assist in the recovery of lost or stolen devices. In addition, some software that allows for remote data deletion (data wipe) in the event of theft or loss of a mobile device can be invaluable to the agency in preventing the release of EPHI.

If a member of an agency is caught accessing EPHI inappropriately or steals a mobile device, the sanctions should be swift and public. Sanctions may range from a warning or suspension with retraining to termination or prosecution, depending on the severity of the security breach. The sanctions must send a clear message to all that protecting EPHI is serious business.

The U.S. Department of Health and Human Services (n.d.) suggests the following strategies for managing remote access:

- Restricting remote access to computers owned or configured by your organization
- Disallowing administrator privileges on remote access computers

---

**BOX 12-3 POKEMON TARGETS HOSPITAL**

Informatics nurse specialists must be aware of the uses of portable devices. In 2016, one hospital in the Pittsburgh area was a site of a popular game, and the administration was upset because it creates a privacy issue for people using their hospital as a search site. This hospital actually contacted the game developer to be removed from their game.

Hospitals must always be concerned about privacy and safety issues within their control, but also be on the alert for those outside their control, such as the Pokemon Go game. Pittsburgh's Action News 4, Marcie Cipriani, reported that Pokemon Go used West Penn Hospital, part of Allegheny Health Network in Pittsburgh, as a real-world location in the game. The game utilizes enhanced reality, which allows players to combine images from the real world with those of the game. The Allegheny Health Network officials stated that the exciting, interactive game created concerns when it brought players inside their hospital. They say hunting Pokemon at the hospital created a patient privacy issue and a safety concern. Administrators warned those who are playing to stay out of their hospitals and contacted the game's developer, who agreed to remove their hospitals from the app. They have asked their employees to be on the lookout for anyone playing the app while they are walking around the hospital and to contact security if they see Pokemon Go players.

Data from Cipriani, M. (2016, July 30). Pokemon Go targets Allegheny Health System hospitals in Pittsburgh. Pittsburgh's Action News 4. Retrieved from http://www.wtae.com /news/pokemon-go-players-not-welcome-at-allegheny-health-network-hospitals/40946828

- Placing restrictions in the VPN and remote access policies
- Configuring the VPN to operate in a "sandbox" or virtual environment that isolates the session from other software running on the remote machine
- Educating users about safe computing practices in remote locations (para. 8)

To protect our patients and their data, nurses must consider the impact of wireless mobile devices (see **Box 12-3**). Data can be stolen by an employee very easily through the use of email or file transfers.

**Malware,** or malicious code that infiltrates a network, can collect easily accessible data. One of the evolving issues is lost or stolen devices that can provide a gateway into a healthcare organization's network and records. When the device is owned by the employee, other issues arise as to how the device is used and secured.

The increase in cloud computing has also challenged our personal and professional security and privacy. Cloud computing refers to storing and accessing data and computer programs on the Internet, rather than the local hard drive of a computer. Common examples of cloud computing for personal use include Google Drive, Apple iCloud, and Amazon. Cloud computing allows for easy syncing of separate devices to promote sharing and collaboration (Griffith, 2016). According to Jansen and Grance (2011), cloud computing "promises to have far reaching effects on the systems and networks of federal agencies and other organizations. Many of the features that make cloud computing attractive, however, can also be at odds with traditional security models and controls" (p. vi). Healthcare organizations are moving to the cloud because cloud computing tends to be cheaper and faster, offers more flexibility for work location, provides nearly immediate disaster recovery, supports collaboration, provides security, and offers frequent software updates (Salesforce UK, 2015). However, there are important security concerns related to cloud computing in health care. Guccione (2015) offers these important considerations for maintaining security in a cloud environment:

> First, a cloud service should be have client-side encryption of data, which both protects files on the local hard drive as well as in the cloud. Second, a secure cloud service should offer multi-factor authentication to add an extra layer of access control for all users. Finally, a secure cloud provider should either provide data loss prevention tools to protect the stored data or allow an organization to extend its DLP protocols to the cloud. In both cases, the organization is alerted immediately the moment a user attempts to send sensitive files to an outside source. (para. 5)

It is clear that healthcare organizations need to be extra vigilant about their data security when using cloud computing. However, as we emphasized several times in this chapter, employee training on security measures may be the most important defense, because "the latest techniques for cyber theft are much less about breaching networks from the outside, such as through the cloud service, than they are exploiting holes inside an organization, particularly from careless employees" (Guccione, 2015, para. 9).

## Summary

Technology changes so quickly that even the most diligent user will likely encounter a situation that could constitute a threat to his or her network. Organizations must provide their users with the proper training to help them avoid known threats and—more importantly—be able to discern a possible new threat. Consider that 10 years ago wireless networks were the exception to the rule, where today access to wireless networks is almost taken for granted. How will computer networks be accessed 10 years from now? The most important concept to remember from this chapter is that the only completely safe network is one that is turned off. **Network accessibility** and **network availability** are necessary evils that pose security risks. The information must be available to be accessed, yet remain secured from hackers, unauthorized users, and any other potential security breaches. As the cloud expands, so do the concerns over security and privacy. In an ideal world, everyone would understand the potential threats to **network security** and would diligently monitor and implement tools to prevent unauthorized access of their networks, data, and information.

### THOUGHT-PROVOKING QUESTIONS

1. Sue is a chronic obstructive pulmonary disorder clinic nurse enrolled in a master's education program. She is interested in writing a paper on the factors that are associated with poor compliance with medical regimens and associated repeat hospitalization of chronic obstructive pulmonary disorder patients. She downloads patient information from the clinic database to a thumb drive that she later accesses on her home computer. Sue understands rules about privacy of information and believes that because she is a nurse and needs this information for a graduate school assignment, she is entitled to the information. Is Sue correct in her thinking? Describe why she is or is not correct.

2. The nursing education department of a large hospital system has been centralized; as a consequence, the nurse educators are no longer assigned to one hospital but must now travel among all of the hospitals. They use their smartphones to interact and share data and information. What are the first steps you would take to secure these transactions? Describe why each step is necessary.

3. Research cloud computing in relation to health care. What are the major security and privacy challenges? Please choose three and describe them in detail.

# References

Caldwell, T. (2011). Ethical hackers: Putting on the white hat. *Network Security, 2011*(7), 10–13. doi:10.1016/S1353-4858(11)70075-7

Degaspari, J. (2010). Staying ahead of the curve on data security. *Healthcare Informatics, 27*(10), 32–36.

Goldsborough, R. (2016). Protecting yourself from ransomware. *Teacher Librarian, 43*(4), 70–71.

Griffith, E. (2016). What is cloud computing? *PCMag.* Retrieved from http://www.pcmag.com /article2/0,2817,2372163,00.asp

Greenberg, A. (2015). Human error cited as leading contributor to breaches, study shows. *SC Magazine.* Retrieved from http://www.scmagazine.com/study-find-carelessness-among -top-human-errors-affecting-security/article/406876

Guccione, D. (2015). Is the cloud safe for healthcare? *Healthcare Informatics.* Retrieved from http://www.healthcare-informatics.com/article/cloud-safe-healthcare

Health Information and Management Systems Society (HIMSS). (2015) 2015 HIMSS Cybersecurity Survey. Retrieved from http://www.himss.org/2015-cybersecurity-survey /executive-summary

Jansen, W., & Grance, T. (2011). National Institute of Standards and Technology (NIST): Guidelines on security and privacy in public cloud computing. Retrieved from https:// cloudsecurityalliance.org/wp-content/uploads/2011/07/NIST-Draft-SP-800-144_cloud -computing.pdf

Mowry, M., & Oakes, R. (n.d.). Not too tight, not too loose. *Healthcare Informatics, Healthcare IT Leadership, Vision & Strategy.* Retrieved from http://www.healthcare -informatics.com/article/not-too-tight-not-too-loose

Ponemon Institute. (2015, May). *Fifth annual benchmark study on privacy & security of healthcare data.* Retrieved from http://media.scmagazine.com/documents/121/healthcare _privacy_security_be_30019.pdf

Salesforce UK. (2015). Why move to the cloud? Ten benefits of cloud computing. Retrieved from https://www.salesforce.com/uk/blog/2015/11/why-move-to-the-cloud-10-benefits-of -cloud-computing.html

Sullivan, T. (2012). Government health IT: DHS lists top 5 mobile medical device security risks. Retrieved from http://www.govhealthit.com/news/dhs-lists-top-5-mobile-device-security-risks

TechTarget (n.d.). Social engineering. Retrieved from http://searchsecurity.techtarget.com /definition/social-engineering

U.S. Department of Health and Human Services. (2006). HIPAA security guidance. Retrieved from https://www.hhs.gov/sites/default/files/ocr/privacy/hipaa/administrative/securityrule /remoteuse.pdf

U.S. Department of Health and Human Services. (n.d.). Implement privacy and security protection measures. Retrieved from http://www.hrsa.gov/healthit/toolbox/healthitimplementation /implementationtopics/ensureprivacysecurity/ensureprivacysecurity_9.html

## Objectives

1. Provide an overview of the purpose of conducting workflow analysis and design.

2. Deliver specific instructions on workflow analysis and redesign techniques.

3. Cite measures of efficiency and effectiveness that can be applied to redesign efforts.

4. Explore meaningful use and beyond with the Medicare Access and Summary CHIP Reauthorization Act.

## Key Terms

- » Alternative Payment Models (APMs)
- » American Recovery and Reinvestment Act (ARRA)
- » Bar-code medication administration (BCMA)
- » Clinical transformation
- » Computerized provider order entry (CPOE)
- » Electronic health records (EHRs)
- » Events
- » Health information exchange (HIE)
- » Health information technology (HIT)
- » Information systems
- » Interactions
- » Lean
- » Meaningful use (MU)
- » Medical home models
- » Medicare Access and CHIP Reauthorization Act of 2015 (MACRA)
- » Merit-Based Incentive Payment System (MIPS)
- » Metrics
- » Process analysis
- » Process map
- » Process owners
- » Qualified Clinical Data Registries (QCDRs)
- » Quality
- » Quality payment program (QPP)
- » Six Sigma
- » Tasks
- » Work process
- » Workflow
- » Workflow analysis

# CHAPTER 13

# Workflow and Beyond Meaningful Use

Dee McGonigle, Kathleen Mastrian, and Denise Hammel-Jones

## Introduction

The healthcare environment has grown more complex and continues to evolve every day. Unfortunately, the complexities that help clinicians to deliver better care and improve patient outcomes also take a toll on the clinicians themselves. This toll is exemplified through hours spent learning new technology, loss in productivity as the user adjusts and adapts to new technology, and unintended workflow consequences from the use of technology.

Despite the perceived negative downstream effects to end users and patients as a result of technology, this very same technology can improve efficiency and yield a leaner healthcare environment. The intent of this chapter is to outline the driving forces that create the need to redesign workflow as well as to elucidate what the nurse needs to know about how to conduct workflow redesign, measure the impact of workflow changes, and assess the impact of meaningful use.

## Workflow Analysis Purpose

According to the American Association for Justice (2016),

> Research has confirmed that 440,000 people die every year because of preventable medical errors. That is equivalent to almost the entire population of Atlanta, Georgia dying from a medical error each year. Preventable medical errors are the third leading cause of death in the United States and cost our country tens of billions of dollars a year. (para. 1)

Not only is there an impact on patients and their families from these errors, but there is also a significant financial impact on healthcare organizations. Clearly, we must minimize these errors, and one of the most important tools for this purpose is the use of electronic health records and **information systems** to provide point-of-care decision support and automation. The key point is that most of these errors are preventable and we must find ways to prevent them.

Technology can provide a mechanism to improve care delivery and create a safer patient environment, provided it is implemented appropriately and considers the surrounding workflow. In an important article by Campbell, Guappone, Sittig, Dykstra, and Ash (2009), the authors suggested that technology implemented without consideration of workflow can provide greater patient safety concerns than no technology at all. **Computerized provider order entry (CPOE)** causes us to focus more specifically on workflow considerations. These workflow implications are referred to as the unintended consequences of CPOE implementation; they are just some of the effects of poorly implemented technology. The Healthcare Information Management Systems Society (HIMSS, 2010) ME-PI Toolkit addressed workflow redesign and considered why it is so critical to successful technology implementations. Thompson, Kell, Shetty, and Banerjee (2016) stated "By partnering clinicians with informaticists we strove to leverage the power of the electronic medical record (EMR) to reduce heart failure readmissions and improve patient transitions back to the community" (p. 380). They concluded that "Partnering with clinical informatics enabled the multidisciplinary team to leverage the power of the EMR in supporting and tracking new clinical workflows that impact patient outcomes" (p. 380). This multidisciplinary team believed that their success could reshape how healthcare providers facilitate patient discharge and the transition home. Leveraging the multidisciplinary team and EMR could provide a model for patient-centered and cost-effective care that could extend beyond their patients with heart failure.

Technology is recognized to have a potentially positive effect on patient outcomes. Nevertheless, even with the promise of improving how care is delivered, adoption of technology has been slow. The cost of technology solutions such as CPOE, **barcode medication administration (BCMA)**, and **electronic health records (EHRs)** remain staggeringly high. The cost of technology, coupled with the lengthy timelines required to develop and implement such technology, has put this endeavor out of reach for many healthcare organizations. In addition, upgrades or enhancements to the technology are often necessary either mid-implementation or shortly after a launch, leaving little time to focus efforts on the optimization of the technology within the current workflow. Furthermore, the existence of technology does not in itself guarantee that it will be used in a manner that promotes better outcomes for patients.

Given the sluggish adoption of technology, in 2009 the U.S. government took an unprecedented step when it formally recognized the importance of **health information technology (HIT)** for patient care outcomes. As a result of the provisions of **American Recovery and Reinvestment Act (ARRA)**, healthcare organizations can qualify for financial incentives based on the level of meaningful use achieved. **Meaningful use (MU)** refers to the rules and regulations established by the ARRA. The three stages of MU were part of an EHR incentive program. During stage 1, the focus was on data capturing and sharing. Stage 2 focused on advanced clinical processes, and stage 3 sought to improve outcomes. Stage 1 was initiated during 2011–2012, stage 2 began in 2014, and stage 3 was to be launched in 2016/2017 and was intended

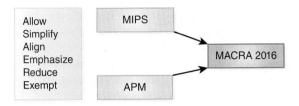

**Figure 13-1** MACRA

to last through 2019 and beyond (Centers for Medicare & Medicaid Services [CMS], 2016a). However, with the new goal of paying for value and better care, the **Medicare Access and CHIP Reauthorization Act of 2015 (MACRA)** reformed Medicare payments by making changes that created a **quality payment program (QPP)** to replace the hodgepodge system of Medicare reporting programs (CMS, 2016b; see **Figure 13-1**). The MACRA QPP has two paths—**Merit-Based Incentive Payment System (MIPS)** or **Alternative Payment Models (APMs)**—that will be in effect through 2021 and beyond (CMS, 2016b). The MACRA requirements for the measure development plan consist of the following:

- Multipayer applicability
- Coordination and sharing across measure developers
- Clinical practice guidelines
- Evidence base for non-endorsed measures
- Gap analysis
- Quality domains and priorities
- Applicability of measures across healthcare settings
- Clinical practice improvement activities
- Considerations for electronic specifications and **Qualified Clinical Data Registries (QCDRs)** (CMS, 2016c, p. 16).

According to Hagland (2016), MACRA, MIPS, and APMs will:

- Allow physicians and other clinicians to choose to select the measures that reflect how technology best suits their day-to-day practice
- Simplify the process for achievement and provide multiple paths for success
- Align with the Office for the National Coordinator for Health Information Technology's 2015 edition Health IT Certification Criteria
- Emphasize interoperability, information exchange, and security measures and give patients access to their information through APIs (application program interfaces)
- Reduce the number of measures to an all-time low of 11 measures, down from 18 measures, and no longer require reporting on the clinical decision support and CPOE measures
- Exempt certain physicians from reporting when EHR technology is less applicable to their practice and allow physicians to report as a group (para. 4).

For an organization that seeks to meet these measures, the data to support these measures must be gathered and reported on electronically—necessitating the use of technology in all patient care areas. The successful implementation of the measurement development plan "depends on a successful partnership with patients, frontline clinicians, and professional organizations and collaboration with other diverse stakeholders to develop measures that are meaningful to patients and clinicians and can be used across payers and health care settings" (CMS, 2016c, p. 64). Many of the **quality** reporting measures rely on nursing and medical documentation. Most healthcare personnel already use EHRs, but MACRA measures will push healthcare organizations to reexamine the use of clinical technologies within their organization and approach implementations in a new way.

Not only is there a potential for patient safety and quality issues to arise from technology implementations that do not address workflow, but a financial impact to the organization is possible as well. All organizations, regardless of their industry, must operate efficiently to maintain profits and continue to provide services to their customers. For hospitals, which normally have significantly smaller profit margins than other organizations, the need to maintain efficient and effective care is essential for survival. Given that hospital profit margins are diminishing, never has there been a more crucial time to examine the costs of errors and poorly designed workflows and the financial burden they present to an organization than now. Moreover, what are the costs to an organization that fails to address the integration of technology? This is an area where few supporting data exist to substantiate the claim that technology without workflow considerations can, in fact, impact the bottom line.

Today, many healthcare organizations are experiencing the effects of poorly implemented clinical technology solutions. These effects may be manifested in the form of redundant documentation, non-value-added steps, and additional time spent at the computer rather than in direct care delivery. For example, Gugerty et al. (2007) studied the challenges and opportunities in nursing documentation and determined that it was possible to decrease the time a nurse spends documenting per shift by 25%. Technology ought not to be implemented for the sake of automation unless it promises to deliver gains in patient outcomes and proper workflow. In fact, the cost to organizations for duplicate/redundant documentation by nursing can range from $6,500 to $13,000 per nurse, per year (Clancy, Delaney, Morrison, & Gunn, 2006). Stokowski (2013) found other issues, such as systems that are slow, freeze, lose data, and "don't dump data from monitors and screening devices into the EHR in real time" slowing the documentation process and increasing the amount of time the nurse must spend on the computer and not in direct patient care (p. 9).

Examining the workflow surrounding the use of technology enables better use of the technology and more efficient work. It also promotes safer patient care delivery. The need to focus on workflow and technology is attracting increasing recognition, although there remains a dearth of literature that addresses the importance of this area. As more organizations work to achieve a level of technology adoption that will enable them to meet MACRA measures and receive financial payments, we will likely see more attention paid to the area of workflow design and, therefore, a greater body of research and evidence (AHRQ, n.d.; Qualis Health, 2011; Yuan, Finley, Long, Mills, & Johnson, 2013).

# Workflow and Technology

**Workflow** is a term used to describe the action or execution of a series of tasks in a prescribed sequence. Another definition of workflow is a progression of steps (**tasks, events, interactions**) that constitute a **work process**, involve two or more persons, and create or add value to the organization's activities. In a sequential workflow, each step depends on the occurrence of the previous step; in a parallel workflow, two or more steps can occur concurrently. The term *workflow* is sometimes used interchangeably with *process* or *process flows*, particularly in the context of implementations. Observation and documentation of workflow to better understand what is happening in the current environment and how it can be altered is referred to as process or **workflow analysis**. A typical output of workflow analysis is a visual depiction of the process, called a **process map**. The process map ranges from simplistic to fairly complex and provides an excellent tool to identify specific steps. It also can provide a vehicle for communication and a tool upon which to build educational materials as well as policies and procedures.

One school of thought suggests that technology should be designed to meet the needs of clinical workflow (Yuan et al., 2013). This model implies that system analysts have a high degree of control over screen layout and data capture. It also implies that technology is malleable enough to allow for the flexibility to adapt to a variety of workflow scenarios. Lessons learned from more than three decades of clinical technology implementations suggest that clinical technologies still have a long way to go on the road to maturity to allow this to be possible. The second and probably most prevalent thought process is that workflow should be adapted to the use of technology. Today, this is by far the most commonly used model given the progress of clinical technology. Bucur et al. (2016) developed clinical models to support clinical decision making that were inserted into the workflow models. This system integrates a workflow suite and functionality for the storage, management, and execution of clinical workflows and for the storage of traces of execution. The knowledge models are integrated and run from the workflow to support decisions at the right point in the clinical process (Bucur et al., p. 152). The ability to track and assess decision making throughout a clinical course of care for a patient will enhance our knowledge and improve patient care.

A concept that has gained popularity in recent years relative to workflow redesign is clinical transformation. **Clinical transformation** is the complete alteration of the clinical environment and, therefore, this term should be used cautiously to describe redesign efforts. Earl, Sampler, and Sghort (1995) define transformation as "a radical change approach that produces a more responsive organization that is more capable of performing in unstable and changing environments that organizations continue to be faced with" (p. 31). Many workflow redesign efforts are focused on relatively small changes and not the widespread change that accompanies transformational activities. Moreover, clinical transformation would imply that the manner in which work is carried out and the outcomes achieved are completely different from the prior state—which is not always true when the change simply involves implementing technology. Technology can be used to launch or in conjunction with a clinical transformation initiative, although the implementation of technology alone is not perceived as transformational.

Before undertaking transformative initiatives, the following guidelines should be understood:

- Leadership must take the lead and create a case for transformation.
- Establish a vision for the end point.
- Allow those persons with specific expertise to provide the details.
- Think about the most optimal experience for both the patient and the clinician.
- Do not replicate the current state.
- Focus on those initiatives that offer the greatest value to the organization.
- Recognize that small gains have no real impact on transformation.

## Optimization

Most of what has been and will be discussed in this chapter is related to workflow analysis in conjunction with technology implementations. Nevertheless, not all workflow analysis and redesign occurs prior to the implementation of technology. Some analysis and redesign efforts may occur weeks, months, or even years following the implementation. When workflow analysis occurs postimplementation, it is often referred to as optimization. Optimization is the process of moving conditions past their current state and into more efficient and effective method of performing tasks. *Merriam-Webster Online Dictionary* (2016) considered optimization to be the act, process, or methodology of making something (as a design, system, or decision) as fully perfect, functional, or effective as possible. Some organizations will routinely engage in optimization efforts following an implementation, whereas other organizations may undertake this activity in response to clinician concerns or marked change in operational performance.

Furthermore, workflow analysis can be conducted either as a stand-alone effort or as part of an operational improvement event. When the process is addressed alone, the effort is termed process improvement. Nursing informatics professionals should always be included in these activities to represent the needs of clinicians and to serve as a liaison for technological solutions to process problems. Additionally, informaticists will likely become increasingly operationally focused and will need to transform their role accordingly to address workflow in an overall capacity as well as respective to technology. As mentioned earlier, hospitals tend to operate with smaller profit margins than other industries and these profits will likely continue to diminish, forcing organizations to work smarter, not harder—and to use technology to accomplish this goal.

If optimization efforts are undertaken, the need to revisit workflow design should not be considered a flaw in the implementation approach. Even a well-designed future-state workflow during a technology implementation must be reexamined postimplementation to ensure that what was projected about the future state remains valid and to incorporate any additional workflow elements into the process redesign.

Exploring the topic of workflow analysis with regard to clinical technology implementation will yield considerably fewer literature results than searching for other topical areas of implementation. More research is needed in the area of the financial implications of workflow inefficiencies and their impact on patient care.

**CASE STUDY**

In my experience consulting, I have seen several examples of organizations that engage in the printing of paper reports that replicate information that has been entered and is available with the electronic health record. These reports are often reviewed, signed, and acted on, instead of using the electronic information. Despite the knowledge that the information contained in these reports was outdated the moment the report was printed and that the very nature of using the report for workflow is an inefficient practice, this method of clinical workflow remains prevalent in many hospitals across the United States.

There is an underlying fear that drives the decisions to mold a paper-based workflow around clinical technology. There is also a lack of the appropriate amount of integration that would otherwise allow this information to be available in an electronic form.

Time studies require an investment of resources and may be subject to patient privacy issues as well as the challenges of capturing time measurements on processes that are not exactly replicable. Another confounding factor affecting the quality and quantity of workflow research is the lack of standardized terminology for this area. A comprehensive literature search was conducted and published through the Agency for Healthcare Quality and Research (AHRQ) in 2008 as an evidence-based handbook for nurses; this literature search yielded findings indicating that a lack of standardized terminology in the area of workflow and publications on this topic have made it a difficult topic to support through research findings.

What all organizations ultimately strive for is efficient and effective delivery of patient care. The terms *efficient* and *effective* are widely known in quality areas or Six Sigma and Lean departments, but are not necessarily known or used in informatics. Effective delivery of care or workflow suggests that the process or end product is in the most desirable state. An efficient delivery of care or workflow would mean that little waste—that is, unnecessary motion, transportation, over-processing, or defects—was incurred. Health systems such as Virginia Mason University Medical Center, among others, have experienced significant quality and cost gains from the widespread implementation of Lean development throughout their organization.

# Workflow Analysis and Informatics Practice

The American Nurses Association (ANA), in *Nursing Informatics: Scope and Standards of Practice* (2015), defined functional areas of practice for the informatics nurse specialist (INS). The functional area of analysis identified the specific functional qualities related to workflow analysis. Particularly, the ANA indicated that the INS should develop techniques necessary to assess and improve human–computer interaction. Workflow analysis, however, is not relevant solely to analysis, but rather is part of every functional area the INS engages in. The functional areas covered by consultants, researchers, and other areas need to understand workflow and appreciate how lack of efficient workflow affects patient care.

A critical aspect of the informatics role is workflow design. Nursing informatics is uniquely positioned to engage in the analysis and redesign of processes and tasks surrounding the use of technology. The ANA (2015) cites workflow redesign as one of the fundamental skills sets that make up the discipline of this specialty. Moreover, workflow analysis should be part of every technology implementation, and the role of the informaticist within this team is to direct others in the execution of this task or to perform the task directly.

Unfortunately, many nurses find themselves in an informatics capacity without sufficient preparation for a **process analysis** role. One area of practice that is particularly susceptible to inadequate preparation is the ability to facilitate process analysis. Workflow analysis requires careful attention to detail and the ability to moderate group discussions, organize concepts, and generate solutions. These skills can be acquired through a formal academic informatics program or through courses that teach the discipline of Six Sigma or Lean, by example. Regardless of where these skills are acquired, it is important to understand that they are now and will continue to remain a vital aspect of the informatics role.

Some organizations have felt strongly enough about the need for workflow analysis that departments have been created to address this very need. Whether the department carries the name of clinical excellence, organizational effectiveness, or Six Sigma/Lean, it is critical to recognize the value this group can offer technology implementations and clinicians.

As we examine how workflow analysis is conducted, note that while the nursing informaticist is an essential member of the team to participate in or enable workflow analysis, a team dedicated to this effort is necessary for its success.

## Building the Design Team

The workflow redesign team is an interdisciplinary team consisting of "process owners." **Process owners** are those persons who directly engage in the workflow to be analyzed and redesigned. These individuals can speak about the intricacy of process, including process variations from the norm. When constructing the team, it is important to include individuals who are able to contribute information about the exact current-state workflow and offer suggestions for future-state improvement. Members of the workflow redesign team should also have the authority to make decisions about how the process should be redesigned. This authority is sometimes issued by managers, or it could come from participation of the managers directly. Such a careful blend of decision makers and "process owners" can be difficult to assemble but is critical for forming the team and enabling them for success. Often, individuals at the manager level will want to participate exclusively in the redesign process. While having management participate provides the advantage of having decision makers and management-level buy-in, these individuals may also make erroneous assumptions about how the process should be versus how the process is truly occurring. Conversely, including only process owners who do not possess the authority to make decisions can slow down the work of the team while decisions are made outside the group sessions.

Team focus needs to be addressed at the outset of the team's assembly. Early on, the team should decide which workflow will be examined to avoid confusion or spending time unnecessarily on workflow that does not ultimately matter to the outcome. In the early stages of workflow redesign, the team should define the beginning and end of a process and a few high-level steps of the process. Avoid focusing on process steps in great detail in the beginning, as the conversation can get sidetracked or team members may get bogged down by focusing on details and not move along at a good pace. Six Sigma expert George Eckes uses the phrase "Stay as high as you can as long as you can"—a good catch phrase to remember to keep the team focused and at a high level. The pace at which any implementation team progresses ultimately affects the overall timeline of a project; therefore, focus and speed are skills that the informatics expert should develop and use throughout every initiative, but particularly when addressing workflow redesign.

The workflow redesign team will develop a detailed process map after agreement is reached on the current-state process's beginning and end points, and a high-level map depicting the major process steps is finalized. Because workflow crosses many different care providers, it may be useful to construct the process map using a swim-lane technique (Figure 13-2). A swim-lane technique uses categories such as functional workgroups and roles to visually depict groups of work and to indicate who performs the work. The resulting map shows how workflow and data transition to clinicians and can demonstrate areas of potential process and information breakdowns.

It may take several sessions of analysis to complete a process map, as details are uncovered and workarounds discussed. There is a tendency for individuals who participate in process redesign sessions to describe workflow as they believe it to be occurring, rather than not how it really is. The informatics expert and/or the process team facilitator should determine what is really happening, however, and capture that information accurately. Regardless of whether a swim-lane or simplistic process map design is used, the goal is to capture enough details to accurately portray the process as it is happening today.

Other techniques (aside from process mapping) may be used to help the team understand the workflow as it exists in the current state. The future-state workflow planning will be only as good as the reliability of the current state; thus it is crucial to undertake whatever other actions are needed to better understand what is happening in the current state. Observation, interviews, and process or waste walks are also helpful in understanding the current state.

## Value Added Versus Non–Value Added

Beyond analysis of tasks, current-state mapping provides the opportunity for the process redesign team to distinguish between value-added and non-value-added activities. A value-added activity or step is one that ultimately brings the process closer to completion or changes the product or service for the better. An example of a value-added step would be placing a name tag on a specimen sample. The name tag is necessary for the laboratory personnel to identify the specimen and, therefore, its placement is an essential or value-added step in the process. Some steps in a process do not necessarily add value but are necessary for regulatory or compliance reasons. These steps are still considered necessary and need to be included in the future process. A non-value-added step, in contrast, does not alter the outcome of a process or product. Activities such as handling, moving, and holding are not considered value-added steps and should be evaluated during workflow analysis. Manipulating papers, moving through computer screens, and walking or transporting items are all considered non-value-added activities.

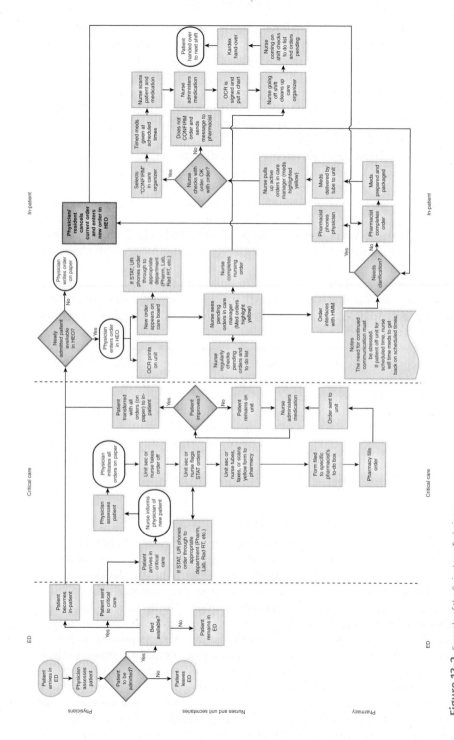

**Figure 13-2**  Example of the Swim Lane Technique

Courtesy of Greencastle Associates Consulting and Atlantic Health. Reprinted by permission.

The five whys represent one technique to drive the team toward identifying value-added versus non-value-added steps. The process redesign facilitator will query the group about why a specific task is done or done in a particular way through a series of questions asking "why?" The goal is to uncover tasks that came about due to workarounds or for other unsubstantiated reasons. Tasks that are considered non–value added and are not necessary for the purpose of compliance or regulatory reasons should be eliminated from the future-state process. The team's purpose in re-designing workflow is to eliminate steps in a process that do not add value to the end state or that create waste by their very nature.

## Waste

A key underpinning of the Lean philosophy is the removal of waste activities from workflow. Waste is classified as unnecessary activities or an excess of products to per-form tasks. The seven categories listed here are the most widely recognized forms of waste:

- Overproduction: pace is faster than necessary to support the process
- Waiting
- Transport
- Inappropriate processing: over-processing
- Unnecessary inventory: excess stock
- Unnecessary motion: bending, lifting, moving, and so on
- Defects: reproduction

## Variation

The nature of the work situation for the nurse is one of frequent interruptions caus-ing the workflow to be disrupted and increasing the chance of error (Yuan et al., 2013). Variation in workflow is considered the enemy of all good processes and, therefore, should be eliminated when possible. Variation occurs when workers per-form the same function in different ways. It usually arises because of flaws in the way a process was originally designed, lack of knowledge about the process, or in-ability to execute a process as originally designed due to disruption or disturbances in the workflow. Examining the process as it exists today will help with identifying variation. A brief statement about variation that cannot be eliminated: Processes that involve highly customized products or services are generally not conducive to stan-dardization and the elimination of variation inherent to the process.

Some argue that delivery of care is subject to variation owing to its very nature and the individual needs of patients. There is little doubt that each patient's care should be tailored to meet his or her specific needs. Nevertheless, delivery of care in-volves some common processes that can be standardized and improved upon without jeopardizing care.

## Transitioning to the Future State

Following redesign efforts, regardless of whether they occurred during or after an im-plementation or as a stand-alone process improvement event, steps must be taken to ensure that change takes hold and the new workflow continues after the support team has disbanded. Management support and involvement during the transition phase is essential, as management will be necessary to enforce new workflow procedures and further define/refine roles and responsibilities. Documentation of the future-state workflow should have occurred during the redesign effort but is not completely finished until after the redesign is complete and the workflow has become operational. Policies and procedures are addressed and rewritten to encompass the changes to workflows and role assignments. Help desk, system analyst, nursing education, and other support personnel need to be educated about the workflow specifics as part of the postimprovement effort. It is considered good practice to involve the operational staff in the future process discussions and planning so as to incorporate specifics of these areas and ensure the buy-in of the staff.

When workflow changes begin to fail and workarounds develop, they signal that something is flawed about the way in which the new process was constructed and needs to be evaluated further. The workflow redesign team is then brought together to review and, if necessary, redesign the process.

The future state is constructed with the best possible knowledge of how the process will ideally work. To move from the current state to the future state, gap analysis is necessary. Gap analysis zeros in on the major areas most affected by the change—namely, technology. What often happens in redesign efforts is an exact or near-exact replication of the current state using automation. The gap analysis discussion should generate ideas from the group about how best to utilize the technology to transform practice. A prudent step is to consider having legal and risk representatives at the table when initiating future-state discussions to identify the parameters within which the group should work; nevertheless, the group should not assume the existing parameters are its only boundaries.

Future-state process maps become the basis of educational materials for end users, communication tools for the project team, and the foundation of new policies and procedures. Simplified process maps provide an excellent schematic for communicating change to others.

## Informatics as a Change Agent

Technology implementations represent a significant change for clinicians, as does the workflow redesign that accompanies adoption of technology. Often the degree of change and its impact are underappreciated and unaccounted for by leadership and staff alike. A typical response to change is anger, frustration, and a refusal to accept the proposed change. All of these responses should be expected and need to be accounted for; thus a plan to address the emotional side of change is developed early on. Every workflow redesign effort should begin with a change management plan (**Figure 13-3**). Engagement of the end user is a critical aspect of change management and, therefore, technology adoption. Without end-user involvement, change is resisted and efforts are subject to failure. Users may be engaged and brought into the prospective change through question-and-answer forums, technology demonstrations, and frequent communications regarding change, and as department-specific representatives in working meetings.

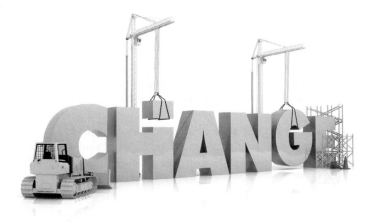

**Figure 13-3**  Change Management
© Digital Storm/Shutterstock

Many change theories have been developed. No matter which change theory is adopted by the informatics specialist, however, communication, planning, and support are key factors in any change management strategy. Informaticists should become knowledgeable about at least one change theory and use this knowledge as the basis for change management planning as part of every effort. John Kotter (1996), one of the most widely recognized change theorists, suggested the following conditions must be addressed to deal with change in an organization:

- Education and communication
- Participation and involvement
- Facilitation and support
- Negotiation and agreement
- Manipulation and co-optation
- Explicit and implicit coercion

In the HIMSS (2015) Nursing Informatics Impact survey, nursing informaticists were identified as the most significant resource in a project team that influences adoption and change management. Nurses bring to such teams their ability to interact with various clinicians, their knowledge of clinical practice, and their ability to empathize with the clinicians as they experience the impact of workflow change. These innate skills differentiate the nursing informaticist from other members of the implementation team and are highly desirable in the informatics community.

Nevertheless, no matter which change management techniques are employed by the informatics specialist and the project team, adoption of technology and workflow may be slow to evolve. Change is often a slow process that requires continual positive reinforcement and involvement of supporting resources. Failure to achieve strong adoption results early on is not necessarily a failure of the methods utilized, but rather may be due to other factors not entirely within the control of the informaticist.

Perhaps a complete alteration in behavior is not possible, but modifications to behaviors needed to support a desired outcome can be realized. This situation is analogous to the individual who stops smoking; the desire for the cigarette remains, but the behavior has been modified to no longer sustain smoking. To manage change in an organization, nurses must modify behavior to produce the intended outcome.

Change takes hold when strong leadership support exists. This support manifests itself as a visible presence to staff, clear and concise communications, an unwavering position, and an open door policy to field concerns about change. Too often, leadership gives verbal endorsement of change and then fails to follow through with these actions or withdraws support when the going gets tough. Inevitability, if leadership wavers, so too will staff.

## Measuring the Results

**Metrics** provide understanding about the performance of a process or function. Typically within clinical technology projects, we identify and collect specific metrics about the performance of the technology or metrics that capture the level of participation or adoption. Equally important is the need for process performance metrics. Process metrics are collected at the initial stage of project or problem identification. Current-state metrics are then benchmarked against internal indicators. When there are no internal indicators to benchmark against, a suitable course of action is to benchmark against an external source such as a similar business practice within a different industry. Consider examining the hotel room change-over strategy or the customer service approach of Walt Disney Company or Ritz Carlton hotels, for example, to determine suitable metrics for a particular project or focus area.

The right workflow complement will provide the organization with the data it needs to understand operational and clinical performance. This area is highlighted through the need for healthcare organizations to capture MACRA measures. Good metrics should tell the story of accomplishment. The presence of technology alone does not guarantee an organization's ability to capture and report on these measures without also addressing the surrounding workflow. Metrics should focus on the variables of time, quality, and costs. **Table 13-1** provides examples of relevant metrics.

MACRA highlights the need for healthcare organizations to collect information that represents the impact of technology on patient outcomes. Furthermore, data are necessary to demonstrate how a process is performing in its current state. In spite of the MACRA mandates, the need to collect data to demonstrate improvement in workflow— though it remains strong—is all too often absent in implementation or redesign efforts. A team cannot demonstrate improvements to an existing

Table 13-1 Examples of Metrics

| Turnaround times | Cycle times | Throughput |
|---|---|---|
| Change-over time | Set-up time | System availability |
| Patient satisfaction | Employee satisfaction | |

process without collecting information about how the process is performing today. Current-state measures also help the process team validate that the correct area for improvement was identified. Once a process improvement effort is over and the new solution has been implemented, postimprovement measures should be gathered to demonstrate progress.

In some organizations, the informatics professional reports to the director of operations, the chief information officer, or the chief operations officer. In this relationship, the need to demonstrate operational measures is even stronger. Operational measures such as turnaround times, throughput, and equipment or technology availability are some of the measures captured.

## Future Directions

Workflow analysis is not an optional part of clinical implementations, but rather a necessity for safe patient care supported by technology. The ultimate goal of workflow analysis is not to "pave the cow path," but rather to create a future-state solution that maximizes the use of technology and eliminates non-value-added activities. Although many tools to accomplish workflow redesign are available, the best method is the one that complements the organization and supports the work of clinicians. Redesigning how people do work will evidentially create change; thus the nursing informaticist will need to apply change management principles for the new way of doing things to take hold.

Workflow analysis has been described in this chapter within the context of the most widely accepted tools that are fundamentally linked to the concepts of Six Sigma/Lean. Other methods of workflow analysis exist and may become commonly used to assess clinical workflow. An example of an alternative workflow analysis tool is the use of radio frequency badges to detect movement within a defined clinical area. Clinician and patient movements may be tracked using these devices, and corresponding actions may be documented, painting a picture of the workflow for a specific area (Vankipuram, 2010).

Another example of a workflow analysis tool involves the use of modeling software. An application such as ProModel provides images of the clinical work area where clinician workflows can be plotted out and reconfigured to best suit the needs of a specific area. Simulation applications enable decision makers to visualize realistic scenarios and draw conclusions about how to leverage resources, implement technology, and improve performance. Other vendors that offer simulation applications include Maya and Autodesk.

Healthcare organizations need to consider how other industries have analyzed and addressed workflow to streamline business practices and improve quality outputs to glean best practices that might be incorporated into the healthcare industry's own clinical and business approaches. First, however, each healthcare organization must step outside itself and recognize that not all aspects of patient care are unique; consequently, many aspects of care can be subjected to standardization. Many models of workflow redesign from manufacturing and the service sector can be extrapolated to health care. The healthcare industry is facing difficult economic times and can benefit from performance improvement strategies used in other industries.

Although workflow analysis principles have been described within the context of acute and ambulatory care in this chapter, the need to perform process analysis on a macro level will expand as more organizations move forward with health information exchanges and **medical home models**. A **health information exchange (HIE)** requires the nursing informaticist to visualize how patients move through the entire continuum of care and not just a specific patient care area.

Technology initiatives will become increasingly complex in the future. In turn, nursing informaticists will need greater preparation in the area of process analysis and improvement techniques to meet the growing challenges that technology brings and the operational performance demands of fiscally impaired healthcare organizations.

# Summary

Meaningful use (MU) reflected the rules and regulations arising from ARRA. MACRA has changed the game and how payment will be determined. EHR adoptions "represent a small step rather than a giant leap forward" (Murphy, 2013, para. 1). Workflows integrating technology provide the healthcare professional with the data necessary to make informed decisions. This quality data must be collected and captured to meet MACRA measures. Nurses must be involved in "meaningful data collection and reporting. Documentation by nurses can tell what's going on with the patient beyond physical exams, test results, and procedures" (Daley, 2013, para. 5).

Workflow redesign is a critical aspect of technology implementation. When done well, it yields technology that is more likely to achieve the intended patient outcomes and safety benefits. Nursing informatics professionals are taking on a greater role with respect to workflow design, and this aspect of practice will grow in light of MACRA-driven measures. Other initiatives that impact hospital performance will also drive informatics professionals to influence how technology is used in the context of workflow to improve the bottom line for their organizations. In an ideal world, nurse informaticists who are experts at workflow analysis will be core members of every technology implementation team.

## THOUGHT-PROVOKING QUESTIONS

1. What do you perceive as the current obstacles to redesigning workflow within your clinical setting?
2. Thinking about your last implementation, were you able to challenge the policies and practices that constitute today's workflow or were you able to create a workflow solution that eliminated non–value-added steps?
3. Is the workflow surrounding technology usage providing the healthcare organization with the data it needs to make decisions and eventually meet MACRA criteria?
4. How does the current educational preparation need to change to address the skills necessary to perform workflow analysis and redesign clinical processes?
5. Describe the role of the nurse informaticist as the payment programs change related to MACRA.

# References

Agency for Healthcare Research and Quality (AHRQ). (n.d.). Workflow assessment for health IT toolkit. Retrieved from http://healthit.ahrq.gov/health-it-tools-and-resources/workflow-assessment-health-it-toolkit

Agency for Healthcare Research and Quality (AHRQ). (2008). Patient safety and quality: An evidence-based handbook for nurses. Retrieved from http://www.ahrq.gov/qual/nurseshdbk

American Association for Justice. (2016). Medical errors. Retrieved from https://www.justice.org/what-we-do/advocate-civil-justice-system/issue-advocacy/medical-errors

American Nurses Association. (2015). *Nursing informatics: Scope and standards of practice* (2nd ed.). Silver Springs, MD: Author.

Bucur, A., van Leeuwen, J., Christodoulou, N., Sigdel, K., Argyri, K., Koumakis, L., . . . Stamatakos, G. (2016). Workflow-driven clinical decision support for personalized oncology. *BMC Medical Informatics & Decision Making, 16*, 151–162. doi:10.1186/s12911-016-0314-3

Campbell, E., Guappone, K., Sittig, D., Dykstra, R., & Ash, J. (2009). Computerized provider order entry adoption: Implications for clinical workflow. *Journal of General Internal Medicine, 24*(1), 21–26.

Centers for Medicare & Medicaid Services (CMS). (2016a). Electronic health records (EHR) incentive programs. Retrieved from https://www.cms.gov/Regulations-and-Guidance/Legislation/EHRIncentivePrograms/index.html

Centers for Medicare & Medicaid Services (CMS). (2016b). MACRA: Delivery system reform, Medicare payment reform. Retrieved from https://www.cms.gov/Medicare/Quality-Initiatives-Patient-Assessment-Instruments/Value-Based-Programs/MACRA-MIPS-and-APMs/MACRA-MIPS-and-APMs.html

Centers for Medicare & Medicaid Services (CMS). (2016c). CMS quality measure development plan: Supporting the transition to the merit-based incentive payment system (MIPS) and alternative payment models (APMs). Retrieved from https://www.cms.gov/Medicare/Quality-Initiatives-Patient-Assessment-Instruments/Value-Based-Programs/MACRA-MIPS-and-APMs/Final-MDP.pdf

Clancy, T., Delaney, C., Morrison, B., & Gunn, J. (2006). The benefits of standardized nursing languages in complex adaptive systems such as hospitals. *Journal of Nursing Administration, 36*(9), 426–434.

Daley, K. (2013). Making HIT meaningful for nursing and patients. *The American Nurse.* Retrieved from http://www.theamericannurse.org/index.php/2011/08/01/making-hit-meaningful-for-nursing-and-patients

Earl, M., Sampler, J., & Sghort, J. (1995). Strategies for business process reengineering: Evidence from field studies. *Journal of Management Information Systems, 12*(1), 31–56.

Gugerty, B., Maranda, M. J., Beachley, M., Navarro, V. B., Newbold, S., Hawk, W., . . . Wilhelm, D. (2007). Challenges and Opportunities in documentation of the nursing care of patients. Baltimore, MD: Documentation Work Group, Maryland Nursing Workforce Commission. Retrieved from http://mbon.maryland.gov/Documents/documentation_challenges.pdf

Hagland, M. (2016). CMS announces long-awaited MACRA proposed rule; Program includes MU makeover for MDs. *Healthcare Informatics.* Retrieved from http://www.healthcare-informatics.com/article/breaking-news-cms-announces-plan-replace-meaningful-use-physicians-new-quality-reporting

Healthcare Information Management Systems Society (HIMSS). (2010). ME-PI toolkit: Process management, workflow & mapping: Tools, tips and case studies to support the understanding, optimizing and monitoring of processes. Retrieved from http://www.himss.org/me-pi-toolkit-change-management

Healthcare Information Management Systems Society (HIMSS). (2015). Nursing informatics impact study. Retrieved from http://www.himss.org/ni-impact-survey

Kotter, J. P. (1996). *Leading change* (pp. 33–147). Cambridge, MA: Harvard Business Press.

*Merriam-Webster Online Dictionary.* (2016). Optimization. Retrieved from http://www.merriam -webster.com/dictionary/optimization

Murphy, K. (2013). Nursing approach to meaningful use, EHR adoption: CIO series. Retrieved from https://ehrintelligence.com/news/nursing-approach-to-meaningful-use-ehr-adoption-cio -series

Qualis Health. (2011). Workflow analysis. Retrieved from http://www.qualishealthmedicare .org/healthcare-providers/improvement-fundamentals/workflow-analysis

Stokowski, L. (2013). Electronic nursing documentation: Charting new territory. Medscape. Retrieved from http://www.medscape.com/viewarticle/810573

Thompson, C., Kell, C., Shetty, R., & Banerjee, D. (2016). Clinical workflow redesign leveraging informatics improves patient outcomes. *Heart & Lung, 45*(4), 380–381.

Vankipuram, K. (2010). Toward automated workflow analysis and visualization in clinical environment. *Journal of Biomedical Informatics.* doi:10.1016/jbi.2010.05.015

Yuan, M., Finley, G., Long, J., Mills, C. & Johnson, R. (2013). Evaluation of user interface and workflow design of a bedside nursing clinical decision support system. *Interactive Journal of Medical Research, 2*(1), e4.

# SECTION IV

# Nursing Informatics Practice Applications: Care Delivery

Nursing information systems must support nurses as they fulfill their roles in delivering quality patient care. Such systems must be responsive to nurses' needs, allowing them to manage their data and information as needed and providing access to necessary references, literature sources, and other networked departments. Nurses have always practiced in a field where they have needed to use their ingenuity, resourcefulness, creativity, initiative, and skills. To improve patient care and advance the science of nursing, clinicians as knowledge workers must apply these same abilities and skills to become astute users of available information systems.

In this section, the reader learns about clinical practice tools, electronic health records, and clinical information systems; informatics tools to enhance patient safety, provide consumer information, and meet education needs; population and community health tools; and telehealth and telenursing.

Information systems, electronic documentation, and electronic health records are changing the way nurses and physicians practice. Nursing informatics systems are also changing how patients enter and receive data and information. Some institutions, for example, are permitting patients to access their own records electronically via the Internet or a dedicated patient portal. Confidentiality and privacy issues loom with these new electronic systems. HIPAA regulations (covered in the Perspectives on Nursing Informatics section) and professional ethics principles (covered in the Building Blocks of Nursing Informatics section) must remain at the forefront when clinicians interact electronically with intimate patient data and information.

The material within this book is placed within the context of the Foundation of Knowledge model (Figure IV-1) to meet the needs of healthcare delivery systems, organizations, patients, and nurses. Readers should continue to assess their personal knowledge progression. The Foundation of Knowledge model challenges us to reflect on how our knowledge foundation is ever-changing and to appreciate that acquiring new information is a key resource for knowledge building. This section addresses the information systems with which clinicians interact in their healthcare environments as affected by legislation, professional codes of ethics, consumerism, and reconceptualization of practice paradigms, such as in telenursing. All of the various nursing roles—practice, administration, education, research, and informatics—involve the science of nursing.

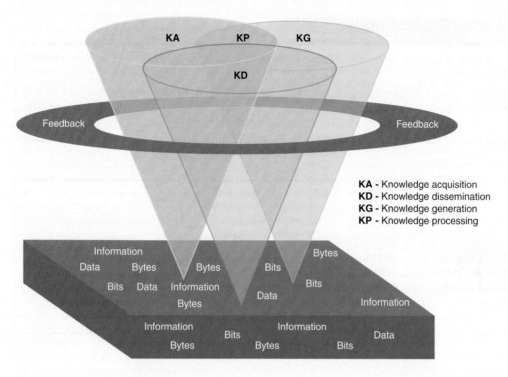

**Figure IV-1** Foundation of Knowledge Model
Designed by Alicia Mastrian

# CHAPTER 14

# The Electronic Health Record and Clinical Informatics

Emily B. Barey, Kathleen Mastrian, and Dee McGonigle

## Introduction

The significance of **electronic health records** (EHRs) to nursing cannot be underestimated. Although EHRs on the surface suggest a simple automation of clinical documentation, in fact their implications are broad, ranging from the ways in which care is delivered, to the types of interactions nurses have with patients in conjunction with the use of technology, to the research surrounding EHRs that will inform nursing practice for tomorrow. Although EHR standards are evolving and barriers to adoption remain, the collective work has a positive momentum that will benefit clinicians and patients alike.

A basic knowledge of EHRs and nursing informatics is now considered by many to be an entry-level nursing competency. Various nursing workgroups have delineated nursing informatics competencies from entry level to nursing informatics specialists, and other groups have identified competencies specific to the EHR. The American Health Information Management Association (AHIMA) collaborated with the Health Professions Network and the Employment and Training Administration to create a graphic depiction of competencies necessary for EHR interaction. The Electronic Health Records Competency Model is divided into six levels: Personal Effectiveness Competencies, Academic Competencies, Workplace Competencies, Industry-Wide Technical Competencies, Industry-Sector Technical Competencies, and a Management Competencies level shared with Occupation Specific Requirements. The EHR Competency Model can be viewed at: www.careeronestop.org/CompetencyModel/competency -models/electronic-health-records.aspx. Hovering over each block in the model provides a definition of each of the competencies covered by the model. For example, the industry-sector technical competencies section includes health information literacy and skills, health informatics skills using the EHR, privacy and confidentiality of health information, and health information data technical security. This drive to adopt EHRs was underscored with the passage of the **Health Information Technology for Economic and Clinical Health Act of 2009 (HITECH)**. It is essential that EHR competency be developed if nurses are to participate fully in the changing world of healthcare information technology.

This chapter has four goals. First, it describes the common components of an EHR. Second, it reviews the benefits of implementing an EHR. Third, it provides an overview of successful ownership of an EHR, including nursing's role in promoting the safe adoption of EHRs in day-to-day practice. Fourth, it discusses the flexibility of an EHR in meeting the needs of both clinicians and patients and emphasizes the need for fully interoperable EHRs and clinical information systems (CISs).

## Setting the Stage

The U.S. healthcare system faces the enormous challenge of improving the quality of care while simultaneously controlling costs. EHRs were proposed as one solution to achieve this goal (Institute of Medicine [IOM], 2001). In January 2004, President George W. Bush raised the profile of EHRs in his State of the Union address by outlining a plan to ensure that most Americans have an EHR by 2014. He stated that "by computerizing health records we can avoid dangerous medical mistakes, reduce costs, and improve care" (Bush, 2004). This proclamation generated an increased demand for understanding EHRs and promoting their adoption, but relatively few healthcare organizations were motivated at that time to pursue adoption of EHRs. The Healthcare Information and Management Systems Society (HIMSS) has been tracking EHR adoption since 2005 through its "Stage 7" award, and in 2013 reported that most U.S. healthcare organizations (77%) were in Stage 3, reflecting only implementation of the basic EHR components of laboratory, radiology, and pharmacy ancillaries; a clinical data repository, including a controlled medical vocabulary; and simple nursing documentation and clinical decision support (HIMSS, 2013). Higher stages of the electronic medical record adoption model include more sophisticated use of clinical decision support systems (CDSSs) and medication administration tools, with HIMSS Stage 7—the highest level—consisting of EHRs that have data sharing and warehousing capabilities and that are completely interfaced with emergency and outpatient facilities (HIMSS Analytics, 2013). Real progress is being made on the adoption of more robust EHRs. HIMSS Analytics (2015) reports that 1,313 hospitals in the United States have achieved Stage 6 with full physician documentation, a robust CDSS, and electronic access to medical images. Healthcare IT News (2015) reported that, to date, over 200 hospitals have achieved Stage 7 and are totally paperless, and that more organizations reach this goal every day.

In President Barack Obama's first term in office, Congress passed the **American Recovery and Reinvestment Act of 2009 (ARRA)**. This legislation included the HITECH Act, which specifically sought to incentivize health organizations and providers to become meaningful users of EHRs. These incentives came in the form of increased reimbursement rates from the Centers for Medicare and Medicaid Services (CMS); ultimately, the HITECH Act resulted in payment of a penalty by any healthcare organization that had not adopted an EHR by January 2015. The final rule was published by the Department of Health and Human Services (USDHHS) in July 2010 for the first phase of implementation. Stage 1 **meaningful use** criteria focused on data capture and sharing (USDHHS, 2010a). Stage 2 criteria, implemented in 2014, advanced several clinical processes and promoted health information exchange (HIE) and more patient control over personal data. Stage 3, which has a target implementation date of 2016, focuses on improved outcomes for individuals and populations, and introduction of patient self-management tools (HealthIT.gov, 2013).

# Components of Electronic Health Records

## Overview

Before enactment of the ARRA, several variants of EHRs existed, each with its own terminology and each developed with a different audience in mind. The sources of these records included, for example, the federal government (Certification Commission for Healthcare Information Technology, 2007), the IOM (2003), the HIMSS (2007), and the National Institutes of Health (2006; Robert Wood Johnson Foundation [RWJF], 2006). Under ARRA, there is now an explicit requirement for providers and hospitals to use a certified EHR that meets a set of standard functional definitions to be eligible for the increased reimbursement incentive. Initially, USDHHS granted two organizations the authority to accredit EHRs: the Drummond Group and the Certification Commission for Healthcare Information Technology. In 2015, there were five recognized bodies for testing and certifying EHRs (HealthIT.gov, 2015a). These bodies are authorized to test and certify EHR vendors against the standards and test procedures developed by the National Institute of Standards and Technology (NIST) and endorsed by the Office of the National Coordinator for Health Information Technology for EHRs.

The initial NIST test procedure included 45 certification criteria, ranging from the basic ability to record patient demographics, document vital signs, and maintain an up-to-date problem list, to more complex functions, such as electronic exchange of clinical information and patient summary records (Jansen & Grance, 2011; NIST, 2010). Box 14-1 lists the 45 certification criteria outlined by NIST in 2010. These criteria have been updated several times since 2010, with the 2015 version developed after going out for public comment (HealthIT.gov, 2015b). Each iteration of certification criteria and testing procedures seeks to make the EHR more robust, interoperable, and functional to meet the needs of patients and users.

Despite the points articulated in the ARRA, the IOM definition of an EHR also remains a valid reference point. This definition is useful because it has distilled all the possible features of an EHR into eight essential components with an emphasis on functions that promote patient safety—a universal denominator that everyone in health care can accept. The eight components are (1) health information and data, (2) results management, (3) order entry management, (4) decision support, (5) electronic communication and connectivity, (6) patient support, (7) administrative processes, and (8) reporting and population health management (IOM, 2003). These initial core components, as well as more recent modifications described by the Health Resources and Services Administration (HRSA, n.d.) and the components of a comprehensive EHR identified by HealthIT.gov (Charles, Gabriel, & Searcy, 2015), are described in more detail here. With the exception of EHR infrastructure functions, such as security and privacy management, controlled medical vocabularies, and interoperability standards, the 45 initial NIST standards easily map into the IOM categories (Jansen & Grance, 2011).

## BOX 14-1 EHR CERTIFICATION CRITERIA

| Criteria # | Certification Criteria |
|---|---|
| §170.302 (a) | Drug–drug, drug–allergy interaction checks |
| §170.302 (b) | Drug formulary checks |
| §170.302 (c) | Maintain up-to-date problem list |
| §170.302 (d) | Maintain active medication list |
| §170.302 (e) | Maintain active medication allergy list |
| §170.302 (f)(1) | Vital signs |
| §170.302 (f)(2) | Calculate body mass index |
| §170.302 (f)(3) | Plot and display growth charts |
| §170.302 (g) | Smoking status |
| §170.302 (h) | Incorporate laboratory test results |
| §170.302 (i) | Generate patient lists |
| §170.302 (j) | Medication reconciliation |
| §170.302 (k) | Submission to immunization registries |
| §170.302 (l) | Public health surveillance |
| §170.302 (m) | Patient-specific education resources |
| §170.302 (n) | Automated measure calculation |
| §170.302 (o) | Access control |
| §170.302 (p) | Emergency access |
| §170.302 (q) | Automatic log-off |
| §170.302 (r) | Audit log |
| §170.302 (s) | Integrity |
| §170.302 (t) | Authentication |
| §170.302 (u) | General encryption |
| §170.302 (v) | Encryption when exchanging electronic health information |
| §170.302 (w) | Accounting of disclosures (optional) |
| §170.304 (a) | Computerized provider order entry |

| §170.304 (b) | Electronic prescribing |
|---|---|
| §170.304 (c) | Record demographics |
| §170.304 (d) | Patient reminders |
| §170.304 (e) | Clinical decision support |
| §170.304 (f) | Electronic copy of health information |
| §170.304 (g) | Timely access |
| §170.304 (h) | Clinical summaries |
| §170.304 (i) | Exchange clinical information and patient summary record |
| §170.304 (j) | Calculate and submit clinical quality measures |
| §170.306 (a) | Computerized provider order entry |
| §170.306 (b) | Record demographics |
| §170.306 (c) | Clinical decision support |
| §170.306 (d)(1) | Electronic copy of health information |
| §170.306 (d)(2) | Electronic copy of health information |
| | Note: For discharge summary |
| §170.306 (e) | Electronic copy of discharge instructions |
| §170.306 (f) | Exchange clinical information and patient summary record |
| §170.306 (g) | Reportable lab results |
| §170.306 (h) | Advance directives |
| §170.306 (i) | Calculate and submit clinical quality measures |

Reproduced from National Institute of Standards and Technology (NIST). (2010). Meaningful use test method: Approved test procedures version 1.0. Retrieved from http://healthcare.nist.gov/use_testing/finalized_requirements.html

## Health Information and Data

**Health information** and data comprise the patient data required to make sound clinical decisions, including demographics, medical and nursing diagnoses, medication lists, allergies, and test results (IOM, 2003). This component of the EHR also includes care management data regarding details of patient visits and interactions with patients, medication reconciliation, consents, and directives (HRSA, n.d.). A comprehensive EHR will also contain nursing assessments and problem lists (Charles, Gabriel, & Searcy, 2015).

## Results Management

**Results management** is the ability to manage results of all types electronically, including laboratory and radiology procedure reports, both current and historical (IOM, 2003).

## Order Entry Management

**Order entry management** is the ability of a clinician to enter medication and other care orders, including laboratory, microbiology, pathology, radiology, nursing, and supply orders; ancillary services; and consultations, directly into a computer (IOM, 2003). A comprehensive EHR will also contain nursing orders (Charles, Gabriel, & Searcy, 2015).

## Decision Support

**Decision support** entails the use of computer reminders and alerts to improve the diagnosis and care of a patient, including screening for correct drug selection and dosing, screening for medication interactions with other medications, preventive health reminders in such areas as vaccinations, health risk screening and detection, and clinical guidelines for patient disease treatment (IOM, 2003).

## Electronic Communication and Connectivity

**Electronic communication** and **connectivity** include the online communication among healthcare team members, their care partners, and patients, including email, Web messaging, and an integrated health record within and across settings, institutions, and telemedicine (IOM, 2003). This component has been expanded to include interfaces and interoperability required to exchange health information with other providers, laboratories, pharmacies (e-prescribing), patients, and government disease registries (HRSA, n.d., para. 2)

## Patient Support

**Patient support** encompasses patient education and self-monitoring tools, including interactive computer-based patient education, home telemonitoring, and telehealth systems (IOM, 2003).

## Administrative Processes

**Administrative processes** are activities carried out by the electronic scheduling, billing, and claims management systems, including electronic scheduling for inpatient and outpatient visits and procedures, electronic insurance eligibility validation, claim authorization and prior approval, identification of possible research study participants, and drug recall support (IOM, 2003).

## Reporting and Population Health Management

**Reporting** and **population health management** are the data collection tools to support public and private reporting requirements, including data represented in a standardized terminology and machine-readable format (IOM, 2003).

NIST has not provided an exhaustive list of all possible features and functions of an EHR. Consequently, different vendor EHR systems combine different components in their offerings, and often a single set of EHR components may not meet the needs of all clinicians and patient populations. For example, a pediatric setting may demand functions for immunization management, growth tracking, and more robust order entry features to include weight-based dosing (Spooner & Council on Clinical Information Technology, 2007). These types of features may not be provided by all EHR systems, and it is important to consider EHR certification to be a minimum standard. See Figure 14-1 for a graphic depiction of EHR functions and communication capabilities.

Another group that focuses on EHR standards and functionality is Health Level Seven International (HL7). Founded in 1987, "Health Level Seven International (HL7) is a not-for-profit, ANSI-accredited standards developing organization dedicated to providing a comprehensive framework and related standards for the exchange, integration, sharing, and retrieval of electronic health information that supports clinical practice and the management, delivery and evaluation of health services" (Health Level Seven International, n.d., para. 1). This group concentrates on developing the

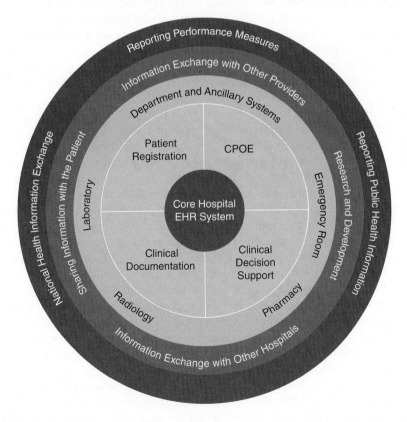

**Figure 14-1** EHR Functions and Communication Capabilities

Reproduced from American Hospital Association. (2010). The road to meaningful use: What it takes to implement EHR systems in hospitals. Retrieved from http://www.aha.org/research/reports/tw/10apr-tw-HITmeanuse.pdf

behind-the-scenes programming standards (Level Seven is the application level of the Open Systems Interconnection model) for interfaces to ensure interoperability and connectivity among systems.

## Advantages of Electronic Health Records

Measuring the benefits of EHRs can be challenging. Possible methods to estimate EHR benefits include using vendor-supplied data that have been retrieved from their customers' systems, synthesizing and applying studies of overall EHR value, creating logical engineering models of EHR value, summarizing focused studies of elements of EHR value, and conducting and applying information from site visits (HealthIT.gov, 2012; Thompson, Osheroff, Classen, & Sittig, 2007).

Early on, the four most common benefits cited for EHRs were (1) increased delivery of guidelines-based care, (2) enhanced capacity to perform surveillance and monitoring for disease conditions, (3) reduction in medication errors, and (4) decreased use of care (Chaudhry et al., 2006; HealthIT.gov, 2012). These findings were echoed by two similar literature reviews. The first review (Dorr et al., 2007) focused on the use of informatics systems for managing patients with chronic illness. It found that the processes of care most positively impacted were guidelines adherence, visit frequency (i.e., a decrease in emergency department visits), provider documentation, patient treatment adherence, and screening and testing.

The second review (Shekelle, Morton, & Keeler, 2006) was a cost–benefit analysis of health information technology completed by the Agency for Healthcare Research and Quality (AHRQ) that studied the value of an EHR in the ambulatory care and pediatric settings, including its overall economic value. The AHRQ study highlighted the common findings already described, but also noted that most of the data available for review came from six leading healthcare organizations in the United States, under-scoring the challenge of generalizing these results to the broader healthcare industry. As noted previously by the HIMSS Stage 7 Awards, the challenge to generalize results persists in the hospital arena, with fewer than 1% of U.S. hospitals or eight leading organizations providing most of the experience with comprehensive EHRs (HIMSS, 2010a). Finally, the literature reviews cited here indicated that there are a limited number of hypothesis-testing studies of EHRs and even fewer that have reported cost data.

The descriptive studies do have value, however, and should not be hastily dismissed. Although not as rigorous in their design, they do describe the advantages of EHRs well and often include useful implementation recommendations learned from practical experience. As identified in these types of reviews, EHR advantages include simple benefits, such as no longer having to interpret poor handwriting and handwritten orders, reduced turnaround time for laboratory results in an emergency department, and decreased time to administration of the first dose of antibiotics in an inpatient nursing unit (HealthIT.gov, 2012; Husk & Waxman, 2004; Smith et al., 2004). In the ambulatory care setting, improved management of cardiac-related risk factors in patients with diabetes and effective patient notification of medication recalls have been demonstrated to be benefits of the EHR (Jain et al., 2005; Reed & Bernard, 2005). Two other unique advantages that have great potential are the ability to use the EHR and decision support functions to identify patients who qualify for research studies or who qualify for prescription drug benefits offered by pharmaceutical companies at safety-net clinics and hospitals (Embi et al., 2005; Poprock, 2005).

The HIMSS Davies Award may be the best resource for combined quantitative and qualitative results of successful EHR implementation. The Davies Award recognizes healthcare organizations that have achieved both excellence in implementation and value from health information technology (HIMSS, 2010a). One winner demonstrated a significant avoidance of medication errors because of bar-code scanning alerts, a $3 million decrease in medical records expenses as a result of going paperless, and a 5% reduction of duplicate laboratory orders by using computerized provider order entry alerting (HIMSS, 2010b). Another winner noted a 13% decrease in adverse drug reactions through the use of computerized physician order entry; it also achieved a decrease in methicillin-resistant *Staphylococcus aureus* (MRSA) nosocomial infections from 9.8 per 10,000 discharges to 6.4 per 10,000 discharges in less than a year using an EHR flagging function, which made clinicians immediately aware that contact precautions were required for MRSA-positive patients (HIMSS, 2009). At both organizations, there was qualitative and quantitative evidence of high rates of end user adoption and satisfaction with use of the EHR.

A 2011 study of the effects of EHR adoption on nurse perceptions of quality of care, communication, and patient safety documented that nurses report better care outcomes and fewer concerns with care coordination and patient safety in hospitals with a basic EHR (Kutney-Lee & Kelly, 2011). In this study, nurses perceived that in hospitals with a functioning EHR, there was better communication among staff, especially during patient transfers, and fewer medication errors. Bayliss et al. (2015) demonstrated that an integrated care system utilizing an EHR resulted in fewer hospital readmissions and emergency room visits for over 12,000 seniors with multiple health challenges.

Without an EHR system, any of these benefits would be very difficult and costly to accomplish. Thus, despite limited standards and published studies, there is enough evidence to embrace widespread implementation of the EHR (Halamka, 2006; HealthIT.gov, 2012), and certainly enough evidence to warrant further study of the use and benefits of EHRs. Box 14-2 describes some of the specific CIS functions of an EHR.

A more recent description of the benefits of an EHR by HealthIT.gov (2014) emphasizes that EHRs hold the promise of transforming healthcare; specifically, EHRs will lead to:

- *Better health care* by improving all aspects of patient care, including safety, effectiveness, patient-centeredness, communication, education, timeliness, efficiency, and equity
- *Better health* by encouraging healthier lifestyles in the entire population, including increased physical activity, better nutrition, avoidance of behavioral risks, and wider use of preventative care
- *Improved efficiencies and lower healthcare costs* by promoting preventative medicine and improved coordination of healthcare services, as well as by reducing waste and redundant tests
- *Better clinical decision making* by integrating patient information from multiple sources (para. 4)

## BOX 14-2 THE EHR AS A CLINICAL INFORMATION SYSTEM

*Denise Tyler*

A CIS is a technology-based system applied at the point of care and designed to support care by providing instant access to information for clinicians. Early CISs implemented prior to the advent of EHRs were limited in scope and provided such information as interpretation of laboratory results or a medication formulary and drug interaction information. With the implementation of EHRs, the goal of many organizations is to expand the scope of the early CISs to become comprehensive systems that provide clinical decision support, an electronic patient record, and in some instances professional development and training tools. Benefits of such a comprehensive system include easy access to patient data at the point of care; structured and legible information that can be searched easily and lends itself to data mining and analysis; and improved patient safety, especially the prevention of adverse drug reactions and the identification of health risk factors, such as falls.

## TRACKING CLINICAL OUTCOMES

The ability to measure outcomes can be enhanced or impeded by the way an information system is designed and used. Although many practitioners can paint a very good picture of the patient by using a narrative (free text), employing this mode of expression in a clinical system without the use of a coded entry makes it difficult to analyze the care given or the patient's response. Free-text reporting also leads to inconsistencies of reporting from clinician to clinician and patient information that is fragmented or disorganized. This can limit the usefulness of patient data to other clinicians and interfere with the ability to create reports from the data for quality assurance and measurement purposes. Moreover, not all clinicians are equally skilled at the free-text form of communication, yielding inconsistent quality of documentation. Integrating standardized nursing terminologies into computerized nursing documentation systems enhances the ability to use the data for reporting and further research.

According to the IOM (2012), "Payers, healthcare delivery organizations and medical product companies should contribute data to research and analytic consortia to support expanded use of care data to generate new insights" (para. 2). McLaughlin and Halilovic (2006) described the use of clinical analytics to promote medical care outcomes research. The use of a CIS in conjunction with standardized codes for patient clinical issues helps to support the rigorous analysis of clinical data. Outcomes data produced as part of these analyses may include length of stay, mortality, readmissions, and complications. Future goals include the ability to compare data and outcomes across various institutions as a means of developing clinical guidelines or best practices guidelines. With the implementation of a comprehensive CIS, similar analyses of nursing outcomes could also be performed and shared. Likewise, such a system could aid nurse administrators in cross-unit comparisons and staffing decisions, especially when coupled with acuity systems data. In addition, clinical analytics can support required data reporting functions, especially those required by accreditation bodies.

## SUPPORTING EVIDENCE-BASED PRACTICE

Evidence-based practice (EBP) can be thought of as the integration of clinical expertise and best practices based on systematic research to enhance decision making and improve patient care. References supporting EBP, such as clinical guidelines, are available for review at the click of a mouse or the press of a few keystrokes. The CIS's prompting capabilities can also reinforce the practice of looking for evidence to support nursing interventions rather than relying on how things have been done historically. This approach enhances processing and understanding of the information and allows the nurse to apply the information to other areas, increasing the knowledge obtained about why certain conditions or responses result in prompts for additional questions or actions.

To incorporate EBP into the practice of clinical nursing, the information needs to be embedded in the computerized documentation system so that it is part of the workflow. The most typical way of embedding this timely information is through clinical practice guidelines. The resulting interventions and clinical outcomes need to be measurable and reportable for further research. The supporting documentation for the EBP needs to be easily retrievable and meaningful. Links, reminders, and prompts can all be used as vehicles for transmission of this information. The format needs to allow for rapid scanning, with the ability to expand the amount of information when more detail is required or desired. Balancing a consistency in formatting with creativity can be difficult but is worth the effort to stimulate an atmosphere for learning.

EBP is supported by translational research, an exciting movement that has enormous potential for the sharing and use of EBP. The use of translational research to support EBP may help to close the gap between what is known (research) and what is done (practice).

## THE CIS AS A STAFF DEVELOPMENT TOOL

Joy Hilty, a registered nurse from Kaweah Delta, came up with a creative way to provide staff development or education without taking staff away from the bedside to a classroom setting. She created pop-up boxes on the opening charting screens for all staff who chart on the computer. These pop-ups vary in color and content and include a short piece of clinical information, along with a question. Staff can earn vacations from these pop-ups for as long as 14 days by emailing the correct answer to the question. This medium has provided information, stimulation, and a definite benefit: the vacation from the pop-up boxes. The pop-up box education format has also encouraged staff to share their answers, thereby creating interaction, knowledge dissemination, and reinforcement of the education provided.

Embedding EBP into nursing documentation can also increase the compliance with Joint Commission core measures, such as providing information on influenza and pneumococcal vaccinations to at-risk patients. In the author's experience at Kaweah Delta, educating staff via classes, flyers, and storyboards was not successful in improving compliance with the documentation of immunization status or offering education on these vaccinations to at-risk patients. Embedding the prompts, information, and related questions in the nursing documentation with a link to the protocol and educational material, however, improved the compliance to 96% for pneumococcal vaccinations and to 95% for influenza vaccinations (Hettinger, 2007).

As more information is stored electronically, nurse informaticists must translate the technology so that the input and retrieval of information are developed in a manner that is easy for clinicians to learn and use. A highly usable product should decrease errors and improve information entry and retrieval. Nurse informaticists must be able to work with staff and expert users to design systems that meet the needs of the staff who will actually use the systems. The work is not done after the system is installed; the system must continue to be developed and improved, because as staff use the system, they will be able to suggest changes to improve it. This ongoing revision should result in a system that is mature and meets the needs of the users.

In an ideal world, all clinical documentation will be shared through a national database, in a standard language, to enable evaluation of nursing care, increase the body of evidence, and improve patient outcomes. With minimal effort, the information will be translated into new research that can be analyzed and linked to new evidence that will be intuitively applied to the CIS. Alerts will be meaningful and will be patient and provider specific. The steps required of the clinician to find current, reliable information will be almost transparent, and the information will be presented in a personalized manner based on user preferences stored in the CIS.

## REFERENCES

Hettinger, M. (2007, March). *Core measure reporting: Performance improvement.* Visalia, CA: Kaweah Delta Health Care District.

Institute of Medicine (IOM). (2012). Best care at lower cost. Retrieved from https://www.nap.edu/catalog/13444/best-care-at-lower-cost-the-path-to-continuously-learning

McLaughlin, T., & Halilovic, M. (2006). Clinical analytics, rigorous coding bring objectivity to quality assertions. *Medical Staff Update Online, 30*(6). Retrieved from http://med.stanford.edu/shs/update/archives/JUNE2006/analytics.htm

# Standardized Terminology and the EHR

As we inch closer to interoperable EHRs that provide for seamless health information exchange among providers and healthcare institutions, the need for standardizing terminologies becomes ever clearer. Consider also the trend toward value-based care reimbursements, in which healthcare data are mined "to demonstrate nursing's contributions to improving the cost, quality, and efficiency of care, key elements of the value equation" (Adams, Ponte, & Somerville, 2016, p. 127). EHR data must be formatted in a machine-readable manner in order to support interoperable exchange of information and data mining. An important distinction that needs to be made here is the difference between interface terminologies (NANDA, NIC, or NOC) and reference terminologies (SMOMED-CT, LOINC).

*While interface terminologies play an important role in promoting direct entry of categorical data by health care providers, both terminology developers and the standards community historically have focused on other types of terminologies, including reference and administrative (rather than on interface) terminologies. Such terminologies are generally designed to provide exact and complete representations of a given domain's knowledge, including its entities and ideas and their interrelationships. For example, reference terminologies can support the storage, retrieval, and classification of clinical data; their contents correspond to the internal system representation storage formats to which interface terminologies are typically mapped. (Rosenbloom, Miller, Johnson, Elkin, & Brown, 2006, p. 278)*

The various interface terminologies and their subsets are coded in the EHR and typically presented to the user in dropdown menus. Users may also be able to use a search function in the EHR to identify the most appropriate term that represents the patient's condition(s). Bronnert, Masarie, Naeymi-Rad, Rose, and Aldin (2012) described the value of an interface terminology for clinician workflow:

*Clinicians interact with interface terminology when documenting diagnoses and procedures in the patient's electronic record. The physician performs searches using the search functionality in designated locations in the EHR, which returns terms to the provider to select the appropriate problem or procedure. The physician [nurse] selects the appropriate term to capture the clinical intent. The term(s) populate predetermined fields in the electronic record. The selected term contains mappings to one or more industry standard terminologies, such as ICD or SNOMED CT. The "behind-the-scenes" mappings allow the physician to focus on patient care while at the same time capturing the necessary administrative and reference codes. (para. 17)*

The National Library of Medicine has been designated as the central coordinating body for clinical terminologies by the USDHHS. (See **Box 14-3** for a list and description of administrative and reference terminologies used in an EHR.) Recall the ongoing work of nursing groups looking to standardize nursing terminologies to capture and codify the work of nursing. (See Chapter 6 for a list of approved nursing terminologies.) In 2015, the American Nurses Association reaffirmed its support for the use of standardized terminologies:

*The purpose of this position statement is to reaffirm the American Nurses Association's (ANA) support for the use of recognized terminologies supporting nursing practice as valuable representations of nursing practice and to promote the integration of those terminologies into information technology solutions. Standardized terminologies have become a significant vehicle for facilitating interoperability between different concepts, nomenclatures, and information systems. (para. 1)*

---

**BOX 14-3 STANDARD EHR ADMINISTRATIVE AND REFERENCE TERMINOLOGIES**

Administrative (Billing) Terminologies
* ICD-10 (International Classification of Diseases, Version 10): Medical diagnosis code set
* CPT (Current Procedural Terminology): Used to code procedures for billing

**CLINICAL TERMINOLOGIES**

- SNOMED CT (Systematized Nomenclature of Medicine—Clinical Terms): Comprehensive clinical terminology (mapping to this terminology is ongoing, including nursing-orders mapping)
- LOINC (Logical Observation Identifier Names and Codes): Universal codes for laboratory and clinical observations
- RxNorm: Terminology system for drug names, providing links to drug vocabularies and interaction software
- Unified Medical Language System (UMLS) and the Metathesaurus: Support terminology integration efforts and online searches (not a terminology system)

See the U.S. National Library of Medicine website for more comprehensive information: www.nlm.nih.gov/hit_interoperability.html

---

Because no single model of standardized terminology for health care or nursing can represent all of the contributions to the health of a patient, work is ongoing to map terminologies to one another. For example, Kim, Hardiker, and Coenen (2014) studied the degree of similarity between the International Classification for Nursing Practice (ICNP) and the Systematized Nomenclature of Medicine–Clinical Terms (SNOMED–CT); while they identified some areas of overlap, they cautioned that there is still more work to be done to truly represent nursing concepts in the EHR. Adams et al. (2016) issued a call to action to Chief Nursing Officers (CNOs): "CNOs must begin partnering with and influencing EHR developers and vendors to ensure the EHRs implemented in their organizations capture nursing content using a standardized taxonomy that is evidence based and mapped to SNOMED-CT and LOINC" (p. 127). Ongoing efforts to map nursing problem lists to SNOMED-CT are evident in the work of Matney and colleagues (2011) and on the National Library of Medicine website (www.nlm.nih.gov/hit_interoperability.html). It is probably safe to say that the number of different types of EHRs and the variability of EHRs are likely to contract and converge as the demand for robust systems supporting interoperability expands. Nurse informatics specialists and CNOs participating in the selection and implementation of EHRs must ask a critical question: To what extent are nursing care contributions visible, retrievable, and accurately represented in this EHR?

## Ownership of Electronic Health Records

The implementation of an EHR has the potential to affect every member of a healthcare organization. The process of becoming a successful owner of an EHR has multiple steps and requires integrating the EHR into the organization's day-to-day operations and long-term vision, as well as into the clinician's day-to-day practice. All members of the healthcare organization—from the executive level to the clinician at the point of care—must feel a sense of ownership to make the implementation successful for themselves, their colleagues, and their patients. Successful ownership of an EHR may be defined in part by the level of clinician adoption of the tool, and this section reviews key steps and strategies for the selection, implementation and evaluation, and optimization of an EHR in pursuit of that goal.

Historically, many systems were developed locally by the information technology department of a healthcare organization. It was not unusual for software developers to be employed by the organization to create needed systems and interfaces between them. As commercial offerings were introduced and matured, it became less and less common to see homegrown or locally developed systems.

As this history suggests, the first step of ownership is typically a vendor selection process for a commercially available EHR. During this step, it is important to survey the organization's level of interest, identify possible barriers to participation, document desired functions of an EHR, and assess the willingness to fund the implementation (Holbrook, Keshavjee, Troyan, Pray, & Ford, 2003). Although clinicians, as the primary end users, should drive the project, the assessment should also include the needs and readiness of the executive leadership, information technology, and project management teams. It is essential that leadership understands that this type of project is as much about redesigning clinical work as it is about technically automating it and that they agree to assume accountability for its success (Goddard, 2000). In addition, this pre-acquisition phase should concentrate on understanding the current state of the health information technology industry to identify appropriate questions and the next steps in the selection process (American Organization of Nurse Executives, 2009). These first steps begin to identify any organizational risks related to successful implementation and pave the way for initiating a change management process to educate the organization about the future state of delivering health care with an EHR system.

The second step of the selection process is to select a system based on the organization's current and predicted needs. It is common during this phase to see a demonstration of several vendors' EHR products. Based on the completed needs assessment, the organization should establish key evaluation criteria to compare the different vendors and products. These criteria should include both subjective and objective items that cover such topics as common clinical workflows, decision support, reporting, usability, technical build, and maintenance of the system. Providing the vendor with these guidelines will ensure that the process meets the organization's needs; however, it is also essential to let the vendor demonstrate a proposed future state from its own perspective. This activity is critical to ensuring that the vendor's vision and the organization's vision are well aligned (Konschak & Shiple, n.d.). It also helps spark dialogue about the possible future state of clinical work at the organization and the change required in obtaining it. Such demonstrations not only enable the organization to compare and contrast the features and functions of different systems, but also are a good way to engage the organization's members in being a part of this strategic decision.

Implementation planning should occur concurrently with the selection process, particularly the assessment of the scope of the work, initial sequencing of the EHR components to be implemented, and resources required. However, this step begins in earnest once a vendor and a product have been selected. In addition to further refining the implementation plan, this is the time to identify key metrics by which to measure the EHR's success. An organization may realize numerous benefits from implementing an EHR. It should choose metrics that match its overall strategy and goals in the coming years and may include expected improvements in financial, quality, and clinical outcomes. Commonly used metrics focus on reductions in the number of duplicate laboratory tests through duplicate orders alerting, reductions in the number of adverse drug events through the use of bar-code medication administration, meaningful use objectives and measures, and the EHR advantages mentioned earlier in this chapter. To ensure that the desired benefits are realized, it is important to avoid choosing so many that they become meaningless or unobtainable, to carefully and practically define those that are chosen, to measure before and after the implementation, and to assign accountability to a member of the organization to ensure the work is completed.

End-user adoption of the EHR is also essential to realizing its benefits. Clinicians must be engaged to use the EHR successfully in their practice and daily workflows so that data may be captured to drive the decision support that underlies so many of the advantages and metrics described. To promote adoption, a change management plan must be developed in conjunction with the EHR implementation plan. The most effective change management plans offer end users several exposures to the system and relevant workflows in advance of its use and continue through the go-live and post-live time periods. Successful pre-live strategies include end-user involvement as subject-matter experts to validate the EHR workflow design and content build, hosting end-user usability testing sessions, shadowing end users in their current daily work in parallel with the new system, and formal training activities. The goal of these pre-live activities is not only to ensure that the EHR implementation will meet end user needs, but also to assess the impact of the new EHR on current workflow and process. The larger the impact, the more change management is required above and beyond system training. For example, simulation laboratory experiences may be offered to more thoroughly dress rehearse a significant workflow change, executive leadership may need to convey their support and expectations of clinicians about a new way of working, and generally more anticipatory guidance is required to communicate to those impacted by the changes.

Training may be delivered in a variety of media. Often a combination of approaches works best, including classroom time, electronic learning, independent exercises, and peer-to-peer, at-the-elbow support. Training must be workflow based and reflect real clinical processes. It must also be planned and budgeted for through the post-live period to ensure that competency with the system is assessed at the go-live point and that any necessary retraining or reinforcements are made in the 30 to 60 days post-live. This not only promotes reliability and safe use of the system as it was designed but also can have a positive impact on end users' morale: Users will feel that they are being supported beyond the initial go-live period and have an opportunity to move from basic skills to advanced proficiency with the system.

Finally, the implementation plan should account for the long-term optimization of the EHR. This step is commonly overlooked and often results in benefits falling short of expectations because the resources are not available to realize them permanently. It also often means the difference between end users of EHRs merely surviving the change versus becoming savvy about how to adopt the EHR as another powerful clinical tool, much as clinicians have embraced such technologies as the stethoscope (HealthIT.gov, 2012). Optimization activities of the EHR should be considered a routine part of the organization's operations, should be resourced accordingly, and should emphasize the continued involvement of clinician users to identify ways that the EHR can enable the organization to achieve its overall mission. Many organizations start an implementation of EHRs with the goal of transforming their care delivery and operations. An endeavor that differs from simply automating a previously manual or fragmented process, transformation often includes steps to improve the process so as to realize better patient care outcomes or added efficiency. Although some transformation is experienced with the initial use of the system, most of this work is done postimplementation and relies on widespread clinician adoption of the EHR. As such, it makes optimization a critical component to successful ownership of an EHR.

## Flexibility and Expandability

Health care is as unique as the patients themselves. It is delivered in a variety of settings, for a variety of reasons, over the course of a patient's lifetime. In addition, patients rarely receive all their care from one healthcare organization; indeed, choice is a cornerstone of the American healthcare system. An EHR must be flexible and expandable to meet the needs of patients and caregivers in all these settings, despite the challenges.

At a very basic level, there is as yet no EHR system available that can provide all functions for all specialties to such a degree that all clinicians would successfully adopt it. Consider oncology as an example. Most systems do not yet provide the advanced ordering features required for the complex treatment planning undertaken in this field. An oncologist could use a general system, but he or she would not find as many benefits without additional features for chemotherapy ordering, lifetime cumulative dose tracking, or the ability to adjust a treatment day schedule and recalculate a schedule for the remaining days of the plan. Some EHRs do a good job of supporting the work of nursing staff and physicians, but are not as supportive of the work of clinicians such as dieticians, physical and occupational therapists, and other healthcare personnel. These systems will continue to evolve and support interprofessional collaboration as more healthcare professionals are exposed to the power of these systems to support their work and become better able to articulate their specific needs.

Further, most healthcare organizations do not yet have the capacity to implement and maintain systems in all care areas. As one physician stated, "Implementing an EMR is a complex and difficult multidisciplinary effort that will stretch an organization's skills and capacity for change" (Chin, 2004, p. 47).

## BOX 14-4 CLOUDY EHRS

A paradigm shift from healthcare facility–owned, machine-based computing to offsite, vendor-owned cloud computing, Web browser–based log-in accessible data, software, and hardware could link systems together and reduce costs. Hospitals with shrinking budgets and extreme IT needs are exploring the successes in this area achieved in other industries, such as Amazon's S3. As providers strive to implement potent EHRs, they are looking for cloud-based models that offer the necessary functionality without having to assume the burden associated with all of the hardware, software, application, and storage issues. However, in the face of the HITECH Act and its associated penalties, how can we overcome the challenges to realize the benefits of this approach? Cloud computing has both advantages and disadvantages, and while they explore this new paradigm, healthcare providers must relinquish control as they continue to strive to maintain security. The vendors that are responsible for developing and maintaining this new environment are also facing challenges originating from both legislatures and healthcare providers. As the vendors and healthcare providers work together to improve the implementation and adoption of the cloud-based EHR, the sky is the limit!

These two conditions are improving every day at both vendor and healthcare organizations alike. Improvements in both areas were recently fueled by ARRA incentives (see Box 14-4).

ARRA has also set the expectation that despite the large number of settings in which a patient may receive care, a minimum set of data from those records must flow or "interoperate" among each setting and the unique EHR systems used in those settings. Today, interoperability exists through what is called a Continuity of Care Document (CCD). This dataset includes patient demographics, medication, allergy, and problem lists, among other things, and the formatting and exchange of the CCD is required to be supported by EHR vendors and healthcare organizations seeking ARRA meaningful use incentives. The document formatted according to HL7 standards is both machine readable and human readable.

Despite this positive step forward, financial and patient privacy hurdles remain to be overcome to achieve an expansive EHR. Most health care is delivered by small community practices and hospitals, many of which do not have the financial or technical resources to implement robust, interoperable EHRs. USDHHS recently loosened regulations so that physicians may now be able to receive healthcare information technology software, hardware, and implementation services from hospitals to alleviate the financial burden placed on individual providers and to foster more widespread adoption of the EHR.

Finally, patient privacy is a pivotal issue in determining how far and how easy it will be to share data across healthcare organizations. In addition to the Health Insurance Portability and Accountability Act privacy rules, many states have regulations in place related to patient confidentiality. An experience of the state of Minnesota foreshadows what all states may encounter. In 2007, Governor Tim Pawlenty announced the creation of the Minnesota Health Information Exchange (State of Minnesota, Office of the Governor, 2007). Although the intentions of the exchange were to promote patient safety and increase healthcare efficiency across the state, it raised significant concerns about security and privacy. New questions arose about the definition of when and how patient consent is required to exchange data electronically, and older paper-based processes needed to be updated to support real-time electronic exchange (Minnesota Department of Health, 2007). For health exchanges such as these to reach their full potential, members of the public must be able to trust that their privacy will be protected, or else the healthcare industry risks that patients may not share a full medical history, or worse yet, may not seek care, effectively making the exchanges useless.

## Accountable Care Organizations and the EHR

EHRs with data-sharing capabilities are central to the support of Accountable Care Organizations (ACOs), a payment incentive program established by the CMS (2015). As discussed elsewhere, this program of shared medical and financial responsibility is designed to provide quality, coordinated care while limiting costs. Some of the core information technology requirements for an ACO are EHRs, HIEs, care management systems, and analytics and reporting systems (Mastagni, Welter, & Holmes, 2015). A robust EHR can support many of these functions:

> *EHR solutions that are interoperable across organizations can significantly reduce the cost and complication of IT infrastructure by creating full EHR visibility between providers. This shared visibility reduces or eliminates the need to participate in HIEs or invest in solutions to integrate data across different EHR platforms. Many EHRs also can serve as a program's care management system, eliminating the need for a separate system to document care management efforts and help care teams engage with patients. (Mastagni et al., 2015, para. 5)*

See Figure 14-2.

## The Future

Despite the challenges, the future of EHRs is an exciting one for patients and clinicians alike. Benefits may be realized by implementing stand-alone EHRs as described here, but the most significant transformation will come as interoperability is realized between systems. As the former national information technology coordinator in the USDHHS David Brailer predicted about the potential of interoperability:

> *For the first time, clinicians everywhere can have a longitudinal medical record with full information about each patient. Consumers will have better information about their health status since personal health records and similar access strategies can be feasible in an interoperable world. Consumers can move more easily between and among clinicians without fear of their information being lost. Payers can benefit from the economic efficiencies, fewer errors, and reduced duplication that arises from interoperability. Healthcare information exchange and interoperability (HIEI) also underlies meaningful public health reporting, bioterrorism surveillance, quality monitoring, and advances in clinical trials. In short, there is little that most people want from health care for which HIEI isn't a prerequisite. (Brailer, 2005, p. W 5-20)*

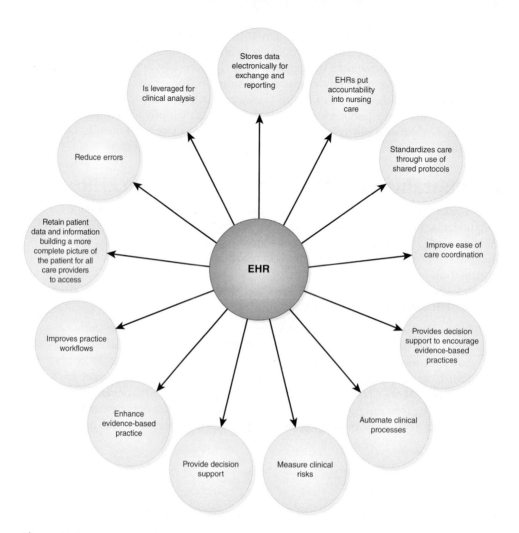

**Figure 14-2**  How EHRs Support Accountable Care
Data from ECG Consultants. (2015). The use of technology in healthcare reform: IT considerations
for accountable care. Retrieved from http://www.ecgmc.com/thought-leadership/articles/the
-use-of-technology-in-healthcare-reform-it-considerations-for-accountable-care

The future also holds tremendous potential for EHR features and functions that will include not only more sophisticated decision support and clinical reporting capacity, but also improved support for all healthcare professionals, improved bio-medical device integration, ease of use and intuitiveness, and access through more hardware platforms.

Implementation of robust and interoperable EHRs is becoming more common-place. More organizations adopting EHRs will facilitate broader dissemination of implementation best practices, with the hope of further shortening the time required to take advantage of advanced EHR features.

In the future, we can expect to see more EHRs housed in the cloud, usable patient portals as we move toward more patient-centered health care, better mobile applications for the EHR, the expansion of telemedicine applications for rural patients and those with chronic illnesses, and precision medicine advances supported by data analytics (Reisenwitz, 2016).

## Summary

It is an important time for health care and technology. EHRs have come to the forefront and will remain central to shaping the future of health care. In an ideal world, all nurses, from entry-level personnel to executives, will have a basic competency in nursing informatics that will enable them to participate fully in shaping the future use of technology in the practice at a national level and wherever care is delivered. Such initiatives as Technology Informatics Guiding Education Reform (TIGER) and the important nursing terminology work are imperative for better integration and, ultimately, more visibility of nursing contributions to health care.

### THOUGHT-PROVOKING QUESTIONS

1. What are the implications for nursing education as the EHR becomes the standard for caring for patients?
2. What are the ethical considerations related to interoperability and a shared EHR?
3. You are asked about a diagnosis with which you are unfamiliar. Where would you start looking for information? How would you determine the validity of the information?
4. Think about the documentation and knowledge management functions of your specialty. If you had the opportunity to create a wish list, what would you include in an EHR to support your work?

## References

Adams, J., Ponte, P. & Somerville, J. (2016). Assuring the capture of standardized nursing data: a call to action for chief nursing officers. *International Journal of Nursing Knowledge*, 27(3), 127–128. doi:10.1111/2047-3095.12136.

American Nurses Association (ANA). (2015). Inclusion of recognized terminologies within ehrs and other health information technology solutions. Retrieved from http://www.nursingworld.org/MainMenuCategories/Policy-Advocacy/Positions-and-Resolutions/ANAPositionStatements/Position-Statements-Alphabetically/Inclusion-of-Recognized-Terminologies-within-EHRs.html

American Organization of Nurse Executives. (2009). *AONE guiding principles for defining the role of the nurse executive in technology acquisition and implementation*. Washington, DC: Author. Retrieved from http://www.aone.org/resources/technology-acquisition-implementation.pdf

Bayliss, E. A., Ellis, J. L., Shoup, J. A., Chan, Z., McQuillan, D. B., & Steiner, J. F. (2015). Effect of continuity of care on hospital utilization for seniors with multiple medical conditions in an integrated health care system. *Annals of Family Medicine*, 13(2), 123–129. doi:10.1370/afm.1739

Brailer, D. J. (2005, January). Interoperability: The key to the future healthcare system. *Health Affairs—Web Exclusive*, W 5-19–W 5-21. Retrieved from http://content.healthaffairs.org/cgi/reprint/hlthaff.w5.19v1

Bronnert, J., Masarie, C., Naeymi-Rad, F., Rose, E., & Aldin, G. (2012, July). Problem-centered care delivery: How interface terminology makes standardized health information possible. *Journal of AHIMA, 83*(7), 30–35.

Bush, G. W. (2004). State of the Union address. Retrieved from http://content.healthaffairs.org/cgi/reprint/hlthaff.w5.19v1

Centers for Medicare and Medicaid Services (CMS). (2015). Accountable care organizations. Retrieved from https://www.cms.gov/Medicare/Medicare-Fee-for-Service-Payment/ACO/index.html

Certification Commission for Healthcare Information Technology. (2007). Certification Commission announces new work group members. Retrieved from Retrieved from http://www.healthimaging.com/topics/health-it/cchit-announces-new-work-group-members

Charles, D., Gabriel, M., & Searcy, T. (2015). Adoption of electronic health record systems among U.S. non-federal acute care hospitals: 2008–2014. *HealthIT.gov*. Retrieved from http://www.healthit.gov/sites/default/files/data-brief/2014HospitalAdoptionDataBrief.pdf

Chaudhry, B., Wang, J., Wu, S., Maglione, M., Mojica, W., Roth, E., . . . Shekelle, P. (2006). Systematic review: Impact of health information technology on quality, efficiency, and costs of medical care. *Annals of Internal Medicine, 144*(10), E-12–E-22.

Chin, H. L. (2004). The reality of EMR implementation: Lessons from the field. *Permanente Journal, 8*(4), 43–48.

Dorr, D., Bonner, L. M., Cohen, A. N., Shoai, R. S., Perrin, R., Chaney, E., & Young, A. (2007). Informatics systems to promote improved care for chronic illness: A literature review. *Journal of the American Medical Informatics Association, 14*(2), 156–163.

Embi, P. J., Jain, A., Clark, J., Bizjack, S., Hornung, R., & Harris, C. M. (2005). Effect of a clinical trial alert system on physician participation in trial recruitment. *Archives of Internal Medicine, 165*, 2272–2277.

Goddard, B. L. (2000). Termination of a contract to implement an enterprise electronic medical record system. *Journal of American Medical Informatics Association, 7*, 564–568.

Halamka, J. D. (2006, May). Health information technology: Shall we wait for the evidence? [Letter to the editor]. *Annals of Internal Medicine, 144*(10), 775–776.

Healthcare Information and Management Systems Society (HIMSS). (2007). Electronic health record. Retrieved from http://www.himss.org/ASP/topics_ehr.asp

Healthcare Information and Management Systems Society (HIMSS). (2009). HIMSS Davies Organizational Award application: MultiCare. Retrieved from http://www.himss.org/multicare-davies-enterpriseorganizational-award

Healthcare Information and Management Systems Society (HIMSS). (2010a). Davies Award. Retrieved from http://www.himss.org/davies

Healthcare Information and Management Systems Society (HIMSS). (2010b). Recipient list. Retrieved from http://www.himss.org/himss-enterprise-davies-award-recipients

Healthcare Information and Management Systems Society (HIMSS). (2013). HIMSS 2013 iHIT Study: Executive summary. Retrieved from http://www.himss.org/library/clinical-informatics/2013-ihitstudy-executive-summary

Healthcare Information and Management Systems Society (HIMSS) Analytics. (2013). Electronic medical record adoption model (EMRAM). Retrieved from http://www.himssanalytics.org/emram/index.aspx

Healthcare Information and Management Systems Society (HIMSS) Analytics. (2014). EMRAM stage criteria. Retrieved from http://www.himssanalytics.org/research/emram-stage-criteria

Healthcare Information and Management Systems Society (HIMSS) Analytics. (2015). Validated Stage 6 & 7 Providers List. Retrieved from http://www.himssanalytics.org/case-study/validated -stage-6-7-providers-list

Healthcare IT News. (2015). 7 tips for EMR success from Stage 7 hospitals. Retrieved from http://www.healthcareitnews.com/news/7-tips-emr-success-stage-7-hospitals

HealthIT.gov. (2012). Benefits of EHRs: Why adopt EHRs? Retrieved from http://www.healthit .gov/providers-professionals/why-adopt-ehrs

HealthIT.gov. (2013). How to attain meaningful use. Retrieved from http://www.healthit.gov /providers-professionals/how-attain-meaningful-use

HealthIT.gov. (2014). What are the advantages of electronic health records? Retrieved from http://www.healthit.gov/providers-professionals/faqs/what-are-advantages-electronic-health -records

HealthIT.gov. (2015a). About the ONC Health IT certification program. Retrieved from http://www.healthit.gov/policy-researchers-implementers/certification-bodies-testing -laboratories

HealthIT.gov. (2015b). 2015 edition test method. Retrieved from http://www.healthit.gov /policy-researchers-implementers/2015-edition-draft-test-procedures

Health Level Seven International (HL7). (n.d.) About HL7 International. Retrieved from http://www.hl7.org

Health Resources and Services Administration (HRSA). (n.d.) Common EHR functions. Retrieved from http://www.hrsa.gov/healthit/toolbox/healthitimplementation/implementationtopics /selectcertifiedehr/selectacertifiedehr_5.html

Holbrook, A., Keshavjee, K., Troyan, S., Pray, M., & Ford, P. T. (2003). Applying methodology to electronic medical record selection. *International Journal of Medical Informatics, 71,* 43–50.

Husk, G., & Waxman, D. A. (2004). Using data from hospital information systems to improve emergency care. *Academic Emergency Medicine, 11*(11), 1237–1244.

Institute of Medicine (IOM). (2001). *Crossing the quality chasm: A new health system for the 21st century.* Washington, DC: National Academies Press.

Institute of Medicine (IOM). (2003). *Key capabilities of an electronic health record system: Letter report.* Washington, DC: National Academies Press.

Jain, A., Atreja, A., Harris, C. M., Lehmann, M., Burns, J., & Young, J. (2005). Responding to the rofecoxib withdrawal crisis: A new model for notifying patients at risk and their healthcare providers. *Annals of Internal Medicine, 142*(3), 182–186.

Jansen, W., & Grance, T. (2011). National Institute of Standards and Technology (NIST): Guidelines on security and privacy in public cloud computing. Retrieved from https://cloudsecurityalliance.org/wp-content/uploads/2011/07/NIST-Draft-SP-800-144 _cloud-computing.pdf

Kelly, T. (2016). Electronic health records for quality nursing & health care. Lancaster, PA: DEStech Publications, Inc.

Kim, T. Y., Hardiker, N., & Coenen, A. (2014). Inter-terminology mapping of nursing problems. *Journal of Biomedical Informatics, 49,* 213–220. doi:10.1016/j.jbi.2014.03.001

Konschak, C., & Shiple, D. (n.d.). System selection: Aligning vision and technology. Retrieved from http://divurgent.com/wp-content/uploads/2013/12/White-Paper.Vendor-Selection .vfinal.pdf

Kutney-Lee, A., & Kelly, D. (2011). The effect of hospital electronic health record adoption on nurse-assessed quality of care and patient safety. *Journal of Nursing Administration, 41*(11), 466–472. doi: 10.1097/NNA.0b013e3182346e4b

Mastagni, E., Welter, T., & Holmes, M. (2015). The use of technology in healthcare reform: IT considerations for accountable care. *ECG Management Consultants*. Retrieved from http://www.ecgmc.com/thought-leadership/articles/the-use-of-technology-in-healthcare -reform-it-considerations-for-accountable-care

Matney, S. A., Warren, J. J., Evans, J. L., Kim, T. Y., Coenen, A., & Auld, V. A. (2012). Development of the nursing problem list subset of SNOMED CT. *Journal of Biomedical Informatics, 45*(4), 683–688. doi:10.1016/j.jbi.2011.12.003

Minnesota Department of Health. (2007, June). *Minnesota Health Records Act—HF 1078 fact sheet*. Minneapolis, MN: Author. Retrieved from http://www.health.state.mn.us /e-health/summit/summit2007/beyerkropuenske07.pdf

National Institute of Standards and Technology (NIST). (2010). Meaningful use test measures: Approved test procedures. Retrieved from http://healthcare.nist.gov/use_testing/finalized _requirements.html

National Institutes of Health. (2006, April). *Electronic health records overview*. McLean, VA: Mitre Corporation.

Poprock, B. (2005, September). *Using Epic's alternative medications reminder to reduce prescription costs and encourage assistance programs for indigent patients*. Presented at the Epic Systems Corporation user group meeting, Madison, WI.

Reed, H. L., & Bernard, E. (2005). Reductions in diabetic cardiovascular risk by community primary care providers. *International Journal of Circumpolar Health, 64*(1), 26–37.

Reisenwitz, C. (2016, January). Top 5 EHR trends for 2016. *Capterra Medical Software Blog*. Retrieved from http://blog.capterra.com/top-5-ehr-trends-for-2016-2/

Robert Wood Johnson Foundation (RWJF). (2006). Health information technology in the United States: The information base for progress. Retrieved from http://www.rwjf.org /programareas/resources/product.jsp?id=15895&pid=1142&gsa=1

Rosenbloom, S. T., Miller, R. A., Johnson, K. B., Elkin, P. L., & Brown, S. H. (2006). Interface terminologies: Facilitating direct entry of clinical data into electronic health record systems. *Journal of the American Medical Informatics Association, 13*(3), 277–288. http://doi.org/10.1197/jamia.M1957

Shekelle, P. G., Morton, S. C., & Keeler, E. B. (2006). *Costs and benefits of health information technology. Evidence report/technology assessment, No. 132* [Prepared by the Southern California Evidence-based Practice Center under Contract No. 290-02-0003]. Agency for Healthcare Research and Quality Publication No. 06-E006. Rockville, MD: Agency for Healthcare Research and Quality.

Smith, T., Semerdjian, N., King, P., DeMartin, B., Levi, S., Reynolds, K.,... Dowd, J. (2004). *Nicholas E. Davies Award of Excellence: Transforming healthcare with a patient-centric electronic health record system*. Evanston, IL: Evanston Northwestern Healthcare. Retrieved from http://www.himss.org/content/files/davies2004_evanston.pdf

Spooner, S. A., & Council on Clinical Information Technology. (2007). Special requirements of electronic health record systems in pediatrics. *Pediatrics, 119*, 631–637.

State of Minnesota, Office of the Governor. (2007). New public–private partnership to improve patient care, safety and efficiency. Retrieved from http://www.governor.state.mn.us /mediacenter/pressreleases/2007/PROD008303.html

Technology Informatics Guiding Education Reform (TIGER). (2006). Evidence and informatics transforming nursing. Retrieved from http://www.amia.org/sites/amia.org/files/Malin-AMIA -Tiger-Team-Testimony.pdf

Thompson, D. I., Osheroff, J., Classen, D., & Sittig, D. F. (2007). A review of methods to estimate the benefits of electronic medical records in hospitals and the need for a national database. *Journal of Healthcare Information Management, 21*(1), 62–68.

Turk, M. (2015). Electronic health records. *Brooklyn Law Review, 80*(2), 565–597.

U.S. Department of Health and Human Services (USDHHS). (2010). Medicare and Medicaid programs: Electronic health record incentive program. Retrieved from http://www.ofr.gov/OFRUpload/OFRData/2010-17202_PI.pdf

U.S. National Library of Medicine. (2016). Supporting Interoperability – Terminology, subsets and other resources from NLM. Retrieved from https://www.nlm.nih.gov/hit_interoperability.html

1. Explore the characteristics of a safety culture.
2. Examine strategies for developing a safety culture.
3. Recognize how human factors contribute to errors.
4. Appreciate the impact of informatics technology on patient safety.

## Key Terms

» Adverse events
» Agency for Health-care Research and Quality (AHRQ)
» Alarm fatigue
» Applications (apps)
» Bar-code medication administration (BCMA)
» Clinical decision support (CDS)

» Computerized physician order entry (CPOE)
» Electronic medication administration system (eMAR)
» Failure modes and effects analysis (FMEA)

» Government Accountability Office (GAO)
» High-hazard drugs
» Human factors engineering
» Just culture
» Never events
» Radio frequency identifier (RFID)

» Root-cause analysis
» Safety culture
» Smart pump
» Smart rooms
» Systems engineering
» Wearable technology
» Workarounds

# CHAPTER 15

# Informatics Tools to Promote Patient Safety and Quality Outcomes

Dee McGonigle and Kathleen Mastrian

## Introduction

Nursing professionals have an ethical duty to ensure patient safety. According to Lavin et al. (2015), "Direct care nurses, at their core, are risk managers. They attach meaning to what is and anticipate 'what might be'" (para. 8). As the media and patients circulate stories about the lack of safety in healthcare institutions, it is no wonder that healthcare consumers are skeptical and providers are wary. A study out of Johns Hopkins University (Johns Hopkins Medicine, 2016) suggested that medical errors are the third-leading cause of death in the United States. Versel (2016) reminded us, however, that "it's not the first time someone has called medical error the No. 3 cause of death in the U.S. John T. James, founder of a group called Patient Safety America, did that in a 2013 report in the *Journal of Patient Safety*." (para. 2). Increasing demands on professionals in complex and fast-paced healthcare environments may lead them to cut corners or develop workarounds that deviate from accepted and expected practice protocols. These deviations are not carried out deliberately to put patients at risk, but rather are often practiced in the interest of saving time or because the organizational culture is such that risky behaviors are commonplace. Occasionally, these inappropriate actions or omissions of appropriate actions result in harm or significant risk of harm to patients. Consider the following case scenario:

> A 19-year-old obese woman who had recently undergone
> C-section delivery of a baby presented in the emergency depart-
> ment (ED) with dyspnea. Believing the patient had developed
> a pulmonary embolism, the physician prescribed an IV hepa-
> rin bolus dose of 5,000 units followed by a heparin infusion at
> 1,000 units/hour. After administering the bolus dose, a nurse
> started the heparin infusion but misprogrammed the pump to run
> at 1,000 mL/hour, not 1,000 units/hour (20 mL/hour). By the time

*the error was discovered, the patient had received more than 17,000 units (5,000 unit loading dose and about 12,000 units from the infusion) in less than an hour since arrival in the ED. A smart pump with dosing limits for heparin had been used. Thus, the programming error should have been recognized before the infusion was started. However, the nurse had elected to bypass the dose-checking technology and had used the pump in its standard mode. It was quite fortunate that the patient did not experience adverse bleeding as her aPTT values were as prolonged as 240 seconds when initially measured and 148 seconds two hours later. (Institute for Safe Medication Practices, 2007, para. 2)*

The smart pump used in this scenario was equipped with dose calculation software that compares the programmed infusion rate to a drug database to check for dosing within safe limits. This technology is particularly important when high-alert or high-hazard drugs are being administered. In this case, however, the available dose-checking technology had been turned off and the pump was operated in standard mode. A subsequent analysis of the error event revealed that many nurses in the institution were bypassing the safety technology afforded by the smart pump to save time. Even though it has been more than a decade since this error occurred, we continue to see alerts and safety checks being worked around, ignored, or turned off. This chapter focuses on some of the recommended organizational strategies used to promote a culture of safety and some of the specific informatics technologies designed to reduce errors and promote patient safety.

## What Is a Culture of Safety?

The 2000 Institute of Medicine report *To Err Is Human* is widely credited for launching the current focus on patient safety in health care. This report was followed in 2001 by the Institute of Medicine's *Crossing the Quality Chasm* report, which brought to national attention healthcare quality and safety. This national attention resulted in a $50 million grant by Congress to the **Agency for Healthcare Research and Quality (AHRQ)** to launch initiatives focused on safety research for patients. Other initiatives prompted by these seminal reports were the Joint Commission's National Patient Safety Goals (2002); the National Quality Forum's **adverse events** and "**never events**" list (2002); the creation of the Office of National Coordinator for Health Information Technology (HIT) to computerize health care (2004); the formation of the World Health Organization's Alliance for Patient Safety (2004); the Institute for Healthcare Improvement's (IHI) 100,000 Lives campaign (2005) and 5 Million Lives campaign (2008); Congressional authorization of patient safety organizations created by the Patient Safety and Quality Improvement Act to promote blameless error reporting and shared learning (2005); the "no pay for errors" initiative launched by Medicare (2008); and the $19 billion Congressional appropriation to support electronic health records (EHRs) and patient safety (Wachter, 2010). In 2013, the Patient Safety Movement Foundation launched the Open Data Pledge, and later announced three new patient safety challenges in 2016 (Patient Safety Movement, 2016). The most pressing challenges they identified—venous thromboembolism, mental health, and pediatric adverse drug events—reflect those where patient death could be prevented with the proper protocols in place during the provision of patient care (Patient Safety Movement).

The AHRQ (2012) safety culture primer laid the foundation for and suggested that organizations should strive to achieve high reliability by being committed to improving healthcare quality and preventing medical errors and to demonstrate an overall commitment to patient safety. That is, everyone and every level in an organization must embrace the safety culture. Key features of a **safety culture** identified by the AHRQ are as follows:

- Acknowledgment of the high-risk nature of an organization's activities and the determination to achieve consistently safe operations
- A blame-free environment where individuals are able to report errors or near misses without fear of reprimand or punishment
- Encouragement of collaboration across ranks and disciplines to seek solutions to patient safety problems
- Organizational commitment of resources to address safety concerns (AHRQ, 2012, para. 1)

An important part of the safety culture is cultivating a blame-free environment. Errors and near misses must always be reported so that they can be thoroughly analyzed. All organizations can learn from mistakes and change their organizational processes or culture to ensure patient safety. The Patient Safety and Quality Improvement Act of 2005 mandated the creation of a national database of medical errors and funded several organizations to analyze these data with the goal of developing shared learning to prevent medical errors. Organizations themselves can engage in **root-cause analysis** or **failure modes and effects analysis (FMEA)** to examine medical errors closely and to determine the system processes that need to be changed to prevent similar future errors (Harrison & Daly, 2009). A tool for implementing root-cause analysis developed by the U.S. Department of Veteran's Affairs National Center for Patient Safety (2015) had three goals: to determine "what happened, why did it happen and how to prevent it from happening again" (para. 4). Everyone is encouraged to submit actual medical errors and/or patient safety issues to the Patient Safety Network (PSNet, 2016a). Similarly, the IHI has a website dedicated to FMEA. "Failure Modes and Effects Analysis (FMEA) is a systematic, proactive method for evaluating a process to identify where and how it might fail, and to assess the relative impact of different failures in order to identify the parts of the process that are most in need of change" (IHI, 2016b, para. 1). If one embraces a blame-free environment to encourage error reporting, then where does individual accountability fit in? According to the AHRQ, one way to balance these competing cultural values (blameless versus accountability) is to establish a "**just culture**" where system or process issues that lead to unsafe behaviors and errors are addressed by changing practices or workflow processes, and a clear message is communicated that reckless behaviors are not tolerated. The "just culture" approach accounts for three types of behaviors leading to patient safety compromises: (1) human error (unintentional mistakes); (2) risky behaviors (**workarounds**); and (3) reckless behavior (total disregard for established policies and procedures).

# Strategies for Developing a Safety Culture

Strategies for achieving a safety culture have been addressed frequently in the literature. The focus here is limited to those strategies described by two key organizations, the AHRQ and the IHI. The AHRQ (2016), based on data from the Hospital Survey on Patient Safety Culture, suggested that teamwork training, executive walk-arounds, and unit-based safety teams have improved safety culture perceptions but have not led to a significant reduction in error rates. The AHRQ recommended seven steps of action planning: "1. Understand your survey results. 2. Communicate and discuss survey results. 3. Develop focused action plans. 4. Communicate action plans and deliverables. 5. Implement action plans. 6. Track progress and evaluate impact. 7. Share what works" (p. 61). Informatics can assist with the analysis, trending, synthesis, and dissemination of the action plan results.

The IHI (2016a) stressed that organizational leaders must drive the culture change by making a visible commitment to safety and by enabling staff to share safety information openly. Some of the strategies suggested by the IHI include appointing a safety champion for every unit, creating an adverse event response team, and reenacting or simulating adverse events to better understand the organizational or procedural processes that failed. Barnet (2016) reported that 49 companies had signed the open data pledge with Patient Safety Movement. Radick (2016) believed that senior leaders must be involved in order to sustain patient safety improvements. Leadership oversight and support is critical to ongoing sharing and, most importantly, collaborative solution development to provide safe care and achieve quality outcomes for all patients.

A **systems engineering** approach to patient safety, in which technology manufacturers partner with organizations to identify risks to patient safety and promote safe technology integration, has been advocated by Ebben, Gieras, and Gosbee (2008). They noted that **human factors engineering** is "[t]he discipline of applying what is known about human capabilities and limitations to the design of products, processes, systems, and work environments," and its application to system design improves "ease of use, system performance and reliability, and user satisfaction, while reducing operational errors, operator stress, training requirements, user fatigue, and product liability" (p. 327). For example, Ebben et al. described the feel of an oxygen control knob that rotated smoothly between settings, suggesting to the user that oxygen flows at all points on the knob, when in fact oxygen flowed only at specifically designated liter flow settings. Human factors engineering testing would most likely reveal this design flaw, and the setting knob could be improved to include discrete audio or tactile feedback (click into place) to the user to indicate a point on the dial where oxygen flows. Ebben et al. also emphasized that testing human use factors provides more objective safety data than the subjective responses gained from user preference testing. "Understanding how the equipment shapes human performance is as important as evaluating reliability or other technical criteria" (p. 329). Organizations that are purchasing medical technology devices should avail themselves of shared safety data on equipment maintained by several key organizations, including the Joint Commission, the Food and Drug

Administration, and the Medical Product Safety Network. Many healthcare practitioners feel that we have not made great strides in either sharing our data or accessing the available data to enhance patient safety interests. According to WISH Patient Safety Forum (2015), the patient safety premises that harms are inevitable, data silos are natural, and heroism is the norm "have inadvertently provided excuses for not addressing patient safety comprehensively" (p. 9). This forum also stated that

> [t]he belief that data silos are acceptable in healthcare settings is an irresponsible view regarding the role of data; it lacks an understanding of the current operational setting. Healthcare is a complex, multidisciplinary environment that requires collaboration and sharing of data across an integrated stakeholder community. (WISH Patient Safety Forum, p. 9)

As HIT evolves, refinements in HIT continue to improve patient safety. Banger and Graber (2015) stated that the

> ONC is involved in a number of initiatives in support of this goal, including plans for a new national Health IT Safety Center to coordinate these efforts. Combined with the active engagement from the private sector, there is every reason to be optimistic that health IT will continue to improve the quality and safety of health care beyond the accomplishments realized to date. (p. 10)

According to the PSNet (2015), "busy health care workers rely on equipment to carry out life-saving interventions, with the underlying assumption that technology will improve outcomes" (para. 2). PSNet provided the following descriptions of equipment issues:

> An obstetric nurse connects a bag of pain medication intended for an epidural catheter to the mother's intravenous (IV) line, resulting in a fatal cardiac arrest. Newborns in a neonatal intensive care unit are given full-dose heparin instead of low-dose flushes, leading to three deaths from intracranial bleeding. An elderly man experiences cardiac arrest while hospitalized, but when the code blue team arrives, they are unable to administer a potentially life-saving shock because the defibrillator pads and the defibrillator itself cannot be physically connected. (para. 1)

See also Figure 15-1.

Once the technology is integrated into the organization, biomedical engineers can become valuable partners in promoting patient safety through appropriate use of these technologies. For example, in one organization, the biomedical engineers helped to revamp processes associated with the new technology alarm systems after they discovered several key issues: slow response times to legitimate alarms and multiple false alarms (promoting **alarm fatigue**) created by alarm parameters that were too sensitive. Strategies for addressing these issues included improving the nurse

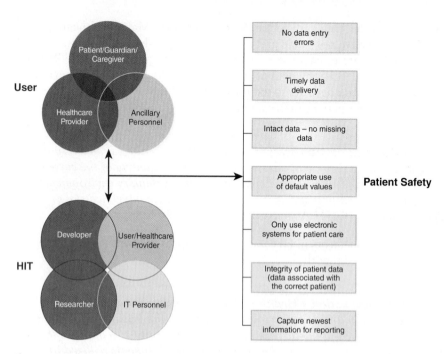

**Figure 15-1** User–Technology–Patient Safety Scheme

call system by adding Voice over Internet Protocol telephones that wirelessly receive alarms directly from technology equipment carried by all nurses, thus reducing response times to alarms; feeding alarm data into a reporting database for further analysis; and encouraging nurses to round with physicians to provide input into alarm parameters that were too sensitive and were generating multiple false alarms (Joint Commission, 2013; Williams, 2009). Research Brief 1 describes three investigations spanning from 2009 to 2016: a study of intelligent agent (IA) technology to improve the specificity of physiologic alarms, an integrative review of alarms, and default alarm setting changes coupled with in-service education. The Case Scenario, *Well-Intentioned Providers*, demonstrates how well-intentioned healthcare providers can cause harm. An audit conducted at one of their customer sites by Philips Healthcare (2013) revealed that a

> *Telemetry Charge Nurse was found to be receiving and responding to an average of 3.7 alarms per minute over the duration of the audit. Even allowing for minimal time to respond to each alarm, it is clear that this situation was problematic. A majority of that nurse's time was spent responding to alarms, and inevitably some were missed. (para. 1)*

The Joint Commission (2016) released the 2016 Hospital National Patient Safety Goals, and one category, Use Alarms Safely, stated that hospitals must "make improvements to ensure that alarms on medical equipment are heard and responded to on time" (para. 4).

## RESEARCH BRIEF 1

The investigators in one study used simple reactive IA technology to develop and test decision algorithms for improving the sensitivity and specificity of physiologic alarms. The IA technology was tested in a 14-bed cardiothoracic unit over 28 days and was implemented in parallel to the usual physiologic patient monitor that provided measures such as systolic blood pressure, mean arterial pressure, central venous pressure, and cardiac index. Alarm data generated by both systems were compared and classified as to whether the alarm represented a true medical event requiring clinician intervention or a false-positive alarm. A total of 293,049 alarms were generated by the usual physiologic monitoring system, and 1,012 alarms were generated by the IA system after raw physiologic data were filtered using rule-based IA technology. The IA filtering system shows promise for improving the specificity of physiologic alarms and decreasing the number of false-positive alarms generated by artifacts, thus reducing the incidence of alert fatigue in clinicians.

The full article appears in Blum, J., Kruger, G., Sanders, K., Gutierrez, J., & Rosenberg, A. (2009). Specificity improvement for network distributed physiologic alarms based on a simple deterministic reactive intelligent agent in the critical care environment. *Journal of Clinical Monitoring and Computing, 23*(1), 21–30.

Another study conducted an integrative review of monitor alarm fatigue. The study's evidence-based practice recommendations for technology included incorporating short delays to increase response rates, creating a set of standardized alarms to enhance the staff's ability to quickly determine what the alarm is for, and animated troubleshooting on monitoring equipment. The author concluded that lack of response to alarms has caused harm and death and stated that, because a focus on patient outcomes is needed, outcomes research must be performed.

The full article appears in Cvach, M. (2012). Monitor alarm fatigue: An integrative review. *Biomedical Instrumentation & Technology, 46*(4), 268–277. doi.org/10.2345/0899-8205-46.4.268

A pilot project was conducted to investigate if "(1) a change in default alarm settings of the cardiac monitors and (2) in-service nursing education on cardiac monitor use in an ICU" would decrease alarm rates and improve the attitudes and practices of nurses in relation to clinical alarms (para. 2). This quality improvement project examined 39 nurses in a 20-bed transplant/cardiac ICU. Nurses received an in-service on monitor use, an audit log of alarms was collected, and the nurses' attitudes and clinical practices were assessed using a pre- and postintervention survey. The authors concluded that "changing default alarm settings and standard in-service education on cardiac monitor use are insufficient to improve alarm systems safety" (para. 5).

The full article appears in Sowan, A. K., Gomez, T. M, Tarriela, A. F., Reed, C. C., & Paper, B. M. (2016). Changes in default alarm settings and standard in-service are insufficient to improve alarm fatigue in an intensive care unit: A pilot project. *JMIR Human Factors, 3*(1), e1.

## CASE SCENARIO: WELL-INTENTIONED PROVIDERS

Even well-intentioned healthcare providers can cause harm. Consider what should have been done differently in the case example below.

Laura, a 25-year-old woman, arrived at the ER complaining of chest pain. She has two young children at home: a 6-year-old boy and a 4-year-old girl. She stated that she has been experiencing severe fatigue and fluttering in her chest for weeks but felt that she needed rest and it was probably nothing. Today, she had the fluttering with chest pain, and even her teeth and jaw hurt. This scared her, so she decided to go to the hospital. However, she had to wait 2 hours for her mother to arrive to watch the children. Her husband is on a business trip and will not be returning for 4 days. The initial ECG revealed normal sinus rhythm and all lab values were normal. The ER physician decided to keep her for observation and sent her to the telemetry unit.

Laura was moved to telemetry and, as she stated, "wired for sound." The nurse described the equipment and told her that in addition to all of the monitoring equipment, they would check her vital signs every hour as well. The nurse no sooner returned to the nurse's station when Laura's cardiac monitor alerted her that Laura was experiencing severe bradycardia (heart rate of less than 40 beats per minute). When the nurse arrived at Laura's bedside, she found Laura sound asleep. She woke her gently and told her that her monitor was alarming and that she was going to check her. Laura stated that she felt tired and was enjoying the peaceful sleep. Laura's vital signs were fine and her heart rate was 72 beats per minute. The nurse reset the monitor, by which point Laura had already fallen back to sleep. The monitor alarmed the same way three more times within the next hour. Each time the nurse woke Laura and everything was fine. The nurse decided to contact the resident. While she was waiting for the resident, it alarmed twice again, but she just reset it and let Laura sleep. The resident came and examined Laura. The resident felt everything was OK and that this young mother needed her rest. The resident suggested that the nurse stop the hourly vitals, call and have the equipment examined by the biomedical department, and in the meantime to turn the alarm off. The nurse agreed, turned off the alarm, placed a call to the biomedical technician on duty, and left a message.

The nurse had another patient who also had frequent alarms, but his corresponded to actual medical events. As a result, the nurse was spending a great deal of time with this elderly gentleman and his wife. Each time she walked by Laura's bed, the nurse noted that Laura was sleeping. She realized that it had been 2 hours since she turned off the alarm and called the biomedical technician, so she decided to check on Laura; however, her other patient's alarm went off and, since Laura was sleeping, the nurse went to the other pateint's bedside. At 4 hours after the alarm had been turned off, the biomedical technician arrived and apologized because there was a call-off in their department and they were running shorthanded. The nurse explained what had happened and the biomedical technician went to check Laura's monitoring equipment. The biomedical technician called for the nurse as the patient was unresponsive. The nurse could not wake Laura, and the monitor was showing asystole. A code was initiated and Laura was pronounced dead 5 hours after she arrived on the telemetry unit.

This situation was assessed by the patient safety officer and the patient safety committee.

Because the monitor was integrated and all functions ran through the same controller, the nurse did not realize she was turning off all of the monitors (pulse oximetry, blood pressure, etc.). This was found to be an issue with the equipment itself because the alarm settings are too close together and not clearly labeled; however, the nurse should never have turned the alarms off. With the hourly checks cancelled and all of the monitoring equipment silenced, Laura was not being monitored at all. Well-intentioned providers were allowing this young mother to sleep, but with fatal consequences.

It is evident from Research Brief 1 and the Case Scenario that we have yet to find a solution to the problem of alarm fatigue and related issues that negatively impact patient safety.

Clearly, there is more work to be done to create safety cultures in complex healthcare organizations and to reduce the incidence of errors. Many organizations are looking to informatics technology to help manage these complex safety issues by using smart technologies that provide knowledge access to users, provide automated safety checks, and improve communication processes. Harrison (2016) stated that "as nurse leaders in a clinical setting where smart tools are leveraged to increase the quality and safety of patient care, we have certain responsibilities to ensure safe implementation, training, and monitoring" (p. 21). To best utilize the available technology, nurse leaders and administrators must be able to use data. More and more graduate programs for nursing administrators are realizing the need for these emerging nursing leaders to be skilled in nursing informatics. These leaders must be able to use data, information, and knowledge efficiently and effectively to assess and manage their clinical settings and ultimately apply these informatics skills to improve patient outcomes and the quality of patient care (Figure 15-2).

On a much higher level, the **Government Accountability Office (GAO)** selected and assessed six hospitals, from which it identified three challenges in implementing patient safety practices. The number one challenge was "obtaining data to identify adverse reactions in their own hospitals" (GAO, 2016, para. 2). Nursing informatics skills and knowledge can address this challenge.

The GAO interviewed patient safety experts and the related literature to identify three key gaps where better information could help guide hospital officials in their continued efforts to implement patient safety practices. These gaps involve a lack of "(1) information about the effect of contextual factors on implementation of patient safety practices, (2) sufficiently detailed information on the experience of hospitals that have previously used specific patient safety implementation strategies, and (3) valid and accurate measurement of how frequently certain adverse events occur" (p. 22). Once again, implementing solid nursing informatics practices, skills, and knowledge can close these gaps.

# Informatics Technologies for Patient Safety

Healthcare technologies are frequently designed to improve patient safety, streamline work processes, and improve the quality and outcomes of healthcare delivery. However, technology is not always the answer to patient safety; as the Joint Commission (2008) cautioned, "the overall safety and effectiveness of technology in health care ultimately depends on its human users, and . . . any form of technology can have a negative impact on the quality and safety of care if it is designed or implemented improperly or is misinterpreted" (para. 2). As we continue to look to HIT to advance patient safety initiatives, we must realize that integrating HIT presents other challenges and can add to the patient safety issues. For example, Singh and Sittig (2016) stated that HIT has the "potential to improve patient safety but its implementation and use has led to unintended consequences and new safety concerns. A key

**Figure 15-2** Data and Quality Connection: There are many ways to obtain data and information. The skill is in knowing how to access, select, and use the data and information, applying nursing informatics to inform practice and improve patient care.

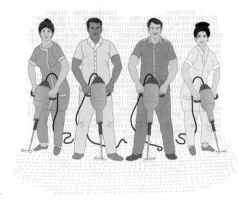

We need to know how to access data and information.

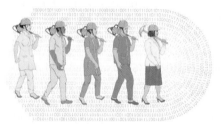

Next, we judiciously select and retrieve the data and information necessary to provide safe, high quality nursing care.

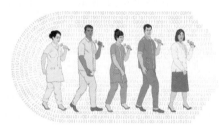

We must be able to search through the available data and information.

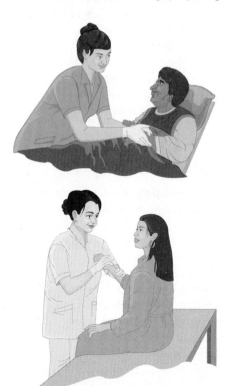

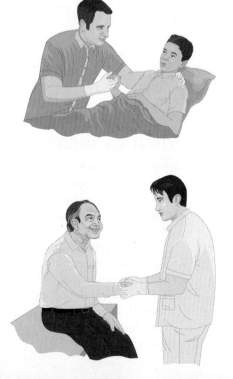

challenge to improving safety in health IT–enabled healthcare systems is to develop valid, feasible strategies to measure safety concerns at the intersection of health IT and patient safety" (p. 226).

Although technology may certainly help to prevent or reduce errors, one must always remember that technology is not a substitution for safety vigilance by the healthcare team in a safety culture. Harrison (2016) stated that "[p]atient safety should always be at the center of the design and adoption of any technology introduced into patient care settings. Technology that's designed to improve patient safety is only as good as the person using the device. It doesn't replace critical thinking, solid nursing practice, and careful patient monitoring" (p. 21).

The Wired for Health Care Quality Act of 2005 began a series of funding streams to promote HIT, promote sharing of best practices in HIT, and help organizations implement HIT (Harrison & Daly, 2009). Many early adopters opted to focus technology and safety initiatives on medication ordering and administration processes. Medication errors are the most frequent and the most visible errors because the medication administration cycle has many poorly designed work processes with several opportunities for human error. Thus **computerized physician order entry (CPOE)**, automated dispensing machines, **smart pump** technologies for IV drug administration, and **bar-code medication administration (BCMA)** frequently preceded the adoption of the EHR in many institutions because of the costs associated with implementing these technologies. In an ideal world, the EHR would be adopted concurrently as part of an interoperable HIT system. In the early EHR systems, clinicians were prompted by electronic alerts reminding them of important interventions that should be part of the standard of care, but these alerts tended to be generalized and not patient specific—for example, "Did you check the allergy profile?" or "Has the patient received a pneumonia immunization?" These early alert and care reminders are now evolving into more sophisticated **clinical decision support (CDS)** systems to promote accurate medical diagnoses and suggest appropriate medical and nursing interventions based on patient data. Ganio and colleagues (2016) stated that

> current EHR software is typically very customizable and may be adapted to multiple purposes. There are often several ways to accomplish a goal using vendor tools already available. Systems analysts should explore the options and weigh the pros and cons of each while consulting with end users to determine which tools meet their needs and are compatible with their workflows. (p. 629)

With the addition of triggers to detect adverse events, diagnostic errors, adverse drug events, hospital-acquired infections, and delays in diagnoses have been identified. "Trigger algorithms are frequently applied to EMRs for automated surveillance, and increasingly to prospectively identify patients at risk" (Rosen & Mull, 2016, p. 3).

The National Patient Safety Foundation (2016) listed the top patient safety issues as wrong-site surgery, hospital-acquired infections, falls, hospital readmissions, diagnostic errors, and medication errors. Many of these issues can be prevented or detected in their early stages using informatics technologies, although we still continue to struggle with these same safety issues. Other technologies designed to promote patient safety include wireless technologies for patient monitoring, clinician alerts, point-of-care applications, apps, and radiofrequency identification applications. Each of these is reviewed here, and the chapter concludes with a section discussing future technologies for patient safety.

## Technologies to Support the Medication Administration Cycle

The steps in the medication administration cycle (assessment of need, ordering, dispensing, distribution, administration, and evaluation) have been relatively stable for many years. Each of the steps depends on vigilant humans to ensure patient safety, resulting in the five rights of medication administration: (1) the right patient, (2) the right time and frequency of administration, (3) the right dose, (4) the right route, and (5) the right drug. Human error can be related to many aspects of this cycle. Distractions, unclear thinking, lack of knowledge, short staffing, and fatigue are a few of the factors that cause humans to deviate from accepted safety practices and commit medication errors. Integration of technology into the medication administration cycle promises to reduce the potential for human errors in the cycle by performing electronic checks and providing alerts to draw attention to potential errors. Research Brief 2 describes high-risk and preventable drug-related complications.

### RESEARCH BRIEF 2

A cluster-randomized, step-wedge trial was conducted involving 33 primary practices that were randomly assigned start dates during a 48-week intervention involving education, informatics, and financial incentives to conduct chart reviews; 33,334 patients in the preintervention period and 33,060 at-risk in the intervention period were included. The main outcome was patient-level exposure to high-risk prescribing of nonsteroidal anti-inflammatory drugs (NSAIDs) or selected antiplatelet agents (e.g., NSAID prescription in a patient with chronic kidney disease or co-prescription of an NSAID and an oral anticoagulant without gastroprotection). Secondary outcomes included the incidence of related hospital admissions. The analyses were conducted based on the intention-to-treat principle, with the use of mixed-effect models to account for clustering in the data.

Targeted high-risk prescribing was significantly reduced, from a rate of 3.7% (1,102 of 29,537 patients at risk) immediately before the intervention to 2.2% (674 of 30,187) at the end of the intervention (adjusted odds ratio, 0.63; 95% confidence interval [CI], 0.57 to 0.68; $P<0.001$). The rate of hospital admissions for gastrointestinal ulcer or bleeding was significantly reduced from the preintervention period to the intervention period (from 55.7 to 37.0 admissions per 10,000 person-years; rate ratio, 0.66; 95% CI, 0.51 to 0.86; $P=0.002$), as was the rate of admissions for heart failure (from 707.7 to 513.5 admissions per 10,000 person-years; rate ratio, 0.73; 95% CI, 0.56 to 0.95; $P=0.02$), but admissions for acute kidney injury were not (101.9 and 86.0 admissions per 10,000 person-years, respectively; rate ratio, 0.84; 95% CI, 0.68 to 1.09; $P=0.19$).

The researchers concluded that their complex intervention combining education, informatics, and financial incentives reduced the rate of high-risk prescribing of antiplatelet medications and NSAIDs and may have improved clinical outcomes.

The full article appears in Dreischulte, T., Donnan, P., Grant, A., Hapca, A., McCowan, C., & Guthrie, B. (2016). Safer prescribing—A trial of education, informatics, and financial incentives. *New England Journal of Medicine, 374*(11), 1053–1064. doi:10.1056/NEJMsa1508955

CPOE is an electronic prescribing system designed to support physicians and nurse practitioners in writing complete and appropriate medication and care orders for patients. When CPOE is part of an EHR with a CDS system, the medication order is electronically checked against specific data in the patient record to prevent errors, such as ordering a drug that might interact with a drug the patient is already taking, ordering a dose that is too large for the patient's weight, or ordering a drug that is contraindicated by the patient's allergy profile or renal function. Because it is impossible for, and unreasonable to expect, a clinician to remember each of the more than 600 drugs that require a dose adjustment in the case of renal dysfunction, for example, safe dosing parameters are provided by the CPOE (Bates & Gawande, 2003). In a stand-alone CPOE system without a CDS system, the medication orders are simply checked by the computer against the drug database to ensure that the dose and route specified in the order are appropriate for the medication chosen. Specific benefits of CPOE include the following:

- Prompts that warn against the possibility of drug interaction, allergy, or overdose
- Accurate, current information that helps physicians keep up with new drugs as they are introduced into the market
- Drug-specific information that eliminates confusion among drug names that look and sound alike
- Reduced healthcare costs caused by improved efficiencies
- Improved communication among doctors, nurses, specialists, pharmacists, other clinicians, and patients
- Improved clinical decision support at the point of care (Steele & DeBrow, n.d.)

CPOE solves the safety issues associated with poor handwriting and unclear or incomplete medication orders. Orders can be entered in seconds and from remote sites, eliminating the use of verbal orders that are especially subject to interpretation errors. Orders are then transmitted electronically to the pharmacy, reducing the potential for the transcription errors commonly encountered in the paper-based system, such as lost or misplaced orders, delayed dosing, or unreadable faxes. Thus CPOE changes workflows for all clinical staff and physicians as well as health team communication patterns (Doshi, 2015). As with any technology integration, introduction of CPOE is associated with a resistance to change and a learning curve to gain proficiency, and users must learn to trust the system. Manor (2010) urges careful planning and training during implementation with plenty of staff support. Manor also reports on the need for a paper-based backup system in the case of network or electrical outages or system maintenance.

The verification and dispensing functions of the pharmacy can also be assisted by technology. The pharmacist begins by verifying the allergy status of the patient and the medication reconciliation information to ensure that the new medication is compatible with other medication in the care regimen. This verification function is computer based, and the medication order is electronically checked via the knowledge database. If the order is verified as safe and appropriate, the pharmacist proceeds to the dispensing process. Bar-code medication labeling at a unit dose level was mandated by the Food and Drug Administration in 2004, with targeted compliance to be achieved by 2006. A bar code is a series of alternating bars and spaces that represents a unique code that can be read by a special bar-code reader. Bar-code technology spans both the medication dispensing and administration steps in the medication administration cycle. In the pharmacy, the bar code helps to ensure that the right drug and the right dose are dispensed by the pharmacy. Medications that are labeled with bar codes can also be dispensed by robots capable of reading the codes or by automated dispensing machines. In this way, bar-code technology helps with the processes of procurement, inventory, storage, preparation, and dispensing (University of Rochester Medical Center, Department of Pharmacy, 2016).

The processes of drug storage, dispensing, controlling, and tracking are easily carried out via automated dispensing machines (also known as automated dispensing cabinets, unit-based cabinets, automated dispensing devices, and automated distribution cabinets). These devices have benefits for both the user and the organization, specifically in the areas of access security (especially with narcotics administration tracking), safety, supply chain, and charge functions (Institute for Safe Medication Practices, 2016).

**Applications (apps)** or mobile apps are being used by and prescribed for patients. The apps used for patient education can engage and inform our patients; an educated patient is believed to be "more likely to understand risks and if there is an adverse event, may less likely file a lawsuit" (Diamond, 2016, para. 2). While there are benefits to their use, we must be judicious in our use of apps. If apps are prescribed for patients, then it is our responsibility to educate the patient and/or family on proper use. It is important that patients and their families understand the benefits and risks of using the app, as well as how to receive help when needed. If data are being exchanged, our patients must comprehend what data will be collected and where, when, and with whom it will be shared.

There are apps for healthcare personnel as well. iScrub is an app used to monitor hand hygiene, which could help prevent healthcare-associated infections (University of Iowa, 2015). The Patient Safety Manual was designed as a resource to treat patients quickly, safely, and effectively (Apkpure, 2016). Apps will continue to be used by providers and patients, so we must all assume the responsibility of making sure the apps are both appropriate to use and used appropriately.

**Radio frequency identifier (RFID)** technology is rapidly gaining a foothold in healthcare technology and may soon be used in the medication administration cycle. Although more expensive than bar coding for packaging, the RFID tags are reprogrammable and issues associated with bar-code printing imperfections and bar-code scanner resolution can be mitigated (Vecchione, 2016). As discussed later in this chapter, RFID technologies may also be an important component of a medication compliance system for patients.

BCMA systems help to ensure adherence to the five rights of medication administration. Whether BCMA is part of the larger EHR or a free-standing **electronic medication administration system (eMAR)**, bar-code technology provides a system of checks and balances to ensure medication safety. The nurse begins by scanning his or her name badge, thereby logging in as the person responsible for medication administration. Next, the bar code on the patient's identification bracelet is scanned, prompting the electronic system to pull up the medication orders. Next, the bar code on each of the medications to be administered is scanned. This technology check ensures that the five rights of medication administration are met. If there is a discrepancy between the order and the medication that was scanned or a contraindication for administration, an alert is generated by the system. For example, in an EHR system with CDS, the nurse may be prompted to check the most recent laboratory results for electrolytes before administering a potassium supplement. In a free-standing eMAR without CDS or EHR links, if the medication orders have recently been changed, the nurse is alerted to the change. When an alert is generated, the nurse must chart the action taken in response to that alert. For example, an early dose might need to be given if the patient is leaving the unit for a diagnostic test.

Despite the promising advances in patient safety afforded by this technology, it is not fail safe (Cochran, Jones, Brockman, Skinner, & Hicks, 2007). Medications that are labeled individually by the in-house pharmacist increase the potential for human error if the medication is given an incorrect bar code, such as one signifying a wrong dose or even the wrong medication. In addition, the bar-code printers themselves may generate unreadable labels, leading to staff workarounds in the interest of saving time. Cochran et al. make the following recommendations to reduce BCMA errors:

- Purchase unit-of-use medications with manufacturer bar codes whenever possible.
- Double-check all hospital-generated bar-code labels, including those for compounded injectable medications, before the product leaves the pharmacy.
- Carefully review all BCMA override reports. Address system workarounds through process change and staff education.
- Minimize false-positive warnings to reduce the likelihood that staff will ignore warnings for real errors.
- Ensure that an urgent need exists for all "stat" orders, as pharmacy review and advantages of bar-code administration are usually circumvented in such cases.
- Establish institutional policies and procedures that can be easily implemented when products fail to scan. Processes in pharmacy will likely be different than processes at the point of care (p. 300).

Smart pump technologies are designed for safe administration of **high-hazard drugs** and to reduce adverse drug events during IV medication administration. Smart pumps have software that is programmed to reflect the facility's infusion parameters and a drug library that compares normal dosing rates with those programmed into the pump. Discrepancies generate an alarm alerting the clinician to a safety issue. A soft alarm can typically be overridden by a clinician at the bedside, but a hard alarm requires the clinician to reprogram the pump so that the dosing falls within the facility's IV administration guidelines for the drug to be infused. All alarms generated by the smart pump are tracked along with the clinician's responses to them (Cummings & McGowan, 2015; Dulak, 2005; University of Alabama at Birmingham, 2013). Smart pumps can be seamlessly integrated into BCMA systems, and data can be fed directly into the EHR. The IHI (2012) recommends the following steps to ensure safe implementation of smart pump technology:

- Prior to deploying these pumps, standardize concentrations within the hospital. Asking the nurse to choose among several concentrations increases the risk of selection error.
- Prior to deploying these pumps, standardize dosing units for a given drug (for example, agree to always dose nitroglycerin in terms of mcg/min or mcg/kg/min, but not both). Asking the nurse to choose among several dosing units increases the risk of selection error.
- Prior to deploying these pumps, standardize drug nomenclature (for example, agree to always use the term KCl, but not potassium chloride, K, pot chloride, or others). Asking the nurse to remember and choose among several possible drug names increases the risk of selection error.
- Perform a failure modes and effects analysis on the deployment of these devices.
- Ensure that the concentrations, dose units, and nomenclature used in the pump are consistent with that used on the medication administration record (MAR), the pharmacy computer system, and the EHR.
- Meet with all relevant clinicians to come to agreement on the proper upper and lower hard and soft dose limits.
- Monitor overrides of alerts to assess whether the alerts have been properly configured or whether additional quality intervention is required.
- Be sure the "smart" feature is utilized in all parts of the hospital. If the pump is set up volumetrically in the operating room but the "smart" feature is used in the ICU, an error may occur if the pump is not properly reprogrammed.
- Be sure there are upper and lower dose limits for bolus doses, when applicable.
- Engage the services of a human factors engineer to identify new opportunities for failure when the pumps are deployed.
- Identify a procedure for the staff to follow in the event a drug that is not in the library must be given or when its concentration is not standard.
- Deploy the pump in all areas of the hospital. If a different pump is used on one floor and the patient is later transferred, this will create new opportunities for failure. Also, there may be incorrect assumptions about the technology available to a given floor or patient.
- Consider using "smart" technology for syringe pumps as well as large-volume infusion devices (para. 7).

Cummings and McGowan (2015) cautioned that we must never solely rely on the pump to identify and alert us to problems. Nurses must always engage in best practices and follow all patient safety practices. There is no substitute for nursing assessment of patients as a key safety tool.

A CDS can enhance the medication administration cycle by promoting safety and improving patient outcomes. The CDS is guided by targeted information delivery, ensuring that the five rights of CDSs are implemented: the right information provided to the right person in the right format through the right channel at the right time in workflow. For example, during medication selection, a CDS helps a clinician select an appropriate medication based on client data, such as clinical condition, weight, renal function, concurrent medications, and cost. This system ensures that the order is complete by performing checks for drug interactions, duplications, or allergy contraindications and ensures the right dose and right route are specified. During the verification and dispensing phase of the medication administration cycle, the CDS provides double checks for interactions, allergies, and appropriate dose orders. Consideration is also given to potential infusion pump programming issues, incompatibilities during infusion, and proper notation and dispensing when portions of a dose must be wasted. During the administration phase, the CDS assists with patient identification and current assessment parameters (i.e., blood pressure, glucose level) that may contraindicate the use of the medication at that point in time. In addition, checks for interactions with foods or other medications and timing and monitoring guidelines are provided to the clinician administering the medication. The CDS has patient education guidelines and printable handouts to assist clinicians in educating patients about their medications. The monitoring functions of the CDS provide a structured data reporting system to track side effects and adverse events across the population (Healthcare Information and Management Systems Society [HIMSS], 2009a).

Several promising technologies may become available in the future to assist patients with medication compliance after discharge. For example, eMedonline collects patient medication compliance data by scanning package bar codes or RFID medication tags and using personal digital assistant or smartphone technology to send compliance data to the server. Clinicians review the medication compliance data and provide education and feedback to patients to increase their compliance with proper medication administration (eMedonline, n.d.). The SIMpill Medication Adherence System uses Web-based technology to monitor patient compliance and provide reminders about taking medications or refilling prescriptions by sending text messages to the patient or caregivers (SIMpill, 2008). Caps of pill bottles may contain RFID tags that monitor and collect data on when the bottle is opened, or that contain flashing time reminders when a dose is due (Blankenhorn, 2010). Smart inhalers track asthma medication compliance using a microprocessor that records and stores medication compliance. They may also include visual and audio reminders to use the inhaler (Adherium, 2010).

In addition, several potential technologies are still being tested. For example, InPen is a smart insulin pen that couples with a smartphone to calculate insulin dosages and track injections (Medgadget, 2016a), PillDrill helps people adhere to a medication schedule and also includes a "mood cube" to track how patients are feeling (Medgadget, 2016b), and Proteus smart pills have sensors attached to medications to track when the pill is actually ingested (Medgadget, 2015). These are just a sampling of the newer technologies for medication adherence; more are expected to emerge in the future.

## Additional Technologies for Patient Safety

CDS systems have safety uses beyond the medication administration cycle. The robust data collection and data management functions help to ensure quality approaches to patient health challenges based on research evidence and clinical guidelines. A CDS may also ensure cost-effectiveness by alerting clinicians to duplicate testing orders, or by suggesting the most cost-effective diagnostic test based on specific patient data (HIMSS, 2009b). Consider this description of the features of a CDS based on screen captures performed by a CDS system:

> The patient is a 75-year-old male with coronary artery disease (CAD), diabetes mellitus (DM), and elevated creatine kinase (CK). Assessment prompts and reminders on the screen for this patient include: no recent LDL test; BP is above goal; patient is due for Pneumovax and influenza vaccines; patient is a current smoker, not thinking of quitting, last counseled with date; patient is overweight; patient is due for eye and ear checks. The patient management prompts include:

> - Lipid management: "No Recent LDL Management" is printed red with a series of check boxes presenting choices to the clinician:
>   * Order lipid panel now
>   * Order lipid panel with direct LDL now
>   * Print instructions for fasting lipid panel (link)
>   * Print orders for outside lab request for lipid panel testing (link)
> - BP management: BP is above goal average over last 2 visits; goal is 130/80
>   * Choices on checkboxes: Start another antihypertensive ("help me choose") link
>   * Series of links listing current medications with opportunities to adjust each
> - Order Chem 7 now or order Chem 7 in (drop-down menu for timing of order)
> - Suggestions for referrals include:
>   * Refer to nutritionist
>   * Refer to cardiac rehabilitation ("help me choose" link)
>   * Refer to BP specialist ("help me choose" link)
>   * Prompts for patient education handouts include Print "control high blood pressure" link
>   * Print DASH diet instructions link
>   * Print exercise prescription (White, Shiffman, Middleton, & Cabán, 2008, Slides 63–65)

The prompts and instructions provided to the clinician by the system in this example are detailed and easy to navigate. As the example suggests, implementation of a CDS has the potential to optimize care by ensuring that all of the details of a patient's health issues are presented to the clinician for management, thereby promoting individualized approaches to the total health of the patient based on best available evidence and clinical guidelines (HealthIT.gov, n.d.). According to the Centers for Medicare and Medicaid Studies (2014),

> [the] CDS is not simply an alert, notification, or explicit care suggestion. CDS encompasses a variety of tools including, but not limited to: computerized

*alerts and reminders for providers and patients; clinical guidelines; condition-specific order sets; focused patient data reports and summaries; documentation templates; diagnostic support; and contextually relevant reference information. These functionalities may be deployed on a variety of platforms. (para. 2)*

RFID technologies have both supply chain and patient care applications to patient safety. An RFID system contains a tag affixed to an object or to a person that functions as a radiofrequency transponder and provides a unique identification code, a reader that receives and decodes the information contained on the tag, and an antenna that transmits the information between the tag and the reader. When RFID tags are embedded in patient identification bracelets, they can help with patient tracking during procedures and testing or function as part of the EHR communicating pertinent information to clinicians at the bedside. RFIDs may be part of the medication administration process, replacing bar-code technologies. They can be used to track medical supplies and equipment, thereby reducing staff time in locating such items. They may also be embedded into surgical supplies to automate supply-counting procedures, thereby reducing the likelihood that sponges or tools will be erroneously left in a patient. RFIDs may also reduce the likelihood of the never events of wrong-patient, wrong-site surgical procedures (PSNet, 2016b; Revere et al, 2010). RFIDs used in the medication supply chain protect patients by reducing the potential that a counterfeit medication might be inadvertently introduced into the supply, and by providing for efficient medication recalls. Potential terrorist manipulation of the medication supply is also thwarted by RFID supply chain tracking technology. Blood and blood products can be efficiently tracked by RFIDs because specialized tags can detect temperature fluctuations and, therefore, ensure that the blood or blood product was stored at the optimal temperature for safe administration; however, RFID technology will probably not replace bar codes in blood banking due to the cost (Wray & Sanislo, 2016).

**Smart rooms** are also being used in healthcare facilities. As a caregiver enters the room, the RFID tag on his or her name badge announces to the patient on a monitor (typically mounted on the wall in the patient's line of sight) exactly who has entered the room and triggers "need to know" data based on caregiver status to be displayed on the monitor in the room. For example, when a dietary aide enters the room, only dietary information is displayed; when a physician or nurse enters, all of the pertinent medical data from the EHR is available. Clinicians can review patient data in real time and chart care at the bedside using touch-screen technology, thereby increasing productivity (Cerner, 2016; Cronin, 2010). Some smart room technologies include workflow algorithms to alert clinicians as they enter the room about procedures that need to be implemented for the patient and can track individual clinician efficiency and effectiveness by aggregating data over time (Foley, 2016; Sharbaugh & Boroch, 2010).

New technologies to improve patient monitoring include **wearable technology** (devices) and wireless area networks, variously called "body area networks" or "patient area networks." The technologies provide the ability to wear a small, unobtrusive monitor that collects and transmits physiologic data via a cell phone to a server for clinician review. Although most of these technologies are designed for monitoring patients with chronic diseases, they also have safety implications because they help to identify early warning physiologic signs of impeding serious health events (California Healthcare Foundation, 2007; Kosir, 2015). A wireless chip on a disposable Band-Aid with a 5- to 7-day battery promises to be able to monitor the patient's heart rate and electrocardiogram, blood glucose, blood pH, and blood pressure, allowing for the collection of important clinical data outside the hospital (Miller, 2008). Wearable stress-sensing monitors detect electrical changes in the skin that may signal increased stress in autistic children who are unable to communicate an impending crisis; caregivers are alerted to the potential crisis via wireless transmission and can intervene to reduce the stress and prevent the crisis (Murph, 2010). Several new technologies promise to aid in early detection of falls in the elderly, including a wearable pendant that triggers a personal emergency response system (Aging in Place Technology Watch, 2012) and smart slippers with pressure sensors in the soles that transmit movement data wirelessly to a remote monitoring site (Mobihealthnews, 2009).

Robotics technologies are also being increasingly tested for safety and efficiency uses. Robotics has been used in minimally invasive surgery for some time; as with most technologies, there are risks and rewards (PSNet, 2016c). Surgical devices include haptic (tactile) feedback to the surgeon, thereby increasing the sense of reality during the procedure and reducing the potential for unsafe manipulation (June, 2010). A robot designed to assist with patient lifting provides increased safety for both patients and clinicians (Melanson, 2010). Finally, laser-guided robots are performing such routine functions as emptying and disposing of trash, cleaning rooms, delivering supplies and meals, and dispensing drugs (Savoy, 2010). Robots are also being used in home care as well as for telehealth (Dahl & Boulos, 2013).

Personalized health care or personalized medicine, which tailors treatment to the specific genetic characteristics of an individual patient and challenges the patient to be more accountable for his or her own health, is rapidly advancing as vendors develop targeted therapies. Its impact is aligned with quality. According to the Armstrong Institute (2012), "personalized medicine and quality improvement are united in a common goal: optimal patient outcomes" (para. 3). Researchers must pursue specific clinical trials and make certain that the data, information, and knowledge generated are captured and disseminated.

The International Medical Informatics Association (IMIA; 2015) has a working group for health informatics for patient safety. This working group is focusing on six areas where health information systems can impact patient safety:

1. Identifying and documenting how health information systems and their associated devices can best be designed, implemented and applied to improve patient safety (e.g., developing usable, integrated workflow solutions that are safe)
2. Identifying and documenting software safety issues involving health information systems (e.g., physician order entry, electronic documentation, decision support tools) and their associated devices
3. Discussing, developing and promoting methodologies that improve patient safety using health information systems and their associated devices
4. Discussing, developing, and promoting methodologies that prevent the occurrence of safety issues involving health information systems and their associated devices

5. Educating health informatics professionals, health professionals, healthcare administrators, and policy makers about how health information systems and medical devices can improve patient safety and the solutions that can be employed to prevent the occurrence of technology-induced errors involving software and medical devices

6. Collecting, analyzing, and disseminating research results about health information systems and medical devices that improve safety as well as those that have been found to inadvertently decrease safety (para. 1)

Many organizations are showing the value of healthcare or clinical informatics methods in improving quality health care and patient safety. We are beginning to see some strides in improving patient safety as these technologies are implemented across healthcare settings, but we still have a long way to go.

## Role of the Nurse Informaticist

The human side of patient safety is paramount. As technologies that can help to reduce errors and increase safety are integrated into caregiving activities, healthcare professionals must also improve their ability to use and manage these technologies. Therefore, not only must the technology be scrutinized and tested routinely, but the users must also be maintained and nurtured so that they are able to use the tools to the patient's benefit, avoiding harm and keeping the patient safe. Even the best CDS systems can contribute to mistakes by providing meaningless or harmful information. Nurse informaticists and the IT team in the facility must ensure that all systems are properly configured and maintained. They should routinely monitor and check these systems while making sure that their human potential—that is, the users—is capable of using the systems accurately to avoid errors. A technology and its user can never be left to their own devices.

As we continue to apply informatics to patient safety, data warehousing and mining, reporting, data trending, and predictive modeling will enhance our ability to improve patient safety and provide quality health care. In order to gather the data and information necessary to analyze safety issues, monitoring systems, software, and hardware will continue to evolve. Risk monitoring and incident reporting software (reporting software specifically generating reports regarding incidents only), patient response monitoring systems, trending and predictive models, and reporting software will provide enhanced data and information to be analyzed.

Human inputting activities must focus on patient safety to raise the appropriate issues and sound out solutions. Nurse informaticists must be involved in all stages of the system development life cycle, while maintaining a focus on safety. Safety concerns and remedies need to be analyzed, synthesized, and integrated throughout the system development life cycle to have a robust tool that provides meaningful information and enhances patient care while preventing errors and promoting patient safety. According to Effken and Carty (2002), "Creating a safe patient environment is a very complex issue that will require the combined knowledge and skill of clinical informaticists, informatics faculty, researchers, and system designers" (para. 16). Research Brief 3 describes the results of a 2009 HIMSS survey on the impact of nurse informaticists on patient safety. Research Brief 4 discusses HIMSS's 2015 follow-up survey.

### RESEARCH BRIEF 3

In 2009, HIMSS conducted an Informatics Nurse Impact Survey sponsored by McKesson. This Web-based survey yielded 432 acceptable responses over a 2-month period from December 2008 to February 2009.

One of the areas assessed was "value and impact of informatics nurse," on a scale of 1 to 7, with 7 being the highest rating:

> *Respondents believe that informatics nurses involved in system analysis, design, selection, implementation and optimization of IT have the greatest impact on patient safety (6.21), workflow (6.17) and user/clinician acceptance (6.15). The area with the least impact was integration with other systems (6.03). These findings suggest the informatics nurse is a driver of quality of care and enhanced patient safety within their organization. (p. 2)*

This demonstrates the belief that nurse informaticists can greatly improve patient safety. The nurse executives who responded rated the positive impact of nurse informaticists on patient safety at 6.36 out of 7.

In their conclusion, the researchers stated that:

> *The role of informatics nurses is not limited to IT; this research also suggests that informatics nurses play an instrumental role with regard to patient safety, change management and usability of systems as evidenced by their impact on quality outcomes, workflow, and user acceptance. These additional areas highlight the value of informatics nurses—their expertise truly translates to the adoption of more effective, higher quality clinical applications in healthcare organizations. (p. 11)*

The full article appears in HIMSS. (2009). Informatics nurse impact survey. Retrieved from http://www.himss.org/files/HIMSSorg/content/files/HIMSS2009NursingInformaticsImpactSurveyFull Results.pdf

### RESEARCH BRIEF 4

This study follows up on research HIMSS conducted in 2009 to evaluate the impact that informatics nurses have on the HIT environment.

Under the heading of Patient Safety,

> *more than three-quarters of respondents (76 percent) indicated that having an informatics nurse involved in the analysis, design, implementation, optimization and selection process for clinical systems results in a high degree of impact with regard to patient safety. . . . Additionally, respondents working for an organization that employs a CMIO [Chief Medical Information Officer] were more likely (79 percent) to report that informatics nurses had a high degree of*

*impact on patient safety derived from clinical systems than were their counterparts at organizations that do not employ a CMIO on staff (73 percent). (p. 15)*

Under the heading of Quality Outcomes, "[n]early two-thirds of respondents (64 percent) indicated that having an informatics nurse involved in the analysis, design, implementation, optimization and selection process for clinical systems has a high degree of impact on quality outcomes" (p. 15).

Under the heading of Reduction of Never Events,

*[n]early two-thirds of respondents (61 percent) indicated that having an informatics nurse involved in the analysis, design, implementation, optimization and selection process for clinical systems had a substantial positive impact on the reduction of never events. Additionally, respondents working for an organization that employ a CNIO [Chief Nursing Informatics Officer] were more likely to indicate that informatics nurses have an impact in this area (72 percent) when compared to respondents that work for an organization that does not have a CNIO (58 percent). (p. 16)*

This showed that the majority of the 576 study participants believed that nurse informaticists positively impact patent safety. It also reinforced the fact that the nurse informaticist's role is not limited to IT, and suggested that informatics nurses play an instrumental role with regard to patient safety, change management, and usability of systems, as evidenced by their impact on quality outcomes, workflow, and user acceptance.

The full article appears in HIMSS. (2015). 2015 impact of the informatics nurse survey. Retrieved from http://www.himss.org/sites/himssorg/files/FileDownloads/2015%20Impact%20of%20the%20Informatics%20Nurse%20Survey%20Full%20Report.pdf

# Summary

Patient safety is an important and ubiquitous issue in health care. This chapter explored the characteristics of a safety culture and technologies designed to promote patient safety. The need to evaluate errors carefully to determine why and how they occurred and how workflow processes might be changed to prevent future errors of the same type was emphasized. Technology is changing rapidly, and the culture of sharing related to technology implementation, error reporting, and troubleshooting should prompt continuous process improvements. The key for organizations is to invest in their users and choose wisely so that the technologies they are adopting will not negatively impact safety and will be interoperable and easily upgradable as technologies and safety practices evolve.

Organizations must make a commitment to a safety culture in which everyone at every level is committed to patient safety at every moment. In an ideal world,

Table 15-1  Patient Safety Websites

| TITLE | URL |
|---|---|
| AHRQ Patient Safety Network | www.psnet.ahrq.gov/primerHome.aspx |
| National Patient Safety Foundation | www.npsf.org |
| National Center for Patient Safety | www.patientsafety.va.gov |
| Institute for Healthcare Improvement | www.ihi.org/explore/patientsafety/Pages/default.aspx |
| Center for Patient Safety | www.centerforpatientsafety.org |
| QSEN Institute (Quality and Safety Education for Nurses) | www.qsen.org |

everyone would first stop and think "Is this safe?" before every action, workarounds would not occur, and everyone would embrace rather than resist the technologies and workflow processes designed to promote patient safety. Table 15-1 provides a list of websites to watch for updates on patient safety technologies. The nurse informaticists, healthcare providers, patients, ancillary team members, administrators, setting/environment, infrastructure, and technologies must all work together to create a safety culture. Every organization must provide safe, quality health care and prevent harm or adverse events for every patient under its care by ensuring that patient safety is critical to the organization's mission.

## THOUGHT-PROVOKING QUESTIONS

1. What are the current patient safety characteristics of your organizational culture? Identify at least three aspects of your culture that need to be changed with regard to patient safety, and suggest strategies for change.
2. Describe a current technology that you use in patient care that would benefit from human factors engineering concepts. What are some ways this technology should be improved?
3. Identify a workaround that you have used and analyze why you chose this risk-taking behavior over behavior that conforms to a safety culture.
4. The GAO (2016) interviewed patient safety experts and the related literature to identify three key gaps in patient safety practice implementation:

   *a lack of (1) information about the effect of contextual factors on implementation of patient safety practices, (2) sufficiently detailed information on the experience of hospitals that have previously used specific patient safety implementation strategies, and (3) valid and accurate measurement of how frequently certain adverse events occur. (p. 22)*

   Select one of these gaps and describe in detail how nursing informatics could help close this gap.

# References

Adherium. (2010). What are smart inhalers? Retrieved from http://www.smartinhaler.com

Agency for Healthcare Research and Quality (AHRQ). (2012). Patient safety primer: Safety culture. Retrieved from http://psnet.ahrq.gov/primer.aspx?primerID=5

Agency for Healthcare Research and Quality (AHRQ). (2016). Hospital survey on patient safety culture: 2016 user comparative database report. Retrieved from http://www.ahrq .gov/sites/default/files/wysiwyg/professionals/quality-patient-safety/patientsafetyculture /hospital/2016/2016_hospitalsops_report_pt1.pdf

Aging in Place Technology Watch. (2012). New more accurate fall detector helps seniors age in place safely. Retrieved from http://www.ageinplacetech.com/pressrelease/new-more -accurate-fall-detector-helps-seniors-age-place-safely

Apkpure. (2016). Patient safety manual APK. Retrieved from https://apkpure.com/patient -safety-manual/com.cranworthmedical.patientsafety?hl=en

Armstrong Institute. (2012). Personalized medicine and patient safety: Two sides of the same coin. Retrieved from https://armstronginstitute.blogs.hopkinsmedicine.org/2012/02/24 /personalized-medicine-and-patient-safety-two-sides-of-the-same-coin

Banger, A. & Graber, M. (2015). Recent evidence that health IT improved patient safety: Issue brief prepared for DHHS Office of the National Coordinator (ONC). *HealthIT*. Retrieved from https://www.healthit.gov/sites/default/files/brief_1_final_feb11t.pdf

Barnet, S. (2016). 49 companies sign Patient Safety Movement's open data pledge. *Becker's Hospital Review*. Retrieved from http://www.beckershospitalreview.com/quality/49-companies -sign-patient-safety-movement-s-open-data-pledge.html

Bates, D., & Gawande, A. (2003). Improving safety with information technology. *New England Journal of Medicine, 348*, 2526–2534.

Blankenhorn, D. (2010). Can better tools overcome the medical compliance crazy? *ZDNet*. Retrieved from http://www.zdnet.com/blog/healthcare/can-better-tools-overcome-the -medical-compliance-crazy/3925

California Healthcare Foundation. (2007). Healthcare unplugged: The evolving role of wireless technology. Retrieved from http://www.chcf.org/~/media/MEDIA%20LIBRARY%20Files /PDF/PDF%20H/PDF%20HealthCareUnpluggedTheRoleOfWireless.pdf

Centers for Medicare and Medicaid Services. (2014). Clinical decision support: More than just "alerts" tipsheet. Retrieved from https://www.healthit.gov/sites/default/files /clinicaldecisionsupport_tipsheet.pdf

Cerner. (2016). Smart room. Retrieved from http://www.cerner.com/solutions/medical_devices /Smart_Room/

Cochran, C., Jones, K., Brockman, J., Skinner, A., & Hicks, R. (2007). Errors prevented by and associated with bar-code administration systems. *The Joint Commission Journal on Quality and Patient Safety, 33*(5), 293–301.

Cronin, M. (2010). SmartRooms from IBM connect hospital staff to patient data. *Cerner*. Retrieved from http://www.cerner.com/uploadedFiles/Content/Solutions/_White_Papers /Medical_Devices/NCH_Smart_Room_Whitepaper.pdf

Cummings, K. & McGowan, R. (2015). "Smart" infusion pumps are selectively intelligent. *U.S. Food and Drug Administration*. Retrieved from http://www.fda.gov/MedicalDevices/Safety /AlertsandNotices/TipsandArticlesonDeviceSafety/ucm245160.htm

Dahl, T., & Boulos, M. (2013). Robots in health and social care: A complementary technology to home care and telehealthcare? *Robotics, 3*, 1–21. doi:10.3390/robotics3010001

Diamond, R. (2016). There's as app for that: Benefits and risks of using mobile apps for healthcare. *The Doctor's Company*. Retrieved from http://www.thedoctors.com/KnowledgeCenter

/PatientSafety/articles/Theres-an-App-for-That-Benefits-and-Risks-of-Using-Mobile-Apps -for-Healthcare

Doshi, D. (2015). Computerized provider order entry (CPOE)—An overview. *International Journal of Innovative Research & Studies, 4*(6), 58–70.

Dulak, S. (2005). Technology today: Smart IV pumps. *Modern Medicine Network.* Retrieved from http://www.modernmedicine.com/modernmedicine/article/articleDetail.jsp?id=254828

Ebben, S., Gieras, I., & Gosbee, L. (2008). Harnessing hospital purchase power to design safe care delivery. *Biomedical Instrumentation & Technology, 42*(4), 326–331. Retrieved from ProQuest Nursing & Allied Health Source (Document ID: 1548954831).

Effken, J., & Carty, B. (2002). The era of patient safety: Implications for nursing informatics curricula. *Journal of the American Medical Informatics Association, 9*(6 suppl 1). http:// www.ncbi.nlm.nih.gov/pmc/articles/PMC419434/

eMedonline. (n.d.). How eMedonline works. Retrieved from http://www.emedonline.com/about .asp?topic=howitworks

Folley, T. (2016). Transforming health—The smart patient room. *Healthcare CommunIT.* Retrieved from http://www.cdwcommunit.com/perspectives/expert-perspectives/transforming-health -the-smart-patient-room/

Ganio, M., Forrey, R., Lopez, B., & Barreto, J. (2016). Adapting an inpatient intervention tool to facilitate cross-encounter communication. *American Journal of Health-System Pharmacy, 73*(10), 627–629.

Government Accountability Office (GAO). (2016). Patient safety report to Congressional requesters. Retrieved from http://www.gao.gov/assets/680/675390.pdf

Harrison, L. (2016). Safely managing smart pumps in the clinical setting. *Nursing Management, 47*(6), 20–21. doi:10.1097/01.NUMA.0000483128.55731.5e

Harrison, J., & Daly, M. (2009). Leveraging health information technology to improve patient safety. *Public Administration and Management, 14*(1), 218–237. Retrieved from ABI/ INFORM Global (Document ID: 1685699891).

Healthcare Information and Management Systems Society (HIMSS). (2009a). Approaching CDS in medication management. Retrieved from http://healthit.ahrq.gov/images/mar09 _cds_book_chapter/CDS_MedMgmnt_ch_1_sec_3_applying_CDS.htm

Healthcare Information and Management Systems Society (HIMSS). (2009b). Clinical decision support (CDS) fact sheet. Retrieved from http://www.himss.org/content/files/CDSFactSheet3 -17-09.pdf

HealthIT.gov. (n.d.). CDS Implementation. Retrieved from http://www.healthit.gov/policy -researcher-simplementers/cds-implementation

Institute of Medicine (IOM). (2000). *To err is human: Building a safer health system.* Washington, DC: National Academies Press.

Institute of Medicine (IOM). (2001). *Crossing the quality chasm: A new health system for the 21st century.* Washington, DC: National Academies Press.

Institute for Healthcare Improvement (IHI). (2012). Reduce adverse drug events (ADES) involving intravenous medications: Implement smart infusion pumps. Retrieved from http://www.ihi.org/knowledge/Pages/Changes/ReduceAdverseDrugEventsInvolving IntravenousMedications.aspx

Institute for Healthcare Improvement (IHI). (2016a). Develop a culture of safety. Retrieved from http://www.ihi.org/knowledge/Pages/Changes/DevelopaCultureofSafety.aspx

Institute for Healthcare Improvement (IHI). (2016b). Failure modes and effects analysis (FMEA) tool. Retrieved from http://www.ihi.org/resources/Pages/Tools /FailureModesandEffectsAnalysisTool.aspx

Institute for Safe Medication Practices. (2007, April 19). Smart pumps are not smart on their own. Retrieved from http://ismp.org/Newsletters/acutecare/articles/20070419.asp

Institute for Safe Medication Practices. (2016). Guidance on the interdisciplinary safe use of automated dispensing cabinets. Retrieved from https://www.ismp.org/Tools/guidelines/ADC/default.asp

International Medical Informatics Association (IMIA). (2015). Health informatics for patient safety. Retrieved from http://imia-medinfo.org/wp/health-informatics-for-patient-safety

Johns Hopkins Medicine. (2016). Study suggests medical errors now third leading cause of death in the U.S. Retrieved from http://www.hopkinsmedicine.org/news/media/releases/study_suggests_medical_errors_now_third_leading_cause_of_death_in_the_us

Joint Commission. (2008). Sentinel event alert #42: Safely implementing health information and converging technologies. Retrieved from https://www.jointcommission.org/sentinel_event_alert_issue_42_safely_implementing_health_information_and_converging_technologies

Joint Commission. (2013). The Joint Commission announces 2014 national patient safety goal. Retrieved from http://www.jointcommission.org/assets/1/18/jcp0713_announce_new_nspg.pdf

Joint Commission. (2016). Hospital national safety goals 2016. Retrieved from https://www.jointcommission.org/assets/1/6/2016_NPSG_HAP_ER.pdf

June, L. (2010). Sofie surgical robot gives haptic feedback for a more humane touch. *Engadget*. Retrieved from http://www.engadget.com/2010/10/11/sofie-surgical-robot-gives-haptic-feedback-for-a-more

Kosir, S. (2015). Wearables in healthcare. *Wearable Technologies*. Retrieved from https://www.wearable-technologies.com/2015/04/wearables-in-healthcare/

Lavin, M., Harper, E., & Barr, N. (2015). Health information technology, patient safety, and professional nursing care documentation in acute care settings. *Online Journal of Issues in Nursing, 20*(2).

Manor, P. (2010). CPOE: Strategies for success. *Nursing Management, 41*(5), 18. Retrieved from ABI/INFORM Global (Document ID: 2044925551).

MedGadget (2015). Proteus swallowable smart pills FDA approved to measure medication adherence. Retrieved from http://www.medgadget.com/2015/07/proteus-swallowable-smart-pills-fda-approved-to-measure-medication-adherence.html

MedGadget. (2016a). InPen: A smart insulin pen that calculates dosage, tracks injections. Retrieved from http://www.medgadget.com/2016/08/inpen.html

MedGadget. (2016b). PillDrill, a smart new medication adherence system. Retrieved from http://www.medgadget.com/2016/04/pilldrill-smart-new-medication-adherence-system-2.html

Melanson, D. (2010). Yurina health care robot promises to help lift, terrify patients. *Engadget*. Retrieved from http://www.engadget.com/2010/08/13/yurina-health-care-robot-promises-to-help-lift-terrify-patients

Miller, P. (2008). Wireless chip on a Band-Aid to monitor patients from home. *Engadget*. Retrieved from http://www.engadget.com/2008/02/05/wireless-chip-on-a-band-aid-to-monitor-patients-from-home

Mobihealthnews. (2009). AT&T develops "smart slippers" for fall prevention. Retrieved from http://mobihealthnews.com/5675/att-develops-smart-slippers-for-fall-prevention

Murph, D. (2010). Affectiva's Q Sensor wristband monitors and logs stress levels, might bring back the snap bracelet. *Engadget*. Retrieved from http://www.engadget.com/2010/11/02/affectivas-q-sensor-wristband-monitors-and-logs-stress-levels/

National Patient Safety Foundation. (2016). Important patient safety issues: What you can do. Retrieved from http://www.npsf.org/?page=safetyissuespatfam

Patient Safety Movement. (2016). Patient Safety Movement announces three new patient safety challenges. Retrieved from http://www.businesswire.com/news/home/20160615006315/en/Patient-Safety-Movement-Announces-Patient-Safety-Challenges

Patient Safety Network (PSNet). (2015). Human factors engineering. Retrieved from https://psnet.ahrq.gov/primers/primer/20/human-factors-engineering

Patient Safety Network (PSNet). (2016a). Submit a case to WebM&M. Retrieved from https://psnet.ahrq.gov/webmm/submit-case

Patient Safety Network (PSNet). (2016b). Wrong-site, wrong-procedure, and wrong-patient surgery. Retrieved from https://psnet.ahrq.gov/primers/primer/18/wrong-site-wrong -procedure-and-wrong-patient-surgery

Patient Safety Network (PSNet). (2016c). Robotic surgery: Risks vs. rewards. Retrieved from https://psnet.ahrq.gov/webmm/case/368/robotic-surgery-risks-vs-rewards-

Phillips Healthcare. (2013). Taking alarm management from concept to reality: A step by step guide. Retrieved from https://www.usa.philips.com/b-dam/b2bhc/us/whitepapers/alarm -systems-management/An-action-Plan.pdf

Radick, L. (2016). Radically redesigning patient safety. *Healthcare Executive, 31*(2), 36–40, 42.

Revere, L., Black, K., & Zalila, F. (2010). RFIDs can improve the patient care supply chain. *Hospital Topics, 88*(1), 26–31. Retrieved from Health Module (Document ID: 2119405721).

Rosen, A. & Mull, H. (2016). Identifying adverse events after outpatient surgery: Improving measurement of patient safety. *BMJ Quality and Safety, 25*, 3–5. doi:10.1136/bmjqs -2015-004752

Savoy, V. (2010). Robots to invade Scottish hospital, pose as "workers." *Engadget.* Retrieved from http://www.engadget.com/2010/06/21/robots-to-invade-scottish-hospital-pose -as-workers

Sharbaugh, D., & Boroch, M. (2010). Hospital smart rooms are ready for rollout. Retrieved from http://www.interiorsandsources.com/article-details/articleid/9675/title/hospital-smart -rooms-are-ready-for-rollout.aspx

SIMpill. (2008). The SIMpill medication adherence solution. Retrieved from http://www.simpill .com/thesimplesolution.htm

Singh, H., & Sittig, D. F. (2015). Measuring and improving patient safety through health information technology: The Health IT Safety Framework [ePub ahead of print]. *BMJ Quality and Safety.* Retrieved from http://qualitysafety.bmj.com/content/early/2015/09/13 /bmjqs-2015-004486.long

Steele, A., & DeBrow, M. (n.d.). Efficiency gains with computerized provider order entry. In K. Henriksen, J. B. Battles, M. A. Keyes, & M. L. Grady (Eds.), *Advances in patient safety: New directions and alternative approaches (Vol. 4: Technology and Medication Safety).* Rockville, MD: Agency for Healthcare Research and Quality. Retrieved from http://www .ahrq.gov/downloads/pub/advances2/vol4/Advances-Steele_100.pdf

Tiase, V. (2015). ANI Emerging Leaders Project: Nurses' perceptions of the use of health information technology tools for patient and family engagement. *CIN: Computers, Informatics, Nursing, 33*(12), 520–522.

University of Alabama at Birmingham (UAB). (2013). UAB Medicine: The connected hospital. Retrieved from http://www.uabmedicine.org/news/news-nursing-the-connected-hospital

University of Iowa. (2015). iScrub Lite 1.5.2. Retrieved from https://compepi.cs.uiowa.edu/iscrub

University of Rochester Medical Center, Department of Pharmacy. (2016). Robotics: Improved efficiency and enhanced accuracy in dispensing drugs for hospital patients at Strong Health. Retrieved from https://www.urmc.rochester.edu/pharmacy/about/safety/robotics.aspx

U.S. Department of Veteran's Affairs National Center for Patient Safety. (2015). Root cause analysis. Retrieved from http://www.patientsafety.va.gov/professionals/onthejob/rca.asp

Vecchione, A. (2015). Patient safety driving increased RFID use in hospitals. *Healthcare IT News.* Retrieved from http://www.healthcareitnews.com/news/patient-safety-driving -increased-rfid-use-hospitals

Wachter, R. (2010). Patient safety at ten: Unmistakable progress, troubling gaps. *Health Affairs*, *29*(1), 165–173. Retrieved from ABI/INFORM Global (Document ID: 194983018).

White, J., Shiffman, R., Middleton, B., & Cabán, T. (2008). A national web conference on using clinical decision support to make informed patient care decisions. Slide 63: Partners CDS services: CAD/DM smart, Form Slides 63–65. Presented at Agency for Healthcare Research and Quality, September 19, 2008. Retrieved from https://healthit.ahrq.gov/events/national-web-conference-using-clinical-decision-support-make-informed-patient-care-decisions

Versel, N. (2016). About that Johns Hopkins study on medical errors (podcast). Retrieved from http://medcitynews.com/2016/05/hopkins-medical-errors-podcast

Williams, J. (2009). Biomeds' increased involvement improves processes, patient safety. *Biomedical Instrumentation & Technology*, *43*(2), 121–3. Retrieved from ProQuest Nursing & Allied Health Source (Document ID: 1692747971).

WISH Patient Safety Forum. (2015). Transforming patient safety: A sector-wide systems approach. Retrieved from https://www.imperial.ac.uk/media/imperial-college/institute-of-global-health-innovation/public/Patient-safety.pdf

Wray, B. & Sanislo, M. (2016). The case for RFID in blood banking. *Medical Laboratory Observer*. Retrieved from http://www.mlo-online.com/the-case-for-rfid-in-blood-banking

1. Define health literacy and e-health.
2. Explore various technology-based approaches to consumer health education.
3. Identify barriers to use of technology and issues associated with health-related consumer information.
4. Imagine future approaches to technology-supported consumer health information.

## Key Terms

- » Blogs
- » Connected health
- » Digital divide
- » Domain name
- » E-brochure
- » E-health
- » eHealth Initiative
- » Empowerment
- » Gray gap
- » Health literacy
- » HONcode
- » Interactive technologies
- » Know–do gap
- » Patient engagement
- » Static medium
- » Trust-e
- » Voice recognition
- » Web quests
- » Weblog

# CHAPTER 16

# Patient Engagement and Connected Health

Kathleen Mastrian and Dee McGonigle

## Introduction

Imagine that you have decided to take up running as your preferred form of exercise in a quest to get in shape. You start slowly by running a half mile and walking a half mile. You gradually build up your endurance and find yourself running nearly every day for longer distances and longer periods of time. But then you notice a nagging pain first in your right hip; over a few weeks, it gradually spreads to the center of your right buttocks and then down your right leg. You try rest and heat, but nothing seems to help. You visit your doctor, and she indicates that you have developed piriformis syndrome and prescribes a series of stretching exercises, ice to the involved area, and rest. You are intrigued by the diagnosis. Upon your return home, you log on to the Internet and begin a search for information about piriformis syndrome. When you type the words into your favorite search engine, you get 371,000 results in response to your query.

Your use of the Internet to seek health information mirrors the behavior of many consumers, who are increasingly relying on the Internet for health-related information. The challenge for consumers and healthcare professionals alike is the proliferation of information on the Internet and the need to learn how to recognize when information is accurate and meaningful to the situation at hand.

This chapter explores consumer information and education needs and considers how patient engagement and connected health technologies, including new trends in wearable technology, may help to meet those needs, yet at the same time create ever increasing demands for health-related information. It begins with a discussion of health literacy, e-health, and health education and information needs, and explores various approaches by healthcare providers to using technology to promote health literacy. Also examined is the use of games, **Web quests**, and simulations as means of increasing health literacy among the school-age population. Issues associated with the credibility of Web-based information and barriers to access and uses for patient engagement are discussed. Finally future trends related to technology-supported consumer information and connectivity are explored.

## Consumer Demand for Information

This is the Knowledge Age; many people want to be in the know. People demand news and information, and they want immediate results and unlimited access. This is increasingly true with health information. More and more people, in a trend known as consumer **empowerment, patient engagement,** and **connected health,** are interested in partnering with healthcare providers to take control of their health. These patients are not satisfied being dependent on a healthcare provider to supply them with the information they need to manage their health. Instead, they are increasingly embracing electronic technologies such as patient portals offering current and past health statuses, lab results, and secure messaging with providers; social media interactions; health-related games; wearable technologies for tracking health; and health management apps.

The most recent Pew Internet and American Life Project Health Online survey report (Fox and Duggan, 2013) indicates that 8 in 10 Americans who are online have searched for health information (these numbers are comparable to the numbers in previous surveys conducted in 2006 and 2011). The most frequent health topic searches (69%) are related to a specific disease or medical problem that the searcher or a member of the family is experiencing. Other frequent topics of health-related searches are weight, diet, and exercise (60%) and health indicators such as blood parameters or sleep patterns (33%). The 2011 survey ($n = 3,001$) reports that consumers also searched for information on food (29%) and drug safety (24%; Fox, 2011). Just over half of "online diagnosers" (those who search online for information about medical conditions) reported that they shared their Internet findings with their healthcare providers, and 41% reported that their findings were confirmed by a clinician (Fox & Duggan, 2013). It is clear that patients are increasingly looking to be partners with their healthcare providers in managing their health challenges and maintaining a level of wellness. All healthcare professionals need to be prepared to listen to the ideas of patients about their personal health and, at the same time, provide direction toward credible health information supplied by electronic provider portals on the Internet. Here is some good news: In an attempt to improve the credibility of the results of online searches about health, in 2015 Google partnered with Mayo Clinic to fact-check the information in a database for 400 of the most-commonly searched for health issues (Lapowsky, 2015). Mayo Clinic (2015) reported that Google

> [has become] part of our daily lives. There's no need to sift through mountains of data and endless links to find the few nuggets we need. So naturally, when people have health concerns, one of their first stops is Google. But anyone who has searched the Internet to self-diagnose knows the dizzying, and sometimes scary, array of results. To help give their users the best health information possible, Google now provides relevant medical facts upfront. (p. 4)

Google intends to "surface these pre-vetted facts at the top of its search results, in hopes of getting people to the right information faster" (Lapowsky, para 2).

It is important to note that surveys of online health behaviors are limited to those individuals who are online and do not reflect the health information needs or demands of those persons who are not online. **Digital divide** is the term used to describe the gap between those who have and those who do not have access to online information. Nurses and healthcare providers need to be aware of the various components of the digital divide to ensure that patients and clients are receiving the health information they need in a format that they are interested in and can comprehend. Notably, persons with chronic diseases are less likely to have Internet connectivity. Fox and Purcell (2010) explain the disparity in that having a chronic disease is associated with age, level of education, ethnicity, and income—all factors also associated with the digital divide. Persons living with a chronic disease who have Internet access are likely to use the Internet for blogging and online discussion forums, activities popularly referred to as peer-to-peer support. A recent issue brief by the Council of Economic Advisers (2015) reiterates digital divide factors as age, education, income, and geographic location. By providing infrastructure investment monies, President Obama's ConnectED program is designed to increase broadband access for schools. A similar initiative is designed to promote competition among Internet providers, thereby lowering costs and making high-speed Internet connections more affordable and accessible across the country.

Missen and Cook (2007) discussed the potential impact that technology-based health information dissemination can have on the know–do gap in developing countries. The **know–do gap** reflects the fact that solutions to global health problems exist but are not implemented in a timely fashion because of the lack of access to important health information. The Internet connections in developing countries are widely scattered and may not be efficient or sufficient for viewing healthcare information. Missen and Cook described the use of a freestanding hard drive loaded with hundreds of CDs of health-related information in a webpage format that responds to a search command. This is a great example of providing technologies that work with the constraints of the situation. Another example of addressing the digital divide is the growing number of health-related websites that support Spanish and other language formats.

# Health Literacy and Health Initiatives

The goal of **health literacy** for all is one that is widely embraced in many sectors of health care; it was a major goal of *Healthy People 2010*, and is being continued in the health communication and health information technology objective of *Healthy People 2020* (Office of Disease Prevention and Health Promotion & U.S. Department of Health and Human Services, 2016). Clinicians who have been practicing for some time recognize that informed patients have better outcomes and pay more attention to their overall health and changes in their health than those who are poorly informed. Some of the earliest formally developed patient education programs, which included postoperative teaching, diabetes education, cardiac rehabilitation, and diet education, were implemented in response to research that suggested the positive impact of patient education on health outcomes and satisfaction with care. Almader-Douglas (2013) updated the National Network Libraries of Medicine webpage on health literacy (http://nnlm.gov/outreach/consumer/hlthlit.html). She concluded from the research on the economic impact of health literacy that those persons with low health literacy have less ability to manage a chronic illness properly and tend to use more healthcare services than those who are more literate. In addition, she used results of health research to demonstrate the impact of low health literacy and the incidence of disease.

The site states that "Health Literacy is defined in the Institute of Medicine report *Health Literacy: A Prescription to End Confusion* as 'The degree to which individuals have the capacity to obtain, process, and understand basic health information and services needed to make appropriate health decisions'" (Almader-Douglas, 2013, para. 2). For example, healthcare providers depend on a patient's ability to understand and follow directions associated with dietary restrictions or exercising at home. It is also assumed, sometimes erroneously, that people will correctly interpret symptoms of a serious illness and act appropriately. The ability to locate and evaluate health information for credibility and quality, to analyze the various risks and benefits of treatments, and to calculate dosages and interpret test results are among the tasks Almader-Douglas identified as essential for health literacy. Other important and less easily learned health literacy skills are the ability to negotiate complex healthcare environments and understand the economics of payment for services. Parker, Ratzan, and Lurie (2003) estimated that at least one third of all Americans have health literacy problems and lament that in a time-is-money economic climate, healthcare practitioners are not always reimbursed for patient education activities. This is still true today. The National Institutes of Health (NIH; 2015) reported that numerous studies concerning health literacy demonstrate that a variety of challenges remain on both the patient and healthcare-provider sides of the equation.

It is increasingly clear that better outcomes result when patients are well informed and engaged in their care. As depicted in **Figure 16-1**, there are a number of effective strategies to promote better health, including strategies for building sound relationships, strategies to ensure that patients are well informed about their health challenges, and strategies to build partnerships with patients.

The **eHealth Initiative** was developed to address the growing need for managing health information and to promote technology as a means of improving health information exchange, health literacy, and healthcare delivery. The eHealth Initiative website (www.ehidc.org) provides more information. Although its scope goes beyond health literacy, a major goal continues to be empowering consumers to understand their health needs better and to take action appropriate to those needs. The eHealth Initiative recently released a 2020 roadmap outlining a vision toward patient-centric care. Poor interoperability among healthcare systems and failure to embrace national data standards for health care continue to be identified as barriers to the eHealth Initiative. Further, concerns about privacy and security of information and the failure to invest appropriately in technology have slowed the development of this important initiative. The Centers for Disease Control and Prevention (CDC, 2016) maintains

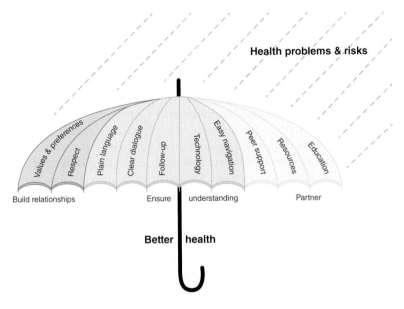

**Figure 16-1** The Health Literacy Umbrella

Developed by the Health Literacy in Communities Prototype Faculty: Connie Davis, Kelly McQuillen, Irv Rootman, Leona Gadsby, Lori Walker, Marina Niks, Cheryl Rivard, Shirley Sze, and Angela Hovis with Joanne Protheroe, and the Ministry of Health, July 2009. IMPACT BC, with funding from the BC Ministry of Health.

an interactive map of the United States that provides access to health literacy and e-health initiatives by state (www.cdc.gov/healthliteracy).

# Healthcare Organization Approaches to Engagement

Healthcare organizations (HCOs) use a wide variety of approaches and tools to engage patients and promote patient education and health literacy. Although the old standby for disseminating information is the paper-based flyer, some HCOs are recognizing that today's consumers are more attracted to a dynamic rather than **static medium**. In addition, the cost of designing and printing pamphlets and flyers becomes prohibitive when one considers the rapidity of change of information; the brochure may be outdated almost as soon as it is printed. One approach to deal with these issues is to have patient education information stored electronically so that changes can be made as needed or information can be better tailored to the specific patient situation and then printed out and reviewed with the patient.

Another old standby approach that is still widely used is the group education class. These classes initially were developed to help people manage chronic health problems (e.g., diabetes) and were typically scheduled while people were hospitalized. Now, many HCOs also sponsor health promotion education classes as a way of marketing their facilities and showcasing some of their expert practitioners.

The movement from static to dynamic presentations began in many HCOs with the use of videotapes, and then DVDs, which were shown in groups or broadcast on demand over dedicated channels via television in patients' rooms. HCOs are now also taking advantage of the fact that patients and families are captive audiences in waiting rooms by promoting education via pamphlet distribution, health promotion programs broadcast on television, and health information kiosks in those locations. The kiosks are typically computer stations and often contain a variety of self-assessment tools (especially those related to risks for diabetes, heart disease, or cancer) and searchable pages of information about specific health conditions. The self-assessment tools represent yet another step forward in technological support for education: In addition to being dynamic, the kiosk is interactive. On the assessment page, the user is asked to respond to a series of questions and then the health risk is calculated by the computer program. One caution, however, is that just because the information is made available, it does not mean that people will participate or that they will understand what they have experienced. Issues related to the level of health literacy, the digital divide, and the **gray gap** (differences in electronic connectivity by age) still exist in these situations.

Many HCOs have invested time and money in developing interactive websites and believe that Web presence is a critical marketing strategy. Sternberg (2002) suggested that many websites began as an **e-brochure** and progressed through various stages to reach a true e-care status. Most offer physician search capabilities, e-newsletters, and call-center tie-ins. As with all patient education materials, there must be a sincere commitment to keeping information current and easily accessible. Web designers must pay particular attention to the aesthetics of the site, the ease of use, and the literacy level of those in the intended audience.

A usability study conducted by Lauterbach (2010) provided some insights into how to measure website usability. Lauterbach compared the usability of the symptom checker functions of two popular websites by asking volunteers to navigate each using four different case scenarios. Users navigated the site to find the symptom checker and then entered the symptoms and evaluated site feedback. Users rated the ease of understanding for each site and completed a short comprehension quiz. Data were collected on descriptions of user site preferences, user satisfaction with the sites, results of the comprehension quiz, and efficiency, which was measured by tracking the number of webpage changes the user performed while navigating the site.

The rapid growth of electronic communication through increased use of computers and access to the Internet, particularly for medical purposes, empowers the clinician as well as the consumer of healthcare information. The integration of information and communication technologies (ICTs) and the growing trend of consumer empowerment have reshaped the delivery of health care. As a result of meaningful use initiatives, many HCOs have developed secure patient portals that allow patients to access their health records, including tracking laboratory results and reviewing the records. Most HCOs, however, do not allow patients to edit these records. In addition, patients are occasionally interested in interacting with others who have the same or similar conditions, and some HCOs are providing the information necessary to help them connect. This so-called peer-to-peer support is especially popular with patients who have cancer diagnoses, diabetes, and other chronic and debilitating conditions (Lober & Flowers, 2011).

**RESEARCH BRIEF**

An exploratory study of social media use among hospitals sought to examine the prevalence of social media use among hospitals, whether hospital structure influenced the choice of social media strategy, and how frequently Facebook was used as an engagement strategy or an information dissemination strategy. The authors examined the websites of 471 randomly selected hospitals to identify the methods that hospitals used to attract customers, such as advertising, personal stories, content related to patient satisfaction, and patient education. Hospital websites were also reviewed for specific links to social media such as YouTube, Twitter, Facebook, LinkedIn, or blogs. The authors examined Facebook usage characteristics in depth.

The authors reported that Facebook is the most commonly used social media site and that all social media use was related to websites that also concentrated on emphasizing quality metrics and education. They report that 70% of the hospitals used some type of social media network and that social media was more likely to be used by larger, urban, nonprofit organizations. In addition, Facebook was more likely to be used as a dissemination strategy rather than a strategy for engagement; only 27% of the sample focused on engagement on Facebook by posing questions, responding to comments, or offering prizes. The authors conclude that social media, and Facebook in particular, is underutilized and that hospitals are missing an important opportunity for low-cost patient engagement.

The full article can be accessed at Richter, J. P., Muhlestein, D. B., & Wilks, C. A. (2014). Social media: How hospitals use it, and opportunities for future use. *Journal of Healthcare Management, 59*(6), 447–460.

Some HCOs are using social media for health education to promote actual engagement of audiences rather than as means of one-way messaging. Neiger, Thackeray, Burton, Giraud-Carrier, and Fagen (2013) suggested "that the use of social media in health promotion must lead to engagement between the health promotion organization and its audience members, that engagement must provide mutual benefit, and that an engagement hierarchy culminates in program involvement with audience members in the form of partnership or participation (as recipients of program services)" (p. 158). The CDC (2014) has an excellent social media tool kit that can be used by health educators to guide the planning and implementation of social media strategies for health promotion. This tool kit can be accessed at the following website: www .cdc.gov/socialmedia/Tools/guidelines/pdf/SocialMediaToolkit_BM.pdf. In addition, the Research Brief provides insights into the potential effectiveness of social media use by HCOs.

# Promoting Health Literacy in School-Aged Children

Promoting health literacy in school-aged children presents special challenges to health educators. There is wide agreement that childhood obesity is a serious and growing issue, which is related not only to poor choice of foods, but also to the sedentary lifestyles promoted by video games and television. In addition, the time once devoted to health and physical education programs in schools has given way to more time spent on core subjects, such as math and science.

The Children's Nutrition Research Center responded early to these challenges by supporting the development of nutrition education programs as interactive computer games, video games, and cartoons referred to as "edutainment" (Flores, 2006). These **e-health** programs are developed specifically to appeal to the generational (highly connected and computer literate) and cultural needs of this group. Flores describes the Family Web project, which uses comic strips to impart nutrition information, and Squires Quest, where the students earn points by choosing fruits and vegetables to fight the snakes and moles that are trying to destroy the healthy foods in the Kingdom of SALot. These are great examples of health education programs that are designed to appeal to this connected generation of learners and their intuitive ability to use **interactive technologies**.

Donovan (2005) described an interdisciplinary Web quest designed to appeal to older school-aged children. The quest is interdisciplinary in that it requires reading comprehension, critical thinking, presentation, and writing; thus, core skills and health literacy skills are learned in a single assignment. Students are directed to the Web to search for information on the pros and cons of low-carbohydrate diets and obesity prevention. Students learn along the way as they search for information, collect and interpret it, and then develop a presentation and final paper.

The Cancer Game (Oda & Kristula, n.d.) was developed by a young man taking a college class on Macromedia software who had previously undergone a bone marrow transplant. Subsequently, he and a professor collaborated and expanded the project to its present form. The game is designed as an arcade-style video game for cancer patients to relieve stress by visualizing the fighting of cancer cells. Although cancer victims of any age can access and play the game, it has a special appeal to children and adolescents. Find the game here: www.cancergame.org. Similarly, Ben's Game (www.wish.org/wishes/wish-stories/i-wish-to-be/ben-video-game-creator) is a video game designed to help relieve the stress of cancer treatment for children (Anderson & Klemm, 2008).

You can access these newer games on the Internet by typing "health games" into a search engine. Be sure to review the information presented in the game for accuracy before you recommend it to parents and children. The National Library of Medicine maintains a site dedicated to health learning games for both children and adults (www.nlm.nih.gov/medlineplus/games.html). You can feel confident in recommending games from this trusted website as they have been vetted for accuracy and credibility.

## Supporting Use of the Internet for Health Education

Nurses and other healthcare providers need to embrace the Internet as a source of health information for patient education and health literacy. Patients are increasingly turning there for instant information about their health maladies. Health-related **blogs** (short for **weblog**, an online journal) and electronic patient and parent support groups are also proliferating at an astounding rate. Clinicians need to be prepared to arm patients with the skills required to identify credible websites. They also need to participate in the development of well-designed, easy-to-use health education tools. Finally, they need to convince payers of the necessity of health education and the powerful impact education has on promoting and maintaining health. Box 16-1 provides more information about patient education.

---

**BOX 16-1 CONSIDERATIONS FOR PATIENT EDUCATION**

*Julie A. Kenney and Ida Androwich*

Nurses need to take many things into account when teaching patients. They need to assess patients' willingness to learn, their reading ability, the means by which they learn best, and their existing knowledge about the subject. These important considerations for patient education are depicted in Figure 16-2.

Nurses also need to take cultural, language, and generational differences into account when teaching their patients. If the nurse chooses to use an electronic method to educate the patient, digital natives (patients who have grown up with technology) need to be taught differently than digital immigrants (those who are late adopters of technology; "Educational Strategies," 2006). Digital natives are typically born after 1982 and may also be referred to as "Generation Y." This generation prefers to learn using technology and learns quite well if information is presented in a format to which they are accustomed, such as an interactive video game to introduce them to a topic. This group is also comfortable using information that they can access via their handheld devices, such as smartphones and tablets, as well as wearable devices such as smartwatches. Those born before 1982 have learning styles that range from preferring to learn in a classroom setting to reading a book about the topic to learning using a hands-on, interactive approach ("Educational Strategies," 2006).

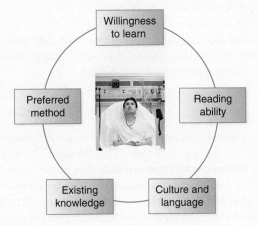

**Figure 16-2** Choosing an Education Strategy
Photo: © ERproductions Ltd/Blend Images/Getty

A systematic review of the literature related to teaching methods (Friedman, Cosby, Boyko, Hatton-Bauer, & Turnbull, 2011) suggested that various modalities ranging from computer technologies to demonstrations and reviews of written materials can all be effective as long as they are structured and specifically designed for and congruent with the patient's culture. More recently, Sawyer (2016) tested a tablet-based education program for patients with heart failure. They sought to demonstrate the value of the tablet-based education approach to staff and, at the same time, find ways to minimize the disruptiveness of the technology-based education on clinical workflow, ensure patent safety by establishing specific procedures for device cleaning, and suggest strategies for maintaining the security of the devices. They conclude that technology-based learning tools may be effective in helping patients manage their disease postdischarge. They also emphasize the need to consider clinician workflow and device security to ensure a successful implementation.

## REFERENCES

Educational strategies in generational designs. (2006). *Progress in Transplantation, 16*(1), 8–9.

Friedman, A. Cosby, R., Boyko, S., Hatton-Bauer, J., & Turnbull, G. (2011). Effective teaching strategies and methods of delivery for patient education: A systematic review and practice guideline recommendations. *Journal of Cancer Education,* 12–21. doi: 10.1007/s13187-010-0183-x.

Sawyer, T. (2016). Implementing electronic tablet-based education of acute care patients. *Critical Care Nurse, 36*(1), 60–70. doi:10.4037/ccn2016541

## PATIENT EDUCATION WEBSITES

American Academy of Family Physicians: www.aafp.org/patient-care.html
American Cancer Society: www.cancer.org
American Heart Association: www.heart.org
Centers for Disease Control and Prevention: www.cdc.gov
Krames (products to purchase): www.staywell.com/patient-education-2
UpToDate (paid subscription): www.uptodate.com

The Health on the Net (HON) Foundation (2005) survey described the certifications and accreditation symbols that identify trusted health sites. The **HONcode** and **Trust-e** were identified as the two most common symbols that power users look for. (Website developers can apply for HONcode certification of Web-based materials. Initial certification is for 1 year, after which the site is reevaluated annually by experts. The HON Foundation also monitors site complaints and factors reported issues into the recertification process [Health on the Net Foundation, 2014].) The survey also indicated that Internet users look at the **domain name** and frequently gravitate toward university sites (.edu), government sites (.gov), and HCO sites (.org). Half of the survey respondents were in favor of the use of a domain name called "health" to identify quality health information websites. In contrast, Anderson and Rainie (2006) indicate that nearly 75% of online searchers do not check the date or the source of information they are accessing on the Web and 3% of online health seekers report knowing someone who was harmed by following health information found on the Web.

The U.S. National Library of Medicine and the NIH jointly sponsor MedlinePlus, a website that has a tutorial for learning how to evaluate health information and an electronic guide to Web surfing that is available in both English and Spanish. This site is found at www.medlineplus.gov. A similar guide explains the major things one should evaluate when accessing health-related resources on the Web (National Center for Complementary and Alternative Medicine, 2014) and can be accessed at http://nccam.nih.gov/health/webresources. Suggest that patients visit these sites to become more adept at identifying whether a website is credible before they adopt the recommendations provided.

Some healthcare professionals have partnered with their organizations to develop patient education materials. These materials must be carefully reviewed for accuracy and usability. The Agency for Healthcare Research and Quality (2013) published an assessment tool for both print and audiovisual patient education materials. Their tool is designed to assess both understandability and actionability by providing a series of review criteria for each of these domains. The tool can be accessed at www.ahrq.gov /professionals/prevention-chronic-care/improve/self-mgmt/pemat/index.html. Clearly, the clinician needs to engage the patient to partner with them in the management of their health. Refer to Boxes 16-1 and 16-2 to review effective education methods used in teaching patients and their families about their health challenges.

## BOX 16-2 A CLINICIAN'S VIEW ON PATIENT EDUCATION

*Denise D. Tyler*

Knowledge dissemination in nursing practice includes sharing information with patients and families so that they understand their healthcare needs well enough to participate in developing the plan of care, make informed decisions about their health, and ultimately comply with the plan of care, both during hospitalization and as outpatients.

There are several effective methods for educating patients and their families. Providing one-on-one and classroom instruction are traditional and valuable forms of education. One-on-one education is interactive and can be adjusted at any time during the process based on the needs of the individual patient or family; it can also be supplemented by written material, videos, and Web-based learning applications. Classroom education can be beneficial because patients and families with similar needs or problems can network, thereby enhancing the individual experience. However, the ability to interact with each member of the group and to tailor the educational experience based on individual needs may be limited by the size and dissimilarities of the group. Individual follow-up should be available when possible.

Paper-based education that is created, printed, and distributed by individual institutions or providers can be very effective because materials can be distributed at any time and reviewed when the patient feels like learning. Many agencies, such as the CDC, have education for patients available on their websites. These documents can be reviewed online, or they can be printed out by healthcare providers or patients. Organizations can also develop and distribute information and instructions specific to their policies and procedures. In addition, printed educational material can be purchased from companies that employ experts in the subject matter and instructional design.

One of the more popular sources of patient education information is the Internet. Many hospitals and HCOs provide proprietary information, such as directions to the facility, information on procedures, and instructions on what to expect during hospitalization, in this manner. Other health organizations, such as the NIH, provide detailed information on their websites. Clinicians should be cautious when recommending websites to patients and families, because not all sites are reliable or valid.

Many companies that provide clinical information systems or electronic health records also include patient education materials linked to the clinical system via an intranet. Thus standardized instructions that are specific to a procedure or disease process can be printed from this computer-based application. Discharge instructions that are interdisciplinary and patient specific can often be modified via drop-down lists or selectable items that can be deleted or changed by the clinician. This ability to modify before printing provides more consistent and individualized instruction. The computer-based generation of instruction is preferable to free text and verbal instruction because it also allows the information to be linked to a coded nursing language and, therefore, easily used for measurement and quality assurance reporting. Relevant triggers may be embedded in the clinical information systems. For example, when a patient answers "yes" to a question about current smoking, smoking cessation information should automatically be printed, or a trigger should remind the nurse to explore this topic with the patient and then provide the patient with preprinted information on smoking cessation.

Integration of standardized discharge instructions and patient education into the clinical system is another way to improve the compliance and documentation of education; it also streamlines the workflow of clinicians. Printing the information to give to the patient should be seamless to the clinician who is documenting in the patient's record. The format should be logical and easy to read. The more transparent the process, the more efficient the system and the easier it is to use for the clinician. What I envision for the future is a system that "remembers" the style of learning preferred by patients and their families, prompts the provider to print handouts, and programs the bedside computer/video education system based on previous selections and surveys. This interactive patient and family education will be integrated into the clinical system and the patient's personal health record.

Some providers have developed a list of credible websites and apps that are shared with patients or family members. Recommendations for websites might include the U.S. Department of Health and Human Services–sponsored healthfinder site (www.healthfinder.gov), a website dedicated to helping consumers find credible information on the Internet. Other excellent sources of reliable information are the National Institutes of Health (www.nih.gov), the Centers for Disease Control and Prevention (www.cdc.gov), Medline Plus (www.medlineplus.gov), NIHSeniorHealth (www.nihseniorhealth.gov), and the National Health Information Center (www.health.gov/nhic). Some of the apps (found on iTunes for iPhones or Google Play for Android devices) that might be recommended include Mayo Clinic on Pregnancy, WebMD Pain Coach, MyFitnessPal, and Understanding Diseases. These are great examples of the wealth of patient information being developed as apps by hospitals and other health-care providers. More apps are being developed every day to engage people in managing and taking control of their health. Perhaps the most important thing that healthcare professionals can stress is that not all apps have credible and valid information. We must encourage our patients to become savvy users of electronic information sources.

## Future Directions for Engaging Patients

Predicting future directions for technology-based health education is somewhat difficult because one may not be able to completely envision the technology of the future. One can predict, however, that some current technologies will be used increasingly to support health literacy, and new technologies will be developed every day. For example, audio and video podcasts may become more commonplace in health education and be provided as free downloads from the websites of HCOs.

**Voice recognition** software used to navigate the Web may reduce the frustration and confusion associated with attempting to spell complex medical terms. However, the confusion and frustration may increase if the patient or client is unable to pronounce the terms. Voice interactivity should help to reduce the digital access disparity associated with those who have limited keyboard or mouse skills. For those persons with visual impairments, some websites may provide both audio and text information and support increased text size for greater ease of reading (Anderson & Klemm, 2008).

Many websites associated with government and national organizations are also providing multiple-language access to health information and decision-support tools (U.S. National Library of Medicine, 2016). The multilanguage access broadens the population to whom education can be provided, and the decision-support programs allow users to access results that are tailored to their age, risk factors, or disease state (Anderson & Klemm, 2008).

As patient engagement strategies become more commonplace, we will also see a movement toward connected health. Those individuals who are frequent email users may be interested in being able to communicate with physicians and other healthcare personnel via email rather than the telephone. This idea may meet with some resistance from physicians who perceive the email correspondence as bothersome and time consuming. However, it is possible that work efficiency might also increase if patients and their needs are screened via secure email before an office or clinic visit. For example, as a result of an email correspondence in lieu of an initial office visit, medications could be changed or diagnostic tests could be performed before the office visit. In addition, patients could be directed to an interactive screening form housed on a secure website where they would answer a series of questions that would help them make a decision about whether they should call for an appointment, head for the emergency room, or self-manage the issue. If self-management is the outcome of the screening tool, then the patient or caregiver could be directed to a credible website for more information. The idea is not to interfere with or replace the face-to-face visit, but rather to supplement the provider–patient relationship and perhaps streamline the efficiency of healthcare delivery. McCray (2005) also suggests that physicians may be resistant to providing email consultations and recommending health-related websites because of the potential for malpractice liability. Other healthcare professionals may share some of these same concerns. There is some evidence that text message reminders delivered via a cell phone are more effective and efficient as appointment reminders than traditional phone calls (Car, Gurol-Urganci, de Jongh, Vodopivec-Jamsek, & Atun, 2012), and text message reminders related to health behaviors such as diet and exercise might also be effective. Similarly, in a descriptive research study by Dudas, Pumilia, and Crocetti (2013), it was found that parents of children who recently visited an emergency department were interested in receiving follow-up communication from healthcare providers by text messaging and/or email. A major barrier to widespread adoption of email and text messaging among American healthcare providers is the fact that reimbursement mechanisms for electronic health care interventions are inadequate or nonexistent. This may be an issue that is resolved in the near future, and other healthcare professionals may soon be a part of these patient engagement and connected health trends. Piette (2007) described the use of interactive behavior change technology to improve the effectiveness of diabetes management. The goal of the interactive behavior change technology is to improve communication between patients and healthcare providers and to provide educational interventions that promote better disease management between office visits. The combination of electronic medication reminders, meters that track glycemic control longitudinally, and personal digital assistant–based calculators was found to support the behavioral interventions necessary to better manage the diabetes.

As a conclusion to their study, Watson, Bell, Kvedar, and Grant (2008) caution that even though patients are part of the digital divide (lacking access or skill in electronic communications and Internet use), one cannot assume that they will be resistant to using other forms of technology to support health. These authors compared Internet users to non-Internet users and found that both groups were willing to learn to use new technology to manage type 2 diabetes, including wireless communication devices for information sharing with physicians.

Healthcare practitioners may soon embrace the use of "information prescriptions" (D'Alessandro, 2010) that direct patients and families to credible websites, including government and HCO websites, and wikis and blogs that may help them understand their health issues or share information with and seek support from others who have similar issues. "Information prescriptions are prescriptions of focused, evidence-based information given to a patient at the right time to manage a health problem" (D'Alessandro, p. 81). The National Health Service in the United Kingdom has developed an information prescription generator that can be used by providers or the public to access Web-based health information (www.nhs.uk/ipg /Pages/IPStart.aspx).

Wearable technologies are becoming increasingly popular among tech-savvy patients. However, their impact on overall health has yet to be realized. Garvin (2016) stated, "As wearables and their applications continue to multiply, a single and familiar question emerges: Where exactly will wearable technology lead us? Is this garnering of such gadgets and their wealth of health data merely a trend, or is there real staying power within these little devices to create substantial impact in healthcare?" (para. 2). The most common consumer-based wearables are fitness trackers, but there are no clear guidelines as to how to integrate the data these devices collect into a patient's health record and make them actionable. Examples of other devices include smart shirts that track anxiety-triggered breathing patterns and promote mindfulness (Garvin); the Smart Stop device, which is designed to detect cigarette cravings and deliver medication to eliminate the craving; and smart contact lenses that measure glucose levels in tears and alert the wearer to a change in glucose level by changing color (Kosir, 2015). For a full discussion of provider prescribed wearables and remote health monitoring, see the telehealth chapter.

Newer technologies designed to engage patients actively in rehabilitation activities were recently reported on MedGadget (2016). For example, to better engage patients in stroke rehabilitation activities, researchers developed a game system that encourages patients to use the affected limb to play the game while restricting the good limb from participation. Another system employs sensors on the affected limbs and the patient's motion is translated into art on the screen. The feedback is immediate and readily apparent, which seems to encourage patients to participate more fully. Along these same lines, a series of neurogaming technologies are being developed to promote cognitive function. "Data generated from these products also provide actionable information to inform care delivery. Therapeutic neurogaming is the use of neurogaming technologies for the purposes of health, wellness, and/or rehabilitation" (Morsy, 2016, para. 2). You can receive free daily updates on medical technologies by subscribing to the newsletter produced by MedGadget (www.medgadget.com).

## Summary

It is clear that the consumer empowerment and connected health movement will continue to drive the need for access to quality health education and support programs. In an ideal world, practitioners will design educational materials that are user friendly, culturally competent, interesting, dynamic, and interactive, and that meet the skills, education needs, and interests of the user.

### THOUGHT-PROVOKING QUESTIONS

1. Choose two patient-engagement or connectivity tools and discuss specifically how you would use these to deliver care in your practice.
2. Formulate a patient education plan for a common chronic health challenge related to your practice. Provide a rationale for each approach and describe a technology tool you would use to engage and educate the patient and his or her family.
3. Reflect on connected health potentials in your practice. What are you doing currently that connects and engages your patients in managing their health? Describe in detail what you plan to do in the next 6 months to 1 year.

# References

Agency for Healthcare Research and Quality (AHRQ). (2013). The Patient Education Materials Assessment Tool (PEMAT) and user's guide. Retrieved from https://www.ahrq.gov/professionals/prevention-chronic-care/improve/self-mgmt/pemat/index.html

Almader-Douglas, D. (2013). Health literacy. Retrieved from http://nnlm.gov/outreach/consumer/hlthlit.html

Anderson, A., & Klemm, P. (2008). The Internet: Friend or foe when providing patient education? *Clinical Journal of Oncology Nursing, 12*(1), 55–63. Retrieved from ProQuest Nursing & Allied Health Source (Document ID: 1430141231).

Anderson, J. Q., & Rainie, L. (2006). The future of the Internet II. *Pew Internet.* Retrieved from http://news.bbc.co.uk/1/shared/bsp/hi/pdfs/22_09_2006pewsummary.pdf

Car, J., Gurol-Urganci, I., de Jongh, T., Vodopivec-Jamsek, V., & Atun, R. (2012). Mobile phone messaging reminders for attendance at healthcare appointments. *Cochrane Database of Systematic Reviews, 7.*

Centers for Disease Control and Prevention (CDC). (2014). The health communicator's social media toolkit. Retrieved from http://www.cdc.gov/socialmedia/Tools/guidelines/pdf/SocialMediaToolkit_BM.pdf

Centers for Disease Control and Prevention (CDC). (2016). Health literacy: Accurate, accessible and actionable health information for all. Retrieved from http://www.cdc.gov/healthliteracy

Council of Economic Advisors. (2015, July). Issue Brief: Mapping the digital divide. Retrieved from https://www.whitehouse.gov/sites/default/files/wh_**digital_divide**_issue_brief.pdf

D'Alessandro, D. (2010). Challenges and options for patient education in the office setting. *Pediatric Annals, 39*(2), 78–83. Retrieved from Health Module (Document ID: 1972816891).

Donovan, O. (2005). The carbohydrate quandary: Achieving health literacy through an interdisciplinary WebQuest. *Journal of School Health, 75*(9), 359–362. Retrieved from Health Module database (Document ID: 924409661).

Dudas, R. A., Pumilia, J., & Crocetti, M. (2013). Pediatric caregiver attitudes and technologic readiness toward electronic follow-up communication in an urban community emergency department. *Telemedicine & E-Health, 19*(6), 493–496. doi:10.1089/tmj.2012.0166

Flores, A. (2006). Using computer games and other media to decrease child obesity. *Agricultural Research, 54*(3), 8–9. Retrieved from Research Library Core database (Document ID: 1005199991).

Fox, S. (2011, February 1). Health topics. *Pew Research Center.* Retrieved from http://www.pewinternet.org/Reports/2011/HealthTopics.aspx

Fox, S., & Duggan, M. (2013). Health Online 2013. *Pew Research Center.* Retrieved from http://www.pewinternet.org/2013/01/15/health-online-2013

Fox, S., & Purcell, K. (2010). Chronic disease and the Internet. *Pew Research Center.* Retrieved from http://www.pewinternet.org/2010/03/24/chronic-disease-and-the-internet

Garvin, E. (2016). The future of wearables for healthcare in 2016 & beyond. *HIT Consultant.* Retrieved from http://hitconsultant.net/2016/01/19/future-wearables-healthcare

Health on the Net (HON) Foundation. (2005). Analysis of 9th HON survey of health and medical Internet users. Retrieved from http://www.hon.ch/Survey/Survey2005/res.html

Health on the Net (HON) Foundation. (2014). HONcode. Retrieved from http://www.hon.ch/HONcode/Pro/Visitor/visitor.html

Kosir, S. (2015). Wearables in healthcare. *Wearable Technologies.* Retrieved from https://www.wearable-technologies.com/2015/04/wearables-in-healthcare

Lapwosky, I. (2015). Google will make health searches less scary with fact-checked results. *Wired.com.* Retrieved from http://www.wired.com/2015/02/google-health-search

Lauterbach, C. (2010). Exploring the usability of e-health websites. *Usability News, 12*(2). Retrieved from http://usabilitynews.org/exploring-the-usability-of-e-health-websites

Lober, W. B., & Flowers, J. L. (2011, August). Consumer empowerment in health care amid the Internet and social media. *Seminars in Oncology Nursing, 27*(3), 169–182. http://dx.doi.org/10.1016/j.soncn.2011.04.002

Mayo Clinic. (2015). Google works with Mayo. *Mayo Clinic Magazine, 29*(1), 4–5.

McCray, A. (2005). Promoting health literacy. *Journal of the American Medical Informatics Association, 12*(2), 152–163. Retrieved from ProQuest Nursing & Allied Health Source database (Document ID: 810410751).

MedGadget. (2016, May 26), Stroke rehab gamification: Hangout with Ohio State Wexner Medical Center's researchers. Retrieved from http://www.medgadget.com/2016/05/stroke-rehab-gamification-hangout-with-ohio-state-wexner-medical-centers-researchers.html

Missen, C., & Cook, T. (2007). Appropriate information-communications technologies for developing countries. *World Health Organization.* Retrieved from http://www.who.int/bulletin/volumes/85/4/07-041475/en/index.html

Morsy, A. (2016, March/April). Blue Marble Game Company. *IEEE Pulse.* Retrieved from http://pulse.embs.org/march-2016/blue-marble-game-company/?trendmd-shared=1

National Center for Complementary and Alternative Medicine (NCCAM), National Institutes of Health. (2014). Finding and evaluating online resources. Retrieved from http://nccam.nih.gov/health/webresources

National Institutes of Health (NIH). (2015). Clear communication: Health literacy. Retrieved from http://www.nih.gov/clearcommunication/healthliteracy.htm

Neiger, B. L., Thackeray, R., Burton, S. H., Giraud-Carrier, C. G., & Fagen, M. C. (2013). Evaluating social media's capacity to develop engaged audiences in health promotion settings: Use of Twitter metrics as a case study. *Health Promotion Practice, 14*(2), 157–162. doi: 10.1177/1524839912469378

Oda, Y., & Kristula, D. (n.d.) The Cancer Game: A side-scrolling, arcade-style, cancer-fighting video game. Retrieved from http://www.cancergame.org

Office of Disease Prevention and Health Promotion & U.S. Department of Health and Human Services (HHS). (2016). 2020 topics and objectives: Objectives A–Z. Retrieved from http://www.healthypeople.gov/2020/topics-objectives

Parker, R., Ratzan, C., & Lurie, N. (2003). Health literacy: A policy challenge for advancing high-quality health care. *Health Affairs, 22*(4), 147. Retrieved from ABI/INFORM Global database (Document ID: 376436551).

Piette, J. (2007). Interactive behavior change technology to support diabetes self-management: Where do we stand? *Diabetes Care, 30*(10), 2425–2432. Retrieved from Health Module database (Document ID: 1360494771).

Sternberg, D. (2002). Building on your quick wins. *Marketing Health Services, 22*(3), 41–43. Retrieved from ABI/INFORM Global database (Document ID: 155769441).

U.S. National Library of Medicine. (2016). MedlinePlus: Health information in multiple languages. Retrieved from https://www.nlm.nih.gov/medlineplus/languages/languages.html

Watson, A., Bell, A., Kvedar, J., & Grant, R. (2008). Reevaluating the digital divide: Current lack of Internet use is not a barrier to adoption of novel health information technology. *Diabetes Care, 31*(3), 433–435. Retrieved from Health Module.

1. Provide an overview of community and population health informatics.

2. Assess informatics tools for promoting community and population health.

3. Explore the roles of federal, state, and local public health agencies in the development of public health informatics.

## Key Terms

- » Agency for Toxic Substances and Disease Registry (ATSDR)
- » Behavioral Risk Factor Surveillance System
- » Bioterrorism
- » Centers for Disease Control and Prevention (CDC)
- » Community risk assessment (CRA)

- » Crowdsourcing
- » Epidemiology
- » National Center for Public Health Informatics (NCPHI)
- » National health information network
- » National Health and Nutrition Examination Survey

- » Public health
- » Public health informatics
- » Public health interventions
- » Quality, research, and public health (QRPH)
- » Regional health information exchanges
- » Risk assessment

- » Social media
- » Suicide Prevention Community Assessment Tool
- » Surveillance
- » Surveillance data systems
- » Syndromic surveillance
- » Youth Risk Behavior Surveillance System

# CHAPTER 17

# Using Informatics to Promote Community/Population Health

Dee McGonigle, Kathleen Mastrian, Margaret Ross Kraft, and Ida Androwich

## Introduction

In late fall of 2002, severe acute respiratory syndrome (SARS) appeared in China. By March 2003, SARS had become recognized as a global threat. According to World Health Organization (WHO) data, more than 8,000 people from 29 countries became infected with this previously unknown virus and more than 700 people died. By 2004, the last SARS cases were caused by laboratory-acquired infections. Because of computerized global data collection, the potentially negative impact of a widespread global epidemic was averted.

Additionally, Renwick (2016) reported that

> [b]y the end of 2015, more than 28,600 people had been infected [with Ebola], killing more than 11,300. That figure was much lower than projections the CDC made a year before, which calculated that as many as 1.4 million people could become infected with Ebola by January 2015. Instead, the disease peaked in late 2014: in Liberia in September, Guinea in October, and Sierra Leone in November. By January 2016, Guinea, Liberia, and Sierra Leone had been declared free of Ebola. (para. 16)

As we lived through the Ebola outbreak, we realized the need for timely information to be shared with the world population, as well as the healthcare workers responsible for caring for them. WHO (2015) stated that "leading international stakeholders from multiple sectors convened at a WHO consultation in September 2015, where they affirmed that timely and transparent pre-publication sharing of data and results during public health emergencies must become the global norm" (para. 1).

More recently, the Zika virus has become a leading public health concern. The Centers for Disease Control and Prevention (CDC; 2016b) reported that their Emergency Operations Center (EOC)

> was activated for Zika on January 22, 2016, and moved to a level 1 activation—the highest level—on February 8, 2016. The EOC is the command center for monitoring and coordinating the emergency response to Zika, bringing together CDC scientists with expertise in arboviruses like Zika, reproductive health, birth defects, and developmental disabilities, and travel health. (para. 1)

The CDC's EOC staff works in collaboration with local, national, and international response partners to analyze, validate, and efficiently exchange information about the outbreak. The CDC (2015) public health surveillance center "refers to the collection, analysis and use of data to target public health prevention. It is the foundation of public health practice" (para. 1). The CDC provides interactive databases and surveys, as well as methods to guide conducting and evaluating surveillance systems and data standardization.

Many **surveillance** systems, loosely termed "syndromic surveillance systems," use data that are not diagnostic of a disease but that might indicate the early stages of an outbreak (see **Figure 17-1**). Outbreak detection is the overriding purpose of **syndromic surveillance** for terrorism preparedness. Enhanced case finding and monitoring the

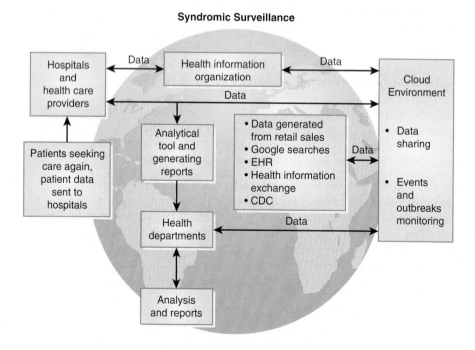

**Figure 17-1** Syndromic Surveillance System

course and population characteristics of a recognized outbreak also are potential benefits of syndromic surveillance. In recent years, new data have been used by public health officials to enhance surveillance, such as patients' chief complaints in emergency departments, ambulance log sheets, prescriptions filled, retail drug and product purchases, school or work absenteeism, and medical signs and symptoms in persons seen in various clinical settings. With faster, more specific, and more affordable diagnostic methods and decision-support tools, timely recognition of reportable diseases with the potential to lead to a substantial outbreak is now possible. Tools for pattern recognition can be used to screen data for patterns needing further public health investigation. For example, during the 2003 SARS epidemic, the **Centers for Disease Control and Prevention (CDC)** worked to develop surveillance criteria to identify persons with SARS in the United States, and the surveillance case definition changed throughout the epidemic, to reflect increased understanding of SARS (CDC, 2013).

Information acquired by the collection and processing of population health data becomes the basis for knowledge in the field of **public health**. There is an ever-increasing need for timely information about the health of communities, states, and countries. Knowledge about disease trends and other threats to community health can improve program planning, decision making, and care delivery. Patients seen from the perspective of major health threats within their communities can benefit from opportunities for early intervention.

This chapter focuses on the application of informatics methods to public health surveillance. The availability of clinical information for public health has been fundamentally changed by the introduction of the electronic health record (EHR) and health information technology (IT), which now give public health "an unprecedented opportunity to leverage the information, technologies and standards to support critical public health functions such as alerting and surveillance" (Garrett, 2010).

## Core Public Health Functions

The core public health functions are as follows:

- The assessment and monitoring of the health of communities and populations at risk to identify health problems and priorities
- The formulation of public policies designed to solve identified local and national health problems and priorities
- To assure that all populations have access to appropriate and cost-effective care, including health promotion and disease prevention services, and evaluation of the effectiveness of that care (Medterms Medical Dictionary, 2007)

Public health focuses on health promotion and disease prevention. According to the CDC Foundation (2016), public health is the

*science of protecting and improving the health of families and communities through promotion of healthy lifestyles, research for disease and injury prevention and detection and control of infectious diseases. Overall, public health is concerned with protecting the health of entire populations. These populations can be as small as a local neighborhood, or as big as an entire country or region of the world. (para. 1–2)*

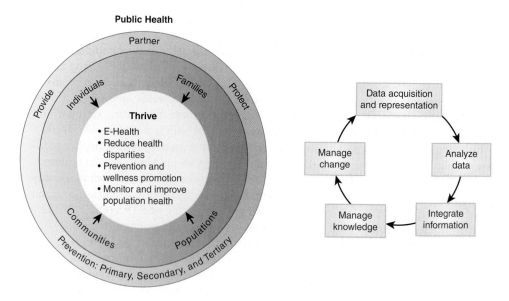

**Figure 17-2** Public Health Informatics

Historically, Dr. John Snow can be designated as the "father" of **public health informatics** (PHI) (**Figure 17-2**). In 1854, he plotted information about cholera deaths and was able to determine that the deaths were clustered around the same water pump in London. He convinced authorities that the cholera deaths were associated with that water pump; when the pump handle was removed, the cholera outbreak ended. It was Dr. Snow's focus on the cholera-affected population as a whole rather than on a single patient that led to his discovery of the source of the cholera outbreak (Vachon, 2005).

Florence Nightingale should also be recognized as an early public health informaticist. Her recommendations about medical reform and the need for improved sanitary conditions were based on data about morbidity and mortality that she compiled from her experiences in the Crimea and England. Her efforts led to a total reorganization of how and which healthcare statistics were collected (Dossey, 2000).

Just as information has been recognized as an asset in the business world, so health care is now recognized as an information-intensive field requiring timely, accurate information from many different sources. Health information systems address the collection, storage, analysis, interpretation, and communication of health data and information. Many health disciplines, such as medicine and nursing, have developed their own concepts of informatics. That trend has reached the field of public and community health. PHI represents "the effective use of information and information technology to improve public health practice and outcomes" (Public Health Informatics Institute, 2015, para. 18). This area of informatics differs from others because it is focused on the promotion of health and disease prevention in populations and communities. PHI efficiently and effectively organizes and manages data, information, and knowledge generated and used by public health professionals to fulfill the core functions of public health: assessment, policy, and assurance (Agency for Toxic Substances and Disease Registry [ATSDR], 2016). Public health changes the social conditions and systems that affect everyone within a given community. It is because of public health initiatives that people understand the importance of clean water, the dangers of second-hand smoke, and the fact that seat belts really do save lives. PHI emphasizes community-based solutions and promotes community empowerment by advancing the state of the art in community benefit projects (Public Health Institute, 2016a). One of the community-based projects—Building Healthy Communities: Hospital Community Benefit Engagement—applies "findings and lessons learned from the collection and analysis of community benefit programming data in the 14 building healthy community sites to create deeper collaboration and partnership-building" (Public Health Institute, 2016b, para. 1). Community empowerment can be realized through the collaborative collection and analysis of data that lead to improved community health outcomes and transformed public health.

The scope of PHI practice includes knowledge from a variety of additional disciplines, including management, organization theory, psychology, political science, and law, as well as fields related to public health, such as **epidemiology**, microbiology, toxicology, and statistics (O'Carroll, Yasnoff, Ward, Ripp, & Martin, 2003, p. 5). PHI addresses the data, information, and knowledge that public health professionals generate and use to meet the core functions of public health. Yasnoff and colleagues (2000) defined four principles that continue to define and guide the activities of PHI: (1) applications promote the health of populations, (2) applications focus on disease and injury prevention, (3) applications explore prevention at "all vulnerable points in the causal changes," and (4) PHI reflects the "governmental context in which public health is practiced" (p. 69).

Functions of public health include prevention of epidemics and the spread of disease, protection against environmental hazards, promotion of health, disaster response and recovery, and providing access to health care.

The initiative of integrating the healthcare enterprise to ensure that healthcare information can be shared more easily and used more effectively has inspired the creation of the domain known as **quality, research, and public health (QRPH)**. Participants in this domain address the repurposing of clinical, demographic, and financial data collected in the process of providing clinical care to the monitoring of disease patterns; incidence, prevalence, and situational awareness of such patterns; and the identification of new patterns of disease not previously known or anticipated. Such data can be incorporated within existing public health population analyses and programs for direct outreach and condition management through registries and locally determined appropriate treatment programs or protocols.

# Community Health Risk Assessment: Tools for Acquiring Knowledge

As the public has become more aware of harmful elements in the environment, **risk assessment** tools have been developed. Such tools allow assessment of pesticide use, exposure to harmful chemicals, contaminants in food and water, and toxic pollutants in the air to determine if potential hazards need to be addressed. A risk assessment may also be called a "threat and risk assessment." A "threat" is a harmful act, such as the deployment of a virus or illegal network penetration. A "risk" is the expectation that a threat may succeed and the potential damage that can occur (PCMag.com Encyclopedia, 2007). "Risk factor assessments complement vital statistics data systems and morbidity data systems by providing information on factors earlier in the causal chain leading to illness, injury or death" (O'Carroll, Powell-Griner, Holtzman & Williamson, 2003, p. 316).

The U.S. Environmental Protection Agency (EPA; 2016) "uses risk assessments to characterize the nature and magnitude of health risks to humans (e.g., residents, workers, recreational visitors) and ecological receptors (e.g., birds, fish, wildlife) from chemical contaminants and other stressors, that may be present in the environment" (para. 3) and are used to weigh the benefits and costs of various program alternatives for reducing exposure to potential hazards. They may also influence public policy and regulatory decisions. Health risk assessment is a constantly developing process based in sound science and professional judgments. There are usually four basic steps ascribed to risk assessment (see also Figure 17-3):

1. *Hazard identification* seeks to determine the types of health problems that could be caused by exposure to a potentially hazardous material. All research studies related to the potentially hazardous material are reviewed to identify potential health problems.
2. *Exposure assessment* is done to determine the length, amount, and pattern of exposure to the potentially hazardous material.
3. *Dose–response assessment* is an estimation of how much exposure to the potential hazard would cause varying degrees of health effects.
4. *Risk characterization* is an assessment of the risk of the hazardous material causing illness in the population (California Environmental Protection Agency, 1998).

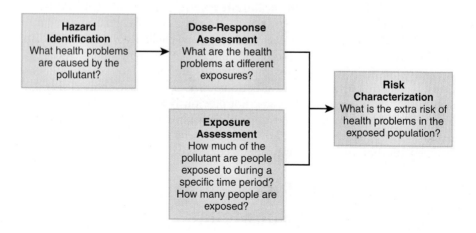

**Figure 17-3**  Four-Step Risk Assessment Process
Modified from U.S. Environmental Protection Agency. (2016). Conducting a human health risk assessment. Retrieved from https://www.epa.gov/risk/conducting-human-health-risk-assessment

The overall question the risk assessment has to answer is, "How much risk is acceptable?" Risk factor systems are used throughout the United States and may be local, regional, or national in scope. Specific risk assessment tools exist for specific health issues, such as the **Suicide Prevention Community Assessment Tool**, which addresses general community information, prevention networks, and the demographics of the target population and community assets and risk factors. Other risk assessment tools include the **Youth Risk Behavior Surveillance System**, the **Behavioral Risk Factor Surveillance System**, and the **National Health and Nutrition Examination Survey**.

Determining the presence of risk factors in a community is a key part of a **community risk assessment (CRA)**. Communities may be concerned about which elements in the environment affect or may affect the community's health, the level of environmental risk, and other factors that should be included in public health planning. Ball (2003) defined value as "a function of cost, service, and outcome" (p. 41). The value of a CRA derives from its ability to provide information crucial to planning, build consensus regarding how to mobilize community resources, and allow for comparison of risks with those of other communities. The goal of a CRA is risk reduction and improved health. A CRA may identify unmet needs and opportunities for action that may help set new priorities for local public health units. It may also be used to monitor the impact of prevention programs.

## Processing Knowledge and Information to Support Epidemiology and Monitoring Disease Outbreaks

There is a need to define the role of federal, state, and local public health agencies in the development of PHI and IT applications. The availability of IT today challenges all stakeholders in the health of the public to adopt new systems that can provide adequate disease surveillance; it also challenges people to improve outmoded processes.

Preparedness in public health requires more timely detection of potential health threats, situational awareness, surveillance, outbreak management, countermeasures, response, and communications. Surveillance uses health-related data that signal a sufficient probability of a case or an outbreak that warrants further public health response. Although historically syndromic surveillance has been used to target investigations of potential infectious cases, its use to detect possible outbreaks associated with **bioterrorism** is increasingly being explored by public health officials (CDC, 2013, 2014). Early detection of possible outbreaks can be achieved through timely and complete receipt, review, and investigation of disease case reports; by improving the ability to recognize patterns in data that may be indicative of a possible outbreak early in its course; and through receipt of new types of data that can signify an outbreak earlier in its course. Such new types of data might include identification of absences from work or school; increased purchases of healthcare products, including specific types of over-the-counter medications; presenting symptoms to healthcare providers; and laboratory test orders (CDC, 2012, 2013). The University of Pittsburgh's Real-time Outbreak and Disease Surveillance Laboratory (RODS), for example, developed the National Retail Data Monitor (NRDM) system. The NRDM collects data on over-the-counter medications and other healthcare products from 28,000 stores and uses computer algorithms to detect unusual purchase patterns that might potentially signal a disease outbreak (RODS Laboratory, 2013). A comprehensive surveillance effort supports timely investigation and identifies data needs for managing the public health response to an outbreak or terrorist event. Informatics tools are becoming increasingly important in these public health efforts.

To appropriately process public health data, PHI has a need for a standardized vocabulary and coding structure. This is especially important as national public health data are collected and data mining performed so that data variables can be understood across systems and between agencies. Health information organizations (HIOs) have been established to support data sharing via health information exchanges (HIE) promoted by the meaningful use criteria of the EHR. Central to these initiatives is the need for standardized codes and terminologies that may be used by the HIOs to map data from disparate sources (Hyde et al., 2013; Shapiro, Mostashari, Hripcsak, Soulakis, & Kuperman, 2011).

In the early 1990s, the CDC launched a plan for an integrated surveillance system that moved from stand-alone systems to networked data exchange built with specific standards. Early initiatives were the National Electronic Telecommunications System for Surveillance and the Wide-ranging Online Data for Epidemiologic Research. Six current initiatives reflect this early vision:

1. PulseNet USA: A surveillance network for food-borne infections.
2. National Electronic Disease Surveillance System: Facilitates reporting on approximately 100 diseases, with data feeding directly from clinical laboratories, which allows for early detection.
3. Epidemic Information Exchange: A secure communication system for practitioners to access and share preliminary health surveillance information.
4. Health Alert Network: A state and nationwide alert system.
5. Biosense: Provides improved real-time biosurveillance and situational awareness in support of early detection.
6. Public Health Information Network: Promotes standards and software solutions for the rapid flow of public health information.

Certainly, the events of September 11, 2001, which indicated the need for the United States to increase its efforts directed toward prevention of terrorism, accelerated the need for informatics in public health practice. Today, response requirements include fast detection, science, communication, integration, and action (Kukafka, 2006). In 2005, the CDC created the **National Center for Public Health Informatics (NCPHI)** to provide leadership in the field. This center aims to protect and improve health through PHI (CDC, 2005; McNabb, Koo, Pinner, & Seligman, 2006). The CDC (2016a) "provides leadership and crosscutting support in developing public health information systems, managing public health surveillance programs and providing health-related data required to monitor, control, and prevent the occurrence and spread of diseases and other adverse health conditions" (para. 1).

Information is vital to public health programming. The data processed into public health information can be obtained from administrative, financial, and facility sources. Included in this data stream may be encounter, screening, registry, clinical, and laboratory and surveillance data. It has been recommended that the functions of population health beyond surveillance be integrated into the EHR and the personal health record. Such an initiative might allow for population-level alerts to be sent to clinicians through these electronic record systems. Systems now being developed allow for automated syndromic surveillance of emergency department records and media surveillance, which in turn supports early detection of potential pandemic occurrences. Such systems were tested during the 2009 H1N1 flu, 2014 Ebola, and 2015 Zika outbreaks. The public health–enhanced electronic medical record can provide immediate detection and reporting of notifiable conditions. The incorporation of geographic information systems allows public health data to be mapped to specific locations that may indicate an immediate need for intervention (CDC, 2016a; Grannis & Vreeman, 2010).

Vital statistics from state and local governments are also used for public health purposes. It should be noted that databases created with public funds are public databases that are available for authorized public representatives for public purposes (CDC, 2016a; Freedman & Weed, 2003).

The widespread implementation of EHRs is facilitating the concept of a public health–enabled record, which can automatically send patient information alerts from the point of care to public health departments when reportable symptoms, conditions, or diseases are encountered. A public health–enabled EHR can be bidirectional, allowing public health information and recommendations for treatment to be accessible at the point of care. One public health EHR prototype addresses the information flow related to newborn screenings (HealthIT.gov, 2013a; Orlova et al., 2005).

Potential applications of HIE to public health have been described by HealthIT.gov (2013b) and Shapiro et al. (2011). They include syndromic surveillance using data generated from mandated and nonmandated laboratory results, physician diagnoses, and emergency or clinic chief complaints; strategies to locate loved ones in mass-casualty events; and public health alerts at the individual and population levels.

## Applying Knowledge to Health Disaster Planning and Preparation

The availability of data and the speed of data exchange can have a significant impact on critical public health functions such as disease monitoring and syndromic surveillance. Currently, surveillance data are limited and historical in nature, although this situation is rapidly changing. Nevertheless, special data collections are needed to address specific public health issues, and investigations and emergencies are still frequently addressed and managed with paper. In the future, PHI will make real-time surveillance data available electronically, and investigations and emergences will be managed with the tools of informatics (Yasnoff et al., 2004). **Surveillance data systems** such as infectious disease trackers that collect data on adverse health effects are invaluable tools for public health officials to tap for planning, evaluation, or implementation of **public health interventions**. The **Agency for Toxic Substances and Disease Registry (ATSDR)**, for example, is a federal agency that acts as a repository for research and data regarding hazardous materials. It "serves the public by using the best science, taking responsive public health actions, and providing trusted health information to prevent harmful exposures and diseases related to toxic substances" (ATSDR, 2016, para. 1). "Syndromic surveillance for early outbreak detection is an investigational approach where health department staff, assisted by automated data acquisition and generation of statistical signals, monitor disease indicators continually (real-time) or at least daily (near realtime) to detect outbreaks of diseases earlier and more completely than might otherwise be possible with traditional public health methods" (Buehler, Hopkins, Overhage, Sosin, & Tong, 2004, para. 7). Traditionally, there has been no common infrastructure to respond to pandemics, but the development of health IT is creating opportunities that go far beyond national boundaries to impact global public health initiatives. In this vein, the U.S. Department of Homeland Security (2015) has a national strategy for pandemic flu that is designed to meet three critical goals:

1. Detecting human or animal outbreaks that occur anywhere in the world
2. Protecting the American people by stockpiling vaccines and antiviral drugs while improving the capacity to produce new vaccines
3. Preparing to respond at the federal, state, and local levels in the event an avian or pandemic influenza reaches the United States (para. 1)

In New York City, a primary care information project funded by the CDC developed a multifaceted initiative, the Center for Excellence in Public Health Informatics, to address issues of measurement of meaningful use, disease and outbreak surveillance, and decision support alerts at the point of care (Buck, Wu, Souliakis, & Kukalka, 2010; Hripcsak, 2015).

## Informatics Tools to Support Communication and Dissemination

The revolution in IT has made the capture and analysis of health data and the distribution of healthcare information more achievable and less costly. Since the early 1960s, the CDC has used IT in its practice; PHI emerged as a specialty in the 1990s. PHI has become more important with improvements in IT; changes in the care delivery system; and the challenges related to emerging infections, resistance to antibiotics, and the threat of chemical and biologic terrorism. Two-way communication between public health agencies, community, and clinical laboratories can identify clusters of reportable and unusual diseases. In turn, health departments can consult on case diagnosis and management, alerts, surveillance summaries, and clinical and public health recommendations. Ongoing healthcare provider outreach, education, and 24-hour access to public health professionals may lead to the discovery of urgent health threats. The automated transfer of specified data from a laboratory database to a public health data repository improves the timeliness and completeness of reporting notifiable conditions.

Public health information systems represent a partnership of federal, state, and local public health professionals. Such systems facilitate the capture of large amounts of data, rapid exchange of information, and strengthened links among these three system levels. Dissemination of prevention guidelines and communication among public health officials, clinicians, and patients has emerged as a major benefit of PHI. IT solutions can be used to provide accurate and timely information that guides public health actions. In addition, the Internet has become a universal communications pathway and allows individuals and population groups to be more involved and take greater responsibility for management of their own health status.

Few public health professionals have received formal informatics training, and many may not be aware of the potential impact of IT on their practice. A working group formed at the University of Washington Center for PHI has published a draft of PHI competencies needed (Karras, 2007). These competencies include the following:

- Supporting development of strategic direction for PHI within the enterprise
- Participating in development of knowledge management tools for the enterprise
- Using standards
- Ensuring that the knowledge, information, and data needs of project or program users and stakeholders are met
- Managing information system development, procurement, and implementation
- Managing IT operations related to a project or program (for public health agencies with internal IT operations)
- Monitoring IT operations managed by external organizations
- Communicating with cross-disciplinary leaders and team members
- Participating in applied public health informatics research
- Developing public health information systems that are interoperable with other relevant information systems
- Supporting use of informatics to integrate clinical health, environmental risk, and population health
- Implementing solutions that ensure confidentiality, security, and integrity, while maximizing availability of information for public health
- Conducting education and training in PHI (Center for Public Health Informatics, 2007)

## Using Feedback to Improve Responses and Promote Readiness

Improvement of community health status and population health depends on effective public and healthcare infrastructures. In addition to information from public health agencies, there is now interest in the capture of information from hospitals, pharmacies, poison control centers, laboratories, and environmental agencies. Timely collection of such data allows early detection and analysis, which can increase the rapidity of response with more effective interventions. Yasnoff et al. (2000) identified the "grand challenges" still facing PHI as the development of national public health information systems, a closer integration of clinical care with public health, and concerns of confidentiality and privacy. Since then, great strides have been made towards a national public health information system, but we currently are still striving to make this a true reality. At present, there is a 10-year vision to achieve an interoperable health IT infrastructure in the United States (Office of the National Coordinator for Health Information Technology, 2014).

Population health data must be considered an important part of the infrastructure of all **regional health information exchanges,** which are the building blocks for a **national health information network.** Organizations and agencies interested in promoting and protecting the public's health must commit to collaboration and seamless data sharing (Office of the National Coordinator for Health Information Technology, 2014). Public health data include data related to surveillance, environmental health, and preparedness systems as well as client information, such as data from immunization registries and laboratory results reporting and analysis. These types of data can provide information about outbreaks, patterns of drug-resistant organisms, and other trends that can help improve the accuracy of diagnostic and treatment decisions and advance public health research (LaVenture, 2005; National Institutes of Health, 2016). A regional health information exchange and national health information network can also support public health goals through broader opportunities for participation in surveillance and prevention activities, improved case management and care coordination, and increased accuracy and timeliness of information for disease reporting (LaVenture).

Much of the information is focused on reaction to issues and timely intervention, rather than harnessing information technology for disease prevention. Fuller (2011) advocated for a shift to prevention informatics by harnessing real-time social data and aggregating and representing these data in a meaningful way so that an appropriate prevention response can be mounted. For example, Internet searches related to flu symptoms might prompt a public health prevention response such as a school closure to minimize spread. Newer software tools to support mapping and real-time data visualization include Riff and Ushahidi, each of which supports "gathering of distributed data from the web and other data streams" (Fuller, p. 40). "Prevention informatics offers a useful paradigm for re-imagining health information systems and for harnessing the vast array of data, tools, technologies and systems to respond proactively to health challenges across the globe" (Fuller, p. 41).

Harnessing data from **social media** such as Twitter and Facebook provides yet another example of using citizen-generated information (**crowdsourcing**) in community health. Merchant and colleagues (2011) described how mining data generated in social media can improve response to mass disasters by helping responders locate people who need help and identify areas where to send resources, build social capital, and promote community resilience postdisaster. "Tweets and photographs linked to timelines and interactive maps can tell a cohesive story about a recovering community's capabilities and vulnerabilities in real time" (Merchant et al., p. 291). These authors caution, however, that social media should be used to augment— not replace—current disaster response and communication systems, as not all communications in social media are entirely trustworthy. In addition to utilizing social media posts, Benforado's (2015) presentation to the EPA on Citizen Science and Crowdsourcing asked the question, "If you had 100,000 people to help you with your work, what would you do?" (slide 2). Enlisting and empowering people can promote volunteerism and advance science. There is power in investing in citizen science approaches and harnessing the efforts of volunteers.

Table 17-1 Important PHI Sites

| Name | Address | Website |
|------|---------|---------|
| American Public Health Association | APHA, 800 I Street, NW Washington, DC 20001 | www.apha.org |
| Center for Public Health Informatics | CPHI, University of Washington, 1100 NE 45th Street, Ste 405, Seattle, WA 98105 | www.washington.edu/research/centers/256 |
| Centers for Disease Control and Prevention | CDC, 1600 Clifton Road, Atlanta, GA 30333 | www.cdc.gov |
| National Center for Public Health Informatics | NCPHI, 1600 Clifton Road, NE Mailstop E-78, Atlanta, GA 30333 | https://web.archive.org/web/20110123075557/http://www.cdc.gov/ncphi |
| Public Health Data Standards Consortium | c/o Johns Hopkins Bloomberg School of Public Health, 624 N Broadway, Room 325, Baltimore, MD 21205 | www.phdsc.org |
| Public Health Institute | PHI, 555 12th Street, 10th Floor, Oakland, CA 94607 | www.phi.org |

# Summary

Public health informatics strives to ensure that evolving health data systems will meet the data needs of all organizations interested in population health as national and international standards are developed for healthcare data collection. This includes standardization of environmental, sociocultural, economic, and other data that are relevant to public health. Table 17-1 provides the names, addresses, and URLs for important organizations dedicated to public health data and informatics. Table 17-2 lists abbreviations commonly used in PHI.

The future of practice in public health depends on how efficiently and effectively public health data are captured, analyzed, and disseminated for regional, national, and global health planning and management. In an ideal world, we would see seamless data collection and sharing with a commitment to prevention and global health planning.

## THOUGHT-PROVOKING QUESTIONS

1. Imagine that you are a public health informatics specialist and that you and your colleagues are concerned about a new strain of influenza. Which public health data are used to determine the need for a mass inoculation? Which data will be collected to determine the success of such a program?
2. What are the advantages and disadvantages of using crowdsourced social media data during a disaster response?

Table 17-2  Abbreviations Used in PHI

| BRFSS | Behavioral Risk Factor Surveillance System |
| --- | --- |
| CDC | Centers for Disease Control and Prevention |
| CEPA | California Environmental Protection Agency |
| CPHI | Center for Public Health Informatics |
| CRA | Community Risk Assessment |
| EPI-X | Epidemic Information Exchange |
| HAN | Health Alert Network |
| IOM | Institute of Medicine |
| IT | Information Technology |
| NCPHI | National Center for Public Health Informatics |
| NEDSS | National Electronic Disease Surveillance System |
| NETSS | National Electronic Technology System for Surveillance |
| NHANES | National Health and Nutrition Examination Survey |
| NHIN | National Health Information Network |
| PH | Public Health |
| PHDSC | Public Health Data Standards Consortium |
| PHI | Public Health Informatics |
| PHIN | Public Health Information Network |
| PHRAP | Pennsylvania's Health Risk Assessment Process |
| QRPH | Quality, Research, Public Health |
| RHIO | Regional Health Information Exchanges |
| SPRC | Suicide Prevention Community Assessment Tool |
| WONDER | Wide-ranging Online Data for Epidemiologic Research |
| YRBSS | Youth Risk Behavior Surveillance System |

# References

Agency for Toxic Substances and Disease Registry (ATSDR). (2016). Homepage. Retrieved from http://www.atsdr.cdc.gov

Ball, M. (2003). Better health through informatics: Managing information to deliver value. In P. O'Carroll, W. L. Yasnoff, M. E. Ward, L. Ripp, & E. Martin (Eds.), *Public health informatics and information systems* (pp. 39–51). New York, NY: Springer-Verlag.

Benforado, J. (2015). Citizen science & crowdsourcing presentation to EPA Tribal Science Council. Retrieved from https://www.epa.gov/sites/production/files/2016-02/documents/citizen-science-crowdsourcing.pdf

Buck, M., Wu, W., Souliakis, N., & Kukalka, R. (2010). *Achieving excellence in public health informatics: The New York City experience*. Washington, DC: AMIA.

Buehler, J. W., Hopkins, R. S., Overhage, J. M., Sosin, D. M., & Tong, V. (2004). Framework for evaluating public health surveillance systems for early detection of outbreaks. *Morbidity and Mortality Weekly Report, 53*, 1–11. Retrieved from http://www.cdc.gov/mmwr/preview/mmwrhtml/rr5305a1.htm

California Environmental Protection Agency (CEPA). (1998). A guide to health risk assessment. Retrieved from http://www.oehha.ca.gov

CDC Foundation. (2016). What is public health? Retrieved from http://www.cdcfoundation.org/content/what-public-health

Center for Public Health Informatics (CPHI). (2007). *Draft competencies V7 for the public health informatician*. Seattle, WA: University of Washington.

Centers for Disease Control and Prevention. (2005). *National Center for Public Health Informatics (CPE)*. Retrieved from http://www.cdc.gov/maso/pdf/ncphifs.pdf

Centers for Disease Control and Prevention (CDC). (2012). Lesson 6: Investigating an outbreak. *Principles of epidemiology in public health practice, third edition: An introduction to applied epidemiology and biostatistics*. Retrieved from http://www.cdc.gov/ophss/csels/dsepd/ss1978/lesson6/section2.html

Centers for Disease Control and Prevention (CDC). (2013). Severe acute respiratory syndrome (SARS). Retrieved from https://www.cdc.gov/sars/index.html

Centers for Disease Control and Prevention (CDC). (2014). Emergency preparedness and response: The history of bioterrorism. Retrieved from https://emergency.cdc.gov/training/historyofbt

Centers for Disease Control and Prevention (CDC). (2015). Surveillance resource center. Retrieved from http://www.cdc.gov/surveillancepractice/index.html

Centers for Disease Control and Prevention (CDC). (2016a). Division of Health Informatics and Surveillance (DHIS). Retrieved from http://www.cdc.gov/ophss/csels/dhis

Centers for Disease Control and Prevention (CDC). (2016b). Zika virus home: What CDC is doing. Retrieved from http://www.cdc.gov/zika/cdc-role.html

Dossey, B. M. (2000). *Florence Nightingale: Mystic, visionary, healer*. Springhouse, PA: Springhouse.

Freedman, M. A., & Weed, J. A. (2003). National vital statistics system. In P. O'Carroll, W. Yasnoff, M. Ward, L. Ripp, & E. Martin (Eds.), *Public health informatics and information systems* (pp. 269–285). New York, NY: Springer-Verlag.

Fuller, S. (2011). From intervention informatics to prevention informatics. *Bulletin of the American Society for Information Science & Technology, 38*(8), 36–41.

Garrett, N. (2010). Leveraging the EHR for public health alerting. CDC Clinician Outreach & Communication Activity (COCA) conference call, June 22, 2010.

Grannis, S., & Vreeman, D. (2010). *A vision of the journey ahead: Using public health notifiable condition mapping to illustrate the need to maintain value sets.* Washington, DC: AMIA.

HealthIT.gov. (2013a). How can electronic health records improve public and population health outcomes? Retrieved from https://www.healthit.gov/providers-professionals/faqs/how-can-electronic-health-records-improve-public-and-population-health-

HealthIT.gov. (2013b). Why is health information exchange important? Retrieved from https://www.healthit.gov/providers-professionals/faqs/why-health-information-exchange-important

Hripcsak, G. (2015). NYC Center of Excellence for Public Health Informatics, #5P01HK000029-03. Retrieved from http://grantome.com/grant/NIH/P01-HK000029-03

Hyde, L., Rihanek, T., Santana-Johnson, T., Scichilone, R., Simmons, C., Turner, J. B., & Zumar, W. (2013). Data mapping and its impact on data integrity. *American Health Information Management Association.* Retrieved from http://library.ahima.org/PdfView?oid=107154

Karras, B. (2007). *Competencies for the public health informatician.* Seattle, WA: University of Washington.

Kukafka, R. (2006). *Public health informatics.* Woods Hole, MA: Medical Informatics Course for Health Professionals.

LaVenture, M. (2005, May). *Role of population/public health in regional health information exchanges.* PHDSC/eHealth Initiative Annual Conference, Washington, DC.

McNabb, S., Koo, D., Pinner, R., & Seligman, J. (2006). Informatics and public health at CDC. *Morbidity and Mortality Weekly Report, 55,* 25–28. Retrieved from http://www.cdc.gov/mmwr/preview/mmwrhtml/su5502a10.htm

Medterms Medical Dictionary. (2007). Public health. Retrieved from http://www.medterms.com

Merchant, R., Elmer, S., & Lurie, N. (2011). Integrating social media into emergency-preparedness efforts. *New England Journal of Medicine, 365*(4), 289–291. doi:10.1056/NEJMp1103591

National Institutes of Health. (2016). Health data resources: Common data types in public health research. Retrieved from http://nihlibrary.campusguides.com/c.php?g=38336&p=244539

O'Carroll, P. L., Powell-Griner, E., Holtzman, D., & Williamson, G. D. (2003). Risk factor information systems. In P. O'Carroll, W. Yasnoff, M. Ward, L. Ripp, & E. Martin (Eds.), *Public health informatics and information systems* (pp. 316–334). New York, NY: Springer-Verlag.

O'Carroll, P., Yasnoff, W., Ward, M., Ripp, L., & Martin, E. (Eds.). (2003). *Public health informatics and information systems.* New York, NY: Springer-Verlag.

Office of the National Coordinator for Health Information Technology. (2014). Connecting health and care for the nation: A 10-year vision to achieve an interoperable health IT infrastructure. Retrieved from https://www.healthit.gov/sites/default/files/ONC10year InteroperabilityConceptPaper.pdf

Orlova, A., Dunnagan, M., Finitzo, T., Higgins, M., Watkings, T., Tien, A., & Beales, S. (2005). *An electronic health record–public health (EHR-PH) system prototype for interoperability in 21st century healthcare systems* (pp. 575–579). AMIA, Annual Symposium Proceedings.

PCMag.com Encyclopedia. (2007). Risk. Retrieved from http://www.pcmag.com/encyclopedia/term/50554/risk

Public Health Informatics Institute. (2015). Public health informatics defined. Retrieved from http://www.phii.org/phii-voices/PH-Info-Defined

Public Health Institute. (2016a). Healthy communities. Retrieved from http://www.phi.org/focus-areas/?focus_area=healthy-communities

Public Health Institute. (2016b). Advancing the state of the art in community benefit. Retrieved from http://www.phi.org/focus-areas/?focus_area=healthy-communities& program=advancing-the-state-of-the-art-in-community-benefit

Renwick, D. (2016). Council on Foreign Relations (CFR) backgrounders: Ebola virus. *Council on Foreign Relations*. Retrieved from http://www.cfr.org/africa-sub-saharan/ebola-virus /p33661

RODS Laboratory. (2013). About the National Retail Data Monitor. Retrieved from http:// www .rods.pitt.edu/site/content/blogsection/4/42

Shapiro, J. S., Mostashari, F., Hripcsak, G., Soulakis, N., & Kuperman, G. (2011). Using health information exchange to improve public health. *American Journal of Public Health, 101*(4), 616–623. doi: 10.2105/AJPH.2008.158980

U.S. Department of Homeland Security (DHS). (2015). National strategy for pandemic flu. Retrieved from https://www.dhs.gov/national-strategy-pandemic-flu

U.S. Environmental Protection Agency (EPA). (2016). About risk assessment. Retrieved from https://www.epa.gov/risk/about-risk-assessment

Vachon, D. (2005). Dr John Snow blames water pollution for cholera epidemic. *Old News, 16*(8), 8–10. Retrieved from http://www.ph.ucla.edu/epi/snow/fatherofepidemiology.html

World Health Organization (WHO). (2015). Developing global norms for sharing data and results during public health emergencies. Retrieved from http://www.who.int/medicines /ebola-treatment/blueprint_phe_data-share-results/en

Yasnoff, W., Humphreys, B., Overhage, J., Detmer, D., Brennan, P., Morris, R., . . . Fanning, J. (2004). A consensus action agenda for achieving the national health information infrastructure. *Journal of the American Medical Informatics Association, 11*(4), 332–338.

Yasnoff, W., O'Carroll, P., Koo, D., Linkings, R., & Kilbourne, E. (2000). Public health informatics: Improving and transforming public health in the information age. *Journal of Public Health Management Practice, 6*(6), 67–75.

# CHAPTER 18

# Telenursing and Remote Access Telehealth

Original contribution by Audrey Kinsella, Kathleen Albright, Sheldon Prial, and Schuyler F. Hoss; revised by Kathleen Mastrian and Dee McGonigle

## Introduction

**Telehealth,** a relatively new term in the medical and nursing vocabulary, refers to a wide range of health services that are delivered by telecommunications-ready tools, such as the telephone, videophone, and computer. The most basic of telecommunications technology, the telephone, has been used by health professionals for many years, sometimes by nurses to counsel a patient or by doctors to change a patient's plan of care. Because of these widespread uses, people are already somewhat familiar with the value of the direct, expedient contact that telecommunications-ready tools provide for healthcare professionals. A 2013 press release by IMS Research reported that telehealth monitoring was used for 308,000 patients in the United States in 2012 and that the demand for services on a worldwide basis is expected to reach 1.8 million patients by 2017. Dorsey and Topol (2016) discussed the state of telehealth and shared that there were over 2 million Department of Veterans Affairs (VA) telehealth visits in 2014, that Kaiser Permanente of California predicted that they will have more virtual visits than face-to-face visits in 2016, and that the Mayo Clinic expects to serve over 200 million patients by 2020 using telehealth technologies globally. The growing field of telehealth is of particular importance to nursing in that there will be many future opportunities for nurses to contribute to care delivery via telehealth services. Let's examine a potential nursing contribution using the Foundation of Knowledge Model.

## The Foundation of Knowledge Model and Home Telehealth

There is much to learn about usual home telehealthcare service delivery, particularly to the elderly and chronically ill patients. Using the Foundation of Knowledge model is key to learning how to use telehealthcare tools with typical patients (elderly patients, patients needing pointed

**CASE STUDY: THE ROLE OF A HOME TELEHEALTH NURSE**

Mrs. A. is an 84-year-old woman who was recently discharged from the hospital with a diagnosis that includes an exacerbation of congestive heart failure (CHF). She also has diabetes and hypertension. Mrs. A. was discharged from the hospital on multiple medications and lives alone.

Home care services were initiated with skilled nursing care visits, some home health aide support, and orders to include daily telemonitoring of her vital signs. The telehealth device will remotely monitor Mrs. A.'s blood pressure, heart rate, oxygen saturation, and weight. In addition, the patient will answer customized questions about her disease on a daily basis. This information will then be transmitted daily to the home care agency, where the telenurse can determine appropriate clinical actions based on the data trends and preset baseline alerts that indicate when set parameters have been exceeded.

care) and operate effectively as telenurses. To understand the mechanics and effectiveness of home telehealth delivery within the Foundation of Knowledge model, one must begin with a typical home telehealth case through which one can explore the telenurse's role in this model.

## Knowledge Acquisition

As the case study illustrates, knowledge acquisition involves the telenurse receiving the information from the telehealth devices via a variety of communication modes. For example, the telenurse receives the patient's vital signs taken in the home and the patient's responses to customized questions. All of this information is transmitted to a remote server or site (a central station or website) that is easily accessible to the telenurse.

## Knowledge Processing

As a result of the telenurse's knowledge acquisition, the next step to be followed is knowledge processing (i.e., understanding a set of information and the ways it can be applied to a specific task). In the case study, the telenurse assesses the patient's vital signs along with subjective data received from the patient as a result of the customized questions that Mrs. A. is asked. For example, she might be asked if she feels more short of breath on a given day as compared to normal. The telenurse then combines this information with the overall patient history and diagnosis to get an up-to-date view of the patient's status and considers where this information fits into the clinical picture being presented for this patient.

As an example, the telenurse notes the following: Postacute heart failure patient shows trended data with weight gain of 5 lb over 2 days, elevated blood pressure, and decreased oxygen saturation, and answers yes to questions about increased shortness of breath and increased fatigue. After processing all of the current information, the telenurse is able to target the appropriate next steps involving knowledge generation and knowledge dissemination.

## Knowledge Generation

By using her own nursing skills and clinical knowledge of the disease process, the telenurse considers all of the data as they apply to Mrs. A. and decides the best course of action to take and acts on the data. The telenurse may, in addition, ask a variety of questions to ensure that a complete and accurate decision about next steps for the patient is made. These questions might include the following:

- Do I need to gather additional data?
- Do I need to call the patient?
- Do I need to call the physician and inquire about a change in the current plan of care?

### Knowledge Dissemination

Finally, the telenurse determines how the knowledge will be used and disseminated. Various questions that were posed in the knowledge generation stage are acted on, including the following possibilities:

- Calling the doctor
- Obtaining a change in medication order
- Calling the patient and instructing her in a medication change
- Reviewing activities that could have led to the changes (e.g., eating salty foods)
- Educating the patient on the disease process, symptom management, and self-management techniques
- Continuing to monitor the patient on an ongoing basis

As the case illustrates, the nurse used various technologies to acquire data; interpreted the meaning of the data, thus generating information and knowledge; and then used that knowledge and wisdom to intervene appropriately.

# Nursing Aspects of Telehealth

Understanding telehealth and the potential use of telehealth technology in nursing practice is necessary in today's changing healthcare arena. As this chapter describes, nurses using telehealth have much greater access to their patients' conditions and needs and are able to respond in a more timely way than is possible using only face-to-face visits. Patients' responses to new medications, for example, can be tracked within hours rather than the several days that elapse between face-to-face visits. The telecommunications-ready tools that can be used to achieve these results are described here, and cases that have demonstrated successful outcomes are highlighted.

Telehealth is still a new and evolving technology; while the offsite interventions or contacts often lead to less time being wasted on non-care-oriented tasks because of the efficiencies offered by the technology applications, its use must never be associated with less care. It is also important to note that nursing activity in telehealth still follows the same best practice standards as those espoused in conventional care. One should simply look at the use of telehealth tools as a means for nurses to do their work better.

As the case study demonstrated, a home healthcare nurse working with telehealth tools was able to detect and respond to a patient's condition more expediently than if the nurse relied solely on scheduled home visits, and thus was able to intervene to prevent a potentially serious deterioration in the patient's condition.

## History of Telehealth

In the early 1960s, President John F. Kennedy gave the National Aeronautics and Space Administration (NASA) the goal of landing an American on the moon. A surprise benefit of the space program was the demonstration of effective remote monitoring of the astronauts—and thus modern telehealth was born.

Although most of the advances in telehealth have taken place in the last 20 to 30 years, Craig and Patterson (2005) described much earlier examples, such as the use of bonfires to alert neighboring villages of the arrival of bubonic plague during the Middle Ages. Postal services and telegraphs were used to transmit health information in the mid-19th century, and 1910 marked the first transmission of stethoscope sounds over a telephone. Radio communications were used to provide medical support for crews on ships; the Seaman's Church Institute of New York (1920) and the International Radio Medical Center (1938) are two examples of organizations founded to provide health support at a distance. These services were later expanded to cover air travel (Craig & Patterson, 2005). The National Institutes of Mental Health supported a program in the mid-1950s that connected seven state hospitals in four different states via a closed-circuit telephone system (Venable, 2005). As technology evolved, its use in health care continued to grow. The first reported use of television to monitor patients in a clinical facility occurred in the 1950s, which then led to the development of interactive closed-circuit applications in the mid-1960s. These early applications of television to health care occurred within the facility but still had the benefit of extending the reach of the caregivers because they did not need to be in the same room to monitor their patients effectively (Prial & Hoss, 2009).

In the 1970s, uses of more advanced forms of telehealth in the medical field, referred to as **telemedicine**, included **teleradiology** and **telepathology**—radiologic and pathologic images transmitted to specialists who were located at some distance (Allan, 2006). As additional specialties, such as dermatology and ophthalmology, entered the telemedicine arena, telehealth use enabled even more physicians to access information about their patients, regardless of the distances between themselves and the patients, and in sites other than conventional healthcare settings.

Success in telehealth was achieved after decades spent refining the technology, which resulted in clearer imaging, more speedy transmissions, and accurate replication of data from remote locations to a central hub. The end results of telehealth interactions today have helped to ensure that professionals, whether working off site or directly with patients, can replicate the usual clinical interactions in all specialties regardless of the distance involved in the contact.

The ability to provide better healthcare access is the number one benefit of using telehealth. By reducing the need for face-to-face interaction with the patient, the nurse, physician, or even technician can be much more productive. When information is collected in the home, it becomes much more convenient for the patient, and the quality and timeliness of the information is improved dramatically. Home **telemonitoring** should be viewed as an enhancement to care, because it allows more direct, physical intervention to occur only when it is actually needed. Care is not directed by prescheduled appointment or subjective perceptions of condition, but instead can be determined by objective measures of physical status. With telehealth, care can also be delivered at the most appropriate site of care, reducing reliance on emergency departments and inpatient facilities (Prial & Hoss, 2009).

# Driving Forces for Telehealth

A significant increase is expected in the use of information technology tools in nursing venues in the coming decades. This use is affected by a number of factors in all of Western society. The following factors are drivers of the growing trend toward telehealth and technology use and will influence nursing practice significantly in the next decades: demographics; nursing and healthcare worker shortages; chronic diseases and conditions; the new, educated consumers; and excessive costs of healthcare services that are increasing in need and kind.

## Demographics

One hears it every day: The baby boomers are getting older and people are living longer. In 2000, 13% of the American population was older than age 65, and the number of older adults is growing significantly. According to the U.S. Bureau of the Census (U.S. Department of Commerce, Bureau of the Census, 2006), 7,918 Americans turn 60 years old every day. Consequently, by 2030, 19% of the U.S. population will be 65 years old or older and the oldest-old (85 years or older) will increase by 3 million

---

### CASE STUDY: EARLY DETECTION OF A CHANGE IN CONDITION

Mrs. C., an independent, 96-year-old woman, has a history of rehospitalization because of atrial fibrillation resulting from CHF and hypertension.

After her most recent hospitalization, Mrs. C. was treated and released into home care at an agency in Washington. A home telemonitoring system that tracks and transmits patients' vital signs was placed in her home. The primary goal of placing this patient on the telemonitor was to provide daily monitoring of her condition, thereby avoiding unnecessary rehospitalizations.

One morning, Mrs. C.'s telenurse detected an alarmingly low oxygen saturation level in the patient's transmitted data. In response, the nurse telephoned Mrs. C. and asked her to retake her oxygen reading. The reading was confirmed and the telenurse contacted the patient's physician, who requested immediate transportation of the patient to the hospital emergency room. Medics were called and Mrs. C. was taken to the hospital, where she was diagnosed with a pulmonary embolism.

The prompt response resulted from early detection and timely intervention enabled by the home telehealth equipment and a home health nurse's oversight. One notable fact in this case is that although the primary goal of monitoring patients is to avoid unnecessary hospitalization, in this case the hospitalization was necessary for the patient as a result of her elevated blood pressure and compromised oxygen saturation levels. The patient was still asymptomatic at the time of detection. However, the telehealth intervention and subsequent hospitalization allowed for the embolism to be treated before any serious damage occurred.

Under the traditional home care model, this patient might have been seen by a nurse only two to three times per week, and the clinician does not have knowledge of the patient's condition in between visits. However, having vital patient data tracked and transmitted daily allowed for rapid response that resulted in a positive outcome, perhaps a life-saving intervention for this patient.

persons between 2010 (5.8 million) and 2030 (8.7 million; U.S. Department of Commerce, Bureau of the Census, 2010). Also on the rise is the number of older Americans living with at least one chronic disease or condition; they account for 4 out of every 5 people older than age 50 (American Association for Retired Persons [AARP], 2009). This trend should alert clinicians to the much greater demand for planned professional care that will arise in the coming years.

## Nursing and Healthcare Worker Shortages

The crisis related to the well-known nursing shortage has two key aspects: a greater need for nurses by more persons, particularly those living with sometimes multiple comorbidities, and a significant decrease in the number of young people entering the nursing profession. Nationwide, the demand for nurses is clearly exceeding the supply. A report by Buerhaus, Auerbach, and Staiger (2009) stated that the recession of the past few years may have helped to ease the RN shortage in the short term, but suggested that the aging of the RN workforce and the aging of the population will likely combine to produce a shortfall of nurses beginning in 2018, with the deficit reaching nearly 260,000 by 2025.

The very serious shortage of healthcare workers in the United States must be addressed with some foresight. Although there is currently more focus on training laypeople, such as aides and other paraprofessionals, to perform certain nursing tasks, this venture certainly cannot replicate the clinical expertise of trained nurses skilled in nursing science. We must begin to look seriously at using effective adjuncts to skilled care, with telehealth being one of these important developments. Some organizations have already begun to do so. For example, a study by the Pennsylvania Homecare Association and Penn State University (2004) looked at how telehealth can be used to address workforce issues in the home healthcare industry and determined that telehealth use may enhance nurses' job satisfaction and help to retain nurses in their current positions.

## Chronic Diseases and Conditions

Chronic conditions are the leading cause of illness, disability, and death in the United States today. The number of elderly persons living with chronic disease is estimated at 140 million in the United States and accounts for more than 80% of healthcare expenditures (Dorsey & Topol, 2016). Both chronic conditions and the number of persons with chronic illnesses are expected to increase dramatically in the United States in the next few decades. Many age groups are also affected by **chronic disease**, not just the elderly. As noted in a report from the Centers for Disease Control and Prevention (CDC; 2005), by the year 2030, 148 million Americans will have a chronic illness, with at least one third of them being limited in their ability to go to school or to live independently. You can follow the CDC's chronic disease surveillance activities at this website: www.cdc.gov/chronicdisease/stats/index.htm. Securing appropriate, adequate, and affordable care services for these populations should be a national concern.

## Educated Consumers

The wave of today's aging baby boomers is steering some of the usual health service practices toward a very different course. Many of these individuals are more educated than their parents and more comfortable with the use of technology. They want to become more informed and involved with their care plans. These empowered consumers will be financially motivated with the introduction of consumer-directed healthcare plans that reward healthier lifestyles and better disease management of chronic conditions. All of these circumstances will further drive the use and the innovation of new technologies to meet consumer need. New plans for this new generation of consumers very much lean toward meeting their demands for when-needed, as-needed care, or care services delivered on their own terms and timing.

## Economics

When one connects the drivers of today's healthcare market—the demographics, nursing shortages, and increased number of persons living with chronic conditions and their extensive use of healthcare services—with excessive costs of this health care, the critical need for solutions becomes obvious. The U.S. healthcare system spends $1.4 trillion per year on conventional medical care. Much more will be spent annually in the coming decades. One must ask: Taking all of the driving factors of today's healthcare market into account, what needs to be done to address healthcare issues in the United States and meet the burgeoning numbers and needs of patients?

One solution is to develop a new clinical model for American health care that includes technology. In particular, telehealth technology should be included to fill the gap resulting from an overabundance of patients and a scarcity of healthcare providers. This concept is indicated in **Figure 18-1**.

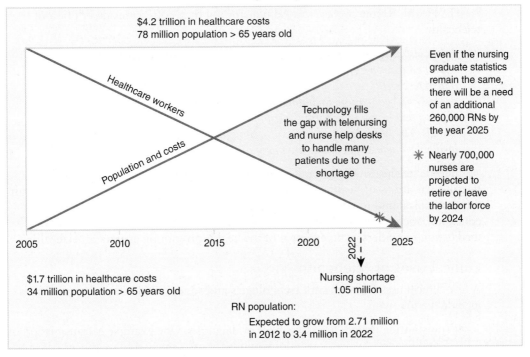

**Figure 18-1** Technology Fills the Gap
Data from Honeywell

Consider the use of technology that might potentially fill the current gaps in the healthcare system. Tools of telehealth can, for example, help render needed services without requiring in-person professional care at all contacts. The remote or virtual visit made by skilled clinicians is just one approach to using the range of health technologies available today. More needs to be learned about what telehealth is, how it works, and which aspects have been successful so that clinicians can plan to incorporate its use into routine clinical care.

## Telehealth Care

Let us start with a basic definition of **telehealth care**. Keep in mind, however, that telehealth is an emerging field, and definitions are subject to change and improvement as technology evolves. The American Telemedicine Association (ATA; 2010) provided the following definition:

> *Telemedicine is the use of medical information exchanged from one site to another via electronic communications to improve patients' health status. Closely associated with telemedicine is the term "telehealth," which is often used to encompass a broader definition of remote health care that does not always involve clinical services. Videoconferencing, transmission of still images, e-health including patient portals, remote monitoring of vital signs, continuing medical education and nursing call centers are all considered part of telemedicine and telehealth. (para. 1)*

The Health Resources Services Administration (n.d.) offers this description of telehealth:

> *Telehealth is the use of technology to deliver health care, health information or health education at a distance. Common applications include: teleradiology, in which test results are forwarded to another facility for diagnosis; continuing professional education, including presentations by specialists to general practitioners; and home monitoring, a supplement to home visits from nursing professionals. The boundaries of telehealth, though, are limited only by the technology available—new applications are being invented and tested every day. (para. 1)*

Indeed, "telehealth" is generally used as an umbrella term to describe all of the possible variations of healthcare services that use telecommunications. Telehealth can refer to clinical and nonclinical uses of health-related contacts. Delivery of patient education, such as menu planning for patients with diabetes or the transmission of medication reminders, is an example of the health-promoting aspects of telehealth.

### Clinical Uses of Telehealth

A few clinical uses for telehealth technologies and some sample clinical applications include the following:

- Transmitting images for assessment or diagnosis. One example is transmission of digital images, such as images of wounds for assessment and treatment consults.

- Transmitting clinical data for assessment, diagnosis, or disease management. One example is remote patient monitoring and transmitting patients' objective or subjective clinical data, such as monitoring of vital signs and answers to disease management questions.
- Providing disease prevention and promotion of good health. Examples include case management provided via telephone or smartphone app and patient education provided through asthma and weight management programs conducted in schools.
- Using telephonic or video interactive technologies to provide health advice in emergent cases. One example is performing teletriage in call centers or real-time stroke consultation between a rural health center and an academic medical center.
- Using real-time video. One example is exchanging health services or education live via videoconference.

## Telehealth Transmission Formats and Their Clinical Applications

Nurses must become familiar with the many and varied clinical and nonclinical transmission formats and applications of telehealth technologies so that they can make informed choices about the tools that are available for their use, as needed. Among these applications are store-and-forward telehealth, real-time telehealth, remote monitoring, telephony, and mHealth. The Center for Connected Health Policy has provided some video overviews of the telehealth transmissions and clinical applications (www.cchpca.org/videos).

### Store-and-Forward Telehealth

In a **store-and-forward telehealth transmission**, digital images, video, audio, and clinical data are captured and stored on the client computer or device; then, at a convenient time, the data are transmitted securely (forwarded) to a specialist or clinician at another location, where they are studied by the relevant specialist or clinician. If indicated, the opinion of the specialist or clinician is then transmitted back. Based on the requirements of the participating healthcare entities, this round-trip interaction could take anywhere from a few minutes to 48 hours. In many store-and-forward specialties, such as teleradiology, an immediate response is not critical. Dermatology, radiology, and pathology are common specialties whose practices are conducive to store-and-forward technologies. Transmission of wound care images for assessment by specialty care nurses or other specialists has become a frequently used and important form of home telehealth nursing practice.

### Real-Time (or Interactive) Telehealth

In **real-time telehealth**, a telecommunications link between the involved parties allows a real-time or live interaction to take place. Videoconferencing equipment is one of the most common forms of technologies used in synchronous telehealth. In addition, peripheral devices can be attached to computers or to the videoconferencing equipment to facilitate an interactive examination. Use of computers for real-time two-way audio and video streaming between centers over ever-improving and cheaper communication channels is becoming common. These developments have contributed to lowering of costs in telehealth. See Figure 18-2 for a depiction of this interaction.

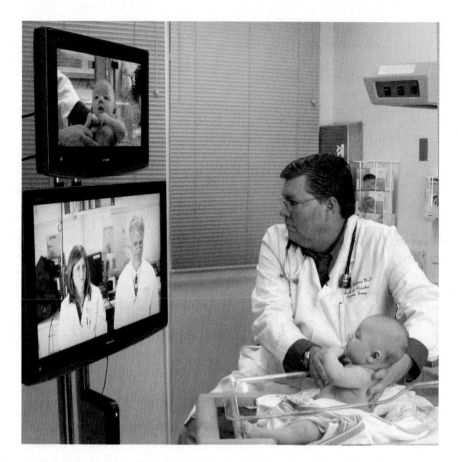

**Figure 18-2** Example of a Physician-to-Physician Consult Using Telehealth
Reproduced from Ohio Supercomputer Center. (2008). Governor Strickland, international panel of experts consider establishing Telehealth Video Resource Center. Retrieved from https://www.osc.edu/press/governor_strickland_international_panel_of _experts_consider_establishing_telehealth_video

Examples of real-time clinical telehealth applications include the following:

- Telemental health, which uses videoconferencing technology to connect a psychiatric nurse with a mental health client.
- Telerehabilitation, which uses videocameras and other technologies to assess patients' progress in home rehabilitation.
- Telehome care, which uses video technologies to observe, assess, and teach patients living in rural areas.
- Teleconsultations, which use a variety of technologies to enable collaborative exchanges or consultations between individuals or among groups that are involved with a case. These teleconsults may be transmitted live using videoconferencing technology. They may, for instance, involve teaching a certain technique to a less-experienced clinician, or they may provide several

clinicians with an opportunity to discuss an appropriate approach to a difficult case.

- Telehospice or telepalliative care, which can use real-time or remote monitoring to provide psychological support to patients and caregivers. Telehealth devices can also play a role in symptom management, in effect helping end-of-life patients achieve an optimal quality of life.

## Remote Monitoring (Telemonitoring or Remote Patient Monitoring)

In remote monitoring, devices are used to capture and transmit biometric data. For example, a tele-electroencephalogram device can monitor the electrical activity of a patient's brain and then transmit those data to a specialist assigned to the case. This interaction could occur either in real time or as a stored and then forwarded transmission. Examples of telemonitoring include the following:

- Monitoring patient parameters during home-based nocturnal dialysis
- Cardiac and multiparameter monitoring of remote intensive care units (ICUs)
- Home telehealth—for example, daily home telemonitoring of vital signs by patients and subsequent transmission of those data that enables offsite nurses to track their patients regularly and precisely and address noticeable changes through education and information suggestions about diet or exercise
- Disease management

## Telephony

Telephone monitoring (**telephony**) is the most basic type of telehealth. It can be described as remote care delivery or monitoring in which scheduled patient encounters via the telephone occur between a healthcare provider and a patient or caregiver (Quality Insights of Pennsylvania, 2005). More details about interaction using telephony are discussed later in this chapter.

## mHealth

The use of mobile phones, tablets, and PDAs for managing health is a rapidly advancing form of telehealth. There are numerous applications (apps) that target specific health behaviors and illnesses and provide a platform for management at a distance. One such management technique is a targeted text message to remind patients to perform a certain behavior, such as monitoring their peak flow to manage asthma or to take medications. Other apps are more specific to public health or provider education. Weinstein and colleagues (2014) explained,

> Current uses of apps on mobile devices include the direct provision of care, real-time monitoring of patient vital signs, delivery of patient information to practitioners and (where appropriate) clinical researchers, and collection of community healthcare data. Specialized sensors and devices that work as accessories to multiple health apps are also seeing tremendous growth and innovation. (p. 185)

## Nonclinical Uses of Telehealth Technologies

There are also many nonclinical uses of telehealth technologies. Currently, these include distance education including continuing medical and nursing education, grand rounds, and patient education; administrative uses including meetings among tele-health networks, supervision, and presentations; and research using the Internet and other online sources for information and health data management.

All of these telecommunications-assisted activities overcome obstacles of distance and provide access to needed health-related information. Clearly, with telehealth, the range of patient care possibilities broadens significantly.

# Telenursing

Where do nurses using telehealth, as in telenursing, fit into today's healthcare delivery arena? As early as 1998, Skiba referred to **telenursing** as the use of telecom-munications and information technology to provide nursing services in health care and enhance care whenever a physical distance exists between patient and nurse or among any number of nurses. As a clinical field, telenursing is part of telehealth and has many points of contact with other medical and nonmedical applications, such as telediagnosis, teleconsultation, and telemonitoring. In their study, St George et al. (2009) concluded, "In terms of the kinds of calls received, the dispositions reached after triage and clinical safety, we could detect no differences between nurses work-ing from home and those working in the call centre" (p. 123). Telenurses serve as an integral part of the healthcare delivery team, no matter their location.

## Applications of Telenursing in Home Care

An early and still-accepted definition of **home telehealth care** was provided by Kinsella (2004): "Home telehealth care is clinician-driven remote care delivery and education services that are delivered to the home via telecommunications-ready tools" (p. 36).

As home telehealth care has evolved, this definition has expanded to include a broader arena of delivery. In fact, some have defined the "home" as anywhere out-side of an acute inpatient setting—a definition that includes nursing homes, assisted living facilities, and other living situations beyond the single-family home or apart-ment. Wherever the home setting may be, people want to be cared for there. Today's burgeoning senior population, in particular, has become quite vocal about this preference, and estimates for preferences of aging in place at home are around 87% (AARP, 2014). Fortuitously, the reach of nurses using telecommunications-ready tools in the home is now remarkably extended. Not only have the settings for home care expanded beyond what was usual (the family home) in the last four decades of home health's formal existence, but the types of services delivered to the home have also become more advanced. The home care industry's newest challenge is to work with sicker patients, many of whom have been discharged from hospitals to home earlier than in the past.

This challenge to extend the range of conventional home care is why telehealth can be and needs to be provided to a wide range of patients, including those who have the following characteristics:

- Are immobilized
- Live in remote or difficult-to-reach places

- Have chronic ailments, such as chronic obstructive pulmonary disease (COPD), diabetes, and congestive heart disease
- Have debilitating diseases, such as neural degenerative diseases (Parkinson disease, Alzheimer disease, amyotrophic lateral sclerosis)

All of these patients may stay at home and be visited and assisted regularly by a nurse via videoconferencing, Internet, videophone, or other telecommunications means. These telecommunications-ready tools enable home telenurses to follow through advanced levels of care, as needed.

Still other varied applications of home telehealth care involve the care of patients in immediate postsurgical situations, those needing care of wounds and ostomies, and handicapped individuals needing physical therapy interventions or telerehabilitation. In addition to this extended range of patients who can be served with telehealth, many more patients can be seen when telehealth is used. For example, in conventional **home health care**, depending on the distances of travel involved, one nurse may be able to visit as many as 7 patients per day. Using telenursing, however, one nurse can remotely visit or televisit 12–16 patients in the same amount of time using interactive telehealth. Over the last decade, the efficiencies of telenursing have been well documented, as have the resulting improved patient care outcomes that can be expected by frequent telecontact.

Another outpatient application of telenursing is telephony-based **call centers**, which may be operated by managed care organizations, hospitals, and other health organizations. Some call centers also include telemonitoring services, which allow the patient to stay at home and use different telehealthcare devices to transmit biometric and other medical information back to the call center. Monitoring can be intermittent or continuous. This use of the teletechnology allows clinicians to evaluate patients' status and use the data to make decisions to better manage patients' health conditions.

Many features of call centers' services are comparable to conventional hands-on care in the home. For instance, call centers are typically staffed by RNs who act as case managers or perform patient triage. These professionals can provide information and counseling to patients as part of a disease management program and as a means to educate them on their disease process. In effect, their goal is to offer appropriate access to care (from nurses at the call centers) and help patients to prevent avoidable emergency room visits and rehospitalizations. An example of this assistance includes a nurse calling (i.e., not waiting for a patient to contact the call center) a recently discharged patient with diabetes on a regularly scheduled basis to evaluate progress at home, activity tolerance, medication compliance, foot care, and diet management. This empowering of patients toward self-management is a very significant and needed part of telenursing.

Home care telenursing can also involve other activities, such as providing customized patient education in dietary or exercise needs, nursing teleconsultations, review of results of medical tests and examinations, and assistance to physicians in the implementation of medical treatment protocols. The work can be wide ranging; for example, some home-based telecardiology programs involve the patient, the family, the physician, and a specialized cardiac monitoring center. A multidisciplinary approach is used along with best practice–defined protocols to manage the patient, improve the patient's quality of life, and reduce healthcare costs, especially hospitalization costs. Nurses play a key role in this network of care.

A relatively new role for advanced practice nurses is that of a tele–intensive care nurse. These nurses provide remote monitoring, oversight, and expert consultation for patients in rural ICUs by examining real-time data collected at the bedside. They look for trends indicating that an intervention is needed and then alert the bedside nurse of the need, thereby providing an extra set of eyes and an advanced level of expertise. "Tele-ICU provides expert-driven, evidence-based, cutting-edge services to the monitoring and treatment of critically ill patients" (Williams, Hubbard, Daye, & Barden, 2012, p. 62). Goran (2011) studied tele-ICU nursing competencies and emphasized that effective listening and collaboration skills and the ability to prioritize patient needs are among the most important attributes of tele-ICU nurses. She also cautions that nurses who function in these collaborative roles need to continue to practice at the bedside to keep their clinical skills sharp. In 2014, the ATA released a clinical care guideline for TeleICU. In this guideline, they identified three practice models:

- Continuous Care Model: Continuous care is monitoring of the patient without interruption for a defined period of time (e.g., on an 8-, 12-, or 24-hour basis).
- Scheduled Care Model: Scheduled care occurs with a periodic consultation on a predetermined schedule (e.g,. during patient rounds).
- Responsive (Reactive) Care Model: In this model, virtual visits are prompted by an alert (e.g., telephone call, page, monitor alarm) and are unscheduled (p. 6).

Access these guidelines, as well as other telehealth guidelines, at www .americantelemed.org/resources/telemedicine-practice-guidelines/telemedicine-practice -guidelines#.V5815vnyCM9. In addition, the American Association of Critical-Care Nurses (AACN, 2013) has developed the TeleICU Model of Success published in the *TeleICU Nursing Practice Guidelines*. This model emphasizes that the patient is central to all of the interactions between providers, and is dependent upon communication and collaboration among providers to promote positive patient outcomes.

By reviewing all of these examples of telenursing practice, one can see that nurses using telenursing can broaden their involvement in the targeted care of their patients. Some sources have predicted that home care will soon become the hub of all patient activity: The home will be where care that is begun in hospitals and other settings will be managed over the very long term and in the most cost-effective healthcare setting. Home care telenurses can expect to play a vital and dynamic role in the changing delivery systems that are likely to be put in place in the coming decades.

# Telehealth Patient Populations*

Any patient who has a condition that must be monitored is a candidate for home tele-monitoring. Patients with chronic illnesses have particularly benefited from ongoing monitoring to prevent acute episodes. Patients who are homebound or who have limited access to transportation are also appropriate candidates for such monitoring.

---

*This section is adapted from Prial & Hoss (2009).

## Patients with Chronic Diseases

Given demographics and advances in medical practice, there has been unprecedented growth in the number of patients with chronic diseases. Those patients are at significant risk of having an acute episode when subtle but significant changes in their medical condition occur. The ability to identify these changes in a timely fashion allows for changes in medication, lifestyle, or treatment to occur. Identification of a 3-lb weight gain over 5 days in a patient with CHF, for example, allows for interventions that could prevent an emergency room visit and subsequent hospitalization. The categories of patients with chronic diseases who are most commonly monitored today include those with CHF, COPD, or diabetes, and those who require long-term wound care.

These patients, particularly those with higher acuity levels, are at significant risk of having a medical crisis that might necessitate emergency or unplanned acute interventions. Many other patients with chronic diseases are less susceptible to a health crisis, but would greatly benefit from home telemonitoring to improve care and reduce costs.

## At-Risk Populations

Telemonitoring can be used effectively on patients who are at greater risk for an episode of acute illness. Patients who have a predisposition to disease are at increased risk of medical problems associated with employment, lifestyle, or location, and those patients who have displayed early signs of potentially serious health problems could be placed on preventive monitoring. In such cases, monitoring is used to ensure that interventions are timely and acute incidents avoided. Such technology could be part of a healthcare early warning system and could support preventive models of care.

## Isolated Patients

Home telemonitoring is effective for patients who cannot physically access healthcare services. The homebound elderly have been among the first to benefit from this technology in conjunction with the home health services they receive. With increasing limits affecting the ability of patients to receive services in the home because of staffing shortages and coverage limitations, telemonitoring technology takes on greater importance in managing homebound patients.

Patients in remote geographic areas have been long-time users of telemedicine interventions, such as robodocs. According to Strauss (2010), "The Remote Presence Robot (RP-7) from InTouch Health is a mobile telemedicine unit that connects physicians and specialists with patients and other doctors who are too distant to consult with them in person" (para. 2). With few rural healthcare facilities being built and access problems becoming more difficult, the use of technology in the home will increase. Even in suburban and rural areas, access is becoming more problematic, requiring greater use of home telemonitoring interventions. A lack of primary care and emergency resources in many urban core areas has prompted many health systems to consider managing certain patients through telemonitoring options and better staging of patient access. Telemedicine also is effective for patients in such institutions as prisons, for whom it is logistically difficult to travel to traditional care sites.

## Incarcerated Patients

Telehealth services are used extensively in seven states to provide mandated medical services for prison populations. These correctional telemedicine programs are cost effective and promote public safety by not having to transport prisoners to healthcare facilities for care (Weinstein et al., 2014).

## Hospitalized Patients

Home telemonitoring has proved effective in managing the flow of patients into and out of hospitals and other inpatient facilities. Patients are monitored to determine when they are admitted, to predict how long they might stay, and to prevent unfunded readmissions. Patients undergoing semielective procedures can be better staged with scheduling options when they are monitored in the home before admission. If deterioration of the patient's condition is observed, a procedure can be accelerated or planned interventions changed.

Monitoring can also be used effectively in length-of-stay reduction strategies. Physicians and surgeons are more confident in discharging patients early when they know that vital signs will be monitored and any decline in condition noted in a timely fashion. Use of monitoring effectively allows for an extension of step-down models of care into the patient's home. These length-of-stay management strategies have been particularly useful when hospital beds are in short supply.

Unplanned readmissions are a serious patient care and financial management issue for hospitals. The use of monitoring in the home has consistently reduced unplanned and unfunded readmissions by enabling healthcare providers to obtain reliable information on the patient and intervene appropriately to keep the patient at home.

## Emergency Response Situations

Telemedicine will likely be a major component of effective patient management in a major disaster, large-scale nuclear or biochemical attack, or outbreak of highly infectious disease. In such a situation, traditional healthcare delivery systems may become overwhelmed, and patients will need to be more effectively triaged and managed by remote providers. Telemedicine applications allow for a dramatic extension of patient management and triaging options and allow offsite providers to be involved in care. If an infectious or communicable disease is involved, patient isolation could be accomplished in the home using telemedicine technology.

## Concerned Patients and Families

Perhaps the largest potential market for home telemonitoring is patients and families who want to have reliable and objective information that allows for their involvement in healthcare decision making. At one extreme is a young person who wants to monitor physiologic data as part of a personal wellness or fitness program. At the other extreme are families that want information on the status of a terminally ill loved one in another city. In between there is a wide range of opportunities for individuals and families to obtain information that promotes realistic and meaningful dialogue with healthcare professionals.

## Assisted Living and Subacute Patients

In assisted living facilities or subacute care centers, a kiosk can be used to obtain vital signs for large groups of people. Vital signs reports can then be forwarded on a regularly established schedule to physicians and others involved in the patient's care. This approach allows for better individual care management and lends itself to developing intervention strategies and education options to benefit the entire population of a facility. Some facilities have even used access to telemonitoring systems as an inducement to attract potential residents.

## Employers and Wellness Programs

Health care is a vital concern for employers. They have a direct financial interest in lowering costs and are financial beneficiaries of long-term-illness preventive strategies. If they can monitor their workers (e.g., offering telehealth options as a wellness program), they will see many benefits for themselves, such as reduced absenteeism and increased productivity. Effective monitoring programs can ultimately lower healthcare costs and associated insurance premiums. Some companies are now exploring the creation of financial incentives for employees who achieve healthcare objectives, such as appropriate weight, reduced blood pressure, and levels of exercise. Monitoring could very well be used as a means of tracking performance in this regard.

# Tools of Home Telehealth

A wide and growing range of telecommunications-ready tools are available for nurses' and patients' use in the home. See Figure 18-3 for a depiction of how these tools are combined to provide home telehealth monitoring.

## Central Stations, Web Servers, and Portals

**Central stations, Web servers,** and **portals** are various terms for the technologies presently used as part of multifunctional telehealthcare platforms and application servers. These clinical management software programs receive and display patients' vital signs and other information transmitted from a medical device, including blood pressure, weight, and glucose information. Such transmission was initially most commonly accomplished over plain old telephone system lines (POTS); however, network access and wireless communication are more commonly used as technology advances and access improves.

Central stations and Web servers are key components of telehealth that can be as minimal as a single screen display or as comprehensive as software applications that provide various functions including triaging the data based on medical alerts, which allows clinicians to quickly identify those patients requiring immediate attention. Other features found in these packages allow clinicians to build personal medical records for patients and provide trended patient data and analysis reports supporting improved patient outcomes using telehealth. In addition, some of the software packages provide remote programming capabilities that allow the clinician to remotely program the medical device in the patient's home. Such an application can change monitoring report times for patients, individualize alert parameters, set up reminders, and send educational content to a patient.

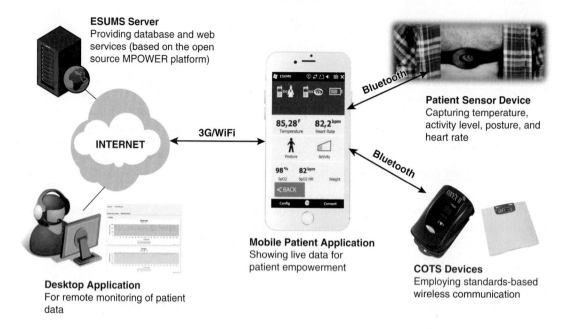

**Figure 18-3** Tools for Home Telehealth Monitoring

Reproduced from Seeberg, T. M., Vedum, J., Sandsund, M., Austad, H. O., Liverud, A. E., Vardøy, A. S. B., . . . Strisland, F. (2014). Development of a wearable multisensor device enabling continuous monitoring of vital signs and activity. Presented at IEEE-EMBS International Conference on Biomedical and Health Informatics (BHI), Valencia, pp. 213–218. doi: 10.1109/BHI.2014.6864342

## Peripheral Biometric (Medical) Devices

**Peripheral biometric (medical) devices** can consist of fully integrated systems, such as a vital signs monitor, or they may be stand-alone telecommunications-ready devices, such as blood pressure cuffs and blood glucose meters. These devices plug directly into the household telephone jack to send data to a central server location or use Bluetooth technology to transmit data.

An ever-increasing number of peripheral devices are being introduced to the market. Examples of other peripheral devices seen in home telehealth today include pulse oximeters; prothrombin time, International Normalized Ratio meters; spirometers; peak flow meters; electrocardiogram monitors; and card readers and writers that use smart card technology and enable multiple users to use one device.

## Telephones

Telephones are already the most familiar household communications tool used in telehealth care. A telephone device can be augmented for easier use by patients, as needed, with a lighted dial pad, an auto-dial system, or a louder ringer. Telephone systems are still and will continue to be important when there is no Internet access in the home.

## Videocameras and Videophones

Videocameras and videophones are readily available consumer items that can be used in telehealth for show-and-tell demonstrations by nurses for patients or to capture wound healing progress, among other applications. Typically, these products operate as a standard telephone or as a video picture telephone, using standard telephone lines to transmit information or interactions.

Currently, the image quality over a POTS is limited by the bandwidth of POTS technology, which favors use of such images for assessment rather than delivering diagnostic-quality images. These imaging capabilities will improve as integrated services digital network lines become more widely available in the home environment. Typically, medical centers and hospitals have access to larger bandwidth capabilities for image transmission and viewing, thus ensuring high-quality diagnostic images and point-to-point consultations in hospital- or medical center-based settings.

## Personal Emergency Response Systems

**Personal emergency response systems** are signaling devices worn as a pendant or otherwise made easily accessible to patients to ensure their safety and to enable them to quickly access emergency care when needed, usually in case of a fall. A preset telephone number is alerted by the patient's pushing a button on the pendant; upon this signal, predesignated emergency help is dispatched. Many newer sensor options for tracking patients at home are being incorporated into multifunctioning personal emergency response systems devices, such as alerting a central call center to water flooding or smoke in a patient's home. The next subsection provides details on these sensors and monitors.

## Sensor and Activity-Monitoring Systems

**Sensor and activity-monitoring systems** can track activities of daily living of seniors and other at-risk individuals in their place of residence. These sensors and monitoring systems can provide insight into behavior changes that might signal changes or deterioration of health status. Such technologies consist of wireless motion sensors that are strategically placed around the residence and can detect motion on a 24-hour basis.

One authority on these technologies, David J. Stern (2007), described their operation further. Data from these sensors are wirelessly sent to a receiver and base station that periodically transmits the information to a centralized server through standard telephone lines. Sophisticated algorithms analyze the data, compiling data on each individual's normal patterns of behavior, including bathroom usage, sleep disturbance, meal preparation, medication interaction, and general levels of activity including fall detection. Deviations from these norms can be important warning signs of emerging health problems and the alerts provided can enable caregivers to intervene early.

In addition to widely used fire, security, and home gas detectors, other sensors can monitor appliances to detect whether a household appliance is turned on or off and can sometimes switch the appliance on and off for the resident. Typical applications for affixing programmable sensors can include lamps, television sets, irons, and kitchen stoves. Such sensors might be very valuable for ensuring the safety of elderly, forgetful persons who live alone. One excellent example of today's sensor use for assistance with the elderly are sensors placed in or on stovetops to alert the user when he or she is standing too close to the equipment or when the kettle or pot has boiled over. Benefits realized from these technologies include enabling people to live independently with an improved quality of life. They can also provide peace of mind for other family members living at a distance.

## Medication Management Devices

**Medication management devices** address a well-recognized major problem in health care: medication management and compliance.

The failure of patients to take medications as prescribed has become a national problem in health care today. This noncompliance can have devastating consequences, particularly for those patients living with chronic illnesses. The National Pharmaceutical Council (2013) estimates that the cost of noncompliance with prescribed medications is $290 billion per year: 3 out of 4 people do not take their medications as prescribed and 1 out of 3 people never fills his or her prescriptions.

To address some of these very pressing problems, a host of telecommunications-ready medication devices have become available, and many more are in development. Some are as simple as a watch that reminds a person to take medications, others are pill organizers with audible reminders, and some can be programmed to dispense prefilled containers with medications and alert a patient or caregiver of a missed dose. Furthermore, some of these medication tools send data from the device back to a central server so that patient's medication compliance can be tracked. These telecommunications-ready devices can organize, manage, dispense, or remind, and they will play an increasingly important role in helping people live independently and manage their disease processes through medication compliance. For more information on these devices, see the *Informatics Tools to Promote Patient Safety and Quality Outcomes* chapter.

## Special Needs Telecommunications-Ready Devices

Special needs telecommunications ready-devices can include preprogrammed, multifunctional infusion pumps for meeting a range of infusion needs, including medications for pain management and other infusion delivery needs, such as hydration and nutrition; peak flow meters; electrocardiogram monitors; and so on. Many such tools are in development to meet the more demanding and challenging needs of today's at-home patients. The common goal of these tools is to increase communications between nurse and patient and to increase the nurse's knowledge of the patient's status in a timely manner. **Figure 18-4** illustrates the process for managing home telehealth.

# Home Telehealth Software*

As important as the gathering of data is the organizing of information to support decision making by clinical professionals. The telehealth software supporting home telehealth programs has become much more sophisticated in recent years, allowing for greater numbers of patients to be better managed by a single clinician. Areas of significant improvement in software include trending, triage, communications protocols, access, and sharing.

---

*This section is adapted from Prial and Hoss (2009).

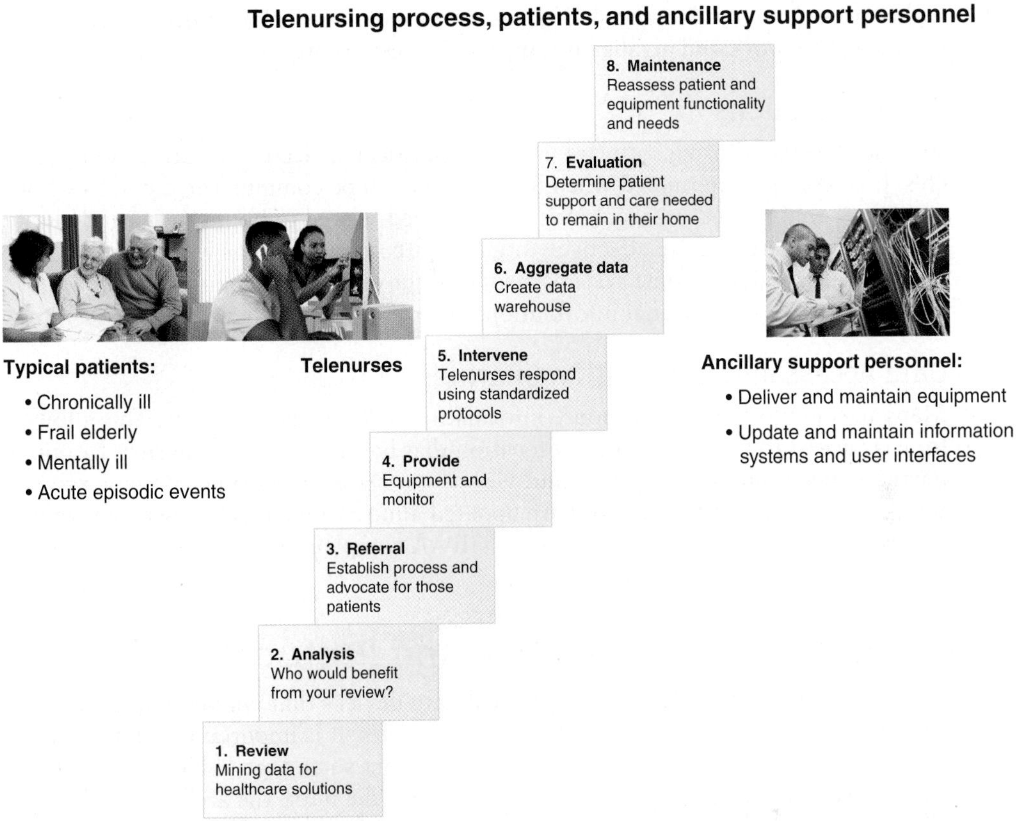

**Telenursing process, patients, and ancillary support personnel**

**8. Maintenance**
Reassess patient and equipment functionality and needs

**7. Evaluation**
Determine patient support and care needed to remain in their home

**6. Aggregate data**
Create data warehouse

**5. Intervene**
Telenurses respond using standardized protocols

**4. Provide**
Equipment and monitor

**3. Referral**
Establish process and advocate for those patients

**2. Analysis**
Who would benefit from your review?

**1. Review**
Mining data for healthcare solutions

**Typical patients:**           **Telenurses**

- Chronically ill
- Frail elderly
- Mentally ill
- Acute episodic events

**Ancillary support personnel:**

- Deliver and maintain equipment
- Update and maintain information systems and user interfaces

**Figure 18-4** Managing Home Telehealth

Elderly patients at a consultation: © Monkey Business Images/Shutterstock; telenurses looking at computer screen: © Rocketclips, Inc./Shutterstock; computer technicians: © dotshock/Shutterstock

## Trending

One of the key advantages of home telemonitoring is the creation of a digital health record that allows information to be recorded over time. If a patient takes his or her weight and blood pressure daily, most software will graphically display these data over time so that subtle trends can be observed. This type of trend data is much more useful in identifying emerging or developing conditions than snapshot data that are collected every 6–8 weeks at a physician's office. Trend information can also be developed for groups of patients or populations, allowing for population-based analyses of interventions. For example, one might gather trend information on patients with COPD, patients of a particular physician, or all patients receiving a certain medication.

## Triage

Most home telemonitoring systems set an acceptable range of values for an individual patient when he or she is enrolled in the monitoring program. For example, if oxygen saturation, blood pressure, or weight values go above or below predetermined amounts, then the software alerts the appropriate party. More sophisticated software looks at readings from multiple pieces of equipment on a single patient and can give higher priority to patients at risk of an acute episode. This helps clinicians better organize their work and arrange for appropriate interventions.

## Communications

Advanced telemonitoring software utilizes sophisticated electronic notification protocols. It is often predetermined when information will be communicated and to whom it is sent. Sophisticated protocols can be developed related to both routine and alert information, thereby more effectively organizing communications with physicians, nurses, and caregivers. Some systems also have the capacity to communicate back to the patient or seek additional information under predetermined circumstances.

## Data Access and Information Sharing

Many telemonitoring systems house information in Web-based formats. This allows for easy access to the data from any location that has access to the Internet. Multiple parties can simultaneously share and view data. Data can also be conveniently transmitted to other clinicians and are updated almost immediately when new values are received. Web-based records are fully HIPAA compliant when appropriate protections and controls are in place.

# Home Telehealth Practice and Protocols

The tools of telehealth described previously are devices that enable remote care delivery, enhance patient care, and improve outcomes. It is important to note that the data received from these tools are useless without some type of clinical oversight. Such tools do not replace the nurse, but rather give the nurse the ability to make more informed clinical decisions based on reliable data and a comprehensive picture of the patient's status. In home care, they also direct the clinical resources to patients based on need. The resulting patient-centered approach to care delivers improved patient outcomes and clinical efficiencies.

Home telehealth is indeed a practice, albeit one that represents a change in the current clinical model of practice for home care. Use of the telehealth tools is integrated into the practice to improve patient outcomes. As with any tool, however, the effectiveness is directly proportional to the appropriateness of the tool's application and use. Home telehealth programs differ depending on the type of technology used and the foci of the telehealth programs. However, every program should have telehealth use criteria established, including provisions for informed consent and assessment of the appropriateness of telehealth use for specific situations. The ATA regularly develops and issues practice guidelines, which can be accessed at the ATA's website: www.americantelemed.org/resources/telemedicine-practice-guidelines/telemedicine-practice-guidelines

Other professional organizations, such as the American Nurses Association (ANA), the Association of Colleges of Nursing (AACN), and the American Academy of Ambulatory Care Nursing (AAACN), also provide telehealth practice guidelines. Patient criteria for telehealth should be governed by established inclusion and exclusion guidelines, detailing who is eligible and appropriate for each type of technology. Other criteria include establishing policies and procedures that address patient enrollment, education,

**CASE STUDY: HOME TELEMONITORING OF MULTIPLE ILLNESSES**

The patient is a 71-year-old male who has stage 4 cardiomyopathy/pulmonary hypertension, atrial fibrillation, COPD, and type 2 diabetes mellitus. He has been an active patient with a home healthcare agency for several years, with an admitting diagnosis of CHF.

Initially, the patient was seen three times a week by an RN for CHF assessment and management. The patient's history included frequent hospitalizations for exacerbation of CHF and uncontrolled atrial fibrillation. He experienced a total of four hospitalizations in the year before placement of a telemonitoring system in his home, after about 6 months of receiving conventional home care.

Ever since the patient was placed on a telemonitoring system for daily tracking more than 8 months ago, he has not been rehospitalized. The telemonitoring interactions with his nurse have made him very conscious of the role that his medications, diet, and fluid restrictions play in his overall health status.

In addition, the telemonitor has proved its benefits to local physicians. The patient's family physician, cardiologist, and pulmonologist all were able to provide better care for the patient by examining the tabular and graphical trends that were elicited from the daily vital signs monitor. This information aided in the titration and addition of the various medications needed to control the patient's CHF and atrial fibrillation. The physicians were able to ascertain the response to the medication adjustments and other treatment modalities, such as oxygen titration. At the start of care, the patient's weight was 196 pounds; it is now at a stable 187 pounds, with the symptoms more controlled than they have ever been.

The patient's nurses, meanwhile, have peace of mind knowing they can keep an eye on their patient daily while making additional visits as needed, with the documentation being provided by the system to justify the additional nursing visit. This tool can also be incorporated into the nurses' care plan, enabling a higher standard of care to the patient.

At present, the patient is being case managed by nursing staff visits that occur once per month. He now enjoys a newfound peace of mind and security and an improved state of health, something this patient has not experienced in more than a year.

and equipment setup; patient and caregiver and home assessment; **patient informed consent**; and privacy and confidentiality rights. In addition, a clinical plan of care that is specific to patient needs should be developed. Telehealth pathways and protocols ensure more focused work with patients and allow for targeted interventions.

Clearly, by using a protocol for patients who regularly use telehealth equipment for tracking their status, nurses receive a good deal more targeted information than can possibly be obtained during scheduled, in-person visits. As a result, the use of telehealth tools, together with clinical oversight and practice, allows for more efficient and effective clinical management by allowing the patient's needs to drive the care. As home telehealth protocols are used more extensively, the improved clinical and operational efficiencies may ultimately affect the home care agency's bottom lines.

One must understand this clinically driven, as-needed approach to care services more fully so that it is not misunderstood as providing less care. In the above case study, a proactive, patient-centered approach enabled a home healthcare agency to identify early exacerbations in a patient's condition and take appropriate action.

## Legal, Ethical, and Regulatory Issues

Telehealth is affected by certain legal, ethical, and regulatory issues of which nurses should be aware. In the United States, interstate practice of telenursing, for example, requires attending nurses to be licensed to practice in all of the states in which they provide telehealth services by directly interacting with patients. This is particularly important when nurses work for health systems that are located near state borders and draw patients from both states. The Telehealth Resource Center provides a nice overview of Licensure and Scope of Practice issues; access it at www.telehealthresourcecenter.org /toolbox-module/licensure-and-scope-practice. In addition, the Center for Connected Health Policy provides an interactive map of current and pending state laws and reimbursement policies; it can be accessed at www.cchpca.org/state-laws-and -reimbursement-policies. There is some evidence that these regulations are slowly changing, so it is important for all licensed professionals to be specifically aware of legislation governing their practice.

In the 2016 report to Congress by the Medicare Patient Advisory Commission (MEdpAC), there was discussion of the need for streamlining interstate licensure for physicians and nurses who provide telehealth services. As an example, one physician had to maintain licenses in 23 states (paid fees and met continuing education [CE] requirements of individual states) in order to provide TeleICU services. A possible solution is the development of the federally sponsored physician Interstate Medical Licensure Compact (IMLC) and Nurse Licensure Compact (NLC) to facilitate portability of licensure across state lines. However, this federal initiative has met opposition from individual states who are unwilling to share licensing authority.

Patient confidentiality and the privacy and safety of clinical data must be given special consideration. Informed consent releases to receive telehealth services are a critical first step. Demiris, Doorenbos, and Towle (2009) suggested that informed consent be treated as a process and not a one-time event. They argue that because telehealth is a completely new experience, patients and families should have the opportunity to revise their consent after they fully understand its implications, especially the intrusiveness of home monitoring. In addition, they suggested that informed consent be obtained from all persons living in the household because there are potential privacy considerations for all who live in the home. When the patient is presented with the informed consent form, the nurse must assure the patient that physiologic data, such as blood pressure readings that will be transmitted over telephone lines or other public communication means, will be kept confidential and protected. In addition, for safety considerations, pointed efforts must be continually undertaken by the nurses' agencies to upgrade their information systems to ensure that a high level of data security is provided at all times. Telehealth providers must adhere to all data privacy and confidentiality guidelines and remain vigilant to ensure that all involved parties, including the technical staff assistants, have appropriate training in privacy and confidentiality issues.

## The Patient's Role in Telehealth

The range and sophistication of home telehealth tools are expanding regularly, and a concern of nurses when choosing appropriate tools for their patients is to ask, Will my patient use this device? Elderly patients may find the monitoring technology that may speak to them in their homes and video cameras to assist in wound care tracking, for example, to be a daunting introduction to home health care. To assuage the possible discomfort, these and other such tools have undergone much iteration so that they are easier to use and patients' ability to turn them on and off is ensured. When patients are scheduled for a televisit, these devices can be turned on and used. This use by patients is critical, of course, so that the necessary information about them will be gathered and transmitted, and so that their needs can be acted on by telenurses.

Demiris et al. (2009) emphasized consideration of usability issues when using telehealth applications with elders who may have sensory, cognitive, and motor disabilities. They suggest rigorous usability testing to maximize the quality of the user experience and special attention to design details for Web-based interfaces, such as font choices and color schemes to improve readability. Similarly, Kaplan and Litweka (2008) emphasize the need for ethical design principles:

- How provider-centric or patient-centric is the technology?
- Does the shift to remote services promote rationality and efficiency at the expense of values traditionally at the heart of caregiving?
- How does the design affect home life and family dynamics?
- To what extent should technology usage involve attempts to manipulate users into different behaviors?
- How might the replacement of human contact by new technologies be ameliorated?
- To what extent is the deployment of technology an end in itself, aimed not toward the improvement of health or well-being, but to create market needs?
- How do we identify the boundaries between genuine solutions and futility in light of technologies that may shift them? (p. 404)

## Telehealth Research

Telehealth research focuses primarily on clinical outcomes, such as effectiveness of telehealth compared to usual care, cost effectiveness of telehealth intervention, and patient and family satisfaction. For example, Dansky, Vasey, and Bowles (2008) studied the effects of home telehealth care on several clinical outcomes in patients with heart failure. They found that patients who received home telehealth care had fewer hospitalizations and costly emergency room visits during the study period and a greater reduction in heart failure symptoms than the control group. These authors suggested that the frequent monitoring of symptoms afforded by telehealth allowed for more frequent encounters than home visits, providing more timely intervention when clinical status changed and more frequent teaching and support by nurses.

Similarly, Jia, Chuang, Wu, Wang, and Chumbler (2009) studied the long-term effects of telehealth on preventable hospital use and found a statistically significant reduction in hospital use for the first 18 months of follow-up, but noted that the effects diminished over the 4-year study period. There were no differences found between telehealth and standard care groups in a study of rates of infection, rejection, and hospitalization in a group of transplant recipients, leading the researchers to conclude that telehealth is as effective as usual care for posttransplant follow-up (Leimig,

Gower, Thompson, & Winsett, 2008). Telehealth was also shown to be effective in providing support and problem-solving assistance for family caregivers of patients who experienced polytrauma (Bendixen et al., 2008) and persons with spinal cord injuries (Elliott, Brossart, Berry, & Fine, 2008).

In a qualitative study of patient and physician perspectives on treating rural depression, Swinton, Robinson, and Bischoff (2009) concluded, "Although an acceptable solution, both patients and PCPs expressed reservations about using telehealth for the treatment of depression because they felt that technology-mediated communication would not lend itself to establishing and maintaining the type of provider–patient relationship that would allow treatment to be effective" (p. 178). However, given the access issues associated with rural communities, telehealth provided an opportunity for intervention in cases where traditional care was challenging. Telehealth was also shown to be an effective alternative to usual care in conducting hearing screenings at rural elementary schools, thereby extending the reach and controlling the costs of conducting hearing screenings (Lancaster, Krumm, Ribera, & Klich, 2008).

Polisena, Coyle, Coyle, and McGill (2009) conducted a meta-analysis of 22 studies that compared telehealth to usual care in patients with chronic diseases; their work included a cost-effectiveness analysis. These authors concluded that in general telehealth can be cost-saving for the health system and insurance providers, but caution that because the overall methodological quality of the studies was low, the societal impact of telehealth remains uncertain.

Research into telehealth interventions clearly demonstrates that telehealth is at least as effective as usual care in managing chronic conditions in the home, and in many cases is more cost-effective than home visits. Demiris et al. (2009) suggested that more studies are needed to focus on the patient–provider relationship changes associated with such care, especially the loss of human touch associated with telehealth interventions. They also caution that researchers who are studying telehealth in remote populations must consider long-term sustainability of telehealth support beyond the study period to ensure that the "research does not exacerbate existing disparities" in access to technologies (p. 132).

The Agency for Healthcare Research and Quality (AHRQ) released a report authored by Totten and colleagues (2016) titled *Telehealth: Mapping the Evidence for Patient Outcomes from Systematic Reviews*. The purpose of the report was to provide a systematic review of evidence related to the impact of telehealth on clinical outcomes. The evidence suggested that

> *telehealth interventions produce positive outcomes when used for remote patient monitoring, broadly defined, for several chronic conditions and for psychotherapy as part of behavioral health. The most consistent benefit has been reported when telehealth is used for communication and counseling or remote monitoring in chronic conditions such as cardiovascular and respiratory disease, with improvements in outcomes such as mortality, quality of life, and reductions in hospital admissions. (p. vi)*

To follow progress in telehealth research, bookmark the sites provided in Box 18-1.

---

**BOX 18-1 TELEHEALTH RESEARCH AND INFORMATION CENTERS**

- Center for Telehealth and E-Health Law: www.ctel.org
- International Society for Telemedicine and eHealth: www.isfteh.org
- Telehealth Resource Centers: www.telehealthresourcecenter.org
- Telemedicine Information Exchange: www.tmhguide.org/site /epage/93994_871.htm
- UTMB Center for Telehealth Research and Policy at University of Texas Medical Branch: http://telehealth.utmb.edu
- Virginia Telehealth Network: www.ehealthvirginia.org

---

# Evolving Telehealth Models

Previous telehealthcare deliveries were largely provider initiated; however, we are beginning to see that consumers will drive the way health care is delivered in the future. Consider that tomorrow's healthcare facility might have no walls. The evolving roles of the Internet, electronic and personal health records, mobile health, health information exchanges, and telehealth all will support a more integrated healthcare model. This convergence of trends and solutions will continue to expand with the introduction of new business practice models, such as retail clinics and direct-to-consumer telehealth services.

Retail clinics, such as CVS's MinuteClinics and Walgreens' Healthcare Clinics, began to emerge in 2001 and have grown steadily to about 1,800 in number (Bachrach & Froelich, 2016). These clinics focus on prevention services such as vaccines; treatment of minor injuries, minor illnesses, and aches and pains; and health monitoring and medication management services for chronic illnesses. The clinics offer affordable, accessible, walk-in, and after-hours care, and are helping to fill the primary care gap created by the Affordable Care Act. Adding telehealth services is allowing these clinics to expand their services. In 2015, CVS announced a partnership with several telehealth organizations—American Well, Teladoc, and Doctor on Demand—to provide onsite telehealth consultations for CVS clinic providers:

> *CVS Health is piloting several different telehealth opportunities, including making telehealth physician care accessible through CVS Health digital properties. CVS Health will also explore enabling MinuteClinic providers to consult with telehealth physicians to expand the scope of care offered at MinuteClinic. In addition, MinuteClinic will continue to provide telehealth care to patients in CVS retail stores and will explore serving as a site for in-person exams to facilitate telehealth medical visits. (CVS Health, 2015, para. 4)*

These telehealth organizations also provide downloadable telehealth apps for consumers to consult directly with board-certified doctors via smartphones, tablets, and computers. For more information, please visit www.amwell.com, www.doctorondemand .com, and www.teladoc.com.

Polinski and colleagues (2015) surveyed 1,734 patients to assess satisfaction and preference for telehealth visits in CVS MinuteClinics. They reported overall satisfaction with telehealth because of its convenience and quality of care, and that one-third of the respondents preferred telehealth to an actual provider visit.

Several new trends include more robust mobile devices that connect with each other (Internet of Things) to provide real-time data on a patient's fitness and exercise to his or her physician's offices. The difficulty with these devices is ensuring security of data transmissions, as well as the possibility of overwhelming physicians with data (TechTarget, n.d.).

The Telemed Tablet is a Food and Drug Administration–approved device that provides access to a pool of specialists for consultation in rural clinics, at the bedside in hospitals, or in emergency rooms. It also allows on-call providers to consult remotely. More information about this product can be found at http://info.americanwell.com /the-telemed-tablet-brochure.

An interesting software application developed by Extreme Health is a motion-tracking technology that enables tracking and analysis of positions assumed by patients in front of a webcam as they perform their prescribed home exercise regimens.

> *Extreme Health's unique technology improves the physiotherapy process for outpatients and care-givers by enabling patients to conducts their exercise sessions at home on their chosen devices while receiving feedback on quality of performance. Meanwhile, the clinician receives the patient's data, configures exercises and monitors performance and progress, allowing the clinic to provide better care for physiotherapy outpatients. (ATA, 2016, para. 2)*

# Parting Thoughts for the Future and a View Toward What the Future Holds

Telehealth is here to stay and will become increasingly important in the future. The barriers to telehealth must be addressed soon. As the ATA (2015) suggested, the following are priorities for the 21st Century Healthcare Package:

- Allow for Medicare payments as a standard benefit without geographic restrictions
- Phase in flexibility for Medicare telehealth at Accountable Care Organizations and provide coverage for:
  * Remote critical care (primarily hospital ICU) services
  * Stroke bundle, including remote diagnosis
  * Home-based remote patient monitoring and physician video visits in home care
  * Home and outpatient telerehabilitation
  * Telemental screening and counseling for depression
- Improve beneficiary access under fee-for-service payments, targeting:
  * Telestroke diagnosis
  * Physician "visual" services by revising the asynchronous restrictions
  * Telehealth for recertifications of need for home health care and durable medical equipment

- Revise the Medicare Chronic Care Initiative to include:
  * Remote patient monitoring
  * Initiatives for hospital readmissions reduction
  * Waivers for telehealth restrictions to allow a state with a Medicaid "health home" project (two or more chronic conditions) to also serve comparable Medicare beneficiaries
  * Promotion of specialty medical homes to provide bundled and coordinated Medicare services for a specific long-term illness, chronic medical condition, or medical subspecialty, such as Parkinson's, multiple sclerosis, or specific cancers
- Consider other federal telehealth improvements, such as:
  * Options for high-risk pregnancy telehealth networks
  * Consolidating U.S. Department of Health and Human Services (USDHHS) telehealth grants, especially for telehealth networks, telehealth resource centers, licensure portability, and evidence-based tele-emergency networks
  * Promoting autism telehealth networks to improve care quality and accessibility
  * License portability for USDHHS health professionals: USDHHS employees and contractors would need only state licenses to provide official services in the United States

The care continuum will need to be supported by a clinical and caregiver structure that uses the data collected from patients to make better and more informed healthcare decisions. Health parameter data could be used by the end user for personal direct care decision making, or it may be used by a member of the healthcare community to determine appropriate healthcare interventions.

The technology of today will be different from the technology of tomorrow, as access to broadband communications systems, acceptance of technology, and mobility and data transfer continue to evolve. As a result of emerging needs, many companies will enter the market and offer a wide range of information technology tools, ranging from embedded and worn sensors to remote monitoring devices. User interfaces will become increasingly sophisticated and more patient-centric.

Clearly, by making key information readily accessible, solutions across all areas (home health, hospitals, and a range of other settings) will facilitate collaboration in care delivery and health information. Products that integrate into consumers' and patients' everyday lives to improve the quality of life will continue to emerge. Telehealth and telenursing will play an important role in improving quality of life and care for the patients served.

Foremost, nurses must be open to change and willing to embrace ever-evolving practice models. Tools should always be used to improve care delivery models so as to make more targeted contact with and about patients. In an ideal world, there will be seamless integration of clinical data systems and robust data exchange to provide quality care for patients no matter their location.

## Summary

Telehealth is a rapidly developing mode of health service delivery in which nurses can expect to play a significant role. The most promising area of concentration for nurses is in home telehealth care, an area that is expected to provide extensive care to the burgeoning numbers of American elderly persons living with challenging chronic diseases and conditions. Many telecommunications-ready tools to assist nurses in delivering this care are currently available, and their effectiveness in maintaining or improving patients' health outcomes is well documented. Today's nurses are providing telehealth services to typical home care patients (elderly patients, patients needing regular and targeted care) and operating effectively as telenurses. The practice of telehealth will provide opportunities for telenurses to become key players in care management across the healthcare continuum.

### THOUGHT-PROVOKING QUESTIONS

1. Will the increased use of telehealth technology tools be viewed as dehumanizing patient care, or will it be viewed as a means to promote more contact with healthcare providers and as new ways for people to stay connected (as in online disease support groups), thereby creating better long-term disease management and patient satisfaction?
2. Which types of resistance to new technologies might be evident among patients, caregivers, and nurses? Which evidence and strategies might help to diminish these resistances?
3. As telehealth technology advances toward seamless data access regardless of distance or health system, how can patient privacy rights and the confidentiality of personal medical data be protected?
4. Consider a recent patient care scenario and describe how it could have been managed at a distance.
   * Which training would be needed?
   * Which equipment would be used?
   * How would the patient and his or her family respond to home telemonitoring?

## References

Allan, R. (2006, June 29). A brief history of telemedicine. *Electronic Design.* Retrieved from http://electronicdesign.com/components/brief-history-telemedicine

American Association of Critical-Care Nurses (AACN). (2013). AACN TeleICU nursing practice guidelines. Retrieved from https://telaacn.nursingnetwork.com/page/31201-aacn -tele-icu-nursing-practice-guidelines

American Association for Retired Persons (AARP). (2009). Chronic conditions among older Americans. Retrieved from http://assets.aarp.org/rgcenter/health/beyond_50_hcr_conditions.pdf

American Association for Retired Persons (AARP). (2014). Livable communities baby boomer facts and figures. Retrieved from http://www.aarp.org/livable-communities/info-2014/livable -communities-facts-and-figures.html

American Telemedicine Association (ATA). (2010). Telemedicine defined. Retrieved from http://www.americantelemed.org/i4a/pages/index.cfm?pageid=3333

American Telemedicine Association (ATA). (2014). Guidelines for TeleICU operations. Retrieved from http://www.americantelemed.org/docs/default-source/standards/guidelines-for-teleicu -operations.pdf?sfvrsn=2

American Telemedicine Association (ATA). (2015). Letter to the Telehealth Workgroup. Retrieved from http://www.americantelemed.org/docs/default-source/policy/ata-comments -on-21st-century-telehealth-package.pdf

American Telemedicine Association (ATA). (2016). 2016 ATA Innovation in Remote Healthcare Award Nominee: Extreme Health. Retrieved from http://www.americantelemed.org/docs /default-source/annual-meeting-2016/extreme-health.pdf

Bacarach, D., & Froclich, J. (2016, May 20). Retail clinics drive new healthcare utilization and that is a good thing. *Health Affairs Blog.* Retrieved from http://healthaffairs.org/blog/2016 /05/20/retail-clinics-drive-new-health-care-utilization-and-that-is-a-good-thing/

Bendixen, R., Levy, C., Lutz, B., Horn, K., Chronister, K., & Mann, W. (2008). A telerehabilitation model for victims of polytrauma. *Rehabilitation Nursing, 33*(5), 215–220. Retrieved from ProQuest Nursing & Allied Health Source (Document ID: 1550211771).

Buerhaus, P., Auerbach, D., & Staiger, D. (2009). The recent surge in nurse employment: Causes and implications. *Health Affairs, 28*(4), 657–668.

Centers for Disease Control and Prevention (CDC). (2005). Chronic disease overview. Retrieved from http://www.cdc.gov/chronicdisease/overview/index.htm

Craig, J., & Patterson, V. (2005). Introduction to the practice of telemedicine. *Journal of Telemedicine and Telecare, 11*(1), 3–9. Retrieved from ProQuest Psychology Journals database (Document ID: 805776671).

CVSHealth. (2015). CVS Health to partner with direct-to-consumer telehealth providers to increase access to physician care. Retrieved from https://cvshealth.com/newsroom/press -releases/cvs-health-partner-direct-consumer-telehealth-providers-increase-access

Dansky, K., Vasey, J., & Bowles, K. (2008). Impact of telehealth on clinical outcomes in patients with heart failure. *Clinical Nursing Research, 17*(3), 182. Retrieved from Health Module (Document ID: 1521037211).

Demiris, G., Doorenbos, A., & Towle, C. (2009). Ethical considerations regarding the use of technology for older adults: The case of telehealth. *Research in Gerontological Nursing, 2*(2), 128–136. Retrieved from ProQuest Nursing & Allied Health Source (Document ID: 1757456631).

Dorsey, E. R., & Topol, E. J. (2016). State of telehealth. *The New England Journal of Medicine, 375*(2), 154–161.

Elliott, T., Brossart, D., Berry, J., & Fine, P. (2008). Problem-solving training via videoconferencing for family caregivers of persons with spinal cord injuries: A randomized controlled trial. *Behaviour Research and Therapy, 46*(11), 1220. Retrieved from Psychology Module (Document ID: 1588 750351).

Goran, S. F. (2011). A new view: Tele-intensive care unit competencies. *Critical Care Nurse, 31*(5), 17–29. doi: 10.4037/ccn2011552

Health Resources Services Administration. (n.d.). What is telehealth? Retrieved from http ://www.hrsa.gov/healthit/toolbox/RuralHealthITtoolbox/Telehealth/whatistelehealth.html

IMS Research. (2013). Telehealth to reach 1.8 million patients by 2017. Retrieved from http://www.imsresearch.com/press-release/Telehealth_to_Reach_18_Million_Patients_by_2017

Jia, H., Chuang, H., Wu, S., Wang, X., & Chumbler, N. (2009). Long-term effect of home telehealth services on preventable hospitalization use. *Journal of Rehabilitation Research and Development, 46*(5), 557–566. Retrieved from Health Module (Document ID: 1884235751).

Kaplan, B., & Litweka, S. (2008). Ethical challenges of telemedicine and telehealth. *Cambridge Quarterly of Healthcare Ethics, 17*(4), 401–416. Retrieved from Health Module (Document ID: 1540615491).

Kinsella, A. (2004). Obesity and new applications for home telehealth care. *Home Health Care Technology Report, 1*(3), 36–45.

Lancaster, P., Krumm, M., Ribera, J., & Klich, R. (2008). Remote hearing screenings via telehealth in a rural elementary school. *American Journal of Audiology, 17*(2), 114–122. Retrieved from ProQuest Nursing & Allied Health Source (Document ID: 1623340331).

Leimig, R., Gower, G., Thompson, D., & Winsett, R. (2008). Infection, rejection, and hospitalizations in transplant recipients using telehealth. *Progress in Transplantation, 18*(2), 97–102. Retrieved from ProQuest Nursing & Allied Health Source (Document ID: 1537443161).

Medicare Patient Advisory Commission (MEdpAC). 2016. Report to the Congress. Medicare and the Healthcare Delivery System. Retrieved from http://medpac.gov/documents/reports/march -2016-report-to-the-congress-medicare-payment-policy.pdf

National Pharmaceutical Council. (2013). Medication compliance/adherence. Retrieved from http://www.npcnow.org/issue/medication-complianceadherence

Pennsylvania Homecare Association & Pennsylvania State University. (2004). *2003–2004 telehealth project evaluation year two: The impact of telehealth on nursing workload and retention* [Unpublished report].

Polinski, J. M., Barker, T., Gagliano, N., Sussman, A., Brennan, T. A., & Shrank, W. H. (2016). Patients' satisfaction with and preference for telehealth visits. *Journal of General Internal Medicine, 31*(3), 269–275. doi:10.1007/s11606-015-3489-x

Polisena, J., Coyle, D., Coyle, K., & McGill, S. (2009). Home telehealth for chronic disease management: A systematic review and an analysis of economic evaluations. *International Journal of Technology Assessment in Health Care, 25*(3), 339–49. Retrieved from ProQuest Nursing & Allied Health Source (Document ID: 1797842261).

Prial, S., & Hoss, S. (2009). Overview of home telehealth. In D. McGonigle & K. Mastrian (Eds.), *Nursing informatics and the foundation of knowledge* (pp. 265–281). Sudbury, MA: Jones and Bartlett.

Quality Insights of Pennsylvania. (2005). *Home telehealth reference 2005* [Unpublished report].

Skiba, D. J. (1998). Health-oriented telecommunications in nursing informatics. In M. J. Ball et al. (Eds.), *Where caring and technology meet* (pp. 40–53). New York, NY: Springer.

St George, I., Baker, J., Karabatsos, G., Brimble, R., Wilson, A., & Cullen, M. (2009). How safe is telenursing from home? *Collegian: Journal of the Royal College of Nursing Australia, 16*(3), 119–123.

Stern, D. J. (2007, January/February). Intuitive system monitors resident behavior patterns. *Assisted Living Consult, 3*(1), 21–25.

Strauss, A. (2010). Robot doctors bring specialty care to rural areas. Retrieved from http://suite101 .com/a/robot-doctors-bring-specialty-care-to-rural-areas-a231775

Swinton, J., Robinson, W., & Bischoff, R. (2009). Telehealth and rural depression: Physician and patient perspectives. *Families, Systems & Health, 27*(2), 172. Retrieved from Health Module (Document ID: 1793129471).

TechTarget. (n.d.) A guide to healthcare IoT possibilities and obstacles. Retrieved from http://searchhealthit.techtarget.com/essentialguide/A-guide-to-healthcare-IoT-possibilities -and-obstacles

Totten, A., Womack, D., Eden, K., McDonagh, M., Griffin, J., Grusing, S., & Hersh, W. (2016). Telehealth: Mapping the evidence for patient outcomes from systematic reviews. Technical Brief No. 26. (Prepared by the Pacific Northwest Evidence-based Practice Center under Contract No. 290-2015-00009-I.) AHRQ Publication No.16-EHC034-EF. Rockville, MD: Agency for Healthcare Research and Quality. Retrieved from http://www.effectivehealthcare.ahrq .gov/reports/final.cfm

U.S. Department of Commerce, Bureau of the Census. (2006). Oldest baby boomers turn 60! Retrieved from http://www.census.gov/newsroom/releases/pdf/cb06-ffse01-2.pdf

U.S. Department of Commerce, Bureau of the Census. (2010). The next four decades: The older population in the United States: 2010 to 2050. Retrieved from http://www.census.gov/prod/2010pubs/p25-1138.pdf

Venable, S. (2005). A call to action: Georgia must adopt a new standard of care, licensure, reimbursement, and privacy laws for telemedicine. *Emory Law Journal, 54*(2), 1183–1217. Retrieved from Law Module database (Document ID: 875322011).

Weinstein, R. S., Lopez, A. M., Joseph, B. A., Erps, K. A., Holcomb, M., Barker, G. P., & Krupinski, E. A. (2014). Telemedicine, telehealth, and mobile health applications that work: Opportunities and barriers. *The American Journal of Medicine, 127*(3), 183–187. doi:10.1016/j.amjmed.2013.09.032

Williams, L., Hubbard, K. E., Daye, O., & Barden, C. (2012). Tele-ICU enhancements: Telenursing in the intensive care unit: Transforming nursing practice. *Critical Care Nurse, 32*(6), 62–69. doi: 10.4037/ccn2012525

# Education Applications of Nursing Informatics

Nursing informatics (NI) provides more tools and capabilities than can at times be imagined. Just as NI has changed the way nursing is administered and practiced, so it has also dramatically affected nursing education practices.

Nursing education is evolving with the increased integration of NI and other technology tools to promote learning. The tools that are available must be used prudently by reflecting on and applying knowledge on teaching styles, learning styles, and other pedagogic concerns. As informatics capabilities continue to expand, a phenomenal amount of potential for virtual reality–embedded education looms on the horizon. Once the purview of gamers and geeks, virtual reality has exploded onto the academic scene. The use of virtual reality has the potential for cross-pollination between fields of inquiry across the curriculum, the university, and even learning systems. Many university departments will experiment with virtual reality in hopes of staying current and appealing to their young and demanding "Generation Next" constituency. However, much of society loves the feel of books too much to dismiss them as archaic. There is room for both books and technology in education. Students, educators, and administrators will ultimately return to a modified form of face-to-face classroom teaching, even with the availability of newer and more adventuresome teaching technologies. Furthermore, after fast, highburn technologies stop flooding the marketplace and big business provides opportunities for proprietary online universities, modified traditions will take their place, creating new spaces for nontraditional students and members of the Net Generation, with both being anxious for technology use in the classroom for very different reasons.

The material in this book is placed within the context of the Foundation of Knowledge model (**Figure V-1**) to meet the needs of healthcare delivery systems, organizations, patients, and nurses. Nursing education promotes scholarship and evidence-based teaching and learning. Through the sound integration of information management and technology tools, teaching and learning strategies promote the social and intellectual growth of the learner. As teachers and learners quest for knowledge, the need for pursuit of lifelong learning is instilled. Teachers and learners involved in the process of education are also involved with all levels of the model. Typically, they acquire and process data and information and generate and disseminate knowledge within the frame of reference of their educational institution. Their knowledge generation remains on a limited, individual/course/school basis unless they become involved with developing publications and educational research that informs others in the nursing profession.

The reader of this section is challenged to ask the following questions: (1) How can I apply the knowledge I gain from my education to benefit my patients and enhance my practice? (2) How can I help my colleagues, patients, and fellow students understand and use the current technologies to promote learning? (3) How can I use my wisdom to help create the theories, tools, and knowledge of the future?

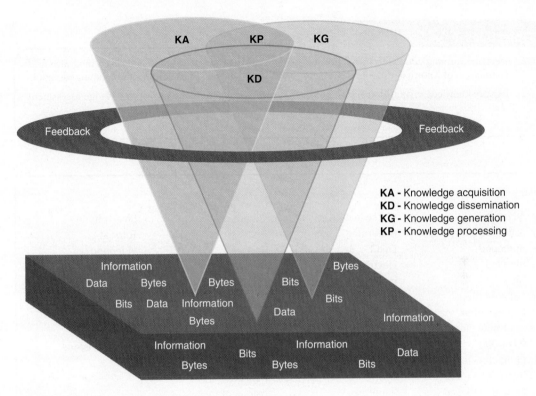

**Figure V-1** Foundation of Knowledge Model
Designed by Alicia Mastrian.

## Key Terms

- Advocate
- Asynchronous
- Audiopod
- Blended
- Blog
- Collaboration
- Compact disk read-only memory (CD-ROM)
- Computer-assisted instruction (CAI)
- Computer-based
- Continuing education
- Copyright
- Digital versatile disk/digital video disk (DVD)
- Distance education
- E-learning
- Email
- Electronic mailing list
- Evidence
- Face-to-face
- Fair use
- Foundation of Knowledge model
- Hybrid
- Hypertext
- Information literacy
- Instant message (IM)
- iPod
- MP3 aggregator
- Multimedia
- Net Generation
- Online chats
- Podcast
- Portal
- Portfolio
- Problem-based
- Professional networking
- Real time
- Really simple syndication (RSS)
- Reflective commentary
- Resource description framework (RDF)
- Role playing
- Scenario
- Simulations
- Smartphone
- Tutorial
- Videopod
- Virtual reality
- Web-based
- Webcast
- Web-enhanced
- Webinar
- Web publishing
- Wiki

# CHAPTER 19

# Nursing Informatics and Nursing Education

Heather E. McKinney, Sylvia DeSantis, Kathleen Mastrian, and Dee McGonigle

## Introduction: Nursing Education and the Foundation of Knowledge Model

Nursing informatics facilitates the integration of information, data, and knowledge to support nurses, patients, and other providers in their various settings and decision-making roles. The **Foundation of Knowledge model** specifically prompts nurses to extend their theoretical and metaphorical knowledge into practical, holistic determinations based on a variety of factors and contexts. Because competencies in informatics include but are not limited to **information literacy**, computer literacy, and the ability to use strategies and system applications to manage data, knowledge, and information, the ability of nursing students to use computer-mediated communication skills is essential to their success in the nursing field and as a means to improve patient safety.

The rise of telecommunications, computer-mediated communications, and virtual technologies has opened up opportunities for improving communication and extending care within the healthcare industry (Barnes & Rudge, 2005). Proponents of instructional applications of computer technology view it as a way to erase geographic boundaries for students, enhance the presentation of content, improve learning outcomes, and even tailor instruction to individual learning needs. When carefully matched with curricular objectives, technology becomes an efficient and affordable avenue through which nursing faculty may provide useful knowledge to their students, thereby facilitating the learning process (Hebda & Czar, 2013). Now going far beyond the simple applications of word processing software or spreadsheets, technology applications have evolved greatly, taking advantage of modern capabilities to provide nursing and related healthcare students with simulations, complex multimedia, virtual reality–assisted clinical scenarios, and a host of information and literature-gathering Internet tools.

# Knowledge Acquisition and Sharing

The shift from computer literacy to information literacy and management has drawn attention to interactivity and design as the most important components of interactive **Web-enhanced** and **Web-based** courses in providing effective learning environments. Thurmond (2003) and Thurmond and Wamback (2002) discussed the four types of interactions related to Web-enhanced courses based on their literature reviews: (1) learner– learner, (2) learner–content, (3) learner–instructor, and (4) learner–interface interactions (Thurmond & Wamback, 2002, para. 1). In traditional learner–learner exchanges, students interact with one another to troubleshoot, work out challenges, and exchange solutions generated from different perspectives. Traditional and familiar, both learner–content and learner–instructor interactions expect students to work directly with course content or the faculty member and then participate in relevant course activities, such as tests and reviews. Learner–interface interaction includes the ways students access their coursework and their ultimate success or failure in finding, retrieving, and using what they need (Thurmond, 2003; Thurmond & Wambach 2002). See Figure 19-1 for a graphic depiction of these interactions. When Web enhanced, these interactions include **online chats**, forum discussions, participation in electronic mailing list groups, instant messaging, blogging, and use of email, all of which ask the student to engage, digest, use, and disseminate information in new ways.

# Evolution of Learning Management Systems

In the 21st century, nursing informatics emphasized technology usability, functionality, and accessibility in education and practice. **Computer-assisted instruction (CAI)** arrived

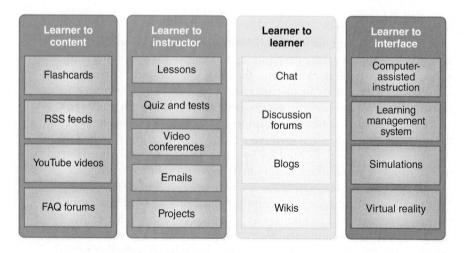

**Figure 19-1** Types of Interactions in Web-Based Courses

Data from Juliano, R. (2016). Best practices guide to converting face to face courses to a distance learning format: Educational technology. Retrieved from http://www.manula.com/manuals/rachael-juliano/best-practices-guide-to-converting -face-to-face-courses-to-a-distance-learning-format/1/en/topic/educational-technology

early on the scene and has had an enormous impact on nursing informatics and nursing education, with many CAI programs offering individualized instruction in the form of customizable scenarios, frameworks, and programs for study. Additionally, CAI contributed to better understanding of material by supporting all learning styles, types, and paces. Consequently, nursing skills–development needs presented endless potential for software development, making the effective use of software and hardware by educators and students a prime necessity (Riley, 1996).

Recall that software comprises the instructions that direct a computer's hardware to work, whereas hardware consists of physical computer components, such as a mouse, keyboard, and monitor. Software essentially translates commands into computer language, allowing the hardware to perform its functions. Without hardware and software, computer technologies are moot; moreover, without software, hardware does not function (McHugh, 2006). Applications software refers to the various programs individuals use to communicate with others, do work, play games, or watch multimedia on a computer. The most common software package sold with computers is an office package, which generally includes a word processing program, spreadsheet capability, a presentation graphics program (e.g., PowerPoint), and some kind of database management system. Software packages are available on **compact disk read-only memory (CD-ROM)**, on **digital versatile disk/digital video disk (DVD)**, or, now most commonly, through the Internet, allowing the user to download the software directly from a vendor's website (McHugh, 2006).

When evaluating software or hardware for purchase, careful assessment of the products and services will help an educator, administrator, or student make the best choices. Most important when evaluating software is to understand how well the software's functionality for computer-assisted learning matches the learning goals and objectives. Although many programs are available for assisting a nurse educator who is evaluating software for particular learning purposes, the main criteria concern content (Is the information accurate? Is it relevant?), format (How is information visually presented? Is it in frames? Does it come with graphics?), documentation style (What is the tone? Is it scholarly and applicable?), and strategies (Is the software useful for all students, including remedial students and accelerated students?) (Edwards & Drury, 2000).

Hardware decisions depend on the way a computer system will be used, in addition to considerations related to cost, ease of use, and durability (Clochesy, 2004). Systems purchased for personal use may differ dramatically from those purchased for online learning laboratories or smart classrooms. Because the technology inherent to workstations, servers, and computers in general tends to change quite rapidly, discussing large system decisions with an information technology expert is likely to yield a better-informed decision. Some factors to consider include where the system will be stationed (e.g., at home for personal use or in a learning laboratory for use by many students), how many desktops there will be (e.g., one or a few dozen), if it will be networked to a school's internal system, if printing will be available, and which level of security is needed (Hebda & Czar, 2013).

As computer-supported learning gained popularity, education innovators realized the need for additional functionality. Integrated learning systems evolved from the earlier uses of computer-based instruction, and offered tracking, content management, and more individualized instruction (Wikipedia, 2016). These early systems primarily supported the administration of the course and content and provided convenience for instructors. According to Brown, Dehoney, and Millichap (2015),

> Higher education is moving away from its traditional emphasis on the instructor, however, replacing it with a focus on learning and the learner. Higher education is also moving away from a standard form factor for the course, experimenting with a variety of course models. These developments pose a dilemma for any LMS [learning management system] whose design is still informed by instructor-centric, one-size-fits-all assumptions about teaching and learning. They also account for the love/hate relationship many in higher education have with the LMS. The LMS is both "it" and "not it"—useful in some ways but falling short in others. (p. 2)

Brown and colleagues also describe the Next Generation Digital Learning Environment (NGDLE) as reimagining the education system. Key characteristics of the NGDLE include:

- *Interoperability and integration:* These allow for seamless exchange, transfer, and utilization of content; the addition of learning tools; and the aggregation, integration, and analysis of learning data.
- *Personalization* supports the ability of instructors, departments, and students to configure the learning environment to meet specific needs.
- *Analytics, advising, and learning assessment:* This component supports learning assessment and assessment of competency-based education and provides data analysis tools for these assessments. It also integrates progress planning and advising functions.
- *Collaboration* may occur within the course among students and instructors, but in the NGDLE collaboration may also occur among disciplines, institutions, and professions, particularly if the system adheres to interoperability standards.
- *Accessibility and universal design:* This component takes into account special needs of persons with disabilities and supports prospective design of accessible features and components.

## Delivery Modalities

Nursing educators are discovering that today's students may not always respond in the same ways the educators did during their own tenure as students. Technology-savvy students from the millennial age demand instant information delivered in an entertaining fashion—an expectation built on extensive exposure to email, text messaging, online chatting, and the Internet (Ridley, 2007). Additionally, many nursing departments are facing an increase in student enrollment and a corresponding growth in faculty. Although new nursing faculty bring significant clinical experience to their academic positions, also apparent for some is an underlying tension and unfamiliarity with technologic advances, outcomes-based accreditation initiatives, and teaching itself. Schools of nursing are scrambling to provide professional development for busy nursing faculty and introducing them to best practices in teaching (Shaffer, Lackey, & Bolling, 2006). See Figure 19-2 for an overview of key digital skills for nurse faculty.

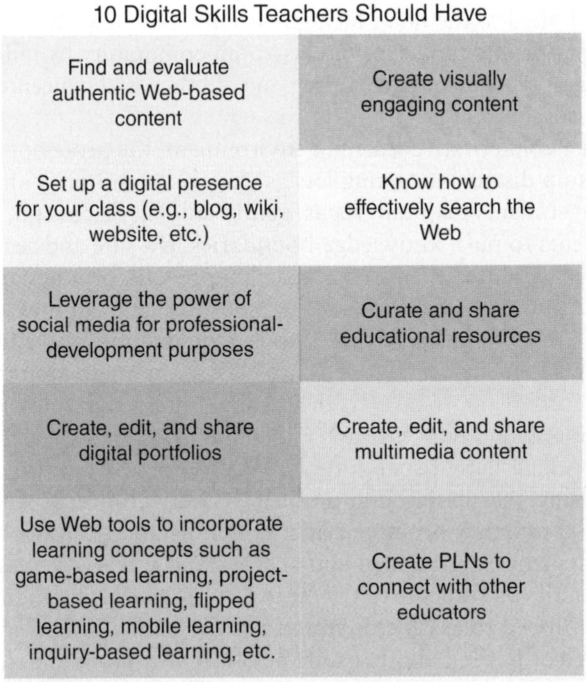

## 10 Digital Skills Teachers Should Have

| | |
|---|---|
| Find and evaluate authentic Web-based content | Create visually engaging content |
| Set up a digital presence for your class (e.g., blog, wiki, website, etc.) | Know how to effectively search the Web |
| Leverage the power of social media for professional-development purposes | Curate and share educational resources |
| Create, edit, and share digital portfolios | Create, edit, and share multimedia content |
| Use Web tools to incorporate learning concepts such as game-based learning, project-based learning, flipped learning, mobile learning, inquiry-based learning, etc. | Create PLNs to connect with other educators |

**Figure 19-2** Ideal Digital Skills for Faculty
Reproduced from Educational Technology and Mobile Learning. (2016). Another excellent poster featuring 10 digital skills for teachers. Retrieved from http://www.educatorstechnology.com/2016/02/another-excellent-poster-featuring-10-digital-skills -for-teachers.html

Learning is a multispatial function, and in the age of technology innovation, instructional delivery can inhabit many forms in both physical and virtual spaces. Spaces in academia are no longer defined by a class or its content, but instead by the learning the class is trying to promote. To this end, learning spaces should support multiple modes of learning and delivery, including reflection, discussion, and experience, and should facilitate face-to-face and online interaction within and beyond classrooms. Truly innovative delivery, whether face-to-face classroom interaction, online engagement, or a blended hybrid of technology and traditional classroom teaching, supports learning activities rather than standing independently of them (Oblinger, 2005).

## Face-to-Face Delivery

Ridley (2007) suggests that although it is the most widely used teaching method among nurse educators, traditional **face-to-face** lecture yields only a 5% information retention rate over a 24-hour period, a rate that compares unfavorably with demonstration (30%), discussion groups (50%), practice activities (75%), and peer teaching (90%; as cited in Sousa, 1995).

Additionally, the inability of physical space to keep pace with evolution of learning models inhibits the benefits gained from face-to-face interaction between teacher and student. For example, collaborative learning grinds to a halt when class is held in a room with chairs bolted to the floor, facing a lectern (Oblinger, 2005); this kind of spatial arrangement prohibits a sense of classroom community by inhibiting easy peer interaction, reducing students' ability to see one another, and concentrating all attention on the professor.

Conversely, in a collaborative learning environment, the professor guides conversation and sets up discussion, acting less as classroom authority and more as facilitator, helping students maintain focus, gently guiding discussion, and ultimately empowering students to push knowledge boundaries in a safe and secure atmosphere of peer support. This inductive, epistemological approach promotes active, critical thinking skills and assists students in learning not just facts, but how to learn. As future healthcare professionals determined to rely on quantification and rationale, nursing students will benefit from face-to-face classroom interaction that hones their ability to manufacture new personal truths through interaction with people and ideas in ways that cannot always be measured and counted.

Ridley (2007) suggests that such interactive, cooperative learning strategies might include gaming, **role playing**, and problem-based learning. Because games are nonthreatening and fun, they promote critical thinking and teamwork by pushing students to work together in groups to find answers and achieve success. Role playing is similar in that it allows students to try on real-life scenarios by filling either pre-scripted or ad-libbed roles (doctor, nurse, patient, clinician, and so forth) without the fear or pressure of putting another's life at risk while trying to determine the best course of action or find a solution for a fictitious patient's health issue.

**Problem-based** learning, a well-accepted form of interactive learning, takes assignments out of a contextual vacuum and applies real-life scenarios to problems or challenges. Students work in groups to solve the dilemma presented by real patient cases and build on prior knowledge, using higher-level thinking skills and progressive inquiry to resolve the problem (Ridley, 2007). This enhances the student's critical skills for acquiring and maintaining knowledge in practice.

## Online Delivery

**E-learning**, online learning, and Web-based education have caused a significant shift in student–teacher relationships in nursing education. According to Oblinger (2005), not only are learning spaces no longer physical or formal, especially on campuses with wireless capabilities, but nursing students also expect to make use of wide ranges of cutting-edge technology during their academic tenure, exchanging the traditional "sage on the stage" for a technologically savvy "guide on the side" (Leasure, Davis, & Thievon, 2000) who gives up the role of gatekeeper and instead promotes and facilitates dialogue as central to teaching–learning (Aquino-Russell, Maillard Strüby, & Reviczky, 2007).

Student-centered and no longer limited to the domain of the classroom, laboratory, or even a patient's bedside, online learning allows educators to translate theory into practice, creating a virtual classroom space that promotes **collaboration**, engagement, discussion, and analysis. Detractors of online learning initiatives suggest, however, that sharing an online space undermines the student–teacher relationship, makes building peer relationships difficult, and generally disrupts the normal classroom dynamic, thereby creating an unfamiliar, uncomfortable atmosphere. Despite these concerns, studies show that not only do Web-based courses continue to gain in popularity, but they also enhance learning in ways that encourage students to share personal experiences and support. Researchers cite many factors that make online learning laudable, with accessibility and convenience being two of the most frequently cited issues (Aquino-Russell, Maillard Strüby, & Reviczky, 2007).

The **asynchronous** and time-independent elements of Web-based courses respond to the huge need for flexible class times among today's growing population of nontraditional learners. Additionally, Web-based and place-independent learning allows participation by anyone, anywhere in the world, with access. Exposure to online learning during healthcare professional education programs will facilitate continuing professional education during the practice tenure. Related to this issue is the democratizing effect of online learning, such that all students have the same opportunity to participate without judgment. Web-based classes provide an easily accessible permanent record, a convenience for both teachers and learners (Aquino-Russell, Maillard Strüby, & Reviczky, 2007).

It is important to use tools that facilitate learning, such as the introduction of social media into nursing education. Twitter (www.twitter.com) can be used to focus and hone student perspectives. Each posting or tweet cannot exceed 140 characters. As they critically think about what they want to add to the discussion, students must act as wordsmiths to express their views succinctly given the character limitation; that is, they must present their viewpoints concisely. Other social media that can be used in education include the following sites:

- Diigo (www.diigo.com), a social bookmarking tool to collect, tag, and share online sources (Meyer, 2015)
- Feedly (www.feedly.com), an online feed aggregator to notify the subscriber of new content on blogs and websites of interest (Meyer, 2015)
- Flickr (www.flickr.com), for photo sharing
- Glogster (www.glogster.com), a graphical blog
- Instagram (www.instagram.com), for customizing and sharing photos and videos (Meyer, 2015)
- Pinterest (www.pinterest.com), a social bookmarking tool used to prime discussions (Meyer, 2015)
- Pixton (www.pixton.com), to create comics or cartoons
- Prezi (www.prezi.com), to create zooming presentations
- Scoop.it (www.scoop.it), an online content curation tool used to collect Web resources, comment on them, and publish the source and commentary (Meyer, 2015)
- Slideshare (www.slideshare.net), a community for sharing presentations
- YouTube (www.youtube.com), to watch and share videos
- VoiceThread (www.voicethread.com), to share images, videos, documents, and commentary (Meyer, 2015)
- Wordle (www.wordle.net), to create word clouds from text

These sites can be used by students to facilitate their presentations and team collaboration. The use of social media not only exposes the students to their use but also promotes the development of skills that will support professional collaboration as students enter the practice arena. Meyer (2015) reported that using social media in education helps students put concepts in context, maintains currency in course content, and fosters a sense of community. **Figure 19-3** demonstrates the purposes and time required for proper use of social media.

## Hybrid or Blended Delivery

Traditional courses are more frequently being offered as online, virtual classes (i.e., **distance education**)—learning that occurs elsewhere than in the traditional classroom and consequently requires special course design, planning, techniques, and communication. A **hybrid** of this delivery mode includes learning in which traditional classroom time is enhanced or broken up with online components, thereby creating a class in which **blended** hybrid learning occurs. Forms of hybrid learning include Web-enhanced learning, such as asking students to **blog** responses to a reading or class discussion, and learning that takes place in and makes use of smart classrooms (e.g., teaching in a wired room equipped with classroom learning technologies, such as the Blackboard Learning System).

Smart classrooms, also known as digital and multimedia classrooms, integrate computer and audiovisual technologies by providing a ceiling-mounted projector with an access point at the front of the room, an instructor podium or workstation, sound, and network access. An enhanced smart classroom also provides networked student workstations instead of traditional desks, allowing students to follow along

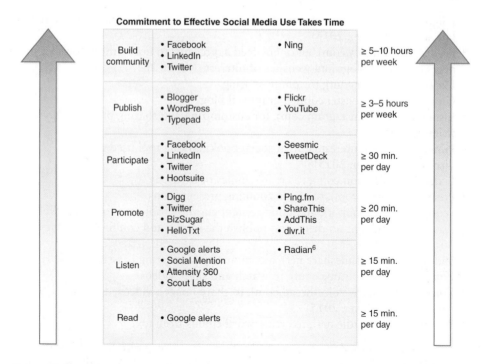

| Commitment to Effective Social Media Use Takes Time | | | |
|---|---|---|---|
| Build community | • Facebook<br>• LinkedIn<br>• Twitter | • Ning | ≥ 5–10 hours per week |
| Publish | • Blogger<br>• WordPress<br>• Typepad | • Flickr<br>• YouTube | ≥ 3–5 hours per week |
| Participate | • Facebook<br>• LinkedIn<br>• Twitter<br>• Hootsuite | • Seesmic<br>• TweetDeck | ≥ 30 min. per day |
| Promote | • Digg<br>• Twitter<br>• BizSugar<br>• HelloTxt | • Ping.fm<br>• ShareThis<br>• AddThis<br>• dlvr.it | ≥ 20 min. per day |
| Listen | • Google alerts<br>• Social Mention<br>• Attensity 360<br>• Scout Labs | • Radian[6] | ≥ 15 min. per day |
| Read | • Google alerts | | ≥ 15 min. per day |

**Figure 19-3** Social Media Time Estimates

Data from The Social Observer. (2016). Find 10 tips that help you take time to be social. Retrieved from http://www.thesocialobserver.com/take-time-to-be-social

online and perform network or Web searches, chat, blog, or myriad other activities as dictated by the professor. For example, at the Penn State College of Nursing, users can access announcements, course materials, faculty information, websites, and other tools through the electronic course management system, enabling the nursing faculty to extend learning beyond the physical classroom walls.

## Competency-Based Learning

More robust learning management systems (LMSs) are particularly well suited to support competency-based learning. Nursing competencies have been well defined by professional and accrediting organizations such as Quality and Safety Education for Nurses (QSEN); the American Association of Colleges of Nursing (AACN), through its Technology Informatics Guiding Education Reform (TIGER) initiative and the essentials of nursing education delineated for undergraduate and graduate study; and informatics competencies promoted by the Healthcare Information and Management Systems Society (HIMSS). As the U.S. Department of Education (2014) explained,

> *Transitioning away from seat time, in favor of a structure that creates flexibility, allows students to progress as they demonstrate mastery of academic content, regardless of time, place, or pace of learning. Competency-based strategies provide flexibility in the way that credit can be earned or awarded, and provide students with personalized learning opportunities. (para. 1)*

Database technologies within LMSs offer the ability to track competency achievement, as Pijl-Zieber, Barton, Konkin, Awosoga, and Caine (2014) explain: "Such technologies could be shared, at least to some degree, between nursing student and nursing instructor, much like clinical evaluation tools are shared on paper, to jointly track skills, knowledge, abilities, critical thinking, clinical reflection, and developing competence" (p. 677).

# Technology Tools Supporting Education

Certain social trends emerging from the morass of both traditional and innovative technology tools include the use of technologies attempting to meet the needs of members of the **Net Generation** or Millennial Generation. These are students who have grown up inside a wired world of instant access and online everything who are connected, digital, experiential, and social learners. Through the use of software, hardware, drivers, dedicated servers, plug-ins, and an Internet connection, students can chat, collaborate, play games, or interact electronically with a peer in some way, all with little to no learning curve or effort. Because visual media are now the vernacular of this highly digital culture, students and faculty are also embracing technology tools that allow for the creation and interpretation of visual images (Oblinger, 2005). Such tools might take the shape of interactive tutorials, a created city within a virtual reality landscape, high-fidelity simulations, serious games, or even a multimedia action maze that prompts users to choose different outcomes within a scenario. Regardless of the particular tool employed, technology can perform only as well as the pedagogy that drives it, thus creating a need for integration, support, and sustainability within nursing education programs willing to implement new instructional and assessment strategies (Bassendowski, 2005).

## Tutorials

The modern **tutorial** mimics lectures by guiding users through a series of objectives or tasks, usually allowing the user to do the work at his or her own pace (Edwards & Drury, 2000). Tutorials generally stand alone as autonomous multimedia that may use animation, text, graphics, sound, questions, and different kinds of interactivity to engage and intrigue the user. They tend to promote active learning by prompting the user to answer sets of questions, follow clickable **hypertext**, or complete quizzes. For example, users might be asked to fill in worksheets after reviewing anatomy concepts, take a quiz, post an answer to a question, or even click through a scenario by choosing the best course of action in a mock clinical situation.

Some tutorials, such as those used by medical students at the Morgan Stanley Children's Hospital of New York, are designed to be brief (10 minutes), interactive, very focused, and immediately relevant. In this case, medical students bustling through a busy clinical rotation who accessed the tutorials actually raised examination grades (Pusic, Pachev, & MacDonald, 2007).

Because most students benefit from being able to contextualize a lesson's framework and purpose, the most effective tutorials provide users with understandable navigation, such as a table of contents at its beginning, or additional navigational aids, such as icons, buttons, or text that indicate where and how they need to progress (Dewald, 1999). Effective tutorials surpass the simple presentation of information in a Web-based format; they instead address certain pedagogic and student-centered needs by identifying and taking into consideration specific factors, such as instructional content, the educator's purpose and teaching goal, the initiative's overall purpose, the potential need for special conceptual input, the learners' ultimate objectives in completing the tutorial, and the standards that determine what qualifies as successful completion of the tutorial (DeSantis, 2002).

Although most tutorials are created to stand alone, some may also benefit and supplement face-to-face instruction, such as the interactive information skills tutorial developed at the Institute for Health and Social Care Research in Salford, United Kingdom. This tutorial divides a traditional lecture series into chunks, incorporating questions that would normally arise during the session into the text, and providing hyperlinks. This organization allows users to browse to different parts of the tutorial, open a database in a new window to perform a practice search, and access other features (Grant & Brettle, 2006). Tutorials in all their iterations urge students to hone and develop effective critical thinking skills. Short tutorials may also be created on an organization's intranet to educate practicing professionals on a new policy, procedure, organizational initiative, or healthcare technology. Since the tutorial is electronic, access and time spent on the tutorial can be easily tracked.

## Case Scenarios

Professional organizations are increasingly recommending performance-based assessments of students in professional degree programs, and enacting case scenarios provides an opportunity for students to practice procedural responses and improve patient safety. The case **scenario**, a form of problem-based learning, has evolved and is now available through simulation software and virtual reality programming. This kind of learning assessment, in which students must respond within context to a perceived situation rather than a theoretical or fact-based question, allows educators to gauge procedural knowledge; it allows them to determine how well a student executes a skill or applies concepts and principles to specific situations (Garavalia, 2002). For example, in a clinical context, a student could explain a specific procedure, but such knowledge is declarative rather than procedural and, therefore, for some evaluators, not as valuable. Conditional knowledge is often also reflected in procedural knowledge, demonstrating a student's ability to know when and why action is or is not taken, and how. As more programs move toward interprofessional education, case scenarios are a great way for students to hone collaboration skills and gain understanding of the roles of other professionals.

## Portfolios

Viewed in the 1980s as realistic evaluative tools of student accomplishment and learning, portfolios in healthcare professional education are growing in popularity as useful tools for documenting students' exposure to educational experiences. A **portfolio** allows a student to document a variety of sometimes unquantifiable skills, such as creativity, communication, and critical thinking. Further, portfolios can reflect achievement of goals, self-evaluation, and professional development, also providing a way for returning students to log and document past work or life experiences in a creative but structured way without taking a standardized test. The usefulness of a portfolio for an undergraduate depends on a structured system of organization: an identification page with a résumé, a table of contents, separate and clearly marked sections, and so forth. In this way, portfolios can monitor program outcomes, positively influence employment and graduate school admission, and provide a clear snapshot of a student's strengths and abilities. See **Box 19-1** for an overview of electronic portfolios, and specific information on developing a professional portfolio.

## Simulations

Used within healthcare circles for more than 15 years, **simulations** in nursing education have experienced a recent upsurge in popularity, in part due to the more widespread availability of high-quality simulation equipment and a reduction in price for this technology. Ranked by fidelity, or the level of realism the equipment resembles, simulation may take various forms: from computer-based simulation, in which software is used to simulate a subject or situation (e.g., an interactive tutorial featuring a nurse–patient situation), to full-scale simulation, in which all the elements of a healthcare situation are recreated using real physiology, people, and interaction to resemble an environment as closely as possible to immerse students in the experience (Seropian, Brown, Gavilanes, & Driggers, 2004). Simulation scenarios aid nursing instructors in assessing competency achievement. For a more comprehensive discussion of simulation as a teaching/learning tool, please see Chapter 20, *Simulation, Gaming Mechanics, and Virtual Worlds in Nursing Education.*

## BOX 19-1 WHAT IS AN ELECTRONIC PORTFOLIO?

*Glenn Johnson and Jeff Swain*

Today's information technology infrastructure allows users to easily build Web-based collections that include **evidence** of their knowledge and skills. Users can upload artifacts that represent evidence of their learning experiences both inside and outside of the classroom. Electronic portfolios (e-portfolios) may also contain a blog element where students reflect on their total experience and demonstrate growth in their areas of study.

E-portfolios can be built using a range of different technologies. Some individuals use PowerPoint presentations to capture and present evidence. Web-based e-portfolios are built using common **Web publishing** tools to create webpages, such as Web 2.0 or open source tools; the webpages are then published on the Internet (Barrett, 2012). In addition, an increasing number of institutional e-portfolio systems have emerged through which users can log in and then upload, enter, and share information or evidence related to their experiences. Examples of such systems include the following:

- Association for Authentic, Experiential and Evidence-Based Learning: www.aaeebl.org
- Digication: www.digication.com
- Facebook: www.facebook.com
- iWebfolio: www.iwebfolio.com
- LiveText: www.livetext.com
- MySpace: www.myspace.com
- PebblePAD: www.pebblepad.com
- TaskStream: www.taskstream.com/pub
- TypePad: www.typepad.com

## WHY CREATE AN E-PORTFOLIO?

Although academic institutions may use e-portfolios for assessment of student learning, for the individual, e-portfolios are all about opportunity. Such opportunities might include supporting a working relationship with a mentor, networking with other professionals, or representing certain qualities and characteristics to prospective employers. In all of these cases, having gone through the process of developing an e-portfolio requires critical examination of which qualities make individuals who they are and why these qualities are important to them and their profession. It is important for all professionals to have a foundational understanding of where they are in their career trajectory and how this fits their long-term professional goals.

Practically speaking, e-portfolios are efficient. When introducing oneself in an email message, a self-starting individual who has taken the initiative to develop and publish an e-portfolio can add this line to the message: "Here is a link to my e-portfolio." The recipient can click on this link, which automatically opens that individual's e-portfolio in a Web browser. Metaphorically, the senders of such messages have just walked into the recipient's office with information that illustrates who they are, what they know, what they can do, and what they value as important; they have just walked in with what could be a multimedia showcase of their qualities. The Internet is a very powerful communication medium, and individuals with professional e-portfolios are simply taking advantage of this fact.

## E-PORTFOLIOS IN HIGHER EDUCATION

As an instructional strategy, portfolios have been around for a long time. Instructionally, portfolios, whether electronic or paper based, require students to demonstrate or provide evidence that they have attained specific learning outcomes. For instance, in the arts, portfolios have been used to demonstrate the depth and breadth of the work of an artist. Although performance-based programs of study are more likely to be familiar with the concept of the portfolio as a demonstration of what a student knows and can do, other areas of study have also begun to adopt this method of assessment.

Portfolios can be particularly helpful in areas where higher-level thinking and analysis are essential. For instance, being a good healthcare professional encompasses much more than simply being able to get high scores on examinations. Professionals need to be able to collect information, analyze the information presented, relate it to past experience, apply related knowledge, and evaluate various options, and from this present a diagnosis and a plan of action. In short, healthcare professionals need to be able to think critically and make informed decisions. In learning to become a healthcare professional, portfolios can be used to capture, support, and improve this type of thinking as it develops.

Like the artist, the healthcare professional student can connect, share, and present cases and findings and include with this evidence the **reflective commentary** that serves to unveil how he or she arrived at a decision, which information or experiences were vital, and how his or her action plan evolved. However, given the vast variety of evidence that individuals might potentially use to represent themselves, what should one select and how should this be shared?

## E-PORTFOLIOS FOR PROFESSIONAL DEVELOPMENT

Using an e-portfolio to support **professional networking** involves a predetermined and focused purpose. This purpose may be to foster better communication between oneself and a mentor, or it may be to establish how what a professional is doing fits with the goals of the institution or perhaps an institution for which the individual would like to work. A professional e-portfolio is evidence based and uses this evidence to make a case that highlights the individual's capacity not only to perform, but also to grow and develop professionally, within his or her chosen field.

## THE E-PORTFOLIO PROCESS

The four steps involved in developing an e-portfolio are recursive in nature, meaning that during the process one can backtrack to fill in missing pieces or reevaluate earlier decisions that were made. The four steps are (1) collect, (2) select, (3) reflect, and (4) connect. See Figure 19-4 for an image of the portfolio creation process.

### Collect

Evidence should demonstrate what a person knows, what he or she can do, or the values that the person holds as being important. When it comes to developing e-portfolios, it is important to think of evidence in very broad terms. This evidence might include the results of what someone has learned in courses taken as a student, especially in terms of demonstrating a new skill or increased knowledge of a subject. More importantly, evidence can come from experiences that take place outside of the classroom. For instance, someone may have been involved in an internship or clinical observation where he or she had the opportunity to connect what was learned in the classroom with how this information is applied in a real-world setting. Not only is such an experience valuable, but it also represents the individual's understanding of how this knowledge can be applied; thus it enhances others' perception of the depth of what the person knows.

Résumés are evidence documents. They are very important, and every professional should have an updated copy available. However, résumés simply list an individual's experiences or accomplishments. E-portfolios, by comparison, go beyond the résumé to emphasize personal attributes that are very important in the specific profession. These attributes include, but are not limited to, interpersonal skills, leadership skills, appreciation of diversity, ability to work in a team, and self-sufficiency. These attributes are difficult, if not impossible, to demonstrate in a résumé. When reflective commentary accompanies evidence of an individual's involvement, these attributes and values can become the highlights of an e-portfolio.

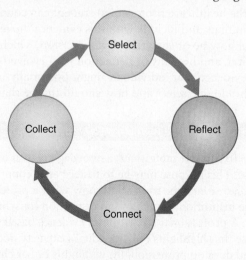

**Figure 19-4** Portfolio Creation Process

### Select

Everyone has his or her own unique pool of evidence from which to pull, and over time this evidence pool can become quite large. What will someone choose to feature and why? Putting together a professional e-portfolio requires that two intertwining questions related to purpose and audience be addressed.

What is the purpose? What is it that someone is attempting to gain by putting an e-portfolio together? Is the purpose related to personal development (i.e., feedback and advice about the professional direction that is being taken)? Is the purpose to connect with colleagues? An individual may, for example, be interested in using his or her e-portfolio to find a job or to gain admission into a graduate program.

Although an e-portfolio can link to everything that a person has accomplished, this may not be the best strategy. Instead, it is essential that an individual consider the audience and establish a plan that enables the person to select the most appropriate pieces of evidence for his or her particular purpose and audience. A helpful way to start is to select the top five pieces of evidence that support the plan. Next, the individual should consider why he or she selected these pieces of evidence. What is it about each piece of evidence that makes it representative of who the individual is, what he or she knows, what he or she can do, and what he or she values as important?

### Reflect

Reflection and reflective commentary take an e-portfolio to the next level. This component may take the form of a single reflective statement, or it may be attached to the evidence throughout the e-portfolio. Reflective comments should open up a window into why an individual thinks this evidence is important, the ways in which the individual values what he or she learned, or why the person thinks it is important for the larger profession. For instance, the individual may present an experience where he or she was challenged to provide assistance. Describing this experience would be important; however, the reflective comments can extend this description, enabling the person to talk about the alternatives considered as the basis for how he or she made a decision to provide the specific type of assistance and the manner in which it was provided. By itself, a description of this experience is good. With reflective comments, readers have a much more thorough perception of and insight into an individual's professional thinking. This is where having a blog element as part of an e-portfolio becomes extremely powerful.

Unlike static webpages, a blog page is a space designed to be interactive. The blog owner posts commentary, thoughts, and experiences for others to read and respond to. Regular entries on a blog give others a reason to return to one's e-portfolio site over and over again. It is an opportunity to share one's perspective on topics of interest and critical to the chosen field. A blog is a place where conversation happens. It provides a nice counterbalance to the static webpages, such as a résumé and project pieces.

Most blogging platforms allow users to select from a range of templates that include a blogging element along with static webpages. Such platforms as WordPress,

Moveable Type, and Google are free for at least the basic service, enabling the user to create a dynamic e-portfolio without having to build webpages. Most platforms allow entries to be in both text and multimedia format, so the blog becomes the perfect place for personal expression. A blog is quickly becoming a standard part of an e-portfolio.

### Connect (Connections) and Feedback

The connection and feedback step is important to validate the assertions someone makes about what it is he or she knows, understands, or values. Individuals may choose to receive feedback from those who are close to them and from here reach out to others who may provide different perspectives. For instance, if a healthcare professional was thinking about using his e-portfolio to apply for a position, he might want to start by first getting feedback from friends and family. He might also share his e-portfolio with a mentor or faculty member, raising the bar by getting professionally grounded feedback before sharing the e-portfolio with a prospective employer.

## CHALLENGES AND ISSUES: PRIVACY AND SECURITY

The ease and popularity of both Web-based social networking and professional e-portfolio tools also raises several challenges and issues for users. Never before has information for individuals been so accessible, and never before has such personal information been so readily made public. For this reason, issues related to privacy and security need to be addressed. What might be appropriate socially can be deadly in a professional context.

## E-PORTFOLIO PROCESS: SUMMARY COMMENTS

In summary, one might think about the process of developing a professional e-portfolio as boiling down to the telling of a rather simple story, albeit a story that has three parts: looking back, looking around, and looking ahead. Readers should think of their own evidence pool as they answer these questions:

1. Looking back: What have you done? In which activities and with which organizations have you been involved? Where have you been? With whom have you worked? How did this help get you where you are today?
2. Looking around: In what are you currently involved? Why are you doing this? What are you getting out of it?
3. Looking ahead: Where would you like to be in 2 years? Where would you like to be in 5 years? Why do you feel this way? What makes you think your goals are realistic?

## REFERENCE

Barrett, H. (2012). ePortfolios. Retrieved from http://www.electronicportfolios.org /eportfolios/index.html

## Virtual Reality

In traditional **virtual reality**, the user receives multiple sensory inputs, either mediated or generated by a computer, through visual stimulation (glasses, goggles, and screens), audio input (earphones, microphones, and synthesizers), and touch (smells, gloves, and bodysuits). A form of simulation training once considered a science fiction technology of the future, the use of virtual reality healthcare training is increasing.

Because virtual worlds foster unintentional learning through gamer-like technology in which students discover and create knowledge to accomplish something, rather than experiencing traditional outcome-based learning, their experiences may result in greater comprehension and deeper knowledge. In a virtual clinical scenario, for example, a simulated, immersive environment presents invaluable learning opportunities for the student who is assuming the role of healthcare provider. Faculty can monitor the inter-action and interrupt as necessary to provide advice or suggestions, while students negotiate the real and virtual world components of the scenario and their avatar patients, thereby becoming aware of how, why, and when to apply specific skills within a clinical setting (EDUCAUSE, 2006).

Because so much of the data nurses rely on are complex, and so many patient cues are lacking in concrete language or responses, the animated, immersive, three-dimensional environment of virtual worlds allows students to practice skills, try new ideas, and learn from their mistakes while receiving feedback from educators within a globally networked classroom environment. Virtual reality tools are a great way to implement competency-based education. Some students may struggle to participate in virtual communities for various reasons. Increasing comfort with multidisciplinary learning among students and educators improves patient safety and encourages the refinement of best practices for effective integration of these tools into mainstream education (EDUCAUSE, 2006). Chapter 20, *Simulation, Gaming Mechanics, and Virtual Worlds in Nursing Education*, provides a more comprehensive discussion of this technology.

# Internet-Based Tools

The general consensus in nursing education suggests that any technology that allows users to interact and engage both materials and one another is useful. More specifically, the Foundation of Knowledge model qualifies this observation with the caveat that technology must display user-friendly capabilities to provide benefits to its users, thereby allowing students not just to find information and one another online, but also to engage, challenge, and institute their discoveries. Providing nursing students with easy-to-use, free Internet tools for reaching the first step in this process (gaining access to materials and peers) has been addressed by the proliferation of communication technologies available to any user with an Internet connection. Beyond the gadgetry, with the development of new strategies, practices, applications, and resources in technology comes the need for instructional strategies that not only appeal to this newer generation of students, but also enhance learning. Such strategies, when coupled with easily accessible and highly functional tools, encourage nursing students to see beyond the right answer and to seek out information that encourages them in developing approaches to issues and resolutions for problems (Bassendowski, 2005).

## Digital Books (eBooks)

While most instructors continue to assign print textbooks for course content reading, there is a clear trend toward the development and use of digital books. As Denoyelles, Raible, and Seilhamer (2015) explained, "While some e-textbooks simply reproduce the print experience, others leverage interactive capabilities such as simulation, polling, discussions, and learning analytics" (para. 1). Affordability is one key advantage of eBooks. There is also the possibility of embedded content in the eBook that could provide a link to a multimedia video or a website. Unfortunately, the availability of quality eTexts in many disciplines is lacking. It is a trend worth following in the future.

## Webcasts and Webinars

A **webcast** is a broadcast of a typically live presentation delivered by way of the Web. Webcasts offer great potential for helping students and faculty to engage both information and one another globally, by tapping into students' multiple intelligences to enable them to access what they need. Because of the growing ease of producing streaming video and subsequently delivering it via larger bandwidth, Webcasts have grown in popularity and are especially favored by programs that feature distance education components. Although some institutions create their own Webcast delivery system, most users rely on a few standard providers that, in turn, present the Webcast online. Although these presentations are often delivered live, allowing audience members to participate in the broadcast, many instructors use Webcasts as an access point for prerecorded archives of lectures and presentations by experts whom their students would not otherwise have the opportunity to see or hear. Studies show that students enthusiastically embrace Webcast technology, accessing archived presentations more repeatedly than traditionally filmed sessions of guest lecturers; this dynamic level of engagement aids students in better grasping the subject matter. Like much dynamic technology, Webcasts are an innovative component that keeps students engaged but tends to work best when learners are provided with learning outcomes before viewing them (Bell, 2003).

A **webinar** is a Web-based seminar that uses Web conferencing software that allows educators to share their computer screen and files and interact with their students. According to Moreau (2013), "depending on what type of webinar service you decide to use, there are interactive sections that the audience can use to ask questions" (para. 5). Webinars are typically delivered live but can be recorded. Moreau equates this presentation form to Skype. In our geographically dispersed, online world of learners, webinars provide another avenue for sharing and collaborating.

There is a key difference between webcasts and webinars. Webcasts present material to the audience with limited or no interactivity. By comparison, webinars are generally live, interactive, educational sessions. Both of these venues provide access to the educator and, depending on the level of interactivity, sometimes to other learners.

## Searching

One of the most common and proliferative search tools in technology today is the **wiki.** Wikis are websites or hypertext document collections that allow users to edit and add content in an open-ended forum. The appeal of (and objection to) wikis resides in their ability to let anyone with an interest and an Internet connection participate in a once-exclusive community of knowledge creators and seekers. As an environment that encourages practice and learning, wikis support learning communities where students collaborate online (Skiba, 2007). Higher education has evolved from a place of straightforward knowledge transmission to a place where one strives to become a member of an expert community, and wikis promise to create opportunities for individuals to participate in this community in heretofore untapped ways.

The most objectionable aspects of wikis are their lack of organizing principle (many are organized alphabetically) and the ability for anyone to edit entries, the latter of which creates new intellectual property right challenges. Wikipedia, for example, is the best-known wiki project on the Web; it is an online encyclopedia of sorts whose open access policy regarding its content keeps educators and professionals wary of inaccurate information to be found there (Skiba, 2007). Wikipedia works well as an initial source of information on a topic or as a quick overview reference, but it should not be relied on as a sole source of information. For more information on the appropriate use of Wikipedia, see this online tutorial: https://libraries.psu.edu/how-use-wikipedia-tutorial.

## Instant Messaging

Instant messaging, one of many collaborative Web chat tools available to any user with a computer and Internet access, continues to establish itself as a working, useful tool for informatics learning, providing instant access to and communication among people, information, and technology. Although some **instant message (IM)** services provide voice and video messages, all instant messaging clients provide text in **real time**, allowing users to interact in the form of an on-screen conversation through a technology that is free, is already quite popular with users, is Web based, does not require additional hardware or software, and has a very low learning curve for those few to whom it is unfamiliar. Beyond having a real-time conversation, instant messaging (IMing) an individual allows the user to share links, pictures, and files. This kind of easy accessibility allows students, when logged on, to collaborate; seek real-time help from professors or librarians; and engage others working on questions, studying for clinical examinations, or reviewing information or notes (Chase, 2007).

## Chats and Online Discussions (Blogs)

Real-time chats occur all over the Internet, at each hour of every day. The best-known chat tools are instant messenger clients, but chatting also refers to real-time discussion venues in which users meet in virtual chat rooms to engage in conversations by posting messages; this provides a comfortable, recognizable way of communicating for Net Generation students used to surfing the Web and interacting online. In a chat, students can meet, discuss, and engage one another over any given topic. Chats take various forms, the most complex of which involve highly evolved virtual communities in which users step into various rooms where they interact with other individuals who are in the room at the same time. Initially the exclusive purview of gamers or hardcore programmers creating private online communities, chat rooms now exist for a wide variety of topics and interests.

Web logs, also known as "blogs," have emerged as low-investment and easy-to-use writing tools that, through their very setup and appearance, enhance health professionals' communication, writing, reading, information-gathering, and collaboration skills (Maag, 2005). Blogs are a kind of online journal, created by individuals who then invite comments from visitors to that Web space. Compared to technically complex online projects, such as tutorials and various multimedia, blogs are immediate, free to set up and access with an Internet connection, and easily negotiable by even the technically ambivalent. By their very nature, blogs present a built-in discussion area to the user, so they are especially useful for study groups interested in reflecting on material and evaluating ideas in a collective, collaborative way (Shaffer, Lackey, & Bolling, 2006). Blogs are a great way for students and professionals to reflect on and share clinical experiences and questions with each other. It is important, however, to be mindful of protecting private health information and share within the confines of HIPAA guidelines.

## Electronic Mailing Lists

One low-investment information-gathering tool for use by nursing professionals is membership in an **electronic mailing list**. These electronic discussion groups use **email** to communicate and promote communication and collaboration with others interested in a particular field of study (Hebda & Czar, 2013). Electronic mailing lists have very few requirements to participate—usually just a free subscription and email capability. Such lists are available on any subject, but most share common features, such as the need to subscribe and then log in to participate. The moderators of an electronic mailing list have specific instructions on how to post messages and how to set subscription controls. Posting information means that when a user replies to a topic thread, he or she generally has sent information to every member of the list. Like other technologies, the capabilities of electronic mailing lists continue to change and expand, providing ongoing viability for use in nursing education.

## Portals

Similar to electronic mailing lists in the way they deliver specific information to one's email, a **portal** allows the personalization of a specific website. Portals organize information from webpages into simple menus so that users may choose what they want to view and how they want to view it (Hebda & Czar, 2013). For example, WebMD is one of the most popular and best-known portals, allowing users to create accounts, bookmark their favorite information, and sign up for email notifications. Portals, like most Web technologies, require an Internet connection and a free subscription that allows the user to log in. Portals rely on the registration of users in order to collect information from them to personalize features for each individual user (Hebda & Czar).

## Podcasts: Audiopods and Videopods

A **podcast** is an audio recording linked to the Web that is then downloaded to an MP3 player (Gordon, 2007), a **smartphone,** or a computer where the listener then accesses the recording or video. An outgrowth of the Apple iPod market, podcasts are developed and delivered by way of the Internet and require minimal investment—namely, a microphone, an Internet connection, and (often free) editing software.

Beyond possibilities for global accessibility to whatever information the user may record, podcasts allow for automatic updates in the form of a **really simple syndication (RSS)** (also known as "**resource description framework (RDF)** site summary") feed that lets subscribers receive automatic notification whenever a podcast is updated (Gordon, 2007). Refer to **Box 19-2** for more information.

---

**BOX 19-2 PODCASTS**

*Jackie Ritzko*

A basic Web search using the search term *free nursing podcast* produced over 1 million hits on one search engine. But what does this mean in the context of nursing informatics? The implication is that there are many resources on the Internet that somehow involve podcasts with a nursing focus. How these sites might be of use to a professional in the nursing field is the focus of this feature. Before any discussion of the educational uses of a technology tool can take place, however, there needs to be an understanding of the hardware, software, training, and support that are required to use the tool, as well as the history of the development of the tool.

*Podcast* is a term coined from the words *iPod* and *broadcast*. **iPod** is the name given to a family of portable MP3 players from Apple Computer. MP3 is a common file format for electronic audio files. Audio files—in particular, MP3 files—can contain verbal speech, music, or a combination of both. MP3 files can be played or listened to using an MP3 player. MP3 players can be portable devices, such as the iPod, or simply software that is installed and used on a computer, tablet, or smartphone. Thus a podcast is simply an MP3 file that can be played on an MP3 player. *Broadcast*, in its simplest usage, refers to the ability to send out. In terms of podcasts, broadcasting is the ability to share MP3 files in such a way that the files are delivered to the user whenever new versions are available through a subscription. This ability to share resources and access the most up-to-date resources is a great advantage, especially for the educational community.

We will now discuss podcasts in terms of function, ranging from the more basic to the more advanced functions: finding podcasts, listening to podcasts, creating podcasts, and sharing podcasts. Finding podcasts at a minimal level requires only an Internet connection and a Web browser. As noted earlier, a basic Web search for the term *nursing podcast* found many sites. Performing a basic Web search, however, may provide a user with only limited search capabilities. An **MP3 aggregator** is a program that can facilitate the process of finding, subscribing to, and downloading podcasts. One popular aggregator is Apple Computer's iTunes, which is a free program available as a download from apple.com. Although iTunes is widely used, it is not the only program of this type. A program such as iTunes gives the user the ability to search for podcasts based on many criteria, including category, author, or title. The iTunes program provides access to audio downloads that may be either songs or podcasts. In both cases, users may find downloads that are free and those that require payment.

Because podcasts are largely MP3 audio files (Advanced Audio Coding [AAC] is a newer format, but is not as widely used), an MP3 player is needed to listen to a podcast. As noted, this can be done on a smartphone, a computer with an MP3 player, or a portable MP3 player. Podcasts can be downloaded in two ways: manually or by subscribing to a podcast. In the case of a subscription, once a new track is added to the podcast, iTunes automatically delivers it to a computer. Continuing to use iTunes as an example, once a podcast is found, it can also be manually downloaded from iTunes to a computer. Once on the computer, it can be listened to or transferred to a portable device, or accessed via a tablet or smartphone.

Users may also choose to produce or record podcasts. As with most technology solutions, hardware and software requirements typically must be met to create podcasts. The hardware for recording a podcast can vary. In a stationary setup, a microphone can be connected to a desktop or laptop computer. Stand-alone audio recorders can also record podcasts, and some MP3 players contain built-in recorders. Free recording software is available for most computer platforms.

Sometimes a podcast is created for the sole use of the creator. More often, however, a podcast is created with the intention of it being shared with and listened to by others. Podcasts can be stored on Web servers for distribution and can also be shared via tools, such as iTunes. Within iTunes, for example, educational institutions are able to host podcasts in the area known as iTunesU.

Podcasts have many uses in education in general and in nursing education in particular. Informal learning can take place when a nursing student listens to nursing podcasts. Listening to or creating podcasts may be a formal class assignment, providing new ways to interact with course material.

Short discussions of what is new in the field may appear as podcasts on the Internet, in particular on news and research sites. Learners may rely on the portability of MP3 players to take learning with them on the road. Commuters and walkers and joggers are often seen listening to MP3 players. Because creating podcasts is relatively easy and inexpensive, such presentations can be produced by students as review files for common terms or used as ways for students to self-assess their ability to discuss topics. The uses of podcasts from an educational perspective are limitless.

Bringing the discussion of podcasts back to the Foundation of Knowledge model, for each task or process in the model, one can see how podcasts fit with that concept. Podcasts can be used to acquire new knowledge from sources on the Web. Listening to podcasts provides learners with another tool for learning in addition to readings and lectures, thereby addressing a wider audience whose members have varying learning styles. Because podcast creation is simple and inexpensive, podcasts are an ideal way to generate and disseminate knowledge.

## Audiopods

**Audiopod** is a term used to describe a traditional or audio-based podcast. Participating in podcasting can exercise not just basic technology skills, but also writing, editing, and speaking skills. Writing scripts for a podcast can be an excellent exercise in critical thinking and information delivery, whereas the technology itself allows global access to information by faculty, teachers, and students anywhere at any time (Gordon, 2007). Both faculty and students can create audiopods with little difficulty, and most use podcasts to share additional class materials, updates, and even entire lectures (Oblinger, 2005).

## Videopods

Similar to an audiopod in setup and accessibility, a **videopod** is a podcast that provides video in addition to audio functionality. Faculty might use videopodcasts to demonstrate concepts, interview experts in the field, and even assess student progress (Gordon, 2007). Libraries and other institutions have even begun using the videopod as a learning alternative to the ubiquitous and often mocked information video, finding that highly mobile students are more readily embracing this technology (Oblinger, 2005).

## Multimedia

As technologically savvy students continue to demand accessible, interactive learning tools to keep them engaged, an increasing number of instructors are experimenting with and incorporating multimedia into their courses. Generally, **multimedia** refers to a **computer-based** technology that incorporates traditional forms of communication to create a seamless and interactive learning environment, such as interactive tutorials, streaming video, and problem-solving programs. Nursing education has long relied on traditional multimedia, such as slide presentations, overhead projections, and training videos, for **continuing education** (CE) of staff, classroom learning, and patient education (Edwards & Drury, 2000). Now, however, new advances in multimedia allow faculty to add such innovations as simulations and virtual reality to their healthcare training, providing a way for students to learn procedural skills, such as insertion of needles and physical assessment, without any risks to an actual patient.

Research suggests that the seeing, hearing, doing, and interacting afforded by multimedia facilitate learning retention, with multimedia being at least as effective as traditional instruction, but offering the benefit of greater learner satisfaction. Authoring software—that is, programs that allow users of varied technical skill to design and create webpages and movies—has greatly facilitated the use of multimedia by faculty (Hebda & Czar, 2013). Nevertheless, the most effective multimedia relies on the careful and pedagogically appropriate combination of textual material, graphics, video, animation, and sound (Edwards & Drury, 2000)—a distinctly separate skill set from teaching and instructing. Some schools of nursing have instructional designers on staff to assist nursing faculty with the development of multimedia to support learning.

Beyond providing a flexible method of delivery for instructional information, multimedia promises to motivate students by requiring them to analyze evidence in ways that require higher-order thinking and problem-solving skills. Similarly, faculty can begin to think about their classes in new ways and accommodate different student learning styles (Oblinger, 2005). **Box 19-3** provides an overview of the capabilities of smartphones and their use in education.

# Promoting Active and Collaborative Learning

Because of the shift within the teaching–learning context from the individual seeking answers to the group trying to construct new knowledge from available information, the most effective learning solutions require new digital communication skills, new

---

### BOX 19-3 SMARTPHONES AND OTHER SMART DEVICES IN NURSING EDUCATION

*Dee McGonigle and Kathleen Mastrian*

Smartphones are another tool for the educational arena. As Yu (2012) stated, "Smart phone technology, with its pervasive acceptance and powerful functionality, is inevitably changing peoples' behaviors" (para. 6).

Our educational uses of a technology such as smartphones cannot only affect the learning episode but also influence how we prepare students to embrace and use technologies appropriately. As educators, we want our students to remain competitive in a highly technologically dependent world. Nursing is a data- and information-driven profession, and nurses must rely on technologies to provide the data and information necessary to provide safe and high-quality care to our patients.

If students have smartphones, we can share text, graphics such as PowerPoint presentations, podcasts, and other audio/video media with them prior to the learning episode. When all students have access to the same information, it enhances the dialogue and topical discussion centered on that information. Nursing educators can use smartphones to distribute announcements, reminders, and even pertinent notes that the students need. Students can also be polled using these devices. Smartphones can even replace huge textbooks with electronic files. Smart devices and their calendars and messaging features help both educators and students organize their lives and keep their hectic schedules straight. The use of smart technologies can facilitate interactions around the world. Students can consult with other students and experts from anywhere on the globe. As this brief list of applications suggests, we have only just begun to think of ways in which to incorporate smartphones into our learning episodes.

In conclusion, we would like to leave you thinking about a money-saving alternative for many schools. Instead of requiring a laptop computer, what if your school required every student to have a smartphone? Could we replace the expensive computer labs on our campuses while better connecting our online and blended students to their educational milieu?

---

### REFERENCE

Yu, F. (2012). Mobile/smart phone use in higher education. Retrieved from http://www.swdsi.org/swdsi2012/proceedings_2012/papers/Papers/PA144.pdf

pedagogies, and new practices (Costa, 2007). A collaborative, student-centered approach uses the best tenets of inductive teaching by imposing more responsibility on students for their own learning than is assumed in the traditional lecture-based deductive approach. These constructivist methods are built on the widely accepted principle that students are constantly constructing their own realities rather than simply absorbing versions presented by their teachers. Collaborative methods often involve students' discussion of questions and in-class problem solving, with much of the work (in and out of class) done by students in groups rather than individually (Felder & Prince, 2007).

Johnson and Johnson (1990) have identified five significant elements for successful collaborative learning that are still pertinent today:

1. Face-to-face interaction between students, allowing them to build on one another's strengths
2. Mutual learning goals that, in turn, prompt students to exhibit positive interdependence rather than individualized competition
3. Equal participation in the work process and personal accountability for the work one contributes
4. Regular debriefing sessions as a group after meetings or presentations during which time feedback is shared and observations analyzed
5. Use of cooperative group process skills learned in the classroom

Although collaborative learning relies heavily on student investment and participation, institutions must ultimately create the best physical and electronic settings where collaboration is encouraged. This can be achieved with a sound educational and technologic infrastructure, reliance on proved working models, adaptable physical spaces, and even pedagogic support in the form of preceptors or mentors.

Especially useful for nursing students is the collaborative fieldwork model in which two or more students share a clinical setting and the same fieldwork educator. In this model, learning happens in a reciprocal fashion, with students constructing knowledge by watching each other and exchanging ideas. The most effective fieldwork experiences are highly structured with clear outlines of responsibilities, duties, and expectations, ensuring that the experience matches the learner's expectations. All activities performed by students, such as conducting evaluations, are done jointly, so that peers provide each other with objective feedback, leading to eventual increased self-confidence (Costa, 2007). In this way, suggests Costa, individuals with different viewpoints and experiences create a space where new knowledge emerges and existing knowledge can be restructured (as cited in Cockrell, Caplow, & Donaldson, 2000).

Libraries have also begun to recognize their role in students' success with and predisposition toward collaborative learning by creating redesigned spaces that reflect students' need to huddle in small groups, sit closely together without barriers, chat about their work, and view digital information without physical hindrances, such as carrels or work stalls. A leader in this movement has been Indiana State University, whose new information commons features completely overhauled furniture, software, monitors, processing power, and wireless access to the university's network. Students can now collect as a group at kidney-shaped tables; better see the information loaded on the flat-screen monitors; make use of brainstorming, design, and planning software;

and discuss their work in a chat-friendly zone. Some faculty members have even scheduled classes at the learning stations, and students, including those in nursing, have responded enthusiastically to the evolved space (Gabbard, Kaiser, & Kaunelis, 2007).

In addition to adaptable physical spaces that encourage discussion and group work, students require a supportive infrastructure that provides essential elements necessary to successful research and scholarship. These include professional development support in the form of workshops that help students acquire or refresh skill sets; presentation opportunities; and hardware, software, and resource support. One such example involves the participation by nursing students at the University of Texas Medical Branch School of Nursing in the Scholarly Talk About Research Series (STARS), in which students and faculty give presentations of their work before presenting those materials at professional conferences (Froman, Hall, Shah, Bernstein, & Galloway, 2003), thereby eliciting collegial feedback, collaborative troubleshooting, and shared research ideas. Imagine how powerful such a process would be in a cross-discipline healthcare education school.

Simply adopting a collaborative, inductive method of learning, however, will not necessarily lead to better learning and more satisfied students. As with any form of instruction, collaborative teaching methods need skilled and careful implementation. Because students are initially often resistant to instruction that makes them more responsible for their own learning, those who attempt to implement an inductive learning method should adhere to best practices, such as providing adequate scaffolding—that is, extensive support and guidance when students are first introduced to the method and gradual withdrawal of that support as students gain more experience and confidence in its use (Felder & Prince, 2007).

Nursing preceptors and mentors, for example, can provide this kind of scaffolded support as clinically active role models (Armitage & Burnard, 1991) and problem-solving **advocates** and collaborators (Gagen & Bowie, 2005). As individuals who are primarily concerned with the teaching and learning aspects of the relationship, preceptors help students learn by acting as clinical practitioner role models from whom the students can copy appropriate skills and behaviors. Kramer (1974) introduced the concept of nurse preceptor to address the theory and practice gap—that is, the difference between what is taught in class and what actually happens in nursing practice. Preceptors enhance clinical competence through direct role modeling, which is especially valuable in a field where competence and clinical ability are paramount (Armitage & Burnard, 1991). Mentors, similar to preceptors, provide equally valuable assistance to nursing students in the form of a facilitator. Mentors are most often used in nursing and education to support new professionals who are trying to fulfill the rigors of a new position while negotiating the stress inherent to a new environment (Gagen & Bowie, 2005). According to Jokelainen, Turunen, Tossavainen, Jamookeeah, and Coco (2011), "student mentoring in nursing clinical placements integrates environmental, collegial, pedagogical and clinical attributes" (para. 6). Mentors tend to address student needs through open conversation, student advocacy, feedback on student progress, facilitation, teaching, and general support (Neary, 2000).

Generally, these and other forms of institutional support promote students' adoption of a meaning-oriented approach to learning, as opposed to a surface or memorization-intensive approach. Collaborative, inductive learning promotes intellectual development that challenges the dualistic thinking that characterizes many entering college students, which holds that all knowledge is certain, professors have it, and the task of students is to absorb and repeat it (Felder & Prince, 2007, p. 55). Further, this kind of learning helps students acquire the self-directed learning and critical thinking skills that characterize the best scientists and engineers (Felder & Prince, 2007). The active, engaging elements of collaborative learning increase self-confidence, promote autonomy in students, and foster a commitment to lifelong learning (Costa, 2007)—all necessities for the success of a new millennial information-literate student.

# Knowledge Dissemination and Sharing

Sharing stories and experience from a clinical point of view accomplishes much more than simply promoting camaraderie or empathy (although this kind of engagement is infinitely valuable in its own way); sharing experiences of clinical learning can help convey life-saving information to other clinicians in a way that is more memorable and palatable and less imposing than warnings delivered outside a social context. Clinical and caring knowledge, often rooted in everyday exchanges, become socially embedded such that those with experience in particular clinical settings share common knowledge and understanding. The social embeddedness of caring and clinical knowledge is a result of shared and shaped collective understanding of practice and sometimes provides an alternative view.

The power of pooled knowledge in combination with knowledge produced in dialogue with others helps to limit tunnel vision and is a powerful strategy for maximizing the clinical knowledge of a group. Whether the nurse is networking, presenting, or seeking CE or recertification, an understanding of socially embedded knowledge coupled with the multiple perspectives of skilled practitioners allows for a rich and vibrant opportunity to apply nursing skill effectively (Benner, Tanner, & Chelsa, 1997).

## Networking

Considered crucial to career development because of opportunities for collaboration and information exchange, networking encourages professional support by making successful professionals accessible to their colleagues. Further, developing interactive professional networks between academic and clinical nurses can benefit practice in diabetes, stroke, and mental health care, and in community nursing—a field where practitioners are encouraged to collaborate (Gillibrand, Burton, & Watkins, 2002).

The value of networking to members of male-dominated professions, such as law, business, and medicine, resides in opportunities to make contact with fellow professionals and, in turn, further one's career. This observation is especially poignant for nursing, a predominantly female profession that, until recently, has rarely reaped the benefits of formal networking (Nicholl & Tracey, 2007).

Because nurses tend to gather their information from personal networks, such as colleagues or professional meetings, the increased availability of technology to assist in networking has greatly facilitated information exchange. Blogs, email, websites, electronic mailing lists, and other communicative technologies have opened up an endless stream of collaboration and networking possibilities, allowing nurses to more easily access and learn from colleagues' experiences. Using the Internet allows for the discovery of information heretofore unavailable through traditional information sources (Pravikoff & Levy, 2006), helping nursing professionals decide whether, for example, pursuing research opportunities or collaboration on specific professional projects seems viable.

Formal networks, such as the International Nurse Practitioner/Advanced Practice Nursing Network (INP/APNN), unveiled in 2000, promote the exchange of knowledge, resources, and expertise in an effort to enhance the presence of nursing in primary health care. Created in response to the globalization of nurse practitioner and advanced practice nursing network (APNN) roles, the network enables the enhancement and advancement of practice both for countries just beginning to initiate advanced practice nursing (APN) roles and for those with experienced practitioners (Affara, Cross, & Schober, 2001).

Membership and participation in professional associations also provide ways to network and advance one's profession. Professional associations represent venues through which members may set standards for professional practice, establish codes of ethics, become involved in advocacy, engage in CE opportunities, access job banks, subscribe to professional journals, and act as a common voice for the profession. For example, the American Nursing Association of Occupational Health Nurses is instrumental in maintaining healthcare issues on the political agenda. There are also several opportunities for nurses to network in specific informatics associations, such as American Nursing Informatics Association (ANIA) and the nursing work group associated with HIMSS. Research shows that nurses sometimes hesitate to join professional organizations because of barriers associated with cost, distance to meetings, lack of activities in their geographic area, and inability to attend meetings. Because networking creates fertile areas for the development of new ideas, partnership, jobs, and strategies, both national and state associations would benefit from creating greater opportunities for healthcare practitioners to earn CE credit and network with others in their field (Thackeray, Neiger, & Roe, 2005).

## Presenting and Publishing

Much in the way the AACN maintains standards for nursing education, professional journals also hold their contributors to similarly rigorous standards and provide a valuable venue in which nursing professionals might share ideology and innovations in the field. With the proliferation of online journals and the availability of nursing information via multiple media, publishing remains an excellent way to participate in the dissemination of professional information. Both nursing magazines and journals reach considerable audiences; journal distinctions lie in their authorship and audience. Although journal articles are written by and for scholars, with refereed or peer-reviewed journals requiring a blind review by a group of reviewers to eliminate bias, magazine articles may be written by a professional in the field, an editor, freelancer, or other author. Publishing provides excellent opportunities to extend knowledge and share research.

Similar to publishing, making presentations at contemporary professional conferences allows nursing educators and students to gain experience and share scholarship with colleagues. Presentations must meet certain standards for an audience to find them credible and effective. Because an audience retains 50% of what they see and hear in a presentation versus 20% if they only hear it, experts suggest the use of audiovisual aids to create the most effective professional presentations (Bergren, 2000). A noteworthy presentation could involve multiple levels of complexity, from a simple PowerPoint slide to an animated tutorial. Because technology and well-designed visuals cannot make up for lack of preparedness or research, however, presenters should be aware of their target audience and details of the research being presented. Regardless of the medium or presentation style, audiovisual presentations should be designed consistently and simply, using colors and fonts that are easy to read and understand and audience-appropriate language.

Conferences often host poster presentations that enable contributors to share research findings, innovations, and exemplar programs in a low-investment but visually captivating way. Because posters are primarily visual, with little or no verbal supplementation, most important for consideration are room elements, such as size, space limitations, and lighting. The best nursing practitioner posters feature consistent visual components, such as appropriately sized, readable font and simple colors, and are based on a research concept or clinical objective (Berg, 2005). A high-tech alternative to a paper poster is an electronic poster—that is, a continuously running PowerPoint presentation either projected for larger audiences or left to run from a laptop or desktop for smaller audiences (Bergren, 2000). Both publishing and presenting provide opportunities for the nursing practitioner to disseminate new knowledge and stay abreast of information in the field. Some educational institutions provide opportunities for undergraduates to showcase projects and research at undergraduate research conferences. These conferences are excellent ways for developing professionals to hone knowledge dissemination skills that will serve them well in their professional practice.

## Continuing Education and Recertification

Nationally, nursing employers and institutions have, because of budgetary constraints, begun to eliminate CE programs traditionally reliant on classes, conferences, and workshops; consequently, reliance on outside agencies and technology has increased to meet this need. The traditional approach to obtaining CE credits has included home study offered by professional journals and organizations in which the client reads articles, answers related questions, and sends in the test form and fee. Although fairly straightforward, this technique provides little in the way of peer interaction (Hebda & Czar, 2013). With the ubiquitous technology influx and the accessibility it affords, obtaining CE credits through e-learning is considered a beneficial delivery method for mandatory educational programs and other programs that provide employees with opportunities to maintain or improve skills. Benefits of e-learning for CE training include the ability to access information at any time (thus creating a flexible schedule) and experience instant feedback and individualized instruction by seeking out specific, additional information as needed.

E-learning can also benefit administrative support of CE credits by providing instantly accessible computerized records and other tracking features, such as records of success and completion, associated costs of program development, and staff productivity. Allowing nursing professionals to complete mandatory training on demand represents a huge benefit of e-learning, with the best programs allowing for customization to accommodate program revisions and regulation changes (Hebda & Czar, 2013).

In some cases, acquiring CE credits may also help the nurse achieve recertification. Available through myriad professional organizations, recertification ensures that nurses are staying current in their fields and some specialties; for example, the field of pediatric nursing requires annual recertification to maintain professional status. During recertification, the Pediatric Nursing and Certification Board offers each certified pediatric nurse (CPN) options for ensuring she or he is maintaining national standards within the specialty of pediatric nursing (Pediatric Nursing Certification Board, 2007).

As an added benefit, some hospitals provide higher salaries to nurses who maintain certification. Additionally, 90% of nurse managers indicate they would prefer to hire a certified nurse over a noncertified nurse. The trend in Magnet hospitals to encourage, reward, and promote certified nurses is spreading to other facilities and healthcare settings, with retirement centers and home health agencies now beginning to seek certified nurses because of the perceived extra benefit to their customers and the marketing advantage obtained from hiring nurses with guaranteed levels of competence (Peterson, 2007). For a comprehensive list of nursing certifications provided by the American Nurses Credentialing Center (ANCC), visit www.nursecredentialing. org/certification.aspx.

## Exploring Information Fair Use and Copyright Restrictions

As we adopt more technology-based tools in education, we need to be mindful of what constitutes fair use of materials and copyright laws. Nurse educators should be careful to model ethical behaviors by attributing works to their rightful authors as they acquire and use education materials. **Fair use** refers to a legal concept that permits the use of copyrighted works for specific purposes without obtaining permission from the author or without paying for the use of the work. Originally, fair use evolved for written work and allowed for uses that include journalists reporting the news, teaching, or scholarly research. As digital technology and the Web burst upon the scene, fair use expanded to apply to the copying and redistribution of digital media, including photographs, graphics, music, videos, audio, and software or computer programs.

Four factors must be considered in determining whether a particular use is fair. These factors are derived directly from the fair use provision (www.copyright.gov/fls /fl102.html) of Section 107 of the U.S. Copyright Law (U.S. Copyright Office, n.d.):

1. The purpose and character of the use, including whether such use is of commercial nature or is for nonprofit educational purposes
2. The nature of the copyrighted work
3. The amount and substantiality of the portion used in relation to the copyrighted work as a whole
4. The effect of the use upon the potential market for, or value of, the copyrighted work

The first factor tends to favor educational institutions and nonprofit entities. The second factor relates to the nature of the work: Courts have consistently protected creative works and those that have not yet been published. The third factor that must be considered relates to the amount of use. Typically you should determine how much of the overall work you are using; if it represents the core or essence of the work, you should not replicate or use it. The fourth and final factor relates to the effect on the creator's market share. If you are using a substantial portion of a text or software work that is offered for sale, you can adversely affect its owner's earning potential. The term itself should make you reflect on all of these factors and decide whether your proposed use is fair.

Copyright refers to the exclusive right of the creator of a work to distribute, sell, publish, copy, lease, or display that work in whatever manner he or she so chooses. Copyright laws are not only misinterpreted, but are constantly being challenged by our advancing technological capabilities. Even though you use American Psychological Association (APA) formatting, for example, and cite the authors, you might be overstepping your rights and infringing on the author's copyright; you might not be accused of plagiarism, but you should always cite where you obtained your information or digital media.

All users of others' work, in whatever medium, must fully understand, be well aware of, and comply with copyright and fair use principles. Typically, you should try to think of what is reasonable use and always make sure that you cite the authors. Reflect on all four fair use factors before making your decision to use another's work for educational purposes. Remember, also, that you are serving as a role model regarding copyright and fair use behaviors for your students.

## The Future

There are several exciting and interesting education technology trends to monitor in the future. Virtual reality–embedded education has exploded onto the academic scene and offers the potential for interdisciplinary inquiry and sharing across the curriculum, university, and globally. Makerspaces are labs provided on university campuses (and in some healthcare institutions) to allow students and healthcare workers to experiment with developing new technologies or modifying existing technologies and equipment to better fit needs. These spaces are frequently equipped with 3D printers and lots of tools and materials that allow for rapid prototyping of ideas. Here is an example of a makerspace innovation from the University of Texas:

> *Taking 10–20 minutes at a time from regular shift work, one nurse demonstrated a prototype he has built over time for a self-operating irrigation system that could be used for burn patients and free up staff to engage in other tasks. Usually a manual task, a patient with a severe burn requiring 11 hours of irrigation prompted this nurse to come up with a better solution. While still in development, the potential of this tool to help alleviate the suffering of a single patient or to free up significant time in the event of a disaster is unquestionable. (Siddiqui, 2016, para. 4)*

Several universities around the country, such as University of South Florida, University of Pittsburgh, Yale University, and Arizona State University, are sponsoring healthcare innovation competitions. Other universities are partnering with industry leaders to sponsor student ideas for healthcare innovations. Another trend, The Internet of Everything (IoE) is touted as the next step beyond the connections of physical things (Internet of Things, or IoT):

> IoT focuses only on sensor networks—machines communicating with other machines, and the data created as a result. As things add capabilities (such as context-awareness, increased processing power, and energy independence), and as more people and new information are connected, IoT becomes IoE, a network of networks where billions, or even trillions, of connections create unprecedented opportunities and new risks. (Selinger, Sepulveda, & Buchan, 2013, p. 3)

Education innovations related to the IoE hold promise for improving education processes, outcomes, and instruction. For example, mobile devices and wearables allow for the collection of learner behaviors, and this data can be translated into targeted, personalized learning. Data generated from the IoE may also be used for professional development to improve teaching and curricular approaches and effectiveness. These are but a few of the education technology trends to watch for in the future.

## Summary

This chapter highlighted the technology tools and delivery modalities that support nursing education. It is clear that nursing education is evolving and will be structured by competency achievement and supported by technologies. In an ideal world, nurses will work against the assumption that technology runs itself and take proactive roles in helping to design the education and technologies necessary best to prepare them for real-world scenarios. Consider that flash is not substance, and drama is not depth; technology performs only as well as the pedagogy that undergirds and sustains it. Plan for and use technology with care so that its best features consequently enrich your experiences as an educator or learner.

### THOUGHT-PROVOKING QUESTIONS

1. What are some of the forces behind the push toward a more wired learning experience in nursing education?
2. Which of the technologies discussed here most appeals to you? Why?
3. Explore one of the newer learning technologies in more depth. How would the use of this technology to benefit you in your practice or education setting? Why do you find this tool useful? From your perspective, how could you enhance this tool?
4. Jean, a diabetes nurse educator, recently read an article in an online journal that she accessed through her health agency's database subscription. The article provided a comprehensive checklist for managing diabetes in older adults, which Jean prints out and distributes to her patients in a diabetes education class. Does this constitute fair use or is it a copyright violation? Explain your answer.

# References

Affara, F., Cross, S., & Schober, M. (2001). Discovering resources: Making global connections, international networking. *Journal of the American Academy of Nurse Practitioners, 13*(10), 445–448.

Aquino-Russell, C., Maillard Strüby, F. V., & Reviczky, K. (2007). Living attentive presence and changing perspectives with a Web-based nursing theory course. *Nursing Science Quarterly, 20*(2), 128–134.

Armitage, P., & Burnard, P. (1991). Mentors or preceptors? Narrowing the theory–practice gap. *Nurse Education Today, 11,* 225–229.

Barnes, L., & Rudge, T. (2005). Virtual reality or real virtuality: The space of flows and nursing practice. *Nursing Inquiry, 12*(4), 306–315.

Bassendowski, S. L. (2005). NursingQuest: Supporting an analysis of nursing issues. *Journal of Nursing Education, 46*(2), 92–95.

Bell, S. (2003). Cyber-guest lecturers: Using webcasts as a teaching tool. *TechTrends, 47*(4), 10–14.

Benner, P., Tanner, C., & Chelsa, C. (1997). The social fabric of nursing knowledge. *American Journal of Nursing, 97*(7), 16BBB–16DDD.

Berg, J. A. (2005). Creating a professional poster presentation: Focus on nurse practitioners. *Journal of the American Academy of Nurse Practitioners, 17*(7), 245–249.

Bergren, M. D. (2000). Power up your presentation with PowerPoint. *Journal of School Nursing, 16*(4), 44–47.

Brown, M., Dehoney, J., & Millichap, N. (2015). The next generation digital learning environment. A report on research. *EDUCAUSE Learning Initiative,* 1–11.

Chase, D. (2007). Transformative sharing with instant messaging, wikis, interactive maps, and Flickr. *Computers in Libraries, 27*(1), 7–56.

Clochesy, J. M. (2004). Hardware and software options. In J. Fitzpatrick & S. Montgomery (Eds.), *Internet for nursing research* (pp. 120–128). New York, NY: Springer.

Cockrell, K., Caplow, J., & Donaldson, J. (2000). A context for learning: Collaborative groups in the problem-based learning environment. *Review of Higher Education, 23*(3), 347–363.

Costa, D. M. (2007). The collaborative fieldwork model. *OT Practice, 12*(1), 25–26.

Denoyelles, A., Raible, J., & Seilhamer, R. (2015). Exploring students' e-textbook practices in higher education. *EDUCAUSEreview.* Retrieved from http://er.educause.edu/articles/2015/7 /exploring-students-etextbook-practices-in-higher-education

DeSantis, S. (2002). *Re-envisioning the pedagogical bridge: The new instructional designer.* Presented at the Pennsylvania Association for Educational Communications and Technology, Hershey, PA.

Dewald, N. H. (1999). Transporting good library instruction practices into the Web environment: An analysis of online tutorials. *Journal of Academic Librarianship, 25*(1), 26–32.

EDUCAUSE Learning Initiative. (2006, June). 7 things you should know about. . . virtual worlds. Retrieved from http://www.educause.edu/library/resources/7-things-you-should-know-about -virtual-worlds

Edwards, M. J. A., & Drury, R. M. (2000). Using computers in basic nursing education, continuing education, and patient education. In M. J. Ball, K. J. Hannah, S. K. Newbold, & J. V. Douglas (Eds.), *Nursing informatics: Where caring and technology meet* (pp. 49–68). New York, NY: Springer.

Felder, R., & Prince, M. (2007). The case for inductive teaching. *Prism, 17*(2), 55.

Froman, R. D., Hall, A. W., Shah, A., Bernstein, J. M., & Galloway, R. Y. (2003). A methodology for supporting research and scholarship. *Nursing Outlook, 51*(2), 84–89.

Gabbard, R. B., Kaiser, A., & Kaunelis, D. (2007). Redesigning a library space for collaborative learning. *Computers in Libraries, 27*(5), 6–12.

Gagen, L., & Bowie, S. (2005). Effective mentoring: A case for training mentors for novice teachers. *Journal of Physical Education, Recreation & Dance, 76*(7), 40–45.

Garavalia, L. S. (2002). Selecting appropriate assessment methods: Asking the right questions. *American Journal of Pharmaceutical Education, 66*, 108–112.

Gillibrand, W. P., Burton, C., & Watkins, G. G. (2002). Clinical networks for nursing research. *International Nursing Review, 49*(3), 188–193.

Gordon, A. M. (2007). Sound off! The possibilities of podcasting. *Book Links,* 16–18.

Grant, M. J., & Brettle, A. J. (2006). Developing and evaluating an interactive information skills tutorial. *Health Information and Libraries Journal, 23*(2), 79–88.

Hebda, T., & Czar, P. (2013). *Handbook of informatics for nurses & health care professionals* (5th ed.). Upper Saddle River, NJ: Prentice Hall.

Johnson, D. W., & Johnson, R. T. (1990). *Learning together and alone: Cooperative, competitive and individualistic learning.* Boston, MA: Allyn & Bacon.

Jokelainen, M., Turunen, H., Tossavainen, K., Jamookeeah, D., & Coco, K. (2011). A systematic review of mentoring nursing students in clinical placements. *Journal of Clinical Nursing, 20,* 2854–2867. doi: 10.1111/j.1365-2702.2010.03571.x

Kramer, M. (1974). *Reality shock.* St. Louis, MO: Mosby.

Leasure, A., Davis, L., & Thievon, S. (2000). Comparison of student outcomes and preferences in a traditional vs. World Wide Web–based baccalaureate nursing research course. *Journal of Nursing Education, 39,* 149–154.

Maag, M. (2005). The potential use of "blogs" in nursing education. *CIN: Computers, Informatics, Nursing, 23*(1), 16–26.

McHugh, M. L. (2006). Computer hardware. In V. Saba & K. McCormick (Eds.), *Essentials of nursing informatics* (4th ed., pp. 517–532). New York, NY: McGraw-Hill.

Meyer, L. (2015). 6 alternative social media tools for teaching and learning. *Campus Technology.* Retrieved from http://campustechnology.com/Articles/2015/01/07/6-Alternative-Social-Media-Tools-for-Teaching-and-Learning.aspx?Page=1

Moreau, E. (2013). What is a webinar? Retrieved from http://webtrends.about.com/od/office20/a/What-Is-AWebinar.htm

Neary, M. (2000). Supporting students' learning and professional development through the process of continuous assessment and mentorship. *Nurse Education Today, 20,* 463–474.

Nicholl, H., & Tracey, C. (2007). Networking for nurses. *Nursing Management, 13*(9), 26–29.

Oblinger, D. G. (2005). Learners, learning, & technology: The EDUCAUSE learning initiative. *EDUCAUSE Review,* 66–75.

Pediatric Nursing Certification Board. (2007). About recertification. Retrieved from http://www.pncb.org/ptistore/control/certs/cpn-cpnp/index

Peterson, T. (2007, November 19). Here's the skinny: What you need to do to become and stay certified. Retrieved from http://www.medscape.com/viewarticle/562945

Pijl-Zieber, E. M., Barton, S., Konkin, J., Awosoga, O., & Caine, V. (2014). Competence and competency-based nursing education: Finding our way through the issues. *Nurse Education Today, 34*(5), 676–678.

Pravikoff, D. S., & Levy, J. R. (2006). Computerized information resources. In V. Saba & McCormick (Eds.), *Essentials of nursing informatics* (4th ed., pp. 517–532). New York, NY: McGraw-Hill.

Pusic, M. V., Pachev, G. S., & MacDonald, W. A. (2007). Embedding medical student computer tutorials into a busy emergency room department. *Academic Emergency Medicine, 14*(2), 138–148.

Ridley, R. T. (2007). Interactive teaching: A concept analysis. *Journal of Nursing Education, 46*(5), 206–209.

Riley, J. B. (1996). Educational applications. In V. K. Saba & K. A. McCormick (Eds.), *Essentials of computers for nurses* (2nd ed., pp. 527–573). New York, NY: McGraw-Hill.

Selinger, M., Sepulveda, A., & Buchan, J. (2013). Education and the Internet of Everything: How ubiquitous connectedness can help transform pedagogy. *Cisco Consulting Services and Cisco EMEAR Education Team.* Retrieved from http://www.cisco.com/web/strategy/docs/education/education_internet.pdf

Seropian, M. A., Brown, K., Gavilanes, J. S., & Driggers, B. (2004). Simulation: Not just a manikin. *Journal of Nursing Education, 43*(4), 164–170.

Shaffer, S. C., Lackey, S. P., & Bolling, G. W. (2006). Blogging as venue for nurse faculty development. *Nursing Education Perspectives, 27*(3), 126–128.

Siddiqui, M. (2016). Making space for innovation in health care. *HHS Idea Lab.* Retrieved from http://www.hhs.gov/idealab/2016/06/21/making-space-for-innovation-in-health-care

Skiba, D. J. (2007). Do your students wiki? *Nursing Education Perspectives, 26*(2), 120–121.

Sousa, D. A. (1995). *How the brain learns.* Reston, VA: National Association of Secondary School Principals.

Thackeray, R., Neiger, B. L., & Roe, K. M. (2005). Certified health education specialists' participation in professional associations: Implications for marketing and membership. *American Journal of Health Education, 36*(6), 337–344.

Thurmond, V. (2003). Defining interaction and strategies to enhance interactions in Web-based courses. *Nurse Educator, 28*(5), 237–241.

Thurmond, V., & Wambach, K. (2002). Understanding interactions in distance education: A review of the literature. *International Journal of Instructional Technology and Distance Learning.* Retrieved from http://www.itdl.org/journal/jan_04/article02.htm

U.S. Copyright Office. (n.d.). Copyright law of the United States of America and related laws contained in Title 17 of the United States code. Retrieved from http://www.copyright.gov/title17/92chap1.html#107

U.S. Department of Education. (2014, October 17). Competency-based learning or personalized learning. Retrieved from http://www.ed.gov/oii-news/competency-based-learning-or-personalized-learning

Wikipedia. (2016). Learning management system. Retrieved from https://en.wikipedia.org/wiki/Learning_management_system

## Objectives

1. Distinguish among learning environments as simulations, virtual worlds, or games.

2. Describe the role of simulation in nursing informatics education.

3. Compare and contrast simulations, virtual worlds, and games as informatics tools for nursing education.

4. Assess strategies for choosing among a simulation, virtual world, or game as the best choice for instructional delivery in a given educational situation.

5. Explore the role of simulation, virtual worlds, and games in nursing education.

6. Differentiate between using a live clinical information system or simulated electronic health records for educational purposes.

## Key Terms

- » Assessment
- » Augmented-reality games (ARGs)
- » Avatar
- » Clinical information systems
- » Database
- » Debrief
- » Dynamic webpage shells
- » Edutainment
- » Enactment
- » Engage
- » Feedback
- » Fidelity
- » Game
- » Game mechanics
- » Gameplay
- » Latex-based simulation
- » Massive multiplayer online role-playing games
- » Multiuser dungeon
- » Nonplayer character (NPC)
- » Object-oriented multiuser dungeon
- » Pre-brief, enactment, debrief, and assessment (PEDA)
- » Pre-brief
- » Scaffolding
- » Second Life
- » Serious game
- » Server
- » Simulated documentation
- » Simulations
- » Simulation scenario
- » Simulator
- » Three-dimensional (3D)
- » Virtual simulation
- » Virtual world

# CHAPTER 20

# Simulation, Game Mechanics, and Virtual Worlds in Nursing Education

Dee McGonigle, Kathleen Mastrian, Brett Bixler, and Nickolaus Miehl

## Introduction

The use of latex-based and virtual simulation (Figures 20-1 and 20-2), virtual worlds, and game mechanics in nursing education continues to increase. Many schools and staff education departments have employed these techniques to provide efficient, effective, and engaging educational experiences for their students and staff. More schools and other educational entities are realizing the benefits of these educational modalities. The monumental National Council of State Boards of Nursing (NCSBN; Hayden, Smiley, Alexander, Kardong-Edgren, & Jeffries, 2014) simulation study brought national attention to the need to enhance, extend, or replace clinical and practicum hours with other effective means such as simulation. In this chapter, we will explore simulated documentation, simulation, virtual worlds, and game mechanics used in teaching nursing informatics competencies and nursing education.

Even though there are many nursing students, nursing educators, and nurses using these technologies, there is not a clear understanding of the terminology associated with these learning modalities. It is important that we are on the same page when we are discussing these technologies and their impact on nursing informatics and nursing education.

- **Simulations** are imitations of real-life events or circumstances; in nursing education, simulations are used to replicate a clinical scenario to provide an opportunity for practice in a mock situation. This can be done via role play, web-based applications, with manikins (**latex-based simulation**), or **virtual simulation** in a virtual world.
- A simulator is a mechanical or electronic device that provides an environment in which a simulation can occur.
- Simulated documentation refers to any simulated electronic format or electronic health record (EHR) that is accessed and used by the learner to actually document simulated nursing care for educational purposes.

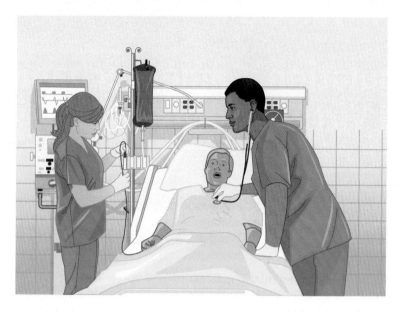

**Figure 20-1** Latex-Based Simulation

- A simulation scenario is a situation or case developed in a simulation setting to mimic an actual practice situation.
- A **game** is a structured activity undertaken for enjoyment.
- In education, **edutainment** is the combination of "education" and "entertainment"; that is, when we make learning fun.
- **Game mechanics** are the rules, instructions, directions, and constructs that the learner interacts with while playing the game. For educators, it is essential that any game mechanics they use are engaging and satisfying for the learner.
- **Gameplay** is how the learner interacts with or plays the game. This is extremely important to understand in order to appreciate how the game functions and how the learners function, play, and learn.

As you progress through the chapter you will delve into simulated documentation, simulation, game mechanics, and virtual worlds.

## Simulation in Nursing Informatics Education

The patient call bell is ringing; you enter the room to find the patient verbalizing complaints of chest tightness. In a moment, the patient becomes unresponsive and a code is called. The team quickly responds, initiating resuscitation measures per

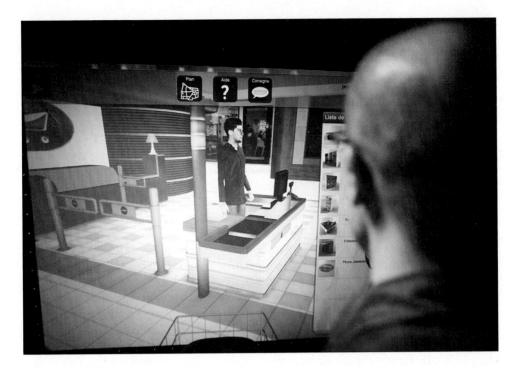

**Figure 20-2** Virtual Simulation
© BSIP/Amelie-Benoist

advanced cardiac life support (ACLS) protocol. You review the EHRs with the attending physician while simultaneously discussing your assessment before the code. After a short while, the resuscitation efforts are successful and the patient is stable enough for transfer to the intensive care unit. You complete your documentation in the patient's EHR, the simulation scenario ends, and the debriefing begins. The instructor provides feedback on not only actions taken within the simulation scenario, but also on the use of the EHR as an important resource for patient information and documentation.

Perhaps it is the first day of a new course and, rather than a lecture-based class with an accompanying textbook, the instructor uses an active learning approach with case studies delivered through an EHR interface to facilitate the learning and application of clinical concepts. In this example, rather than being part of an entire simulation scenario, the EHR itself is the learning tool providing learners with a hands-on learning opportunity centered on accessing and using the information contained within the patient record. Choi, Park, and Lee (2016) concluded that academic EMRs (AEMRs) would improve students' understanding of clinical practice; "the findings of this study will provide important developments by applying an AEMR, which will augment students' informatics competencies and critical thinking, into the nursing curricula to better prepare the future workforce" (p. 264).

## Nursing Informatics Competencies in Nursing Education

In the late 1990s, it was identified that healthcare professionals needed to possess both skill and knowledge of informatics (American Association of Colleges of Nursing, 1997; Gassert, 1998; Pew Health Professions Commission, 1998). Additionally, information technology has been identified as a key measure in improving patient safety and quality of care (American Academy of Nursing, 2003; Institute of Medicine, 2000). In response to this increasing demand for practitioners to become skilled in this area, coupled with the absence of research-based informatics competencies, a Delphi study was used to identify informatics competencies for nurses at four different levels of practice (Staggers, Gassert, & Curran, 2002). In essence, this seminal study created informatics competencies for entry-level nurses through informatics specialists and innovators, with a focus on computer skills, informatics knowledge, and informatics skills.

Although informatics competencies for nurses have been identified, the degree to which schools of nursing have woven them into the curriculum varies greatly (Carty & Ong, 2006). In a study conducted by Fetter (2009), a survey of graduating senior nursing students ranked the following competencies with which they had no experience or minimal skill: (1) using applications to document, (2) creating an electronic care plan, (3) valuing informatics knowledge for practice, (4) valuing informatics knowledge for skill development, and (5) using applications for data entry. Hunter, McGonigle, and Hebda (2013) developed the online self-assessment tool, TIGER-based Assessment of Nursing Informatics Competencies (TANIC); this instrument assesses the Level I: Beginning Nurse and Level 2: Experienced Nurse competencies. McGonigle, Hunter, Hebda, and Hill (2014) developed the Nursing Informatics Competency Assessment (NICA) for Level 3 (L3): Informatics Nurse Specialist and Level 4 (L4): Informatics Innovator based on the seminal work of Staggers, the current literature, and expert input. This online self-assessment was noted in the 2015 American Nurses Association (ANA) *Nursing Informatics: Scope and Standards of Practice, Second Edition*. These self-assessment tools are discussed in Chapter 7, *Nursing Informatics as a Specialty*.

The question then becomes, which best practices will ensure that students become prepared in informatics? In a position statement by the National League for Nursing (2008), results from a survey of nursing educators and administrators indicated that only 50–60% of respondents said that informatics was integrated throughout the curriculum and that experience with nursing informatics was provided during clinical rotations. Findings also suggested that little clinically related informatics content and few such learning experiences were provided in nursing programs. Use of technology tools containing care-planning software and clinical information systems were least likely to be incorporated into the courses. This continues to be an issue, and one area of concern is the nursing informatics preparation of the faculty. Rajalahti, Heinonen, and Saranto (2014) made several recommendations, including the following:

"A description of nursing informatics competencies for nurse educators is needed at a national and global level. Advanced nursing informatics programmes are needed in the nurse educators' training programme" (p. 64). Nursing faculty must be prepared to use these technologies. With emerging technologies in nursing and healthcare education, the use of these technologies, including simulation, to allow students to use informatics in an active manner, and in an authentic and realistic learning context, is one potential approach to remedy these shortcomings.

## A Case for Simulation in Nursing Informatics Education and Nursing Education

A simulation recreates a real-life set of conditions or events with as much fidelity as possible (Alessi, 1988). Aldrich (2010) contended that simulations develop cognition (learning-to-know skills), ethics and roles (learning-to-be skills), and application capabilities (learning-to-do skills). Unlike games, however, simulations are not necessarily designed to be fun.

Simulations contain four major components: **pre-brief, enactment, debrief,** and **assessment** (**PEDA**; refer to Table 20-1). Every simulation should have these elements in order to prepare and assess students while also facilitating learning through doing and reflection. The most important translational PEDA component is the debrief. When done well, debriefing helps the learner reflect on the authentic experience and solidifies the learning by facilitating the transfer of theory and skills to their real practice setting. Harris, Shoemaker, Johnson, Tompkins-Dobbs, and Domian (2016) believed that simulation could assist family nurse practitioner (FNP) students with their role transition from generalist to advanced practice by

- "Allowing FNP students opportunities to gain confidence in a risk-free environment.
- Providing FNP students an entire comprehensive office-based or acute patient care experience.
- Reinforcing classroom content and bridging the theory to practice gap" (p. 14).

Table 20-1 Simulation PEDA (Pre-brief, Enactment, Debrief, Assessment)

| Each simulation must have four components: | |
|---|---|
| 1. Pre-brief<br>2. Enactment<br>3. Debrief<br>4. Assessment | |
| Pre-brief | The student receives the simulation information: goal, educational outcomes, and related course/program outcomes. The simulation should be explained and focused for the student. They should know how to prepare for the activity and be told what is expected, provided with the background necessary to be able to fully enact their role in the activity, and given specifics about how they will be assessed. They must also be provided with the timeframe within which the simulation must be completed. |

| | |
|---|---|
| Enactment | The simulation area is prepared to facilitate the activity. The student enacts the role assigned and/or completes their assigned activities during the established timeframe. |
| Debrief | Debriefing is "a student-centered discussion during which the participants and observers reflect on performance during the scenario and make recommendations for future practice" (Mastrian, McGonigle, Mahan, & Bixler, 2011, p. 351). The debriefing can be done one-on-one and/or with entire teams. Faculty can help students during and after their activities by focusing on breakdowns and areas of growth to hone future learning episodes (Tanner, 2006).<br><br>Objectives:<br>Following the completion of each activity, it is important to:<br><br>1. Answer student questions.<br>2. Address student perspectives, perceptions, and concerns.<br>3. Emphasize and reinforce specific learning outcomes.<br>4. Create authentic linkages to the "real world."<br>5. Assess student learning: What did they learn?<br>6. Validate what they learned.<br><br>Questions for Discussion<br><br>Ask the student to reflect on the simulation activity: both how they felt during the activity and how they feel now that the activity is completed.<br><br>1. What did the student enjoy the most and the least about the activity?<br>2. What were the student's perceptions regarding the activity?<br>  a. Can students describe the emotions they experienced while completing the activity?<br>  b. How do the students describe the interpersonal interactions or the enactment of their role?<br>3. What were the major points of the activity?<br>4. Did the student experience any problems that impacted their ability to make the necessary decisions during the activity?<br>  a. How could you prevent these problems in the "real world"?<br>  b. If you cannot prevent them, how could you avoid them in the "real world"?<br>5. What did the student learn?<br>  a. What did the student learn that was new to them?<br>  b. Did things that the student already knew take on new meanings after the activity?<br>  c. Was there a specific aspect of the activity where the student learned the most?<br>  d. Reflect on their perceived learning and validate what was learned.<br>6. Would the student recommend any changes to enhance the activity? If yes, what changes and how would each change enhance the activity?<br>7. What will the student take away with them after having completed this activity? |
| Assessment | The student should be provided with a detailed explanation of how they will be assessed and graded that relates to the goal, educational outcomes, and if applicable, course/program outcomes. Detailed rubrics are recommended. The assessment process must be shared during pre-briefing. If the activity is not being graded, a self-assessment should be provided for the students so they know how to evaluate their own performance. |

Developed by Dee McGonigle.

Simulations may be experiential and task based, where the learner takes on a first-person role and executes a self-chosen series of decisions, manipulating the variables in the simulation toward a desired outcome (Gredler, 1996; Weatherford, n.d.). Simulations may also be symbolic scenarios, where the learner directly manipulates variables, sees the results of changes, and then makes decisions on how to continue in the simulation. Spreadsheets are often used for this type of simulation. Symbolic simulations are good choices for discovering principles, misconceptions, and relationships, and for fostering understanding, prediction, and solution development (Mastrian et al., 2011).

Simulations may use a process known as **scaffolding** (Jonassen, 1999; Podolefsky, Moore, & Perkins, 2013) to assist in acquiring the accepted level of proficiency. An example of scaffolding is when corrective **feedback** is initially used, correcting user mistakes and ensuring success, and then the feedback fades away when it is no longer needed.

Medical simulations use realistic three-dimensional computer models of humans to investigate new medical possibilities and to test assumptions (learning-to-know skills). Simulations of drawing blood and complex medical operations are used to teach learning-to-do skills.

In general terms, a **simulator** can perhaps best be described as a tool designed to emulate some aspect of the clinical practice environment, which may be focused on a single task or designed to mimic a complete patient care situation (Gaba & DeAnda, 1998). At its essence, it is any device that is used to create a realistic learning experience for the learner but that removes the risk associated with learning during hands-on patient care. A simulator offers the unique ability to create a realistic learning environment that is safe, structured, and supportive for the learner (Bligh & Bleakley, 2006).

Simulators encompass a broad range of devices, such as partial task trainers (e.g., an IV insertion arm); screen-based simulations, including simulated EHRs, simulated documentation, and simulated environments replicating a realistic patient care area (virtual simulation); and complex computer-driven human patient simulation manikins (latex-based simulation). Web-based virtual standardized patients are also increasing in use. It is important to understand which of these products you are using: one in which you enter and interact in a virtual world, access a web-based product, or interact in a latex-based lab. Although each of these simulation modalities can be used alone, collectively they can be powerful learning tools when used together to create a realistic patient care scenario. When designing simulation learning environments, "[i]nnovative educators design learning environments that encourage active engagement in the learning process. . . . Active engagement creates a personal connection with the learning experience and motivates the learner to take greater responsibility in the learning process" (Fisher, 2016, p. 9). The goal of simulation, according to Gaba (2004), is a seamless immersion into the simulated practice environment during which learners are drawn into the reality of the environment or task at hand. Hertel and Millis (2002) noted that this is a cooperative process whereby learners come together in an authentic setting and begin to learn from one another. Darragh et al. (2016) recommended realistic scenarios that elicit autonomous problem solving and decision making to immerse and **engage** the participants in active learning and critical thinking. Refer to Figure 20-3.

Considering the realistic nature of simulation and its hands-on active approach to learning, it seems that the use of simulation modalities can be a powerful tool in moving student nurses—indeed, any practitioners— toward achieving the informatics competencies. Recall the examples given at the beginning of this chapter. In the first example, the EHR is part of a larger simulation scenario that mimics a real-life clinical case. In the second example, the EHR itself functions as a simulator and becomes a true-to-life learning tool. In either case, simulation is used to incorporate nursing informatics into the con-text of patient care, thereby giving students an authentic learning experience that can be applied in clinical practice.

According to the NCSBN National Simulation Study (Hayden et al., 2014), 50% simulation can be effectively used in various program types, in different geographic areas, and in urban and rural settings with good educational outcomes. The NCSBN study results and the lack of available or quality clinical/practicum placements are prompting the move to integrate more simulation into nursing education. Virtual and latex-based simulations are valuable educational assets at all levels of nurs-ing education. They provide a safe, authentic environment to develop knowledge, skills, and attitudes prior to interacting with actual patients. There is no risk to pa-tients, and students can practice and receive assessment and feedback for controlled

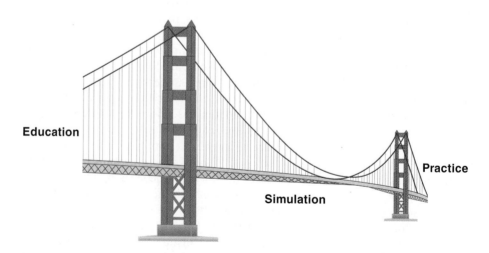

**Figure 20-3** Simulation Can Bridge the Gap

episodes, including unusual events. Simulation relates well to adaptive learning methods, such as branching logic, that allow the learner to guide the learning. The nurse educator can tailor the simulation to the learning needs of the students, providing deliberate practice with feedback. The learner can learn, relearn, and hone skills while safely practicing in dynamic and complex situations with a view to decreasing and eliminating mistakes.

# Incorporating EHRs into the Learning Environment

There are two main approaches to the incorporation of an EHR into the learning environment, whether used within a simulated clinical environment as part of a patient care scenario or as a stand-alone learning tool. First, the EHR can be created specifically for simulation purposes; options range from a well-developed Microsoft Access database to commercially available products designed specifically for simulation purposes. Second, the simulation may use a real EHR system, either within a hospital-based simulation center or through a partnership with a healthcare facility or an EHR vendor.

There are certain advantages and disadvantages to each **simulated documentation** solution (see **Figure 20-4**). As Brown (2005) noted, whereas "live" documentation systems provide learners with a realistic experience and can be incorporated into the learning environment, they also present certain drawbacks: (1) they are designed for the patient care environment, not the learning environment, and therefore lack an efficient feedback mechanism for learners; (2) they are designed to work in real time, not simulated time, creating issues with data recall, especially when a record may be used repeatedly over a period of months or years; and (3) if a system is overly complex, it may unintentionally focus the learning on the specific system, rather than the process of data retrieval and documentation. Refer to Research Brief 1 for more on the challenges of teaching clinical documentation skills in an EHR.

One system designed specifically for simulation is the Web-based medical chart (WMC), as described by Brown (2005). This system requires four components: (1) a database, (2) **dynamic webpage shells**, (3) a **server**, and (4) computers with access to the Internet. With this system, a Microsoft Access **database** is created to hold administrative information about the simulation scenario and other pertinent overview information accessible only by the instructor, as well as simulated patient data, simulated patient documentation, student documentation entries, and learner feedback from instructors. Each time a learner logs into the WMC system via the Internet, the server custom-creates the requested page using the existing database information, user-specific information, and the webpage shells to create a realistic EHR for use by the student. Although this type of system offers a great deal of flexibility, because it is custom created by the end user (but is certainly a cost-effective solution), it requires that the simulation instructor have a strong background in computer science and information technology to create and maintain the database and supporting materials.

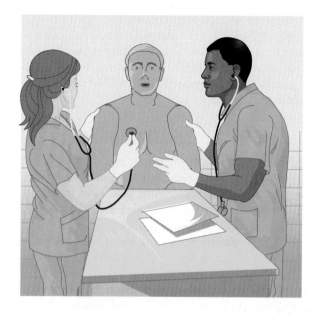

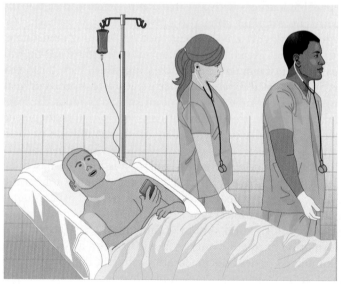

**Figure 20-4** Simulated Documentation Nurse/Patient

You are working as a team. This is Mr. Poli and as your simulated patient, you will be saving him from falling when you assist him to the restroom and determining why he is unsteady. At the end of your shift, you will document the nursing care you provided to this patient. When you leave, Mr. Poli will Tweet about his experience with each of you as his nurse and post comments about the care you provided. Not only is it important to simulate what the nurse must document, but also what our patients document and how they use social media to describe their care experience. It is important that you realize that patients take note of our actions and use social media to share their opinions and observations. Think about your best and worst experiences in health care. It might be something you experienced yourself or with a loved one. Where and what would you share through social media?

**RESEARCH BRIEF 1**

Faculty perceptions of the challenges of teaching undergraduate students proper clinical documentation in both paper-based and electronic systems are described in a qualitative research study by Mahon, Nickitas, and Nokes (2010). In this study, participants ($N = 25$) were interviewed using both open- and closed-ended questions, and results were analyzed using a constant comparative method. The most common method of teaching documentation skills was some variation of demonstration–return–demonstration method. Faculty were concerned about the amount of time taken honing documentation skills in the actual clinical area, indicating a median of 2 hours of an 8-hour clinical day was taken up with this task, and shared that there was seemingly little documentation taught in the classroom or laboratory. Faculty relied heavily on experts in the clinical setting and used their documentation as models for students to emulate. In the case of the electronic health record documentation, on-site nursing experts proficient in the use of the system were especially useful as role models. However, faculty remained concerned that using the electronic system and the endless drop-down menus might actually interfere with the development of nursing expertise and critical thinking.

One critical issue that was shared by faculty with regard to electronic documentation was that the clinical facility provided the instructor with only one access code, so that all of the students in the clinical group used the same code to document, and there was limited access to computers on the clinical unit. The faculty was very concerned about the legal and ethical issues for appropriate documentation and for the provision of care, such as on-time medication administration in a group of 8–10 students with one access code.

The authors suggested the need to integrate information competencies throughout the curricula and to provide opportunities for faculty development in informatics. They suggested that "faculty competencies in the area of informatics must be identified and standardized" and that faculty must learn to "model self-efficacy: the patience, support and persistence that characterize individual development within a professional discipline" (p. 620).

The full article appears in Mahon, P. Y., Nickitas, D. M., & Nokes, K. M. (2010). Faculty perceptions of student documentation skills during the transition from paper-based to electronic health records systems. *Journal of Nursing Education, 49*(11), 615–621.

A qualitative research study by Kennedy, Pallikkathayil, and Warren (2009) described the experiences and development of nursing process skills in nursing students ($N = 5$) using the Simulated E-hEalth Delivery System (SEEDS) learning innovation. In the SEEDS learning innovation, students were given written case studies and asked to enter the patient data in a simulated electronic health record and generate a care plan for the patient and family. The authors concluded, "The technology provided an interactive venue for developing nursing process skills by linking assessment data from case studies with foundational concepts in nursing" (p. 99). "The exercise was authentic, dynamic, and learner centered" (p. 99).

As a result of the themes discovered in this qualitative study, the authors proposed two hypotheses for future research to explore learning outcomes resulting from the use of a simulated e-health system:

- There is greater interaction among technologically competent students who use electronic documentation for patient data during clinical conferences. These students interact more freely with other students and their faculty members and experience enhanced learner satisfaction. These students also demonstrate superior nursing process skills than students using traditional postclinical group discussion about patient care.
- Technologically competent students also have higher test scores on specific topics than students who use paper and pencil means to organize the assessment data and develop care plans.

The full article appears in Kennedy, D., Pallikkathayil, L., & Warren, J. J. (2009). Using a modified electronic health record to develop nursing process skills. *Journal of Nursing Education, 48*(2), 96–102.

Note: The SEEDS project began in 2002 and continues at time of writing; according to the University of Kansas Medical Center (2016), "The impetus for this partnership arises from the Institute of Medicine (IOM) reports published in late 1999 and early 2001 addressing the quality, error and waste in the U.S. health care system" (para. 1).

One example of a commercially available solution is Elsevier's Simulation Learning System (2010). This system includes all of the elements needed for preparing, programming, running, and debriefing a **simulation scenario**, including a fully functional EHR. The EHR is linked to the simulation scenario and contains all of the pertinent patient information for learners to access before or during the simulation scenario. This system also incorporates the ability for learners to document just as they would in an actual clinical setting, with the capability of submitting the documentation to the instructor for evaluation and feedback. A major strength of this type of system is that it is a prepackaged Web-based solution that does not need to be created from scratch.

Additionally, there are many learning systems designed for simulation that contain all of the necessary tools for the instructor or simulation center staff to build the simulation scenario, including (but not limited to) programming guides, staging and scripting information for the scenario, and debriefing guides. Two potential disadvantages with any commercially available solution, however, are the cost to purchase it, which varies depending on the product and vendor, and the ability for or cost associated with customization.

Although the main disadvantages of a live system were discussed at the beginning of this section, the use of a real EHR system clearly provides learners with a truly authentic experience. One innovative solution to bridge this gap was developed out of an academic–business partnership between the Cerner Corporation and the University of Kansas School of Nursing. The Simulated E-hEalth Delivery

System (SEEDS) incorporated the use of Cerner Corporation's clinical information system and PowerChart application (Connors, Weaver, Warren, & Miller, 2002; University of Kansas Medical Center, 2016). This system was specifically adapted for educational purposes to address the learner's informatics needs. Similar to the WMC system discussed previously, instructors developed the patient data stored within the Cerner Corporation's clinical information system database, creating virtual patients within the system. Students could navigate through the system and view pertinent patient data and then document assessment information and create a plan of care within the PowerChart application. Additionally, the instructor could access student documentation for evaluation and feedback. According to the University of Kansas Medical Center (2016), "[SEEDS] marks the first time that a live-production, clinical information system designed for care delivery is being used in a simulated way for teaching curriculum content to health professional students" (para. 1). Refer to the Research Brief 1 for a discussion of a study on the use of the SEEDS approach.

## Challenges and Opportunities

The adoption and use of simulation technologies present unique advantages and disadvantages. Using simulated medical records, either as a stand-alone learning tool or in conjunction with a complete simulation scenario, provides the learner with an opportunity for a realistic, hands-on learning experience. Major considerations when looking to adopt a simulated EHR include (1) cost, (2) ease of use for the instructor and learner, (3) technical support from the vendor, (4) time to build or develop the patient database, (5) additional simulation materials included with the package, (6) flexibility of the system to be customized and used as a stand-alone tool or in the setting of a full-scale simulation scenario, and (7) overall fidelity or realism.

In 2006, a coalition consisting of experts from the fields of health care, informatics, business and industry, and nursing proposed the Technology Informatics Guiding Education Reform (TIGER) initiative (TIGER, 2007). The aim of this group is to advance the integration of informatics core competencies into nursing education so as to provide better and safer care to patients. Seven key steps were established to meet the 10-year vision of the TIGER initiative. Of particular interest is the call to take an active role in the design and integration of informatics tools that are "intuitive, affordable, usable, responsive and evidence-based" (p. 5). This approach will promote truly new and innovative strategies for informatics education and create significant opportunities for collaboration between industry, academia, and clinical practice.

## The Future of Simulation in Nursing Informatics Education

Simulation will clearly play an important role in the development of informatics competencies for student nurses and practitioners. One theme of simulation-based learning is practicing just as a nurse would in the actual clinical setting. With regard to facilitating the growth of informatics competencies, it is no different. If there are expectations regarding the use of clinical information systems and EHRs in the clinical setting, then the opportunity also exists for the incorporation of such tools into the classroom and simulated clinical setting.

Aside from using the simulated EHR in the setting of a clinical simulation scenario, there are also opportunities to incorporate the simulated EHR into the classroom in new and innovative ways. As mentioned in the beginning of the chapter in the second scenario, the EHR can be used as an active learning tool within the classroom. Rather than requiring students to absorb information from a book, the EHR can become a powerful way for learners to make important connections about caring for patients with a specific disease process or to learn concepts of pathophysiology or pharmacology.

# Game Mechanics and Virtual World Simulation for Nursing Education

## Introduction

The use of game mechanics in educational games and virtual world simulation for education continues to grow, with a great deal of research effort and funds directed toward the discoveries of their best uses. Educational games and virtual world simulations all share some characteristics, and it is difficult to find a pure experience in any of the genres. Simulations may have game-like qualities, and virtual worlds may be used to present a simulation.

## Case Scenario

Joe sits down at the computer and logs into StratWorld, a virtual world that enables the user to create his or her own team, then compete against other teams created by other StratWorld players. The developers of StratWorld create interesting challenges, part intellectual and part brute force, which teams strive to solve before other, competing teams solve them first.

After Joe logs on, he is presented with a **three-dimensional (3D)** view of a forest. Directly in front of him is a 3D figure that looks very much like Joe, except for broader shoulders, a more rugged face, and better skin complexion. This is Joe's **avatar**, his representation of self in StratWorld. Joe can change his avatar's appearance as he wishes, but he likes to stick to something close to the real thing. The members of one of his opposing teams in StratWorld all prefer to appear as masses of glowing tubes. Joe thinks they are strange.

Today, he is recruiting for his virtual team, so he ducks into his inventory (a place to store items his avatar can wear and use) and dons his manager's jacket. "Joe's Team" is proudly displayed on the back. Joe is proud of the jacket; he created the lettering himself in a graphics program and uploaded it to StratWorld, then added it to a plain jacket and gave a copy to all new members of his team. As in many virtual worlds, clothes do make the man, woman, or thing.

Using the arrow keys and the mouse to manipulate his avatar, Joe begins to make his avatar walk down the forest trail. He is looking to recruit an Ogre for his team to beef up their physical offensive capabilities and replace the recent loss of Charlie the Unicorn. Ogres are big and strong, perfect for the task. Joe is a little nervous. He has never been to this part of StratWorld before, and explorations in new areas can be fraught with peril. After a brief sojourn, Joe comes upon an Ogre sitting in a daisy-strewn clearing, picking his teeth with a small sapling ripped from the ground. "Ogre!" Joe shouts. "I need someone to smash through things for my team. Interested?"

"What in it for me?" the Ogre asks, thumping his chest with the remains of the sorry sapling, splintering it in oblivion. "Darn! That was good toothpick!" The chirps of birds, the drone of insects in the foliage, all normal background noise here, suddenly stop. Joe picks up on this environmental clue and, just as in the real world when this happens, knows he is in danger.

Joe ponders the question. He knows he is talking to a **nonplayer character (NPC)**, one that seems to have a brain behind the 3D façade, but in reality has very clever programming attached to it so that it can seem to carry on an intelligent conversation. Some companies call this artificial intelligence, but both the creators of these environments and the scholars who study them hotly debate the proper use of that term. Joe also knows that the world is constructed so that he has to balance his profits from game wins with overhead costs, such as player salaries and equipment maintenance. He needs to make an offer to the Ogre. An offer of too little will insult the Ogre, and a fight between it and Joe is the probable result. Joe's avatar could die, an inconvenience that will cost him time and loss of reputation with other StratWorlders. A generous offer will probably be accepted, but might bankrupt Joe over time. Joe needs to balance his needs and costs, and also think outside the box. It is a complex problem-solving situation!

"Okay, Ogre, here's the deal. Pay is $900 a month, and . . ." Joe attempts to continue, but the Ogre quickly rises in an aggressive manner. "Wait! Let me continue! I know that's a little less than normal, but I'll throw in a nice, new sapling each week for tooth maintenance! How about it?"

The Ogre sits back down and eyes Joe warily. "Just need to pick tooths, not maintain ants. Contract for . . ." (the Ogre pauses to quickly count his fingers) "10 months?"

"Sure, sure, but if you are injured, you go to half-pay until you can play again," Joe answers.

"I still get toothpick each week, even if hurt?"

"Absolutely. I mean, yes."

The Ogre leans forward on its haunches. "Sound good! You go. I follow."

"One more thing, Ogre. What do I call you?" Joe asks.

"Daisy! You managers sure stupid!"

Joe takes Daisy back to his office by teleporting there, a way to move from one place to another with a simple click of a button. Joe pulls up a map of StratWorld, locates the land he owns, and clicks on it for instantaneous transport. Joes sends Daisy the Ogre down to practice smashing down walls in his training field, and then pauses for a moment to admire his recreation of his grandfather's old roll-top desk. He recreated it from an old photograph just for his office in StratWorld. Looking out the window, he sees Daisy running out on the training field. He sits down at his desk to go over his team's statistics. With the addition of Daisy to the team, Joe needs to recalculate all his strategies. He needs to determine how he can acquire a sapling each week for Daisy: Where will he get one, and how much will it cost? Then he needs to send out an acceptance to a recent invitation from the game developers to participate in next week's challenge. A win will be sweet, but it will be a busy week of preparation!

Before Joe hunkers down to work, he sends an instant message to Kathy, an admirable opponent in StratWorld against whom he has competed several times. Typing furiously and with a certain glee, he writes, "Hi, Kathy, guess what? I'm gonna DUST your team in the next challenge!" Kathy's reply is swift: "Bring it on, Joe, bring it on!"

## Case Scenario Discussion

This is a brief description of what occurs in many online virtual environments today. People create a presence in the environment, then manipulate events for a desired outcome. They explore, build things, interact with others, and try to achieve goals. The story is fictional; there is no StratWorld, but games do exist where people build teams and compete against one another. So, is StratWorld a simulation, a virtual world, or a game? What do you think? Think about simulations you have experienced or heard of, games you have played, and anything you have read about virtual worlds. Try looking up some definitions online. Write down your thoughts and come up with some justifications that back your decision.

# Game Mechanics and Educational Games

Game mechanics are, simply put, the rules and limitations in which a game takes place. It is imperative that the rules are clearly stated in the instructions so the players know what is expected of them and the rules that the game itself much follow. The mechanics determine how the players or learners interact with the rules and how the game responds to the players' or learners' moves or behaviors within the game, thus connecting the players' or learners' actions to the purpose of the game. People voluntarily play games because they are fun and embody many motivational aspects (Mastrian et al., 2011). Great games provide an optimally challenging state between boredom and frustration (Csikszentmihalyi, 1990). Games exist within a set of rules (Kelley, 1988; Salen & Zimmerman, 2003), and players receive feedback from their interactions in the game and rule space.

An educational game—one designed for learning—is a subset of both play and fun, and is sometimes referred to as a "**serious game**" (Zyda, 2005). It is a melding of educational content, learning principles, and computer games (Prensky, 2001) that should emphasize the value of the experience (Nemerow, 1996). Mungai, Jones, and Wong (2002) stated that the flow of an educational game may be under the designer's control more than a noneducational game, and feedback should be used to stress competency, not just achievement. The trick in designing an educational game is to maintain the same fun state found in noneducational games (Koster, 2004). "Contemporary teachers wishing to incorporate game-based learning whether doing so within a virtual environment, through video games, or by leveraging mobile apps and other technologies are at the forefront of a paradigm shift" (Bauman, 2016, p. 110)

Many different types of games exist, and each type has a different potential for educational use (Mastrian et al., 2011). To learn to respond quickly and hone reflexes, action games may be used. Adventure games may be used to discover the unknown, such as diagnosing a patient's illness. Construction and building games could be used for building complex mental constructs that can be understood only through knowledge of their constituent parts and the ways in which they interrelate. Strategy games are great for nursing education teaching moments where careful, up-front planning is critical and on-the-fly adjustments to one's plan may be needed to ensure its success.

In role-playing games, the player takes on the role of one or more characters and improves them while progressing through a storyline. Today, **massive multiplayer online role-playing games** are very popular, using the Internet to provide a shared, simultaneous experience for dozens or even hundreds of players. Role-playing games are an excellent way for nursing educators to guide students through any situation where a sequenced step-by-step introduction to the parts of the job or skill is required.

Fairly new are casual games, also known as mini-games. These games are designed to be played in a short time span, or for a few minutes a day over several days, weeks, or even months. Many online browser–based games fit this category. Casual games may be useful for continuous reinforcement of basic concepts, for emulating a slowly changing environment, and for modifying the player's attitudes on a given topic over a period of time. To date, these games remain largely untapped as educational tools.

There are also gaming simulations. A simulation game uses game mechanics to imitate or copy real-ife activities or actions in the form of a game. Refer to Research Brief 2 for a mixed methods, quantitative, and qualitative study on the health and safety of home healthcare professionals, including nurses.

## RESEARCH BRIEF 2

Darragh et al. (2016) stated that the rapid increase in home healthcare services is driving a need for additional trained home healthcare professionals. The training must be effective for managing personal health and safety hazards encountered when providing healthcare services in the home environment. The process of developing and evaluating an interactive virtual simulation training system to educate home healthcare professionals, including nurses, was described.

Sixty-eight home healthcare professionals participated in the study, with the majority being white (71%), female (95%), and with an average age of 49 years (with a standard deviation of 11.8 years). Sixty-seven percent worked in Ohio and Kentucky. The participants represented RNs, aides and homemakers, administrators, educators, occupational therapists, and physical therapists.

A mixed-methods design, qualitative and quantitative, using an interdisciplinary, participatory design methodology was used to develop a virtual simulation training system to train home healthcare professionals to identify and manage health and safety hazards in the home using a gaming simulation learning approach. The participants identified the layout and features of a typical client home to the interdisciplinary research team. Once the working version of the virtual simulation training system was created, ongoing assessment of usefulness, usability, and desirability continued to develop and modify the system.

Quantitatively, the researchers used the Modified Home Healthcare Worker Questionnaire (MHHWQ), and the usefulness, usability, and desirability (UUD) survey. Qualitative data collection consisted of structured focus groups and individual interviews. The participants described 353 hazard management dilemmas and explained multiple types of "making do" solutions for the hazards, most of which were classified as "less-than-optimal."

The simulation game facilitated active learning and critical thinking processes crucial for these professionals as they are typically highly autonomous professionals who work independently in unpredictable environments where they must problem solve to create solutions to unforeseen or complex events that affect their health and safety, as well as the health and safety of their clients.

In order to prepare professionals using health and safety trainings, the training must focus on realistic scenarios, flexible solutions, and independent problem-solving activities. The virtual simulation training system includes immersion and engagement through a process of identification, response, problem solving, and feedback. The professionals had to assess the environment for hazards in multiple rooms, then received feedback both about correct identification and right and wrong answers, problem-solving about potential strategies, and assessment of progress in both a training and evaluation environment; this facilitated deliberate practice, which is a powerful component of skill acquisition.

The researchers concluded that participatory methods are a useful and effective way to design a virtual simulation training system that is interactive, engaging, and informative. Since this project is ongoing, their long-term goal was to improve the health and safety of home healthcare professionals who work in client homes.

The full article appears in Darragh, A., Lavender, S., Polivka, B., Sommerich, C., Wills, C., Hittle, B., . . . Stredney, D. (2016). Gaming simulation as health and safety training for home health care workers. *Clinical Simulation in Nursing, 12*(8), 328–335. doi:10.1016/j.ecns.2016.03.006

# Virtual Worlds in Education

Cohen and colleagues (2013) define a **virtual world** as follows:

> *Virtual worlds are live, online, interactive 3-dimensional environments in which users interact using speech or text via a personalised avatar. Access requires a modern computer and Internet connection. Healthcare practitioners are increasingly utilising virtual worlds and other web-based technologies for educational purposes, including resuscitation training, conferences, surgical education and team-working for multidisciplinary healthcare providers. (p. 79)*

A 3D virtual world often mimics a real-world environment, although it may also include impossible abilities, such as flying unaided (Mastrian et al., 2011). Users of virtual worlds are often quick to stress that these creations in and of themselves are not games, although this confusion is easy to understand because virtual worlds share many of the same interface characteristics as 3D action and role-playing games.

The best use of virtual worlds for educational purposes may occur when there is a need for an immersive experience coupled with a need for social interaction. For example, in the virtual world of **Second Life**, one university has developed a virtual hacienda for students learning Spanish (Clark, 2009). Students interact with the environment and the objects in the hacienda while speaking to one another in Spanish, thereby participating in authentic learning activities. Some of the Second Life scenarios used by another college of nursing include a real human resources representative whom the student must call; the pair must discuss the situation and the student then determines a solution based on the representative's input. This activity immerses the students in their role and fully engages them in the learning episode. Cohen et al. (2013) tested the use of a virtual world as a training site for emergency preparedness and coordination for first responders in major incidents (such as a terrorist attack), and concluded that

> *[m]ajor incident exercises are complex in nature and expensive and they thereby require novel methodologies to aid training and preparation. This study has established the feasibility of developing low-cost, immersive, accessible virtual environments for major incident preparation using a systematic approach. Both the environment and scenarios were deemed realistic and acceptable for training and testing of existing plans by clinicians. (pp. 83–84)*

Virtual worlds need not be 3D. Predecessors to the 3D environment include the **multiuser dungeon**, **object-oriented multiuser dungeon**, and multiuser shared hallucination. All of these environments are text based, so that the user receives environmental information as passages of text and manipulates objects and talks to others by typing text commands. Multiuser dungeons, object-oriented multiuser dungeons, and multiuser shared hallucinations are still in use today.

## Choosing Among Simulations, Educational Games, and Virtual Worlds

Simulations, educational games, and virtual worlds all have a great deal of overlap. Games may be placed in virtual worlds, and simulations may have game-like elements. Yet, these three tools also have distinctive characteristics. By examining several of these key characteristics (goal orientation, competition, the fun factor, and exploratory learning and social interaction affordances), it becomes easier to choose the correct tool for teaching purposes.

Games are goal oriented and may be competitive in nature. They should be fun and perhaps a bit fantastical and light-hearted. A particular game may or may not include exploratory learning and social interaction. Although simulations are also goal oriented, the competition is generally subdued. Simulations are generally more realistic and are not necessarily fun to use. A particular simulation may or may not include exploratory learning and social interaction. Virtual worlds in and of themselves do not have goals or competition; it is up to the player to construct them and add them to the world. Virtual worlds are not by default fun, although they may include the fantastical. Virtual worlds generally lend themselves to exploratory learning and social interaction. When educators develop virtual worlds for education, they can control the scenarios or activities experienced by the learners. Virtual worlds used for simulation also include a debrief for their learners and this debriefing process solidifies the learning.

## The Future of Simulations, Games, and Virtual Worlds in Nursing Education

The use of simulations, games, and virtual worlds in Western society continues to increase. The combination of best practices supported by sound research, the ever-growing power of technology, and learners who grew up using these environments will lead to greater use of these tools for learning (New Media Consortium, 2007).

In addition, games are becoming less expensive to produce and consume. Game development engines, which were long in the hands of only major game development companies, are now available at a cost that many users and organizations can afford. Some games come with built-in development tools, an attempt by the game producers to use free labor to extend their product (Dyer-Witheford & de Peuter, 2009). The growth of indie (independent) game companies is leading to a plethora of cheap, yet high-quality, games. The same holds true for virtual worlds. New virtual worlds spring up all the time. Many offer free, if limited, accounts, and educators are exploring these spaces with increasing regularity, building fantastic learning environments.

Companies are tapping mobile devices as another avenue to push out their games. These devices are already used for a variety of communication and social functions, so why not build on that with casual games that rely on social interactions? Expect to see much more happening in this space in the near future.

Another related area of growth is in **augmented-reality games (ARGs)**. Augmented reality occurs when one uses a device, such as a smartphone, to overlay additional information on the real world (Klopfer & Squire, 2008). For example, one might use the camera in the phone to view the stars at night and see on the phone's screen both the stars and the constellation labels and linking lines between the stars in a constellation. ARGs exploit this concept in game-like ways, bringing people together physically and virtually to solve a series of challenges. In education, ARGs may be used to provide a fun way to collect and analyze data, to collaborate with other students, to access information resources, and to provide a new way to look at the world.

Serious games may also have a place in helping practicing nurses maintain or hone skills. Baker (2009) suggested that gaming has a place in continuing education. The science of nursing practice encourages us to ask questions, promote dialogue, share lessons learned willingly and openly, and make the outcomes of our patients constructive and positive. Rigorous or high-quality evaluation and research into the teaching and learning techniques offered by serious games can offer insight into future changes not conceived of at this moment. For example, if a serious game could effectively assist nurses in maintaining the skill set required to care for a patient who is experiencing hypothermia, would that be worth the investment? If a game could reduce medication errors in the operating room by 50–75% compared to what has been demonstrated in the past, would that have value? If it were found that after implementation of a serious game, a facility experienced zero errors in right-site, right-procedure, and right-patient events during a 10-year period, would this be of value (Baker, 2009, p. 173)?

Other new games that can be used to educate health professionals have been discussed by Skiba (2008). She described Foldit, a game that challenges players to fold proteins as part of a research experience for Life and Death in the Age of Malaria, a game that simulates advice nurses would give to world travelers on health maintenance strategies, and 3dMD, designed to facilitate skills training in teamwork for military environments.

Best uses of all of these technologies and approaches related to nursing education remain a bit murky (Bauman, 2016, p. 110). Fortunately, a great deal of research, whose findings will guide future educators toward the most effective uses of educational games, simulations, and virtual worlds, is under way. In an ideal world, educators would have a plethora of available, well-designed, and educator-certified games to choose from that mesh with the educational objectives of their classes, courses, and curricula.

## Summary

Simulated experiences in nursing education contain the PEDA elements to provide important opportunities for students to hone critical-thinking and clinical skills in a safe and supportive environment. Simulation scenarios may also provide a better variety of clinical and practicum experiences than those available in a real setting, and they also provide nursing faculty the opportunity to track student progress and development against specific learning objectives. Nurse educators can share simulation scenarios and experiences and thus contribute to the body of nursing education knowledge to improve education practice. Simulations, games, and virtual worlds have a great deal of potential as educational tools that can augment, supplement, or even replace traditional methods of teaching. As educators become more skilled in the use of these tools, and as designers share their creative works with others, we can expect to see these tools used more frequently in the coming decade.

## THOUGHT-PROVOKING QUESTIONS

1. Consider your experience and learning with regard to EHRs. If you were to design a learning program centered on the use of EHRs, what would it look like? Consider this from the viewpoint of an educator, a student, a clinician, and a healthcare administrator.
2. Think about the clinical courses you have taken as a student. Which opportunities and challenges exist regarding the use of an EHR as a major learning tool in conjunction with, or perhaps even replacing, the required textbook?
3. If you were to design a simulation scenario incorporating the use of an EHR, which informatics competencies would you focus on and why?
4. Games are supposed to be fun and voluntary. How can educators force a game on a student and expect it to remain fun and engaging?
5. It can take several hours of gameplay to learn the mechanics of some games, and even longer for the more complex games. If subject-matter learning can occur only after this initial game-mechanics learning occurs, how can educators justify the amount of time a learner must spend within the game just to get to the point where learning begins?
6. If you were choosing between a latex-based simulation and a virtual simulation, what would you list as each of their advantages and disadvantages? Would PEDA elements be present for both?
7. How do educators acquire the training needed not just to get by in these new environments, but rather flourish, thrive, and mold the environments for their purposes?

# References

Aldrich, C. (2010, August). *Virtual worlds, simulations and games for online educators.* Manga Online Seminar presented at Penn State University, University Park, PA.

Alessi, S. M. (1988). Fidelity in the design of instructional simulations. *Journal of Computer-Based Instruction, 15*(2), 40–47.

American Academy of Nursing. (2003). Proceedings of the American Academy of Nursing conference on using innovative technology to decrease nursing demand and enhance patient care delivery. *Nursing Outlook, 51,* 1–41.

American Association of Colleges of Nursing. (1997). *A vision of baccalaureate and graduate nursing education: The next decade.* Washington, DC: Author.

American Nurses Association (ANA). (2015). *Nursing informatics: Scope and standards of practice* (2nd ed.). Silver Spring, MD: Nursesbooks.org.

Baker, J. (2009). Serious games and perioperative nursing. *AORN Journal, 90*(2), 173–175. Retrieved from Health Module (Document ID: 1853293981).

Bauman, E. (2016). Games, virtual environments, mobile applications and a futurist's crystal ball. *Clinical Simulation in Nursing, 12,* 109–114.

Bligh, J., & Bleakley, A. (2006). Distributing menus to hungry learners: Can learning by simulation become simulation of learning? *Medical Teacher, 28*(7), 606–613.

Brown, M. C. (2005). Internet-based medical chart for documentation and evaluation of simulated patient care activities. *American Journal of Pharmaceutical Education, 69*(1–5), 204.

Carty, R., & Ong, I. (2006). The nursing curriculum in the information age. In V. K. Saba & K.A. McCormick (Eds.), *Essentials of nursing informatics* (4th ed., pp. 517–531). New York, NY: McGraw-Hill.

Choi, M., Park, J., & Lee, H. (2016). Assessment of the need to integrate academic electronic medical records into the undergraduate clinical practicum. *Computers, Informatics, Nursing (CIN), 34*(6), 259–265.

Clark, G. (2009). These horses can fly! and other lessons from Second Life: The view from the virtual hacienda. In R. Oxford & J. Oxford (Eds.), *Second language teaching and learning in the Net Generation* (pp. 153–172). Honolulu, HI: National Foreign Language Resource Center.

Cohen, D., Sevdalis, N., Taylor, D., Kerr, K., Heys, M., Willett, K., . . . Darzi, A. (2013). Emergency preparedness in the 21st century: Training and preparation modules in virtual environments. *Resuscitation, 84*(1), 78–84. doi:10.1016/j.resuscitation.2012.05.014

Connors, H. R., Weaver, C., Warren, J., & Miller, K. L. (2002). An academic–business partnership for advancing clinical informatics. *Nursing Education Perspectives, 23*(5), 228–233.

Csikszentmihalyi, M. (1990). *Flow: The psychology of optimal experience.* New York, NY: Harper Collins.

Darragh, A., Lavender, S., Polivka, B., Sommerich, C., Wills, C., Hittle, B., . . . Stredney, D. (2016). Gaming simulation as health and safety training for home health care workers. *Clinical Simulation in Nursing, 12*(8), 328–335. doi:10.1016/j.ecns.2016.03.006

Dyer-Witheford, N., & de Peuter, G. (2009). *Games of empire: Global capitalism and video games.* Minneapolis, MN: University of Minnesota Press.

Fetter, M. (2009). Graduating nurses' self-evaluation of information technology competencies. *Journal of Nursing Education, 48*(2), 86.

Fisher, R. (2016). Designing the simulation learning environment: An active engagement model. *Journal of Nursing Education and Practice, 6*(3), 6–14. doi: 10.5430/jnep.v6n3p6

Gaba, D. (2004). The future vision of simulation in health care. *Quality and Safety in Healthcare, 13*, 2–10.

Gaba, D., & DeAnda, A. A. (1998). A comprehensive anesthesia simulation environment: Recreating the operating room for research and training. *Anesthesiology, 69*, 387–393.

Gassert, C. A. (1998). The challenge of meeting patients' needs with a national nursing informatics agenda. *Journal of the American Medical Association, 3*, 263–268.

Gassert, C. A., & Sward, K. A. (2007). Phase I implementation of an academic medical record for integrating information management competencies into a nursing curriculum. *Studies in Health Technology and Informatics, 129*(Pt 2), 1392–1395.

Gredler, M. E. (1996). Educational games and simulations: A technology in search of a (research) paradigm. In D. H. Jonassen (Ed.), *Handbook of research for educational communications and technology* (pp. 521–540). New York, NY: Simon & Schuster Macmillan.

Harris, J., Shoemaker, K., Johnson, K., Tompkins-Dobbs, K., & Domian, E. (2016). Qualitative descriptive study of family nurse practitioner student experiences using high-fidelity simulation. *Kansas Nurse, 91*(2), 12–15.

Hayden, J. K., Smiley, R. A., Alexander, M., Kardong-Edgren, S., & Jeffries, P. R. (2014). The NCSBN national simulation study: A longitudinal, randomized, controlled study replacing clinical hours with simulation in prelicensure nursing education. *Journal of Nursing Regulation, 5*(2 suppl.). Retrieved from https://www.ncsbn.org/JNR_Simulation _Supplement.pdf

Hertel, J. P., & Millis, B. J. (2002). *Using simulations to promote learning in higher education: An introduction.* Sterling, VA: Stylus.

Hunter, K., McGonigle, D., & Hebda, T. (2013). TIGER-based measurement of nursing informatics competencies: The development and implementation of an online tool for self-assessment. *Journal of Nursing Education and Practice (JNEP), 3*(12), 70–80. doi: 10.5430/jnep.v3n12p70

Institute of Medicine. (2000). *To err is human: Building a safer system.* Washington, DC: National Academic Press.

Jonassen, D. H. (1999). Designing constructivist learning environments. In C. M. Reigeluth (Ed.), *Instructional design theories and models: A new paradigm of instructional theory* (Vol. 2, pp. 215–239). Mahwah, NJ: Lawrence Erlbaum Associates.

Kelley, D. (1988). *The art of reasoning.* New York, NY: W. W. Norton.

Klopfer, E., & Squire K. (2008). Environmental detectives: The development of an augmented reality platform for environmental simulations. *Education Technology Research and Development, 56,* 203–228.

Koster, R. (2004). *A theory of fun for game design.* Scottsdale, AZ: Paraglyph Press.

Mastrian, K. G., McGonigle, D., Mahan, W. L., & Bixler, B. (2011). *Integrating technology in nursing education: Tools for the knowledge era.* Sudbury, MA: Jones & Bartlett Learning.

McGonigle, D., Hunter, K., Hebda, T., & Hill, T. (2014). *Self-Assessment of Level 3 and Level 4 NI Competencies Tool Development.* Retrieved from http://www.himss.org /self-assessment-level-3-level-4-ni-competencies-tool-development

Mungai, D., Jones, D., & Wong, L. (2002, August). *Games to teach by.* Paper presented at the 18th Annual Conference on Distance Teaching and Learning, Madison, WI.

National League for Nursing. (2008). *Preparing the next generation of nurses to practice in a technology-rich environment: An informatics agenda* [Position statement]. New York, NY: Author.

Nemerow, L. G. (1996). Do classroom games improve motivation and learning? *Teaching and Change, 3*(4), 356–361.

New Media Consortium. (2007). Massively multiplayer educational gaming. *The Horizon Report,* 2007 Edition. Retrieved from http://www.nmc.org/horizonproject/2007 /massively-multiplayer-educational-gaming

Pew Health Professions Commission. (1998). *Recreating health professional practice for a new century: The fourth report of the Pew Health Professions Commission.* San Francisco, CA: Author.

Podolefsky, N. S., Moore, E. B., & Perkins, K. K. (2013). Implicit scaffolding in interactive simulations: Design strategies to support multiple educational goals. Retrieved from: https:// arxiv.org/pdf/1306.6544.pdf%3B

Prensky, M. (2001). *Digital game-based learning.* New York, NY: McGraw Hill.

Rajalahti, E., Heinonen, J., & Saranto, K. (2014) Developing nurse educators' computer skills towards proficiency in nursing informatics. *Informatics for Health and Social Care, 39*(1), 47–66.

Salen, K., & Zimmerman, E. (2003). *Rules of play: Game design fundamentals.* Cambridge, MA: MIT Press.

Simulation Learning System. (2010). Retrieved from https://evolve.elsevier.com/education /nursing/simulation-learning-system/?pageid=10705

Skiba, D. (2008). Games for health. *Nursing Education Perspectives, 29*(4), 230–232. Retrieved from ProQuest Nursing & Allied Health Source (Document ID: 1538660701).

Staggers, N., Gassert, C. A., & Curran, C. (2002). A Delphi study to determine informatics competencies for nurses at four levels of practice. *Nursing Research, 51*(6), 383–390.

Technology Informatics Guiding Education Reform (TIGER). (2007). The TIGER initiative: Evidence and informatics transforming nursing 3-year action steps toward a 10-year vision. Retrieved from http://www.aacn.nche.edu/education-resources/TIGER.pdf

University of Kansas Medical Center. (2016). Simulated E-hEalth Delivery System (SEEDS). Retrieved from http://www.kumc.edu/health-informatics/seeds.html

Weatherford, J. (n.d.). Instructional simulations: An overview. Retrieved from http://www.etc.edu.cn/eet/Articles/instrucsimu/start.htm

Zyda, M. (2005). From visual simulation to virtual reality to games. *Computer, 39*(9), 25–32.

# Research Applications of Nursing Informatics

**Nursing informatics (NI) provides more tools and capabilities than can at times be imagined.** Just as NI has changed the way nursing is administered and practiced, so it has also dramatically altered research practices.

Nursing research has evolved with technology. In the era of evidence-based practice, clinicians must continue to think critically about their actions. What is the science behind interventions? Things must no longer be done a certain way just because they have always been done that way. Instead, one should research the problem, use evidence-based resources, critically select electronic and non-electronic references, consolidate the research findings and combine and compare the conclusions, present the findings, and propose a solution. The nurse may be the first to ask *why*, thereby becoming a key player in making change happen.

NI enhances and facilitates collaboration; improves access to online libraries; provides research tool transparency for collection, analysis, and dissemination of research knowledge; and facilitates the development of a common data language. It provides organizational and informational support to advance translational research, helping to fill the gap between research findings and practice implementation. Repeat studies are needed to provide meaningful meta-analyses and systematic reviews of evidence to advance practice. Technology advancement in the area of incorporating evidence into clinical tools must continue. Removing the barriers to knowledge-seeking behavior and providing access to evidential resources promotes knowledge use and, in the end, improves patient outcomes. In addition, NI provides support for powerful research techniques such as data mining and research involving biological processes and genomics that hold the promise of discovering new knowledge to improve clinical practices.

The material in this book is placed within the context of the Foundation of Knowledge model (**Figure VI-1**). Nursing research is conducted to generate knowledge that is used to meet the needs of healthcare delivery systems, organizations, patients, and nurses. In relation to the model, the nurse researcher is involved with every aspect—from acquiring (collecting) and processing (analyzing) data and information, to generating knowledge, to disseminating the results or findings (knowledge). Through this work, the researcher generates knowledge for the nursing profession. Knowledge generation is extremely important in the advancement of nursing science.

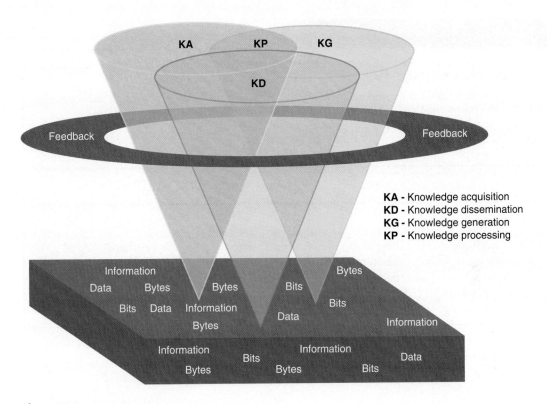

**Figure VI-1** Foundation of Knowledge Model
Designed by Alicia Mastrian.

1. Describe nursing research in relation to the Foundation of Knowledge model.

2. Explore the acquisition of previous knowledge through Internet and library holdings.

3. Explore information fair use and copyright restrictions.

4. Assess informatics tools for collecting data and storage of information.

5. Compare tools for processing and analyzing quantitative and qualitative data.

## Key Terms

- » American Library Association
- » Copyright
- » Cumulative Index to Nursing and
- Allied Health Literature
- » Educational Resources Information Center
- » Fair use
- » Foundation of Knowledge model
- » Handheld devices
- » Information literacy
- » MEDLINE
- » PsycInfo

# CHAPTER 21

# Nursing Research: Data Collection, Processing, and Analysis

Heather E. McKinney, Sylvia DeSantis, Kathleen Mastrian, and Dee McGonigle

## Introduction: Nursing Research and the Foundation of Knowledge Model

The **Foundation of Knowledge model** suggests that the most important aspect of information discovery, retrieval, and delivery is the ability to acquire, process, generate, and disseminate knowledge in ways that help those managing the knowledge reevaluate and rethink the way they understand and use what they know and have learned. These goals closely reflect the Information Literacy Competency Standards for Higher Education, published by the **American Library Association** (ALA) in 2003 in response to changing perceptions of how information is created, evaluated, and used.

According to the ALA (2000), an information-literate individual is able to do the following:

- Determine the extent of information needed
- Access the needed information effectively and efficiently
- Evaluate information and its sources critically
- Incorporate selected information into one's knowledge base
- Use information effectively to accomplish a specific purpose
- Understand the economic, legal, and social issues surrounding the use of information and access and use information ethically and legally

In addition, new challenges arise for individuals seeking to understand and evaluate information because information is available through multiple media (graphical, aural, and textual). The sheer quantity of information does not by itself create a more informed citizenry without complementary abilities to use this information effectively. Most significantly, information literacy forms the basis for lifelong learning, serving as a commonality among all learning environments, disciplines, and levels of education (Association of College and Research Libraries [ACRL], 2000, 2016). These standards and challenges are still applicable today.

During rounds, Charles encounters a rare condition he has never personally seen and only vaguely remembers hearing about in nursing school. He takes a few moments to prepare himself by searching the Internet. That evening, he does even more research so that he can assess and treat the patient safely. He searches clinical databases online and his own school textbooks. Most of the information seems consistent, yet some factors vary. Charles wants to provide the highest quality of patient care and safety. He wonders which resources are best, which are the most trusted, and which are the most accurate.

# Knowledge Generation Through Nursing Research

**Information literacy** is an intellectual framework for finding, understanding, evaluating, and using information (refer to Figure 21-1). These activities are accomplished in part through fluency with information technology and sound investigative methods, but most importantly through critical reasoning and discernment. The ACRL (2016) has suggested that "information literacy initiates, sustains, and extends lifelong learning through abilities which may use technologies but are ultimately independent of them" (para. 8).

As nursing informatics (NI) combines all four nursing practice areas (clinical, research, administration, and education), the ability to recognize the need for a specific kind of information and then locate, evaluate, and effectively use that information within the NI paradigm will catapult nurses ahead of other healthcare professionals in applying and engaging various facets of technology (ACRL, 2016). However, because so few nurses have formal training in technology but still represent a disproportionate number of users, the ways in which nursing research integrates healthcare technology within NI creates an unseen challenge (McHaney, 2007). This potentially enormous impact on the future of health care and technology will determine the success of information-literate nurses: those who have learned how to learn and who understand the intricacies of how knowledge is organized, retrieved, and used in such a way that others can learn from them (ACRL, 2016). It is important that nurse educators prepare nursing students for information-literate practice in technology-laden healthcare environments. Stephens-Lee and colleagues (2013) stressed that "[n]ursing students require opportunities to help them develop NI skills and abilities to prepare them for contemporary workplaces" (para. 39). Nash (2014) stated,

> If we desire nurses who practice the art of nursing as well as the science of nursing, we must make it a priority to address the issue of integrating those interpersonal and critical thinking skills we value into an increasingly complex, high-tech, fast-paced healthcare system that often works against us practicing at our very best. (p. 13)

Nursing students today use technology in their personal lives, and they know that

> technology allows them to share photos (Flickr), exchange files and images, send videos (YouTube, Snapchat), bookmark (Quorum or Diigo, Pinterest), micro-blogs or short postings (Twitter, Tumblr, MySpace), blog (Blogger),

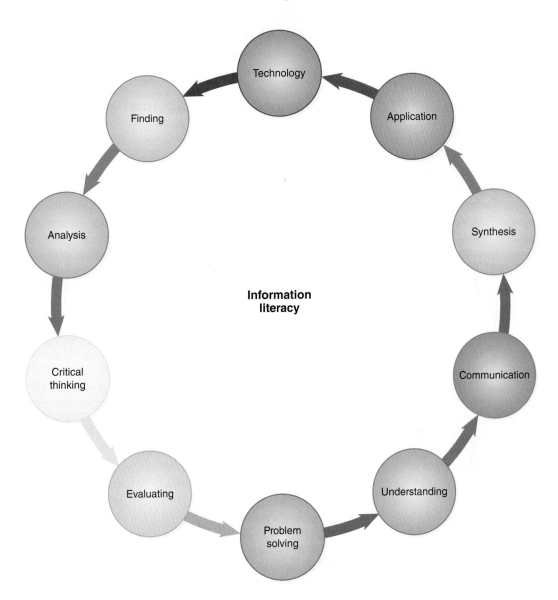

**Figure 21-1** Information Literacy

*socialize (Facebook, Vimeo, Instagram), search (Google, Google+), and network professionally (Altogether, LinkedIn, Yahoo Groups). (Merrill, 2015, p. 72)*

Nursing faculty must be able to adapt their teaching in this new technology era so that they engage their students and help them assimilate technology as they prepare for their professional nursing roles. Focusing on nurses providing direct patient care, Piscotty et al. (2015) stated that "finding methods that can help nurses offer safe and effective care using technology is an absolute necessity" (p. 287). As nurses enact their role as administrators, researchers, educators, and/or clinical staff members, integrating technology in the current technology-laden information era is paramount.

# Acquiring Previously Gained Knowledge Through Internet and Library Holdings

In an environment characterized by rapid technological change coupled with an overwhelming proliferation of information sources, nurses face an enormous number of options when choosing how and from where to acquire information for their academic studies, clinical situations, and research. Because information is available through so many venues, libraries, special-interest organizations, media, community resources, and the Internet in increasingly unfiltered formats, healthcare practitioners must inevitably question the authenticity, validity, and reliability of information (ACRL, 2016).

Often, the retrieval of reliable research and information may seem to be a daunting task in light of the seemingly ubiquitous amount of information found on the Web. Focusing on specific information venues not only aids this search but also assists in negotiating the endless maze of resources, allowing a nursing practitioner to find the best and most accurate information efficiently.

## Professional Online Databases

Professional databases represent a source of online information that is generally invisible to all Internet users except those with professional or academic affiliations, such as faculty, staff, and students. These databases, which range from specific to general, act as collection points by aggregating information, such as abstracts and articles from many different journals; two such databases include the **Cumulative Index to Nursing and Allied Health Literature** (CINAHL) and **MEDLINE**. CINAHL, for example, specifically includes information from all aspects of allied health, nursing, alternative medicine, and community medicine. The MEDLINE database contains references to more than 22 million journal articles and is maintained and produced by the National Library of Medicine. Other databases, such as **PsycInfo** from the American Psychological Association and the **Educational Resources Information Center** (ERIC) database, may also benefit nursing. Many databases also offer full-text capabilities, meaning that entire articles are available online. The articles and abstracts contained within these databases have already withstood the rigors of publication in professional journals and, therefore, are considered viable and authentic peer-reviewed sources.

Libraries with subscriptions to databases often employ library professionals who are able to help patrons sift through the vast amounts of available electronic information; using the expert research capabilities of a health science librarian at one's local university is the best way to learn how to conduct database searches that yield the most efficient and useful results. Also useful are websites that provide tutorials on best searching practices specifically for medically oriented databases, such as the tutorials provided by EBSCO support to search the CINAHL database.

## Search Engines

Search engines allow users to surf the Web and find information on nearly anything, although many researchers steer clear of search engines because of the vast amounts of unsubstantiated information they are likely to uncover. Because no legitimacy needs to be provided for any information that appears on the Web, an author can make claims, substantiated or not, and still use the Web as a publishing venue. Despite the pitfalls associated with search engines in general, they can yield a bounty of useful information when used with discretion.

Different search engines will produce different results when used for the same research. For example, one popular search engine ranks its results by number of hits a page or site has received. Whereas the most popular research results are likely to be relevant, the order in which results appear does not indicate quality or viability of the source.

Different Web address (domain) suffixes (.com, .edu, .org, .gov, and so forth) indicate who is responsible for creating the website. Although a .edu site is hosted by an educational institution and for that reason may seem legitimate, consider that it could also belong to a student stating personal opinion, gossip, or guesswork. In contrast, .gov sites are maintained by the government and nearly always have professional contact information. Web hosts develop new domain suffixes constantly, so although looking at the suffix can be useful, it should not be the sole deciding factor when choosing to trust information.

One should never blindly trust information found on a webpage. When possible, check the date of the most recent update (How old is the page?), contact information (Is a bibliography or list of sources provided?), links to external sources (Do they seem relevant?), and previous attained knowledge from other reputable sources (Is the information too unbelievable?).

Fees and information retrieval charges should be approached with skepticism. Private companies do offer information aggregation services for a fee. In these cases, users pay a flat monthly fee for access to collections of articles in a particular field. What users (especially those affiliated with an academic institution) may not realize is that they are likely to have free access to the same, if not more complete, information through their institution's library system.

Some legitimate databases and traditional newspapers that maintain a Web presence do provide access for a small fee, but just as many others simply ask users to register to see articles for free. Many nursing students and professionals affiliated with a university may find that their university library has already purchased access for the student body.

## Electronic Library Catalogs

Nearly all higher education institutions have placed their library catalogs online. Although this is an obvious convenience for many students, some nursing professionals unused to working completely online may be intimidated by an e-catalog. Library professionals at the tiniest university and the busiest community college are available to demonstrate how to navigate a basic search of their library's catalog. Asking for assistance in learning how to access the vast assortment of journals, books, databases, and other resources available at one's college library is an excellent idea. Students in nursing programs at larger universities will likely find free classes that specifically teach users how to navigate and use the online catalog. If smaller colleges and universities do not offer these services, one should take advantage of the library's online tutorials, help pages, frequently asked questions pages, and online reference service (if available). Local public libraries often have subscriptions to popular databases and offer free classes on searching techniques to patrons, providing yet another free access point to the best information for one's research needs. Making full use of available library resources serves to strengthen information literacy skills, enabling learners to master content and extend their investigations, become more self-directed, and assume greater control over their own learning (ACRL, 2016).

# Fair Use of Information and Sharing

**Copyright** laws in the world of technology are notoriously misunderstood. The same copyright laws that cover physical books, artwork, and other creative material apply in the digital world. Have you ever given a friend a flash drive that contains a computer game or some other type of software that you paid for and registered? Have you ever downloaded a song from the Internet without paying for it? Have you ever copied a section of online content from a reference site and used that content as if it was your own? Have you ever copied a picture from the Internet without asking permission from the photographer who took the picture? Have you ever copied and pasted information about a disease or drug from a website and then printed out the information to give to a patient or family member? These are all examples of the type of copyright infringements enabled by technology that occur almost without thought.

The value of creative material—whether it is written content, a song, a painting, or some other type of creative work—lies not in the physical medium on which it is stored, but rather in the intangibles of creativity, skills, and labor that went into creating that item. The person who created the material should be properly credited and possibly reimbursed for the use of the material. How would musicians be reimbursed for their music if everyone just downloaded their songs illegally from the Internet? Imagine that you created a game to teach patients with type 1 diabetes how to manage their diet, and other nurses copied and distributed that game without getting your permission to do so. How would you feel?

Almost all software, music, and movies (either digital or in hard copy [CDs or DVDs] form) come with restrictions on how and why copies can be made. The license included with the software clarifies exactly which restrictions are applicable. The most common type of software license is a "shrink wrap" license, meaning as soon as the user removes the shrink wrap from the CD or DVD case, he or she has agreed to the license restriction. Most computer software developers allow for a backup copy of the software to be made without restriction. If the hard drive fails on the user's computer, the software can usually be reinstalled through this backup copy. Some software companies even allow the purchaser of a software package to transfer it to a new user. In this case, the software typically must be uninstalled from the original owner's computer before the new owner is free to install the software on his or her computer. Most of these restrictions depend on the honesty of the user in reading and following the licensing agreement. As a result of widespread abuses, however, the music and film industries commonly include hardware security features in their products that block users from making a working copy of a music CD or movie DVD.

The bottom line: Copyright laws also apply to the digital world, and copyright violations can lead to prosecution. Advances in technology have made the sharing of information easy and extremely fast. A scanner can convert any document to digital form instantly, and that document can then be shared with people anywhere in the world. Nevertheless, the person who originally created that document has the right to approve of the sharing of the work. Carefully read the fine print of any software purchased and be sure to clarify any questions regarding how that software can be copied. Avoid downloading music illegally from the Internet, and do not use information from the Internet without permission to do so or without citing the reference appropriately. Healthcare organizations that allow access to the Internet from a network computer should ensure that users are well aware of and compliant with all copyright and **fair use** principles.

# Informatics Tools for Collecting Data and Storage of Information

Nurses are already intimately familiar with data collection as daily agents of patient care documentation, patient monitoring, and interview data (Chang, 2001; International Council of Nurses, 2012). In this way, formal nursing datasets are actually made up of gathered information, such as healthcare definitions, classification, and nursing information. Before data can be analyzed or critically reviewed to determine outcomes or assessment, they must be collected and aggregated. According to the Cleveland Clinic (2010):

> [C]ollaborative nursing-led research is enhanced by the ability to support these projects with patient data that is more easily extracted electronically. Supporting these efforts and initiatives is a dedicated team of clinical and system analysts who provide support for the development and management of information databases, systems and processes to bring efficiency to nursing-driven quality and research endeavors through informatics. (para. 12–13)

Nurses may generate and record data from their own observations or with the assistance of various devices. Free text (informational data, such as drug dosages administered, resources used, and problems diagnosed) is recorded electronically. Free text is then interpreted and organized by some standardizing principle, either manually or by computer. In this way, data (often qualitative data that cannot be traditionally measured in a numeric sense) can be organized and processed. A central issue to the generation and analysis of free text data is the lack of a generally accepted set of terminology to capture nursing data. Data actually become information when these separate components are interpreted, organized, combined, and structured within a specific context to convey particular meanings (Hovenga & Sermeus, 2002; Kempe, 2013).

Database management systems consist of software designed to collect, sort, organize, store, retrieve, select, and aggregate data. Nursing and health data may be classified into four basic types: (1) resource data (e.g., financial information); (2) patient and client demographics; (3) activity data (clinical data); and (4) health service provider data. These primary data may be either recorded manually or collected electronically, with manual collection providing a greater opportunity for error. When data are electronically recorded, this process follows a programmed set of instructions built into the software, thereby cutting down substantially on collection error. Of paramount importance in the collection process are the data collection form and the computer interface used for inputting the data; these affect the completeness, consistency, and accuracy of the resulting data (Hovenga & Sermeus, 2002; Kempe, 2013).

Quantitative data collection tools or instruments include questionnaires, interviews, surveys, quizzes, assessments, email interviews, and Web-based surveys, all of which generate numerical data rather than text-based data. Questionnaires—one of the most popular means of data collection—can be administered in hard copy, on paper, or programmed into a website where individuals may answer the questions electronically (Chang, 2001; Statistics Canada, 2014). Other electronic data collection tools include handheld devices and onsite laptops. A key benefit of using electronic data collection is the ability to transmit data to another computer directly for compilation and analysis, thereby cutting down on the risk of error (Hebda, Czar, & Mascara, 2005; Kania-Richmond, Weeks, Scholten, & Reney, 2016; Teale, Young, & Sleigh, 2013).

Of course, one must always be cognizant of the need to protect the privacy of participants by deidentifying data collected for research and by having tools in place to provide secure transmission and storage of private information. Some researchers are finding rich qualitative data on public and freely available patient support sites and blogs. An important issue associated with such Internet-based data collection is whether participants actually are who they say they are, and whether they actually have the variable of interest or are just pretending to be someone or something they are not. Remember that the same rules for protecting human subjects apply no matter where the data are accessed or collected, and that all research involving human subjects should be formally approved by the appropriate institutional review board (IRB). Many IRBs have specific policies in place that govern electronic data collection and storage to ensure that the rights and privacy of research participants are protected (Office of the Vice President for Research at Penn State, n.d.).

An excellent example of innovative electronic data collection is the system used by participants in the Nightingale Tracker System pilot study, in which nursing students traveling to rural clinical sites submitted information via handheld devices while miles away from their preceptor-supervisors. The results of this study suggest that, despite some technical challenges associated with the hardware, using the handheld technology enhanced students' learning (especially in the area of physical assessment), increased their confidence in practicing in community-based settings, and provided efficient data input capabilities (Black & Merrill, 2015; Ndiwane, 2005).

Harder-to-measure, nonnumerical qualitative data can be collected electronically in the form of a narrative or diary-like entry. Much in the way free text is analyzed and sorted, this narrative dialogue is assessed and then coded, looking for patterns and themes that represent the phenomenon under study. For example, a nurse researcher may be interested in studying the lived experiences of women recently diagnosed with breast cancer and, therefore, may ask them to keep a diary of their thoughts, questions, and treatment experiences.

# Tools for Processing Data and Data Analysis

Data analysis is the process by which data collected during the course of a study are processed to identify trends and patterns of relationships. Descriptive statistics allow the researcher to organize information meaningfully, thereby facilitating insight by describing what the data show (Hebda, Czar, & Mascara, 2005). Figure 21-2 describes the importance of descriptive statistics. There exist a range of tools to facilitate such analysis, including specialized databases, word processing/spreadsheet/database applications, and statistical packages (Hovenga & Sermeus, 2002; Latinen, 2014).

## Quantitative Data Analysis

Quantitative data focus on numbers and frequencies, with the goal of describing a situation or looking for more robust relationships such as correlations and specific variable contributions to an outcome. This aim stands in contrast to qualitative analysis, which focuses on experiences and meaning. Although the kind of data generated by

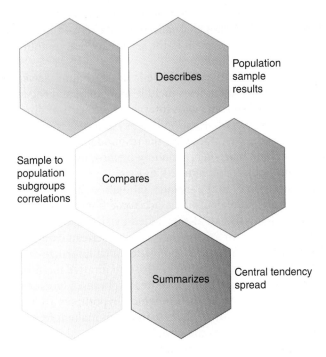

**Figure 21-2** The Importance of Descriptive Statistics

quantitative collection is fairly straightforward and easy to analyze (responses to questionnaires, experiments, and psychometric tests), quantitative data analysis has come under criticism. Psychologists, for example, prefer to use a combination of quantitative and qualitative data, backing up research participants' explanations with statistically reliable information obtained by numerical measurement (Holah.co.uk, n.d.).

In quantitative studies, variables represented by data are collected in numerical form. These values are then entered into specific fields that have predetermined meanings or are coded. Various quantitative data analyses can be applied to nursing research, such as intervention research, quality improvement studies, and outcomes research. One of the most popular statistical packages for this kind of analysis is the Statistical Package for Social Sciences (SPSS). Depending on the research goal, the researcher may use different types of analysis. Different statistical goals may require hypothesis testing, model building, descriptive and exploratory analyses, and others. For example, hypothesis testing is based on assumptions regarding the relative truth of the hypothesis, so a data analysis would compare actual outcomes with purported hypotheses.

## Qualitative Data Analysis

Extremely varied in nature, qualitative data can include nearly any information that can be captured and is not numerical (Trochim, 2006a). Qualitative data are more concerned with describing meaning than with drawing statistical inferences; what is lost in reliability (faulty transcription, forgotten details, and so forth) is gained in validity (Holah.co.uk, n.d.). Although qualitative data rely on judgments, they can still be manipulated numerically, much in the same way that quantitative data can be open to judgment (Trochim, 2006b).

Some major types of qualitative data include in-depth interviews, direct observation, and written documents. Interviews include individual and focus group interviews and may be recorded in some way. Interviews differ from direct observation in their interactive nature. Direct observation differs from case to case and often means the researcher does not make contact with the respondent. Written documents might include a variety of written materials, including memos, newspaper clippings, conversation transcripts, and books (Trochim, 2006a).

Computers can aid greatly in the storage, tabulation, and retrieval of qualitative data by acting as the equivalent of an electronic filing cabinet (Hebda, Czar, & Mascara, 2005). Data analysis can also be aided by simple data management programs, such as Excel, Access, or NVivo, in which a user can categorize data and link categories with key words. Data can be converted into information and knowledge by either inductive or deductive reasoning. Most qualitative methods use an inductive approach in which the researcher generates hypotheses (versus the deductive approach typical of quantitative studies, in which hypotheses are tested). Data analysis in quantitative studies may allow the researcher to make inferences to a population beyond the sample, as long as the sample was representative of the population. In contrast, generalizing to a larger population is not a goal of qualitative research. Rather, in qualitative research the goals are exploration and deeper understanding of a phenomenon that has not been widely studied (see Figure 21-3).

Two relatively new approaches to quantitative research are cohort research and case control research. Cohort research is a type of study in which two groups of

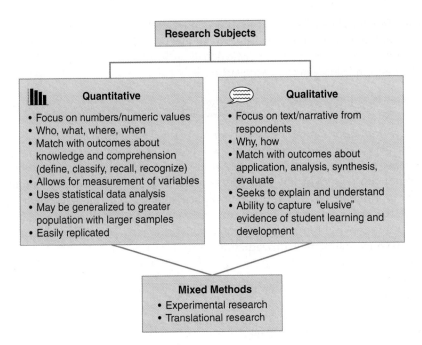

**Figure 21-3** Quantitative Versus Qualitative Research

people are identified, one with an exposure of interest and another without the exposure. The two groups are followed forward to determine whether the outcome of interest occurs. Groups are defined based on whether they have had an exposure to a particular risk factor. Case control research, in contrast, is a type of study in which patients who have an outcome of interest and patients who do not have the outcome are identified; the researcher then looks back in time (typically using health records) to determine exposures and experiences that could have contributed to the outcome occurring or not occurring (Brown, 2014).

## The Future

The future of NI is growing as fast as technology itself. The more nurses participate in the development process of healthcare technology, the more efficient and effective NI may become. Nurses are urged to take an active role in the profession by providing real-world feedback during the design process and after implementation. Such practical insights will provide valuable data for technology evaluation and advancement in the field of nursing informatics.

## Summary

This chapter discussed the value of information literacy as an essential research tool and its relationship to knowledge generation and lifelong learning. The reader is now acquainted with informatics tools useful for acquiring new knowledge and assessing previous knowledge and tools useful for collecting and storing and analyzing information to generate knowledge. In an ideal world, information literacy and informatics tools will be used as a critical skill set for increasing healthcare efficiency, effectiveness, and safety in the 21st century.

## THOUGHT-PROVOKING QUESTIONS

1. How does information literacy affect NI in the 21st century?
2. Provide a detailed description of how NI facilitates both qualitative and quantitative research.
3. Reflect on copyright law and why it is needed. Suppose you determine that photographs or other images can be replicated based on your assessment of fair use, but your administrative assistant refuses to photocopy them because he feels that it is copyright infringement and against company policy. Describe in detail how you would handle this situation.

# References

American Library Association (ALA). (2000). *Information literacy competency standards for higher education.* Chicago, IL: Author.

Association of College and Research Libraries (ACRL). (2000). Information literacy competency standards for higher education. Retrieved from https://arizona.openrepository.com/arizona/handle/10150/105645

Association of College and Research Libraries (ACRL). (2016). Information literacy competency standards for higher education. Retrieved from http://www.ala.org/acrl/standards/information literacycompetency

Black, C., & Merrill, E. (2015, Fall). Using mobile devices in nursing education. *The ABNF Journal,* 78–84.

Brown, S. (2014). *Evidence-based nursing: The research–practice connection* (3rd ed.). Burlington, MA: Jones & Bartlett Learning.

Chang, B. L. (2001). Computer use in nursing education. In V. Saba & K. McCormick (Eds.), *Essentials of computers for nurses: Informatics for the new millennium* (3rd ed., pp. 445–456). New York, NY: McGraw-Hill.

Cleveland Clinic. (2010). Nursing informatics. Retrieved from http://my.clevelandclinic.org/nursing/informatics.aspx

Hebda, T., Czar, P., & Mascara, C. (2005). *Handbook of informatics for nurses & health care professionals* (3rd ed.). Upper Saddle River, NJ: Prentice Hall.

Holah.co.uk. (n.d.). Quantitative and qualitative data. Retrieved from http://www.holah.karoo.net/quantitativequalitative.htm

Hovenga, E. J. S., & Sermeus, W. (2002). Data analysis methods. In J. Mantas & A. Hasman (Eds.), *Textbook in health informatics: A nursing perspective* (pp. 113–125). Amsterdam, Netherlands: IOS Press.

International Council of Nurses. (2012). *Closing the gap: From evidence to action.* Retrieved from http://nursingworld.org/MainMenuCategories/ThePracticeofProfessionalNursing/Improving-Your-Practice/Research-Toolkit/ICN-Evidence-Based-Practice-Resource/Closing-the-Gap-from-Evidence-to-Action.pdf

Kania-Richmond, A., Weeks, L., Scholten, J., & Reney, M. (2016). Evaluating the feasibility of using online software to collect patient information in a chiropractic practice-based research network. *Journal of the Canadian Chiropractic Association, 60*(1), 93–105.

Kempe, S. (2013). The data – information – knowledge cycle. *Dataversity.* Retrieved from http://www.dataversity.net/the-data-information-knowledge-cycle

Latinen, H., Kaunonen, M., & Astedt-Kurki, P. (2014). Methodological tools for the collection and analysis of participant observation data using grounded theory. *Nurse Researcher, 22*(2), 10–15.

McHaney, D. F. (2007, June–August). Embracing the integration of technology and care. *Alabama Nurse, 34*(2), 1.

Merrill, E. (2015). Integrating technology into nursing education. *The ABNF Journal, 26*(4), 72–73.

Nash, B. (2014, November/December). Maintaining the art of nursing in an age of technology. *Ohio Nurses Review*, 12–13.

Ndiwane, A. (2005). Teaching with the Nightingale Tracker technology in community-based nursing education: A pilot study. *Journal of Nursing Education, 44*(1), 40–42.

Office of the Vice President for Research at Penn State. (n.d.). IRB guideline X: Guidelines for computer- and Internet-based research involving human participants. Retrieved from https://www.research.psu.edu/irb/policies/guideline10

Piscotty, R., Kalisch, B., & Gracey-Thomas, A. (2015). Impact of healthcare information technology on nursing practice. *Journal of Nursing Scholarship, 47*, 287–293.

Statistics Canada. (2014). Data collection and questionnaire. Retrieved from http://www.statcan.gc.ca/eng/cs/questions-3

Stephens-Lee, C., Lu, D., and Wilson, K. (2013). Preparing students for an electronic workplace. *Online Journal of Nursing Informatics (OJNI), 17*(3). Retrieved from http://ojni.org/issues/?p=2866

Teale, E., Young, J., & Sleigh, I. (2013). A point of care electronic stroke data collection system. *British Journal of Healthcare Management, 19*(1), 10–15.

Trochim, W. M. K. (2006a). Qualitative data. *Research Methods Knowledge Base.* Retrieved from http://www.socialresearchmethods.net/kb/qualdata.php

Trochim, W. M. K. (2006b). Types of data. *Research Methods Knowledge Base.* Retrieved from http://www.socialresearchmethods.net/kb/datatype.php

# CHAPTER 22

# Data Mining as a Research Tool

Dee McGonigle and Kathleen Mastrian

## Introduction: Big Data, Data Mining, and Knowledge Discovery

Data mining methods have been developed over time using research. As data mining evolves, we have not only become able to navigate our data in real time, but have also progressed beyond mere access to retrospective data with navigational improvements. Using data warehousing and decision support, we could, for example, answer the question, "What was the most commonly diagnosed disease in our nine-hospital system last April?" We could then drill down to one hospital. As we have developed big data collection capabilities, data capture, data transmission, storage capabilities, powerful computers, statistics, artificial intelligence, high-functioning relational database engines with data integration, and advanced algorithms, we have realized the ability to data mine our big data to predict and deliver prospective and proactive information. We can begin to predict by answering a question such as "What is likely to be the most commonly diagnosed disease next month and why?" Data mining includes tools for visualizing relationships in the data and mechanizes the process of discovering predictive information in massive databases.

Pattern discovery entails much more than simply retrieving data to answer an end user's query. Data mining tools scan databases and identify previously hidden patterns. The predictive, proactive information resulting from data mining analytics then assists with development of business intelligence, especially in relation to how we can improve. Much of our big data is **unstructured data**; unstructured big data reside in text files, which represent more than 75% of an organization's data. Such data are not contained in databases and can be easily overlooked; moreover, it is difficult to discern trends and patterns in such data. Data mining is an iterative process that explores and models big data to identify patterns and provide meaningful insights.

As we evolve the tools with which we can collect, access, and process data and information, it is necessary to concomitantly evolve how we analyze and interpret the data and information. IBM (2013) describes **big data** in a way that is easy to understand:

> Every day, we create 2.5 quintillion bytes of data—so much that 90% of the data in the world today has been created in the last two years alone. This data comes from everywhere: sensors used to gather climate information, posts to social media sites, digital pictures and videos, purchase transaction records, and cell phone GPS signals to name a few. This data is big data. (p. 1)

According to Tishgart (2012), "More data means more knowledge, greater insights, smarter ideas and expanded opportunities for organizations to harness and learn from their data" (para. 2). **Data mining** is the process of using software to sort through data to discover patterns and ascertain or establish relationships. This process may help to discover or uncover previously unidentified relationships among the data in a database with a focus on applications. This information can then be used to increase profits or decrease costs, or a combination of the two. In health care, it is being used to improve efficiency and quality, resulting in better healthcare practices and improved patient outcomes. As we hone our analytical skills, we will be able to clarify and explain patterns in our big data related to improved patient responses to select treatments for optimal patient outcomes. We can then drill down for each treatment to examine the conditions the patient presented with and the number of visits they made. The data can then be explored to refine the output. For example, it would be very important to know more about each patient, such as if they had other conditions or diseases (comorbidities) that could affect their outcomes as well as their age, gender, educational level, and so on. Moskowitz, McSparron, and Celi (2015) stated,

> Beyond simple user principles, trainees do not learn the skills and concepts necessary for the optimal use of EMRs, including knowledge creation and personalized clinical decision making through analysis of large data sets. To date, this is largely because such systems have not been designed or implemented with these goals in mind. In the coming era of "Big Data," our community of medical educators and researchers must leverage digital systems for this purpose and find a way to prepare trainees for this critical role. (para. 9)

Their next steps concluded that "[t]he time has come to leverage the data we generate during routine patient care to formulate a more complete lexicon of evidence-based recommendations and support shared decision making with our patients" (para. 19).

Data mining projects help organizations discover interesting knowledge. These projects can be predictive, exploratory, or focused on data reduction. Data mining focuses on producing a solution that generates useful forecasting through a four-phase process: (1) problem identification, (2) exploration of the data, (3) pattern discovery, and (4) knowledge deployment, or application of knowledge to new data to forecast or generate predictions. Data mining is an analytic, logical process with the ultimate goal of forecasting or prediction. It mines or unearths concealed predictive information, constructing a picture or view of the data that lends insight into future trends, actions, or behaviors. This data exploration and resulting knowledge discovery foster proactive, knowledge-driven decision making. See **Figure 22-1**, which illustrates how raw data is transformed to knowledge.

*Problem identification* is the initial phase of data mining. The problem must be defined, and everyone involved must understand the objectives and requirements of the data mining process they are initiating.

*Exploration* begins with exploring and preparing the data for the data mining process. This phase might include data access, cleansing, sampling, and transformation; based on the problem you are trying to solve, data might need to be transformed into another format. To assure meaningful data mining outcomes, you must comprehend and truly understand your data. The goal of this phase is to identify the relevant or important variables and determine their nature.

Sometimes known as model building or pattern identification, *pattern discovery* is a complex phase of data mining. In this phase, different models are applied to the same data to choose the best model for the dataset being analyzed. It is imperative that the model chosen should identify the patterns in the data that will support the best predictions. The model must be tested, evaluated, and interpreted. Therefore, this phase ends with a highly predictive, consistent pattern-identifying model.

The final phase, *knowledge deployment*, takes the pattern and model identified in the pattern discovery phase and applies them to new data to test whether they can

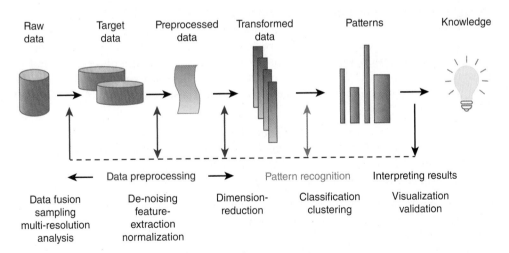

**Figure 22-1** Transforming Raw Data into Knowledge
Reproduced from Login Works. (2016). The process of data mining. Retrieved from http://www.loginworks.com/data-mining-services-various-type

achieve the desired outcome. In this phase, the model achieves insight by following the rules of a decision tree to generate predictions or estimates of the expected outcome. This deployment provides the organization with the actionable information and knowledge necessary to make strategic decisions in uncertain situations.

Data mining develops a model that uses an algorithm to act on **datasets** for one situation where the organization knows the outcome and then applies this same model to another situation where the outcome is not known—an extension known as **scoring**. Data mining is concerned with extracting what is needed, and it applies statistics so that organizations can gain an advantage by manipulating information for practical applications. In our information-overloaded healthcare world, all too often we find ourselves grasping for knowledge that is currently nonexistent or fleeting. Data mining is a dynamic, iterative process that is adjusted as new information surfaces. It is a robust, predictive, proactive information and knowledge tool that, when used correctly, empowers organizations to predict and react to specific characteristics of and behaviors within their systems.

Data mining is also known as knowledge discovery and data mining (KDD), knowledge discovery in data, and knowledge discovery in databases. The term "knowledge discovery" is key, as data mining looks at data from different vantage points, aspects, and perspectives and brings new insights to the dataset. This analysis then sorts and categorizes the data, and finally summarizes the relationships identified. In essence, then, data mining is the process of finding correlations or patterns among the data.

Health care, as noted earlier, generates big data. Data mining tools, in turn, are able to analyze enormous databases to determine patterns and establish applications to new data. Healthcare organizations clearly need to invest more in big data and data mining analysis: The "big data market [reached an estimated] $2.2 billion in 2011, [but] only 6% of that investment came from health care" (Tishgart, 2012, para. 2).

The healthcare sector has discovered data mining through the realization that knowledge discovery can help to improve healthcare policy making, healthcare practices, disease prevention, detection of disease outbreaks, prevention of sequelae, and prevention of in-hospital deaths. On the business side, healthcare organizations use data mining for the detection of falsified or fraudulent insurance claims. According to Manyika et al. (2011),

> If US healthcare were to use big data creatively and effectively to drive efficiency and quality, the sector could create more than $300 billion in value every year. Two-thirds of that would be in the form of reducing US healthcare expenditure by about 8 percent. (para. 2)

If they are to develop a successful data mining process, organizations must have the data needed to create meaningful information. In health care, we are honing our ability to analyze our data by making sure that those data are comprehensive and complete, meet our needs, and are cleansed and prepared for the data mining process. Many facilities are using data warehouses to store data and facilitate this pre–data mining process. We are learning to ask the right questions during the data mining process to gain a thorough understanding of our data. The following pages introduce the concepts, techniques, and models used in data mining.

# KDD and Research

According to IBM (2013), big data does not just refer to size, but rather "is an opportunity to find insights in new and emerging types of data and content, to make your business more agile, and to answer questions that were previously considered beyond your reach" (p. 6). Data mining for knowledge discovery is not new; it has been used for some time in research. However, we now have advanced analytical software designed to facilitate data mining. The knowledge discovery capabilities continue to evolve. Goodwin et al. (1997), for example, reported on their collaborative data mining research, which explored the relationship between clinical data and adult respiratory distress syndrome (ARDS) in critically ill patients. DeGruy (2000) indicated that big data in health care needed to be analyzed using KDD tools and applications to determine trends and relationships, with the ultimate goal of decreasing healthcare costs while improving quality. Berger and Berger (2004) suggested that nurse researchers are positioned to use data mining technologies to transform the repositories of big data into comprehensible knowledge that will be useful for guiding nursing practice and facilitating interdisciplinary research.

Madigan and Curet (2006) described the **classification and regression trees (CART)** data mining method for analyzing the outcomes and service use in home health care for three conditions: chronic obstructive pulmonary disease, heart failure, and hip replacement. They found that four factors—patient age, type of agency, type of payment, and ethnicity—influenced discharge destination and length of stay.

Over the last several decades, the KDD capability has improved as the analytical power of data mining tools has increased, thereby facilitating the recognition of patterns and relationships in big data. Trangenstein, Weiner, Gordon, and McNew (2007) described how their faculty used data mining to analyze their students' clinical logs, which enabled them to make programmatic decisions and revisions and rethink certain clinical placements. Zupan and Demsar (2008) described the open source tools developed by data mining researchers that they felt were ready to be used in biomedical research. Fernández-Llatas et al. (2011) described workflow mining technology as a means to facilitate relearning in dementia processes. Lee et al. (2011) discussed the application of data mining to identify critical factors such as nursing interventions related to patient fall outcomes. Lee, Lin, Mills, and Kuo (2012) used data mining to determine risk factors related to each stage of pressure ulcers and identified five predictive factors: hemoglobin level, weight, sex, height, and use of a repositioning sheet. Based on the results of this data mining analysis, nurses can better target their interventions to prevent pressure ulcers. Green et al. (2013) identified differences in limb volume patterns in breast cancer survivors; their results have the potential to influence clinical guidelines for the assessment of latent and early-onset lymphedema.

As these examples suggest, we must continue to employ data mining and interprofessional collaboration to reduce inefficiencies, improve quality, and support transformations using data-driven models of care.

In a large teaching hospital, there is a high rate of readmission for patients with congestive heart failure (CHF) who are being treated at the facility. The chief nursing officer (CNO) wants to know the cause of the readmissions, as the rate at this facility is almost twice that of competing healthcare entities in the area. The CNO works with the nursing researchers at the university to address this situation.

The researchers begin to scour the electronic health records (EHRs) of more than 15,000 CHF hospitalizations in the past 4 years to determine the cause of the situation. As they begin to understand this dataset, they are able to build a data mining model using algorithms to discover patterns and relationships in the data. Based on the old data, they determine that the key factor for readmission was the length of time it took to follow up at home with discharged patients.

In response to this new knowledge, a program in which nurses contact patients with CHF the day after their discharge by phone was developed, and a home visit is scheduled for the second day post-discharge to ensure a smooth transition to home or an assisted living facility. This follow-up within the first 4 days of discharge has reduced readmissions by 40%. The model that was used with the old data is being applied to the new data.

# Data Mining Concepts

**Bagging** is a term for the use of voting and averaging in predictive data mining to synthesize the predictions from many models or methods or the use of the same type of a model on different data. This term can also refer to the unpredictability of results when complex models are used to mine small datasets.

**Boosting** is what the term infers—a means of increasing the power of the models generated by weighting the combinations of predictions from those models into a predicted classification. This iterative process uses voting or averaging to combine the different classifiers.

Data reduction shrinks large datasets into manageable, smaller datasets. One way to accomplish this is via aggregation of the data or clustering.

**Drill down** analysis typically begins by identifying variables of interest to drill down into the data. You could identify a diagnosis and drill down, for example, to determine the ages of those diagnosed or the number of males. You could then continue to drill down and expose even more of the data.

**Exploratory data analysis (EDA)** is an approach or philosophy that uses mainly graphical techniques to gain insight into a dataset. Its goal varies based on the purpose of the analysis, but EDA can be applied to the dataset to extract variables, detect outliers, or identify patterns.

Feature selection reduces inputs to a manageable size for processing and analysis, as the model either chooses or rejects an attribute based on its usefulness for analysis.

**Machine learning** is a subset of artificial intelligence that permits computers to learn either inductively or deductively. Inductive machine learning is the process of reasoning and making generalizations or extracting patterns and rules from huge datasets—that is, reasoning from a large number of examples to a general rule. Deductive machine learning moves from premises that are assumed true to conclusions that must be true if the premises are true.

**Meta-learning** combines the predictions from several models. It is helpful when several different models are used in the same project. The predictions from the different classifiers or models can be included as input into the meta-learning. The goal is to synthesize these predicted classifications to generate a final, best-predicted classification—a process also referred to as **stacking**.

Predictive data mining identifies the data mining project as one with the goal of identifying a model that can predict classifications.

Stacking or stacked generalization synthesizes the predictions from several models.

# Data Mining Techniques

It is important to understand your data before you begin the data mining process so that you can choose the best technique and get the most from the data mining. The commonly used techniques in data mining are neural networks, decision trees, rule induction, algorithms, and the nearest neighbor method.

A **neural network** represents a nonlinear predictive model. These models learn through training and resemble the structure of biological neural networks; that is, they model the neural behavior of the human brain. Computers are fast and can respond to instructions or programs over and over again. Humans use their experience to generalize the world around them. Neural networks are a way to bridge the gap between computers and humans. Neural networks go through a learning process or training on existing data so that they can predict, recognize patterns, associate data, or classify data.

A **decision tree** is so named because the sets of decisions form a tree-shaped structure. The decisions generate rules for classifying a dataset. CART and chi square automatic interaction detection (CHAID) are two commonly used types of decision tree methodologies. See **Box 22-1** and **Figure 22-2** for an overview of decision tree analysis.

---

**BOX 22-1 DECISION TREE ANALYSIS**

*Steven L. Brewer, Jr.*

Decision trees are a statistical technique based on using numerous algorithms to predict a dependent variable. These predictions are determined by the influence of independent variables. Decision trees help researchers understand the complex interactions among variables generated from research data. The entire dataset is split into child nodes based on the impact of the independent predictors. The most influential variable is situated at the top of the tree; the subsequent nodes are ranked by the significance of the remaining independent predictors.

Graphically, decision trees produce a tree (as illustrated in **Figure 22-2**) that consists of a root node and child nodes. The tree is an inverted, connected graphic. The graphic representation of the decision tree helps general users, such as practitioners, understand the complex interrelationships between the independent and dependent variables in a large dataset.

Within the graphical display, there are three major components: the root node, the child node, and the terminal node. The root node represents the dependent variable, and the child nodes represent the independent variables. The root node is essentially the base of the tree or the top node. It contains the entire sample, while each child node contains a subset of the sample within the node directly above it. In Figure 22-2, the root node represents a sample of women who were either reassaulted or not reassaulted in a domestic violence database. Data in the root node are then partitioned and passed down the tree.

The number of child nodes will vary depending on the **classification** procedure that is used to determine how the data are split. In Figure 22-2, the first child node is "women's perception of safety." This node suggests that the most influential predictor in domestic violence reassault for this sample is the women's perception of safety. The tree produces additional child nodes based on the responses to that variable. Node 1 represents the women who responded "no" when asked whether they felt safe in the relationship. For this node, women had a 90% chance of being reassaulted. In contrast, node 2 represents the women who responded "yes" when asked whether they felt safe in the relationship. These women had only a 72% chance of being reassaulted.

The decision tree in Figure 22-2 splits the entire sample into subsamples, which in turn allows for different predictions for different groups within the sample. For example, women who felt safe in their relationship (node 2) and experienced controlling behaviors (node 6) had an 80% chance of being reassaulted. In contrast, women who did not feel safe (node 1) and were in a relationship characterized by controlling behaviors (node 4) had a 97.3% chance of being reassaulted. The splitting of the data continues until the data are no longer sufficient to predict the remaining variables or there are no additional cases to be split.

Classification trees share commonalities with nonlinear traditional methods such as discriminant analysis, cluster analysis, nonparametric statistics, and nonlinear estimation; however, the technique differs significantly from linear analyses. In general, the decision tree technique does not rely on "multiplicative" or "additive" assumptions such as regression to predict the outcome of $y$. The flexibility of classification trees is one characteristic that makes them attractive to researchers. The trees are not bound or limited to examining all predictor variables simultaneously. Therefore, each predictor variable can be examined as a singularity to produce univariate splits in the tree. Additionally, classification trees can handle a mixture of categorical and continuous variables when univariate splits are used. While this flexibility offers advantages over traditional methods, classification trees are not limited to univariate splits.

Decision trees have become a popular alternative to methods such as regression and discriminate analysis for data mining big data. Such trees use algorithms from one of the numerous classification procedures to separate the data into different branches or child nodes that predict $y$. The dependent variable ($y$) is represented by the root node.

These algorithms have three main functions: (1) they explain how to separate or partition the data at each split, (2) they decree when to stop or end the splitting of data, and (3) they determine how to predict the value of $y$ for each $x$ in a split. The child nodes are separated into homogenous groups by the algorithms from different classification procedures. This process of partitioning is the main purpose of classification procedures. First, the procedure clusters and creates child nodes. Second, it ranks them based on their predictive values of $y$. Hence, the most influential variable(s) will be located at the base of the tree. From this point, the classification procedures further expand the child nodes by finding the next best factor. The tree is expanded until the algorithm is unable to find a clearly distinguishable split within the data.

Based on the results of the sample decision tree analysis presented in Figure 22-2, practitioners would conclude that women should be attuned to their perception of safety in a relationship, as those who feel unsafe have a much higher chance of another assault.

Decision trees are a powerful tool that can be used to mine large datasets and discover previously unknown relationships among the data. The predictive relationships uncovered by the decision tree analysis may be useful in directing approaches to future care interventions.

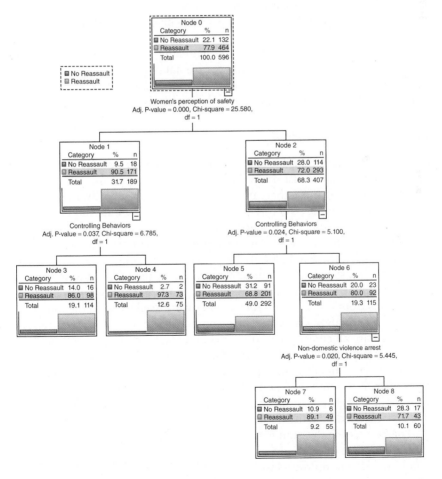

**Figure 22-2** Decision Tree Analysis Output

Rule induction is based on statistical significance. Rules are extracted from the data using *if-then* statements, which become the rules.

**Algorithms** are typically computer-based recipes or methods with which data mining models are developed. To create the model, the dataset is first analyzed by the algorithm, looking for specific patterns and trends. Based on the results of this analysis, the algorithm defines the parameters of the data mining model. The identified parameters are then applied to the entire dataset to mine it for patterns and statistics.

Nearest neighbor analysis classifies each record in a dataset based on a select number of its nearest neighbors. This technique is sometimes known as the *k*-nearest neighbor.

Text mining for text is equivalent to data mining for numerical data. Because text is not always consistent in health care owing to the lack of a generally accepted terminology structure, it is more difficult to analyze. Text documents are analyzed by extracting key words or phrases.

**Online analytic processing (OLAP)** generates different views of the data in **multidimensional databases**. These perspectives range from simplistic views such as descriptive statistics, frequency tables, or comparative summaries to more complicated analyses requiring various forms of cleansing the data such as removing outliers. OLAP is also known as fast analysis of shared data.

**Brushing** is a technique in which the user manually chooses specific data points or observations or subsets of data on an interactive data display. These selected data can be visualized in two-dimensional or three-dimensional surfaces as scatterplots. Brushing is also known as graphical exploratory data analysis.

## Data Mining Models

To generate predictions and infer relationships, the dataset, statistics, and patterns identified in existing data must be applied to new data. A data mining model is developed by exercising more than algorithms on data. Specifically, the data mining model consists of a mining structure plus an algorithm. The data mining model remains empty until it applies the algorithm or processes and analyzes the data provided by the mining structure. This model stores the information obtained from a statistical analysis of the data, identifying patterns and gaining insights. It then contains metadata that specify the name and definition of the model, the server location or other place where it is stored, definitions of any filters applied when processing the model, columns from the mining structure that were used to build the model, and the algorithm used to analyze the data. The columns, their data types, any filters, and the algorithm used are all choices that are made in the data mining process, and each of these decisions can greatly influence the data mining results. The same data can be used to create many models; one type of model could organize the data into trees, for example, whereas another type of model might cluster the data in groups based on the rules applied. Different results can be achieved from the same mining structure, even though it is used in many models, based on the filtering method or analysis conducted. Therefore, each decision made along the way is very important.

There are many models. In this chapter, we will review the following models: Cross-Industry Standard Process for Data Mining (CRISP-DM), Six Sigma/Lean, and SEMMA (Sample, Explore, Modify, Model, Access).

## CRISP-DM

The CRISP-DM model follows a path or series of steps to develop a business understanding by gaining an understanding of the business data collected and analyzed. The six steps are business understanding, data understanding, data preparation, modeling, evaluation, and deployment.

The CRISP-DM model begins with an understanding of the business. The situation must be assessed to establish the data mining goals and produce the project plan. You must be able to answer the following questions: What are the business objectives? What are the requirements? Have we specifically defined the problem? The answers to these questions help transform the business perspective knowledge into a data mining problem definition and initial plan to meet the objectives.

Data understanding begins with the preliminary data collection and assimilation of the data. It is during this step that the data will be described and explored to facilitate the user's comprehension of the data. As the user gains familiarity with the data, data quality issues are identified and the quality of the data is verified.

The data are cleansed and transformed during the data preparation step. First, one must select the data, attributes, and records to be used. These data are then cleansed, constructed, integrated, and properly formatted. At this point, the final dataset is constructed from the data; this dataset will be processed by the model.

Modeling involves selection of the modeling methods and their application to the prepared dataset. Parameters are calibrated, a test design is generated, and the model is built and assessed. This step might require you to revisit data preparation if the format of the data does not meet the specific requirements of the methods.

During the evaluation step, the degree to which the objectives were met is assessed from a business perspective. A key question: Were any important business issues not considered? The model was built for high-quality data analysis. To see whether this goal has been met, the process is reviewed, results evaluated, and the model interpreted. This is where you determine whether the model should be implemented or whether more iterations must occur before its deployment. The project may not be completed, or a new data mining project might be initiated. If the project is deployed, this step is when you must decide how the results from the data analysis will be used.

Deployment is the final step, in which the model is finally implemented. The plan must be monitored and maintained and the project reviewed. The six-step process should yield a reliable, repeatable data mining process. The knowledgeable insights gained from the implementation of the model must be organized and presented in such a way that they can be used. The final project report is generated to document the process and share this enhanced knowledge of the data.

The CRISP-DM model employs a process that has been proven to make data mining projects both more rapid and more effectual. Using this model helps to avoid typical mistakes while assessing business problems and detailing data mining techniques.

## Six Sigma

Six Sigma/Lean are data-driven methods to eliminate defects, avoid waste, or assess quality control issues. (Although they are often considered in tandem, we will be discussing only Six Sigma here.) It aims to decrease discrepancies in business and manufacturing processes through dedicated improvements. Six Sigma uses the DMAIC steps: define, measure, analyze, improve, and control.

The first step defines the goals of the project or the goals for improvement. During this step, you can use data mining techniques to discover prospective ideas for implementing the project.

In the measure step, exploratory and descriptive data analyses are used on the existing system to enhance the understanding of the data. Reliable, valid, and accurate metrics with which to measure goal achievement in each of the steps are identified.

The analysis step should assess the system to identify discrepancies between the current big data and the goal. Statistical methods guide this analysis.

Improvements must be made to the current system to attain the organizational goals. The use of project management skills facilitates the application of the new methodology and processes. Statistical methods assess the improvements and any deficiencies that exist.

The final step of the model is control. Controlling the system is important so discrepancies are remedied before they cause a disruption.

The Six Sigma model applies a different mentality to the same old business model or way of thinking. The DMAIC steps that are implemented typically result in success.

## SEMMA

According to SAS (n.d.), "The acronym SEMMA—sample, explore, modify, model, assess—refers to the core process of conducting data mining" (para. 1). This model is similar to Six Sigma but concentrates more on the technical activities characteristically involved in data mining.

The first step is to sample the data. Sampling is optional but creates a more robust data mining effort. Using "[a] statistically representative sample of your data, SEMMA makes it easy to apply exploratory statistical and visualisation techniques, select and transform the most significant predictive variables, model the variables to predict outcomes, and confirm a model's accuracy" (SAS, n.d., para. 1). Creating a target dataset shrinks the data to a manageable size, yet maintains the important information necessary to mine.

The exploration of the data seeks to discover discrepancies, trends, and relationships in the data. It is at this point that ideas about the data should emerge to help the organization understand the data and its implications for the organization's business. In health care, for example, it would be important to determine how many people use the emergency department each year and how many of those people are admitted, released, and return, and to identify any disparities in care and diagnoses. What did you discover? What are the trends and relationships that emerge from the data mining?

After exploring, you should modify your data based on the information discovered. It might be important to modify the data based on groupings such as "all people who are diagnosed with congestive heart failure who present with shortness of breath" if the trending and relationships indicate that this subgroup is significant. Other variables can also be introduced at this time to help gain a further understanding of the data.

The data are modeled to predict outcomes based on analytically searching the data. Combinations of data must be identified to predict desired outcomes.

During the assessment phase, the data as well as the models are assessed for not only the reliability of the discoveries, but also the usefulness of the data mining process. Assessment is key to determine the success of the data mining approach.

SEMMA focuses on the tasks of modeling. This approach has been praised for its ability to guide the implementation of data mining. Conversely, it has been criticized for omitting the critical features of the organization's business. SEMMA is logical and can be robust from sampling through assessment.

Based on the needs of the organization, a variety of models can be used in combination. A coordinated, cooperative environment is necessary for complicated data mining projects, because they require organizational commitment to ensure their success. As described in this section, models such as CRISP-DM, Six Sigma, and SEEMA have been designed as blueprints to deal with the dilemma of how to integrate data mining techniques into an organization. They facilitate the gathering of data, the analysis of those data, the conversion of the data into information, and the dissemination of this information in a format that is easy to digest and understand so as to inform organizational decision making. It is imperative that the results of the data mining process be implemented and any resultant improvements monitored and evaluated.

## Benefits of KDD

KDD can enhance the business aspects of healthcare delivery and help to improve patient care. Some examples of how KDD can be applied effectively follow:

- A durable medical equipment company analyzed its recent sales and enhanced its targeting of hospitals and clinics that yielded the highest return on investment (ROI).
- Several plastic surgery suites were bought by the same group of surgeons. They wanted to know how those organizations were the same and how they were different. They ran analytics for disparities while looking for patterns and trends that led them to develop standardized policies and modify treatment plans.
- Analytic techniques were used in the clinical trials of a new oral contraceptive to aid in monitoring trends and disparities.
- Hidden patterns and relationships between death and disease in selected populations can be uncovered.
- Government spending on certain aspects of health care or specific disease conditions can be analyzed to discover patterns and relationships and to distinguish between the real versus desired outcomes from the investment.
- Patient data can be analyzed to identify effective treatments and discover patterns or relationships in the data to predict inpatient length of stay (LOS).
- Data can be analyzed to help detect medical insurance fraud.

Even though KDD can be complex, this process tends to yield a potent knowledge representation. As analytics evolve, KDD will almost certainly become easier to use, more efficient, and more effective in facilitating data mining in health care.

# Data Mining and Electronic Health Records

As EHRs become more prevalent, the data contained therein can be mined for many different clinical and organizational purposes. We have already established the use of data-driven decision making in patient care as supported by sophisticated EHR functions such as clinical decision support and clinical pathways. Looking beyond the management of individual patient health care, however, we see that EHR data mining can help with managing population health, assist with and inform administrative processes, provide metrics for quality improvement, support value-based reimbursement, and provide data for registry software that helps with population health management. O'Connor (2015) stated, "Analytics is driving innovative solutions that extract, aggregate and 'interpret' the massive volume of data stored within EHR systems into actionable, useful information physicians can use to improve quality of care and make better-informed decisions in the exam room" (para. 3). He also suggested the following uses of EHR data in physician practices:

1. Demographic analytics support efficient diagnosing.
2. Combining disparate data types creates opportunities to strengthen financial planning.
3. Tracking the patient flow enables productivity improvements.
4. Improving system performance in an interconnected world. Information in an EHR comes from diverse sources, hospitals, prior doctors, third-party payers, and other organizations.
5. Comparing your organization's performance to peers and national standards allows you to discover strengths and weaknesses in your operation (para. 4).

Registries are also being used to identify care gaps in patient populations in a physician practice or other healthcare organization. As Terry (2015) explained, some EHRs have a built-in registry function, while others interface with third party registries. Registries are designed to:

- Provide lists of subpopulations, such as patients with hypertension and diabetes
- Identify patients with care gaps, based on evidence-based guidelines
- Support outreach to patients who have care gaps
- Provide feedback on how each physician is doing on particular types of care, such as the percentage of their diabetic patients who have their Hba1c levels or blood pressure under control
- Generate quality reports for the practice (para. 17)

Another type of clinical data mining designed to improve patient outcomes is a retrospective look at clinical data in an EHR, known as temporal event analysis (Gotz, Wang, & Perer, 2014). As Gotz et al. explained,

> Our approach consists of three key components: a visual query module, a pattern-mining module, and an interactive visualization module. We combine these three technologies together within a single framework that enables ad hoc event sequence analysis. With this capability, users are able to discover patterns of clinical events (e.g., sequences of treatments or medications) that

*most impact outcome. Moreover, our approach allows users to better under-
stand how those associations change as patients progress through an episode
of interest. (p. 150)*

In addition, data in an EHR can be used for administrative process improvement.
Rojas, Munoz-Gama, Sepúlveda, and Capurro (2016) conducted a literature review
on administrative process mining. "The application of process mining in healthcare
allows health experts to understand the actual execution of processes: discovering
process models, checking conformance with medical guidelines, and finding improvement opportunities" (p. 234). Process mining is a relatively new use of data generated
in hospital information systems and is dependent on event logs generated in the system. As Rojas and colleagues explained,

> *Activities are recorded in event logs for support, control and further analy-
> sis. Process models are created to specify the order in which different health
> workers are supposed to perform their activities within a given process, or to
> analyze critically the process design. Moreover, process models are also used
> to support the development of [health information systems], for example, to
> understand how the information system is expected to support the process
> execution. (p. 225)*

It is clear that we have only begun to imagine how EHR data mining can inform
healthcare practices and support quality improvement.

## Ethics of Data Mining

Data mining in health care is dependent on the use of private health information
(PHI). Practitioners engaging in data mining must ensure that such data are deidentified and that confidentiality is maintained. Because most data mining depends on the
aggregation of data, maintaining individual patient confidentiality should be relatively
straightforward. You can follow changes and specific requirements for compliance
with HIPAA at this website: http://www.hhs.gov/ocr/privacy/hipaa/understanding
/special/research/index.html

## Summary

Big data is everywhere—we collect and store data every second of every day. The data
in big clinical datasets can get lost, however, diminishing its value. Therefore, in health
care, it is imperative that we use KDD to analyze these datasets and discover meaningful information that will influence our practice. Our existing data repositories are ripe
for the picking; they contain hidden patterns, trends, and undiscovered nuggets that
we must mine to continue to hone our understanding and improve health care.

Data management is essential so that this process can begin with clean, good data.
The decisions that are made when conducting the analysis and when developing the
model and algorithms enable us to predict and discover patterns and trends in the
data, thereby making them meaningful. We must be able not only to extract meaningful information and knowledge, but also to share and disseminate what we are learning
and the new knowledge we are generating.

## THOUGHT-PROVOKING QUESTIONS

1. Reflect on these terms: database, data warehouse, and data mining. What do they have in common? How do they differ?
2. Describe an issue associated with healthcare data that impedes the construction of meaningful databases and inhibits the data mining process. Which strategies would you use to remedy this situation? Thoroughly describe one strategy and its potential outcomes.
3. Suggest a data mining project for your practice. Which information would you like to have about your practice area that could be extracted using data mining strategies?
4. Data mining is associated with numerous techniques and algorithms. How can you make sure that you select and develop those that best fit your data?

# References

Berger, A. M., & Berger, C. R. (2004). Data mining as a tool for research and knowledge development in nursing. *Computers Informatics Nursing, 22*(3), 123–131. PubMed ID: 15520581

DeGruy, K. B. (2000). Healthcare applications of knowledge discovery in databases. *Journal of Healthcare Information Management, 14*(2), 59–69. PubMed ID: 11066649

Fernández-Llatas, C., Garcia-Gomez, J. M., Vicente, J., Naranjo, J. C., Robles, M., Benedi, J. M., & Traver, V. (2011). Behaviour patterns detection for persuasive design in nursing homes to help dementia patients. *Conference Proceedings IEEE Engineering in Medicine & Biology Society,* 6413–6417. PubMed ID: 22255806

Goodwin, L., Saville, J., Jasion, B., Turner, B., Prather, J., Dobousek, T., & Egger, S. (1997). A collaborative international nursing informatics research project: Predicting ARDS risk in critically ill patients. *Studies in Health Technology Informatics, 46,* 247–249. PubMed ID: 10175406

Gotz, D., Wang, F., & Perer, A. (2014). A methodology for interactive mining and visual analysis of clinical event patterns using electronic health record data. *Journal of Biomedical Informatics, 48,* 148–159. doi:10.1016/j.jbi.2014.01.007

Green, J., Paladugu, S., Shuyu, X., Stewart, B., Shyu, C., & Armer, J. (2013). Using temporal mining to examine the development of lymphedema in breast cancer survivors. *Nursing Research, 62*(2), 122–129. PubMed ID: 23458909

IBM. (2013). Big data at the speed of business. Retrieved from http://www-01.ibm.com/software/data/bigdata

Lee, T., Lin K., Mills, M., & Kuo, Y. (2012). Factors related to the prevention and management of pressure ulcers. *Computers Informatics Nursing, 30*(9), 489–495. PubMed ID: 22584879

Lee, T., Liu, C., Kuo, Y., Mills, M., Fong, J., & Hung, C. (2011). Application of data mining to the identification of critical factors in patient falls using a Web-based reporting system. *International Journal of Medical Informatics, 80*(2), 141–150. PubMed ID: 21115393

Madigan, E., & Curet, O. (2006). A data mining approach in home healthcare: Outcomes and service use. *BMC Health Services Research, 6,* 18. PubMed ID: 16504115

Manyika, J., Chu, M., Brown, B., Bughin, J., Dobbs, R., Roxburgh, C., & Byers, A. (2011). Big data: The next frontier for innovation, competition, and productivity. *McKinsey Global Institute.* Retrieved from http://www.mckinsey.com/insights/business_technology/big_data_the_next_frontier_for_innovation

Moskowitz, A., McSparron, J., & Celi, L. (2015). Preparing a new generation of clinicians for the era of big data. *Harvard Medical Student Review, 2*(1), 24–27. Retrieved from http://hmsreview.org/issue/2015/1/preparing-a-new-generation-of-clinicians-for-the-era-of-big-data

O'Connor, S. (2015). 5 EHR data analytics you aren't paying attention to. *Advanced Data Systems Corporation.* Retrieved from http://healthcare.adsc.com/blog/5-ehr-data-analytics-you-arent-paying-attention-to

Rojas, E., Munoz-Gama, J., Sepúlveda, M., & Capurro, D. (2016). Process mining in healthcare: A literature review. *Journal of Biomedical Informatics, 61*, 224–236. doi:10.1016/j.jbi.2016.04.007

SAS. (n.d.). SAS enterprise miner. Retrieved from http://www.sas.com/offices/europe/uk/technologies/analytics/datamining/miner/semma.html

Terry, K. (2015). Mining EHR data for quality improvement. *Medical Economics.* Retrieved from http://medicaleconomics.modernmedicine.com/medical-economics/news/mining-ehr-data-quality-improvement?page=full

Tishgart, D. (2012). Why security matters for big data and health care: Data integrity requires good data security. *Microservices Expo Journal.* Retrieved from http://soa.sys-con.com/node/2389698

Trangenstein, P., Weiner, E., Gordon, J., & McNew, R. (2007). Data mining results from an electronic clinical log for nurse practitioner students. *Studies in Health Technology Informatics, 129*, 1387–1391. PubMed ID: 17911941

Zupan, B., & Demsar, J. (2008). Open-source tools for data mining. *Clinics in Laboratory Medicine, 28*(1), 37–54. PubMed ID: 18194717

# CHAPTER 23

# Translational Research: Generating Evidence for Practice

Jennifer Bredemeyer, Ida Androwich, Dee McGonigle, and Kathleen Mastrian

## Introduction

Mr. James is an 87-year-old man with osteoarthritis in his knees. He is frail and very thin and requires assistance getting out of bed. Mary, a new registered nurse, is making her rounds with her team members and nurse's aide. Realizing Mr. James is at risk for skin breakdown and falls, she reviews the agency policy manual regarding pressure ulcer prevention and fall prevention. Which other resources could Mary consult if she wanted more information on preventing these issues? If Mary wanted to know what the current research suggests about preventing each of these conditions, how would she obtain this information?

This chapter introduces the concept of translational research and its role in evidence-based practice with specific emphasis on nursing informatics. Before pursuing the content in this chapter, the reader should already have an understanding of nursing research, the Foundation of Knowledge model, and knowledge generation through nursing research. Key words and definitions used in this chapter are described briefly next. Classic sources (5 years or older) are used to enhance the reference base.

> *If I limit what I speak about to what I know from experience to be true rather than what I think I am expected to say or what I am pressured to say, then I will have a contribution to make. (Camus, 1943)*

## Clarification of Terms

*Evidence-based practice*, *translational research*, and *research utilization* are all terms that have been used to describe the application of evidential knowledge to clinical practice. The following paragraphs explore the definitions of each term. Although these terms are related, they have slightly different meanings and applications.

Evidence-based practice (EBP), developed originally for its application to medicine, is defined by Sackett et al. (1996) as "The conscientious, explicit and judicious use of current best evidence in making decisions about the care of individual patients" (p. 71). The "best evidence" in this context refers to more than just research. Goode and Piedalue (1999) stated that evidence-based practice should be combined with other knowledge sources and "involves the synthesis of knowledge from research, retrospective or concurrent chart review, quality improvement and risk data, international, national, and local standards, infection control data, pathophysiology, cost effectiveness analysis, benchmarking data, patient preferences, and clinical expertise" (p. 15). EBP starts with a clinical question to resolve a clinical problem (see Figure 23-1). For example, published research studies are used in healthcare quality initiatives as the evidence behind the development of practice algorithms designed to decrease practice variability, increase patient safety, improve patient outcomes, and eliminate unnecessary costs. Use of EBP promotes the use of clinical judgment and knowledge in relation to the patient's contextual situation and preferences, with procedures and protocols being linked to scientific evidence rather than based on what is customary practice or opinion.

Research utilization is the use of findings from one or more research studies in a practical application unrelated to the original study (Polit & Beck, 2008, p. 29), resulting in the generation of new knowledge. Stetler (2001) defines research utilization as the "process of transforming research knowledge into practice" (p. 274). Research utilization can be self-limiting if research is inconsistent or not enough

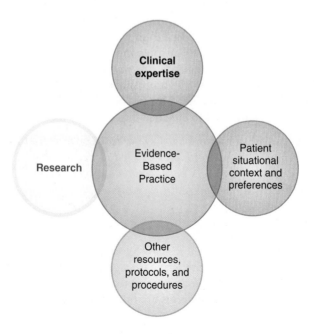

Figure 23-1 Evidence-Based Practice

research is available to develop a consensus regarding the answer to the clinical question (Kirchhoff, 2004).

**Translational research** (science) describes the methods used in translating medical, biomedical, informatics, and nursing research into bedside clinical interventions. Refer to **Figure 23-2**. Woolf (2008) described translational research in two ways:

- T1: the transfer of clinical research to its first testing on humans
- T2: the transfer of clinical research to an everyday clinical practice setting

Difficulties in translating research to the T2 setting exist when research applications do not fit well within the clinical context or practical considerations constrain the application in a clinical setting. Translational research is complicated by the follow-up analysis, practice, and policy changes that occur when adopting research into practice; consequently, available evidence-based healthcare practices are often not fully incorporated into daily care (Titler, 2004, 2010). Organizational culture influences the changes made to a clinical application and establishes the groundwork and the support for change-making activities (Titler, 2004). The study of ways to promote the adoption of evidence in the healthcare context is called "translation science" (Titler, 2010).

**Translational bioinformatics** is the "development of storage, analytic, and interpretive methods to optimize the transformation of increasingly voluminous biomedical data, and genomic data, into proactive, predictive, preventive, and participatory health (American Medical Informatics Association [AMIA], 2016c, para. 1). It integrates biological and clinical data and the evolution of clinical informatics methodology to include biological observations. "The end product of translational bioinformatics is newly found knowledge from these integrative efforts that can be disseminated to a variety of stakeholders, including biomedical scientists, clinicians, and patients" (AMIA, 2016c, para. 1).

**Clinical informatics** is the "application of informatics and information technology to deliver healthcare services. It is also referred to as applied clinical informatics and operational informatics" (AMIA, 2016a, para. 1).

**Clinical research informatics** is defined by AMIA (2016b) as involving the use of informatics in the discovery and management of new knowledge relating to health

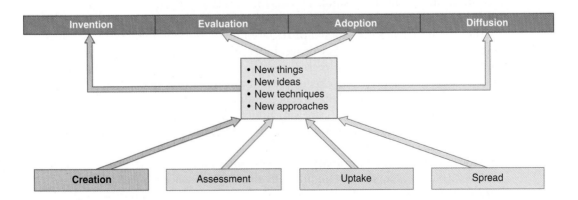

**Figure 23-2** Translational Research Pathway

and disease. "It includes management of information related to clinical trials and also involves informatics related to secondary research use of clinical data. Clinical research informatics and translational bioinformatics are the primary domains related to informatics activities to support translational research" (para. 1).

## History of Evidence-Based Practice

Research results are crucial to furthering EBP. The concept of using randomized controlled trials and systematic reviews as the gold standard against which one should evaluate the validity and effectiveness of a clinical intervention was introduced in 1972 by Archie Cochrane, a scientist and a physician (Cochrane, 1972). Cochrane's experiences as a prisoner of war and medical officer while interning during World War II led to his belief that not all medical interventions were needed and some caused more harm than good. Cochrane viewed the randomized clinical trial as a means of validating clinical interventions and limiting the interventions to those that were scientifically based, effective, and necessary (Dickersin & Manheimer, 1998).

Cochrane's colleague, Iain Chalmers, began compiling a comprehensive clinical trials registry of 3,500 clinical trial results in the field of perinatal medicine. In 1988, after being published in print 3 years earlier, the registry became available electronically. Chalmers's methods for compiling the trials databases became a model for future registry assembly. Eventually, the National Health Service in the United Kingdom, recognizing the value of and need for systemic reviews for all of health care, developed the Cochrane Center. The Cochrane Collaboration was initiated in 1993 and expanded internationally to maintain systematic reviews in all areas of health care (Dickersin & Manheimer, 1998). Many universities subscribe to the Cochrane Collaboration database, making this information easily accessible to students, faculty, and nurses who work for university hospital systems. Visit www.cochrane.org for a link to the latest Cochrane evidence.

## Evidence

The **randomized controlled trial (RCT)** is considered the most reliable source of evidence. Yet, RCTs are not always possible or available; consequently, nurses must use critical analysis to base their clinical decision making on the best available evidence (Baumann, 2010). The updated Stetler model of research utilization (Stetler, 2001) identified internal and external forms of evidence. External evidence originates from research and national experts, whereas internal forms of evidence originate from nontraditional sources, such as clinical experience and quality improvement data.

**Evidence** includes standards of practice, codes of ethics, philosophies of nursing, autobiographic stories, esthetic criticism, works of art, qualitative studies, and patient and clinical knowledge (Melnyk, Fineout-Overholt, Stone, & Ackerman, 2000). French (2002) summarizes evidence as "truth, knowledge (including tacit, expert opinion and experiential), primary research findings, meta-analyses and systematic reviews" (p. 254). Nurses may additionally draw on evidence from the **context of care**, such as audit and performance data, the culture of the organization, social and professional networks, discussion with stakeholders, and local or national policy (Rycroft-Malone et al., 2004, p. 86).

Concern has been voiced by nurse theorists that nurses are being influenced too much by the medical model in accepting the RCT as the only true source of evidence, thereby "reverting to the medical perspective" rather than incorporating "theory-guided evidence and diverse ways of knowing" (Fawcett, Watson, Walker, & Fitzpatrick, 2001, p. 115). The context change from medicine to nursing requires nurses to apply other knowledge and nursing theory. The use of research results as the sole basis for clinical decision making ignores other types of evidence inherent in nursing practice (Scott-Findlay & Pollock, 2004).

To use evidence in practice, the weight of the research, also called **research validity**, must be determined. Evidence hierarchies have been defined to grade and assign value to the information source. For example, an evidential hierarchy developed by Stetler et al. (1998) prioritized evidence into six categories:

1. Meta-analysis
2. Individual experimental studies
3. Quasi-experimental studies
4. Nonexperimental studies
5. Program evaluations, such as quality improvement projects
6. Opinions of experts

The hierarchy identifies **meta-analysis** as the highest-quality evidence because it uses multiple individual research studies to reach a consensus. It is interesting to note that opinions of experts are considered the least significant in this hierarchy, yet nurses most often seek the opinion of a more experienced colleague or peer when searching for information regarding patient care (Pravikoff, Tanner, & Pierce, 2005).

Qualitative research allows one to understand the way in which the intervention is experienced by the researcher and the participant and the value of the interventions to both parties (O'Neill, Jinks, & Ong, 2007). Qualitative research is not always considered in EBP, because methods for synthesizing the evidence do not currently exist. The Cochrane Qualitative Research Methods Group (CQRMG) has developed search, appraisal, and synthesis methodologies for qualitative research (Joanna Briggs Institute, n.d.) and provides a database of articles related to methodological research (Cochrane Collaboration, 2016).

# Bridging the Gap Between Research and Practice

The time between research dissemination and clinical translation may be significant, and this delay may adversely affect patient outcomes. Bridging the gap between research and practice requires an understanding of the key concepts and barriers, access to research findings, access to clinical mentors for research understanding, a reinforcing culture, and a desire on the part of the clinician to implement best practices (Melnyk, 2005; Melnyk, Fineout-Overholt, Stetler, & Allen, 2005). In the **Iowa model** of EBP, research and other evidential sources are adopted directly in the practice setting with the goal of developing a standard of care and team decision making (Schaffer, Sandau, & Diedrick, 2013; Titler, 2007). Additionally, the groundwork required to create a conceptual framework supportive of an EBP includes workplace culture change and support of the change through leadership (Stetler et al., 1998). Beliefs and attitudes, involvement in research activities, information seeking, professional characteristics, education, and other socioeconomic factors are potential determinants of research utilization (Estabrooks, Floyd, Scott-Findlay, O'Leary, & Gushta, 2003); however, meta-analysis points out that too much original research and not enough repetition of previous studies fails to advance the knowledge base.

Developing countries are often constrained economically from accessing research sources. Such organizations as the Cochrane Collaboration provide free reviews to fill this void. Even so, knowledge dissemination strategies and education are required to take advantage of these resources (Cochrane Collaboration, 2004).

## Barriers to and Facilitators of Evidence-Based Practice

Tacia and colleagues (2015) concluded there were six challenges or barriers to the application of EBP: "institutional and/or cultural barriers, lack of knowledge, lack of motivation, time management, physician and patient factors, and limited access to up to date, user-friendly technology and computer systems" (p. 93). Nurses may also see the job of interpreting research as too complex or see the organizational culture as a barrier to implementation of EBP (Kieft, de Brouwer, Francke, & Delnoij, 2014; McCaughan, Thompson, Cullum, Sheldon, & Thompson, 2002). Many believe that inpatient direct care nurses lack basic knowledge of EBP and must have access to and assistance with technical resources.

Yet, Melnyk and colleagues (2009) noted that a number of factors also facilitate the use of EBP. These driving forces include knowledge and skills in EBP; having a conviction that there is a value to using evidence in practices; and practicing in a supportive culture with tools available to sustain evidence-based care, including access to computers and databases, evidence-based content at the point of care, and the presence of EBP mentors. Tacia et al. (2015) noted that interprofessional collaboration, mentorship, and administrative support were necessary for the adoption of EBP. It is imperative that we remove the barriers and support nurses using EBP, as well as continuing to mentor and work with those who are just beginning to initiate EBP in their practice.

## The Role of Informatics

Computers are used in all areas of research: (1) literature search databases, such as CINAHL; (2) online literature reference lists, such as RefWorks; (3) data capture, collection, and coding; (4) data analysis; (5) data modeling; (6) meta-analysis; (7) qualitative analysis; and (8) dissemination of results (Saba & McCormick, 2006). The context for nursing informatics has expanded to support dramatic changes in the way science is accomplished. Information need and the collaborative component of inter-disciplinary research rely heavily on technology and informatics. Technologies such as social networking have also improved collaboration. The use of technology and infor-matics in facilitating interdisciplinary and translational research is a key architectural component of the National Institutes of Health's (NIH's) reengineering of the clini-cal research enterprise as part of its road map initiative for medical research (NIH,

2009). As technology continues to advance, so do the informatics tools available to researchers. The Institute of Translational Health Sciences (2016) offers a deidentified clinical data repository, data quest, and research electronic data capture (REDCap), which is

> *a rapidly evolving web tool developed by researchers for researchers in the translational domain. REDCap features a high degree of customizability for your forms and advanced user right control. It also features free, unlimited survey functionality, a sophisticated export module with support for all the popular statistical programs, and supports HIPAA compliance. (para. 1)*

Clinical research informatics at the Oregon Clinical & Translational Research Institute (2016) accelerates translational research "by providing informatics tools to leverage clinical data (Epic) for research and to develop state-of-the-art clinical research data collection and management software and expertise. These tools support a diverse array of research including bench-to-bedside, clinical, and healthcare systems research" (para. 1). **Translational informatics** refers to the application of research informatics to translational research in order to close the gap from research to the bedside to improve the health of patients and the community.

An informatics infrastructure is critical to EBP. Bakken, Stone, and Larson (2008) discussed expanding the context of informatics to genomic health care, shifting research paradigms, and social Web technologies. Ensuring the global collaborative nature of nursing research for 2010–2018 requires an expansion of the nursing research agenda to user information needs, data management, information support for nurses and patients, practice-based knowledge generation, and design evaluation methodologies. Giuse et al. (2005) described the evolving role of the clinical informationist (informaticist) as being a partner on the healthcare team who provides timely clinical evidence for the clinical workflow. Although not specific to nursing informatics, the NIH provides awards under its Clinical and Translational Science Award (CTSA) program to accelerate the transfer of research to the clinical setting (NIH, 2016). The Quality and Safety Education for Nurses (QSEN; 2013) cites key competencies (knowledge, skills, and attitudes) in both EBP and informatics. With the goal of promoting the use of research findings and tool use based on these findings, the **Agency for Healthcare Research and Quality (AHRQ)** became an active participant in pushing evidence forward into practice. The AHRQ is a government-sponsored organization with the mission of reducing patients' risk of harm, decreasing healthcare costs, and improving patient outcomes through the promotion of research and technology applications focused on EBP. In 1999, AHRQ implemented its Translating Research into Practice Initiative (TRIP) to generate knowledge about evidence-based care (AHRQ, 2001). In the second Translating Research into Practice Initiative (TRIP-II), the focus shifted to improving health care for underserved populations and using information technology to shape translational research and health policy. AHRQ, in partnership with the American Medical Association and the American Association of Health Plans, developed the **National Guideline Clearinghouse (NGC)**. NGC is a comprehensive database of evidentially based clinical practice guidelines and related documents that are regularly published through the NGC electronic mailing list and are available on the NGC website (https://guideline.gov). The NGC website allows users to browse for the clinical guidelines, view abstracts and full-text links, download full text clinical guidelines to personal digital assistant (PDA) devices and smartphones, obtain technical reports, and compare guidelines. PubMed4Hh (PubMed for handheld devices) is a powerful and free application for smartphones that provides access to the national Library of Medicine and supports PICO searches, clinical queries, and multilanguage searches with links to consensus abstracts.

In addition, a growing number of printed and electronic resources are available to assist in creating guidelines and offering information about EBP. A selection of existing websites is shown in Table 23-1.

Table 23-1  The Role of Informatics: Online Evidence-Based Resources

| Website | Description |
| --- | --- |
| Academic Center for Evidence-Based Practice (ACE) www.acestar.uthscsa.edu | The School of Nursing at the University of Texas Health Science Center at San Antonio sponsors the Academic Center for Evidence-Based Practice. The center's ultimate goal is to bring research to practice to improve patient care, outcomes, and safety. The center is also home to the ACE star model of knowledge transformation. |
| The Agency for Healthcare Research and Quality www.ahrq.gov | The Agency for Healthcare Research and Quality contains a wealth of information regarding healthcare quality. There is no charge for access to the site or its resources. |
| BMJ Clinical Evidence http://clinicalevidence.bmj.com/x/index.html | The BMJ publishing group provides clinical databases by prescription. The BMJ Clinical Evidence site allows the download of some clinical papers and some interesting risk tools without charge. |
| The Center for Evidence-Based Practices (CEBP) www.evidencebasedpractices.org | The Center for Evidence-Based Practices of the Orelena Hawks Puckett Institute focuses on research to practice initiatives related to early intervention, early childhood education, parent and family support, and family-centered practices. |
| Centre for Evidence-Based Medicine www.cebm.net | The Centre for Evidence-Based Medicine, located in Oxford in the UK, is devoted to developing and promoting evidence-based resources for healthcare professionals. In addition to free articles, the site also provides free teaching resources and presentation. |
| CINAHL www.cinahl.com | CINAHL information systems offers a multitude of online services, which include website link sources, CINAHL's online nursing and allied health database, document delivery, and search services. |
| The Cochrane Collaboration www.cochrane.org | The Cochrane Collaboration provides reviews for free, but full-text articles are by subscription. |
| Entrez PubMed www.ncbi.nlm.nih.gov/pubmed | Entrez PubMed is a service provided by The National Library of Medicine (NLM). The NLM was developed by the National Center for Biotechnology Information (NCBI), which provides access to life science journals and MEDLINE citations. Some of the journal links are free, and some require a subscription. |

| Information & Resources for Nurses Worldwide www.nurses.info/specialty_evidenced_based_orgs .htm | This website provides searchable links to evidence-based practice organizations by specialty. |
|---|---|
| The Iowa Model of Evidence-Based Practice www.nnpnetwork.org/ebp-resources/iowa-model | This website provides a brief overview of the Iowa Model for Evidence-Based Practice (for members only). |
| The Joanna Briggs Institute www.joannabriggs.org | The Joanna Briggs Institute was established in 1996 as a resource for best care practices. Joanna Briggs was first matron of the Adelaide Hospital in Australia and is recognized for her financial and organizational support. The Joanna Briggs Institute is a leader in developing evidence-based practices. |
| The Johns Hopkins Bloomberg School of Public Health, Evidence-Based Practice Center www.jhsph.edu/research/centers-and-institutes /johns-hopkins-evidence-based-practice-center | The Johns Hopkins Evidence-Based Practice Center was established in 1997 and is one of 14 such centers producing comprehensive, systematic reviews for the AHRQ. |
| PubMed Central www.ncbi.nlm.nih.gov/pmc | PubMed Central (PMC) is a free digital archive of science-related articles managed by the NCBI. BioMed Central (an open-source online archive) may be accessed here. |
| Trip database www.tripdatabase.com | The Trip database is a clinical search tool to allow clinicians to identify the best evidence for clinical practice. |
| World Views on Evidence-Based Nursing http://onlinelibrary.wiley.com/journal/10.1111 /(ISSN)1741-6787 | Through Blackwell Publishing, this magazine, sponsored by Sigma Theta Tau International, is dedicated exclusively to evidence-based nursing articles. The magazine is also offered online by subscription. |

# Developing EBP Guidelines

Several models have been developed to guide organizations into translating research into practice. Brief descriptions of these models are provided in Table 23-2. As an example, Titler (2007) identified the steps in the Iowa model for translating research into practice as (1) identifying the problem, issue, or topic in nursing practice; (2) research and critique of related evidence; (3) adaptation of the evidence to practice; (4) implementation of the EBP; and (5) evaluation of patient outcomes and care practices. Careful analysis and discussion of the research or other forms of evidence in this scenario may reveal that given the context, implementation may not be practical. Following implementation, results must be monitored to determine whether the application works for the context. Thoughtful discussion of the findings will help the clinical team determine if further research is warranted or if further change is needed. As a practical application, evidence-based standards for care are developed by hospitals to meet the American Nurses Association/American Nurses Credentialing Center standards for achieving Magnet hospital recognition.

Information technology is important in synthesizing the research regardless of the model. Bakken (2001) recommended (1) standardized nomenclature required for the electronic health record (standardized terminologies and structures); (2) digital

Table 23-2 Comparison of Model Approaches to Evidence-Based Practice

| Stetler Model (Stetler, 2001) | ACE Star Model (Stevens, 2004) | The Iowa Model of Evidence-Based Practice to Promote Quality Care (Titler et al., 2001) |
| --- | --- | --- |
| 1. Preparation | 1. Discovery | 1. Select the trigger as impetus for practice (knowledge focused or practice focused) change. |
| 2. Validation | 2. Evidence summary | 2. Determine if the topic is worth pursuing for the organization and if not, pursue new trigger. |
| 3. Cooperative evaluation | 3. Translation | 3. Determine if there is significant research base. If so, change, otherwise conduct research or seek more research. |
| 4. Decision making | 4. Integration | |
| 5. Translational application | 5. Evaluation | 4. If change is appropriate for practice, implement change. |
| 6. Evaluation | | 5. Monitor results. |
| | | 6. Disseminate results. |

Data from Stetler, C. B. (2001). Updating the Stetler model of research utilization to facilitate evidence-based practice. *Nursing Outlook, 49*(6), 272–279; Stevens, K. R. (2004). *ACE star model of EBP: Knowledge transformation*. Retrieved July 2010 from http://www.acestar.uthscsa.edu/Learn_model.htm; Titler, M. G., Kleiber, C., Steelman, V., Rakel, B., Budreu, G., Everett, L., . . . Goode, T. (2001). The Iowa model of evidence-based practice to promote quality care. *Critical Care Nursing Clinics of North America, 13*(4), 497–509.

sources of evidence; (3) standards that facilitate healthcare data exchange among heterogeneous systems; (4) informatics processes that support the acquisition and application of evidence to a specific clinical situation; and (5) informatics competencies (p. 1999). Bakken's recommendations encouraged the development of an infrastructure that creates a database of experiential clinical evidence.

# Meta-Analysis and Generation of Knowledge

Systematic reviews combine results from multiple primary investigations to obtain consensus on a specific area of research. Studies are discarded from the review if they are not considered sound, thereby creating a reliable end result. The strength of the systematic review is its ability to corroborate findings and reach consensus. Systematic reviews show the need for more research by revealing the areas where quantitative results may be lacking or minimal. Bias may occur if the selected studies are inadequate, if all sources of evidence are not investigated, or if the publications selected are not adequately diverse (Lipp, 2005). The BMJ Clinical Evidence Blog (http://blogs.bmj.com/ce) has stressed the importance of getting evidence into health service decision making, but to beware of evidence spin that adds bias to the reporting of the evidence.

Meta-analysis, a form of systematic review, uses statistical methods to combine the results of several studies (Cook, Mulrow, & Haynes, 1997). Quantitative studies are typically used. According to Glass (1976), meta-analysis is the statistical analysis of a large collection of analysis results from individual studies for the purpose of integrating the findings (p. 3).

Kraft (2006) described the documentation search strategy for meta-analysis as beginning with the identification of the studies through a search of bibliographic databases, identification of meta-analysis articles that match the search criteria, elimination of those articles that do not match the search criteria, review of the reference lists in the meta-analysis for other articles that may relate to the topic, and review of each article for quality and content. Additional sources should include unpublished works, such as conferences and dissertation abstracts, with the goal of obtaining as many relevant articles as possible. Gregson, Meal, and Avis (2002) identified the steps of a meta-analysis as (1) defining the problem, followed by protocol generation; (2) establishing study eligibility criteria, followed by literature search; (3) identifying the heterogeneity of results of studies; (4) standardizing the data and statistically combining the results; and (5) conducting sensitivity testing to determine whether the combined results are the same. The often-cited criticism of meta-analysis is that emphasis is on **quantitative studies**, not **qualitative studies**. Additionally, the analysis is only as good as the studies used (Gregson, Meal, & Avis). Collection and dissemination of these meta-analysis and systematic reviews are available in paper and on the Internet, although many such databases require a subscription.

The term "open access" refers to a worldwide movement to make a library of knowledge available to anyone with Internet access. The **Open Access Initiative** came about in response to the tremendous cost of research library access. Libraries pay large fees for journal subscriptions, and the richness of library references is limited to what the budget allows. The cost of keeping current with research has caused library subscriptions to decline (Yiotis, 2005). Open access adds to the controversy, with some journals charging authors for publication of their work, which in itself may provide a financial barrier to publication in this form.

According to Suber's (2015) open access overview, open access refers to digital literature that is available to anyone with Internet access free of charge. There are two vehicles for open access: archives and journals. Open access journals are generally peer reviewed and freely available. The publishers of open access journals do not charge the reader, but rather obtain funds for publishing elsewhere. Open access journals may charge the author or depend on other forms of funding, such as donations, grants, and advertising, to publish.

## The Future

Our future depends on a prepared workforce ready to meet the challenges of tomorrow. This will require a focus on informatics, bioinformatics, clinical research, translational research, other research methods, and evidence-based practice. In this data-driven healthcare delivery system in which we work, we must adopt data standards. Given the vast amounts of data, Bakken et al. (2008) identified areas of focus for nursing informatics in knowledge representation, data management, analysis, and predictive modeling in genomic health care and the need for policies and procedures to protect data acquisition, dissemination, privacy, security, and confidentiality, as well as education in these areas. Informatics tools support nursing practice, education of healthcare consumers, and knowledge generation. The technology is available now to incorporate evidence into reference links embedded in electronic clinical care plans. Incorporation of personalized clinical desktops to allow each clinician to have appropriate references (similar to Internet ad bot technology) provided to him or her may be possible. The other challenge includes developing and maintaining interprofessional collaborative environments that truly operate in a cooperative and open manner. Time, research, and technology will tell.

## Summary

These are amazing times. Technology has taken us faster and further than we ever thought possible. Healthcare jobs have become more technical and more complicated. In some ways, technology has increased the margin for error. Some healthcare practitioners will continue to rely on little scraps of paper and nonsystematic methods to keep themselves and their patients safe. Unfortunately, individuals who become so tied to these things close their mind to new innovations. The evolving quality culture and increased patient safety concerns are dragging healthcare workers forward. For the benefit of our patients, health care must move forward.

Collaboration, improved access to online libraries, research tool transparency, a common data language, organizational and informational support, and continued research are a short list of needed items to advance translational research. Repeat studies are needed to provide meaningful meta-analysis and systematic reviews. Technology advancement in the area of incorporating evidence into clinical tools must continue. Removing the barriers to knowledge-seeking behavior and providing access to evidential resources will promote knowledge and, in the end, improve patient outcomes.

### THOUGHT-PROVOKING QUESTIONS

1. Twelve-hour shifts are problematic for patient and nurse safety, yet hospitals continue to keep the 12-hour shift schedule. In 2004, the Institute of Medicine (Board on Health Care Services & Institute of Medicine, 2004) published a report that referred to studies as early as 1988 that discussed the negative effects of rotating shifts on intervention accuracy. Workers with 12-hour shifts experienced more fatigue than workers on 8-hour shifts. In another study done in Turkey by Ilhan, Durukan, Aras, Turkcuoglu, and Aygun (2006), factors relating to increased risk for injury were age of 24 years or younger, less than 4 years of nursing experience, working in surgical intensive care units, and working for more than 8 hours. As a clinician reading these studies, what would your next step be?

2. The use of heparin versus saline to maintain the patency of peripheral intravenous catheters has been addressed in research for many years. The American Society of Health System Pharmacists (ASHSP) published a position paper in January 2006 advocating its support of the use of 0.9% saline in the maintenance of peripheral catheters in nonpregnant adults. It seems surprising that this position paper references articles that advocate the use of saline over heparin dating from 1991. What do you believe are some of the barriers that would have caused this delay in implementation?

In the era of EBP, healthcare providers must continue to think critically about their actions. What is the science behind their interventions? Healthcare workers must no longer do things one way just because they have always been done that way. Research the problem; use evidence-based resources; critically select electronic and non-electronic references; consolidate the research findings and combine and compare the conclusions; present the findings; and propose a solution. One will be the first to ask why and may be a key player in making change happen.

# References

Agency for Healthcare Research and Quality. (2001). AHRQ profile: Quality research for quality healthcare. Retrieved from http://www.ahrq.gov/about/profile.htm

American Medical Informatics Association (AMIA). (2016a). Clinical informatics. Retrieved from https://www.amia.org/applications-informatics/clinical-informatics

American Medical Informatics Association (AMIA). (2016b). Clinical research informatics. Retrieved from https://www.amia.org/applications-informatics/clinical-research-informatics

American Medical Informatics Association (AMIA). (2016c). Translational bioinformatics. Retrieved from https://www.amia.org/applications-informatics/translational-bioinformatics

American Society of Health System Pharmacists. (2006). ASHSP therapeutic position statement on the institutional use of 0.9% sodium chloride injection to maintain patency of peripheral indwelling intermittent infusion devices. *American Journal of Health System Pharmacy, 63*, 1273–1275.

Bakken, S. (2001). An informatics infrastructure is essential for evidence-based practice. *Journal of American Medical Informatics Association, 8*, 199–201.

Bakken, S., Stone, P. W., & Larson, E. L. (2008). A nursing informatics research agenda for 2008–18: Contextual influences and key components. *Nursing Outlook, 56*, 206–214.

Baumann, S. (2010). The limitations of evidence-based practice. *Nursing Science Quarterly, 23*(3), 226–230.

Board on Health Care Services & Institute of Medicine. (2004). *Keeping patients safe.* Washington, DC: National Academies Press.

Camus, A. (1943). *The stranger.* London, UK: Penguin.

Cochrane, A. L. (1972). *Effectiveness and efficiency: Random reflections on health services.* London, UK: Nuffield Provincial Hospitals Trust.

Cochrane Collaboration. (2004). Bridging the gaps across the income divide: A review of the collaboration's efforts to date and recommendations for the future. Retrieved from https://abstracts.cochrane.org/2004-ottawa/bridging-gaps-across-income-divide-review -collaborations-efforts-date-and

Cochrane Collaboration. (2016). Methodology register. Retrieved from http://methods.cochrane .org/qi/methodology-register

Cook, D. J., Mulrow, C. D., & Haynes, R. B. (1997). Systematic reviews: Synthesis of best evidence for clinical decisions. *Annals of Internal Medicine, 126*(5), 376–380.

Dickersin, K., & Manheimer, E. (1998). The Cochrane Collaboration: Evaluation of health care services using systematic reviews of the results and randomized control trials. *Clinical Obstetrics and Gynecology, 41*(2), 315–331.

Estabrooks, C. A., Floyd, J. A., Scott-Findlay, S., O'Leary, K. A., & Gushta, M. (2003). Individual determinants of research utilization: A systematic review. *Journal of Advanced Nursing, 42*, 73–81.

Fawcett, J., Watson, J., Walker, P. H., & Fitzpatrick, J. J. (2001). On nursing theories and evidence. *Journal of Nursing Scholarship, 33*(2), 115–119.

French, P. (2002). What is the evidence on evidence-based nursing? An epistemological concern. *Journal of Advanced Nursing, 37*(3), 250–257.

Giuse, N. B., Koonce, T. Y., Jerome, R. N., Gahall, M., Sathe, N. A., & Williams, A. (2005). Evolution of a mature clinical informationist model. *Journal of the American Medical Informatics Association, 12*(3), 249–255.

Glass, G. V. (1976). Primary, secondary and meta-analysis of research. *Educational Research, 5*(10), 3–8.

Goode, C. J., & Piedalue, F. (1999). Evidence-based clinical practice. *Journal of Nursing Administration, 29*(6), 15–21.

Gregson, P. R., Meal, A. G., & Avis, M. (2002). Meta-analysis: The glass eye of evidence-based practice? *Nursing Inquiry, 9*(1), 24–30.

Ilhan, M. N., Durukan, E., Aras, E., Turkcuoglu, S., & Aygun, R. (2006). Long working hours increase the risk of sharp and needlestick injury in nurses: A need for new policy implication. *Journal of Advanced Nursing, 56*(5), 563–568.

The Institute of Translational Health Sciences. (2016). REDCAP. Retrieved from https://www.iths.org/investigators/services/bmi/redcap

Joanna Briggs Institute. (n.d.). Homepage. Retrieved from http://www.joannabriggs.org/index.html

Kieft, R., de Brouwer, B., Francke, A., & Delnoij, D. (2014). How nurses and their work environment affect patient experiences of the quality of care: A qualitative study. *BMC Health Services Research, 14*, 249–267. doi: 10.1186/1472-6963-14-249

Kirchhoff, K. T. (2004). State of the science of translational research: From demonstration projects to intervention testing. *Worldviews on Evidence-Based Nursing, 1*(suppl 1), S6–S12.

Kraft, M. R. (2006). Meta-analysis: A research tool. *SCI Nursing Journal, 23*(2). Retrieved from http://www.unitedspinal.org/publications/nursing/2006/08/27/research-corner

Lipp, A. (2005). The systematic review as an evidence-based tool for the operating room. *Association of Operating Room Nurses Journal, 81*(6), 1279–1287.

McCaughan, D., Thompson, C., Cullum, N., Sheldon, T. A., & Thompson, D. R. (2002). Acute care nurses' perceptions of barriers to using research information in clinical decision-making. *Journal of Advanced Nursing, 39*(1), 46–60.

Melnyk, B. M. (2005). Advancing evidence-based practice in clinical and academic settings. *Worldviews on Evidence-Based Nursing, 3*, 161–165.

Melnyk, B. M., Fineout-Overholt, E., Stetler, C., & Allen, J. (2005). Outcomes and implementation strategies from the first U.S. evidence-based practice leadership summit. *Worldviews on Evidence-Based Nursing, 2*(3), 113–121.

Melnyk, B. M., Fineout-Overholt, E., Stillwell, S., & Williamson, K. (2009). Igniting a spirit of inquiry: An essential foundation for evidence-based practice. *American Journal of Nursing, 109*(11), 49–52.

Melnyk, B. M., Fineout-Overholt, E., Stone, P., & Ackerman, M. (2000). Evidence-based practice: The past, the present, and recommendations for the millennium. *Pediatric Nursing, 26*(1), 77–80.

National Institutes of Health (NIH). (2009). Re-engineering the clinical research enterprise. https://web.archive.org/web/20100527150048/http://commonfund.nih.gov/clinicalresearch/overviewtranslational.asp

National Institutes of Health (NIH). (2016). Clinical and Translational Science Awards (CTSA) Program. Retrieved from http://www.ncats.nih.gov/ctsa

O'Neill, T., Jinks, C., & Ong, B. N. (2007). Decision-making regarding total knee replacement surgery: A qualitative meta-synthesis. *BMC Health Services Research, 7*(52).

Oregon Clinical & Translational Research Institute. (2016). Clinical research informatics. Retrieved from http://www.ohsu.edu/xd/research/centers-institutes/octri/about/organizational-structure/programs/clinical-research-informatics.cfm

Polit, D. F., & Beck, T. C. (2008). *Nursing research: Generating and assessing evidence for nursing practice* (8th ed.). Philadelphia, PA: Lippincott Williams & Wilkins.

Pravikoff, D. S., Tanner, A. B., & Pierce, S. T. (2005). Readiness of U.S. nurses for evidence-based practice. *American Journal of Nursing, 105*(9), 40–51.

Quality and Safety Education for Nurses (QSEN). (2013). EBP and informatics. Retrieved from http://qsen.org/competencies/pre-licensure-ksas/#evidence-based_practice

Rycroft-Malone, J., Seers, K., Titchen, A., Harvey, G., Kitson, A., & McCormack, B. (2004). What counts as evidence in evidence-based practice? *Journal of Advanced Nursing, 47*(1), 81–90.

Saba, V. K., & McCormick, K. A. (2006). *Essentials of nursing informatics* (4th ed.). New York, NY: McGraw-Hill.

Sackett, D. I., Rosenberg, W. M., Gray, J. A., Haynes, R. B., & Richardson, W. S. (1996). Evidence based medicine: What it is and what it isn't. *British Medical Journal, 312*, 71–72.

Schaffer, M., Sandau, K., & Diedrick, L. (2013). Evidence-based practice models for organizational change: Overview and practical applications. *Journal of Advanced Nursing, 69*(5), 1197–1209.

Scott-Findlay, S., & Pollock, C. (2004). Evidence, research, knowledge: A call for conceptual clarity. *Worldviews on Evidence-Based Nursing, 1*(2), 92–97.

Stetler, C. B. (2001). Updating the Stetler model of research utilization to facilitate evidence-based practice. *Nursing Outlook, 49*(6), 272–279.

Stetler, C. B., Brunell, M., Giuliano, K. K., Morse, D., Prince, L., & Newell-Stokes, V. (1998). Evidence-based practice and the role of nursing leadership. *Journal of Nursing Administration, 28*(7/8), 45–53.

Stevens, K. R. (2004). *ACE star model of EBP: Knowledge transformation.* Retrieved from http://www.acestar.uthscsa.edu/Learn_model.htm

Suber, P. (2015). A very brief introduction to open access. Retrieved from http://legacy.earlham.edu/~peters/fos/overview.htm

Tacia, L., Biskupski, K., Pheley, A., & Lehto, R. (2015). Identifying barriers to evidence-based practice adoption: A focus group study. *Clinical Nursing Studies, 3*(2), 90–96. doi:10.5430/cns.v3n2p90

Titler, M. G. (2004). Methods in translation science. *Worldviews on Evidence-Based Nursing, 1*, 38–48.

Titler, M. G. (2007). Translating research into practice: Models for changing clinician behavior. *American Journal of Nursing, 107*(6), 26–33.

Titler, M. G. (2010). Translation science and context. *Research Theory and Nursing Practice: An International Journal, 24*(1), 35–55.

Titler, M. G., Kleiber, C., Steelman, V., Rakel, B., Budreu, G., Everett, L., . . . Goode, T. (2001). The Iowa model of evidence-based practice to promote quality care. *Critical Care Nursing Clinics of North America, 13*(4), 497–509.

Woolf, S. H. (2008). The meaning of translational research and why it matters. *Journal of the American Medical Association, 299*(2), 211–213.

Yiotis, K. (2005). The Open Access Initiative: A new paradigm for scholarly communications. *Information Technology and Libraries, 24*(4), 157–162. Retrieved from http://ejournals.bc.edu/ojs/index.php/ital/article/view/3378/2988

# CHAPTER 24

# Bioinformatics, Biomedical Informatics, and Computational Biology

Dee McGonigle and Kathleen Mastrian

## Introduction

The National Center for Biotechnology Information (NCBI; 2004) states that "Biology in the 21st century is being transformed from a purely lab-based science to an information science as well" (para. 5). What must be remembered when delving into the new informatics frontier is that biological systems are information systems. Consider that DNA essentially is a storehouse of information. Unlocking that information and learning how that information is transcribed to RNA and ultimately expressed as proteins promises interesting and cutting-edge developments in understanding diseases and managing them at the molecular level. This chapter introduces the reader to the exciting world of bioinformatics and provides a beginning understanding of the frontiers unleashed by the collection, mapping, storage, and sharing of genetic data.

## Bioinformatics, Biomedical Informatics, and Computational Biology Defined

Three terms are frequently used: (1) **bioinformatics**, (2) **biomedical informatics**, and (3) **computational biology**. As terms continue to be bandied about, it is important to comprehend what they mean to understand better these evolving fields. According to the University of Texas at El Paso (2010) website, "Bioinformatics is an interdisciplinary science with a focus on data management and interpretation for complex biological phenomena that are analyzed and visualized using mathematical modeling and numerical methodologies with predictive algorithms" (para. 1). A website operated by the University of Minnesota (2012) stated:

> Bioinformatics is defined here as an interdisciplinary research area that applies computer and information science to solve biological problems. However, this is not the only definition. The field is

*being defined (and redefined) at present, and there are probably as many definitions as there are bioinformaticians (bioinformaticists?). (para. 1)*

The myriad of definitions for the "moving target named bioinformatics" (University of Minnesota, 2012, para. 2) is reflected in those developed from 2000 to 2009. According to NCBI (2004), "Bioinformatics is the field of science in which biology, computer science, and information technology merge to form a single discipline. The ultimate goal of the field is to enable the discovery of new biological insights" (para. 5). Network Science (2009) believed that

*[a]n absolute definition of bioinformatics has not been agreed upon. The first level, however, can be defined as the design and application of methods for the collection, organization, indexing, storage, and analysis of biological sequences (both nucleic acids [DNA and RNA] and proteins). The next stage of bioinformatics is the derivation of knowledge concerning the pathways, functions, and interactions of these genes (functional genomics) and proteins (proteomics). (para. 14)*

Mulligen et al. (2008) wrote that

*BioInformatics (BI) is a less mature scientific discipline which aims to research and develop algorithms, computational and statistical techniques which solve biological problems. Significantly, BI has experienced an exponential growth as a result of its importance to the understanding and interpretation of data generated by "omics" technologies. (para. 6)*

The complete sequencing of the human genome has led to systems biology referred to as "omics" and has elevated scientists' ability from studying one gene or protein to studying fundamental biological processes (Box 24-1).

---

### BOX 24-1 OMICS

Kelly (2008) describes that "'ome' and 'omics' are suffixes that are derived from genome" (para. 1). National Public Radio (2010) credits botanist Hans Winkler with merging "the Greek words 'genesis' and 'soma' to describe a body of genes" (para. 1) in 1920. The term "genome" was born from this combination, and genomics arose as the study of the genome.

Kelly (2008) continues to explain:

*Scientists like to append these to any large-scale system (or really, just about anything complex), such as the collection of proteins in a cell or tissue (the proteome), the collection of metabolites (the metabolome), and the collection of RNA that's been transcribed from genes (the transcriptome). High-throughput analysis is essential considering data at the "omic" level, that is to say considering all DNA sequences, gene expression levels, or proteins at once (or, to be slightly more precise, a significant subset of them). (para. 1)*

The National Human Genome Research Institute (NHGRI; 2015) describes bioinformatics as a branch of biology concerned with the acquisition, storage, display, and analysis of the information found in nucleic acid and protein sequence data. Computers and bioinformatics software are the tools of the trade. Based on these definitions, one can get a flavor for what bioinformatics entails. It is clear that the definition of bioinformatics varies, and that there is no single definition that everyone agrees with at the present time.

Biomedicine applies bioinformatics to promote health. According to the website of the Ohio State University Medical Center (2010), "Biomedical informatics is the study and process of efficiently gathering, storing, managing, retrieving, analyzing, communicating, sharing, and applying biomedical information to improve the detection, prevention, and treatment of disease" (para. 2). The Vanderbilt University (2016) website suggested that

> *Biomedical Informatics is the interdisciplinary science of acquiring, structuring, analyzing and providing access to biomedical data, information and knowledge. As an academic discipline, biomedical informatics is grounded in the principles of computer science, information science, cognitive science, social science, and engineering, as well as the clinical and basic biological sciences. (para. 1)*

Oregon Health & Science University (OHSU; 2016) defined biomedical informatics as "the field that is concerned with the optimal use of information, often aided by the use of technology, to improve individual health, health care, public health, and biomedical research" (para. 1). Bioinformatics can be viewed as a biological science or computer science. According to the Bioinformatics Organization (2011), bioinformatics as a biological science can be defined as "any use of computers to characterize the *molecular* components of living things" (para. 2). As a computer science, bioinformatics is the use of "computers to store, retrieve, analyze or predict the composition or the structure of biomolecules" (Bioinformatics Organization, para. 3).

Biomedical informatics is a growing field, with significant applications and implications throughout the biomedical and clinical worlds. The authors believe that biomedical informatics is the application of bioinformatics to health care.

Computational biology is the action complement of bioinformatics and, therefore, biomedicine. NCBI (2004) stated:

> *Ultimately, however, all of this information must be combined to form a comprehensive picture of normal cellular activities so that researchers may study how these activities are altered in different disease states. Therefore, the field of bioinformatics has evolved such that the most pressing task now involves the analysis and interpretation of various types of data, including nucleotide and amino acid sequences, protein domains, and protein structures. The actual process of analyzing and interpreting data is referred to as computational biology. Important subdisciplines within bioinformatics and computational biology include:*
>
> - *The development and implementation of tools that enable efficient access to, and use and management of, various types of information*

- *The development of new algorithms (mathematical formulas) and statistics with which to assess relationships among members of large data sets, such as methods to locate a gene within a sequence, predict protein structure and/or function, and cluster protein sequences into families of related sequences. (para. 6)*

In 2000, the National Institutes of Health's (NIH) Biomedical Information Science and Technology Initiative Consortium defined bioinformatics and computational biology. Members of the consortium believed that no definition could completely eliminate overlap with other activities or preclude variations in interpretation by different individuals and organizations. Ultimately, they defined bioinformatics as the research, development, or application of computational tools and approaches for expanding the use of biological, medical, behavioral or health data, including those to acquire, store, organize, archive, analyze, or visualize such data. The same group defined computational biology as the development and application of data-analytical and theoretical methods, mathematical modeling and computational simulation techniques to the study of biological, behavioral, and social systems. The Biomedical Information Science and Technology Initiative (BISTI) continues "as the focus of biomedical computing issues at the NIH" (NIH, 2016b, para. 1).

Bioinformatics tools help biomedical **informaticists** and healthcare personnel tackle the analysis of large datasets. The authors believe that biomedical informatics uses bioinformatics, whereas computational biology is its action complement. By using bioinformatics and computational biology to analyze and interpret intricate biological events, biomedical informaticists promote health and improve patient care. Biomedical informatics and bioinformatics may seem similar but if one thinks of biomedical informatics as focusing on health care and patients, it helps distinguish between the two. Biomedical informaticists use bioinformatics methods to integrate large biological and medical **datasets** to facilitate understanding of the human body and its biological functioning; these efforts are geared toward improving health by defeating disease.

## Why Are Bioinformatics and Biomedical Informatics So Important?

The future of health care is based on **genomics**. Bioinformatics and computational biology have provided the tools to make it possible to analyze and interpret complex biological processes. Through these developments, several projects have advanced understanding of the human **genome, haplotypes**, and the genomic changes related to disease.

In 2006, the Cancer Genome Atlas Project began (NIH, 2016a). This pilot cost $100 million to map the genomic changes in brain, lung, and ovarian cancers to assess the feasibility of a full-scale effort to systematically explore the entire spectrum of genomic changes involved in every major type of human cancer. The goal of this project is to develop a resource that will be used to develop new strategies for preventing, diagnosing and treating the disease.

The goal of the International **HapMap** Project (2006) is to

*develop a haplotype map of the human genome, the HapMap, which will describe the common patterns of human DNA sequence variation. The*

*HapMap is expected to be a key resource for researchers to use to find genes affecting health, disease, and responses to drugs and environmental factors. The information produced by the Project will be made freely available. (para. 1)*

This international partnership of scientists has taken blood samples from clusters of related people, such as parents and children, from different international regions. Using these samples, the researchers have been able to catalog some of the common variations in DNA and investigate inherited **alleles**. As the name implies, a haplotype map identifies a set of closely linked alleles on a chromosome that tend to be inherited together. Refer to **Figure 24-1**.

The International HapMap Project states:

*Most common diseases, such as diabetes, cancer, stroke, heart disease, depression, and asthma, are affected by many genes and environmental factors. Although any two unrelated people are the same at about 99.9% of their DNA sequences, the remaining 0.1% is important because it contains the genetic variants that influence how people differ in their risk of disease or their response to drugs. Discovering the DNA sequence variants that contribute to common disease risk offers one of the best opportunities for understanding the complex causes of disease in humans. (para. 3)*

A major contribution has been the **Human Genome Project** (HGP), which began in 1990 and was completed in 2003 (HGP, 2010). The U.S. Department of Energy and the NIH coordinated this program, which had the following goals:

- Identify all of the approximately 20,000–25,000 genes in human DNA
- Determine the sequences of the 3 billion chemical base pairs that make up human DNA
- Store this information in databases

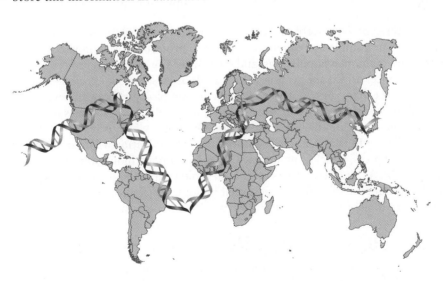

**Figure 24-1** International HapMap Project

Modified from National Human Genome Research Institute. (2012). International HapMap project. Retrieved from https://www.genome.gov/10001688/international-hapmap-project

- Improve tools for data analysis
- Transfer related technologies to the private sector
- Address the ethical, legal, and social issues (ELSI) that may arise from the project (para. 2)

According to NHGRI (2015), "One of the most important aspects of bioinformatics is identifying genes within a long DNA sequence" (para. 1). It was clear that the speed of DNA sequencing would have to be realized sooner in order to decrease costs. The process was refined so the sequencing was improved. It took 4 years to sequence the first billion bases but just 4 months to sequence the second billion bases.

During the month of January 2003, 1.5 billion bases were sequenced. As the speed of DNA sequencing increased, the cost decreased from $10 per base in 1990 to $0.10 per base at the conclusion of the project in April 2003 (NHGRI, 2015).

One of the most important aspects of bioinformatics is identifying genes within a long DNA sequence. Until the development of bioinformatics, the only way to locate genes along the chromosome was to study their function in the organism (in vivo) or to isolate the DNA and study it in a test tube (in vitro). Bioinformatics allows scientists to make educated guesses about where genes are located simply by analyzing sequence data using a computer (in silico) (NHGRI, 2015).

The other major piece brought out through the HGP was the realization that ESLI arise from studying human genomes. The participants in the HGP set aside a percentage of their annual budgets to research ESLI (HGP, 2008). **Box 24-2** and Figure 24-2 identify some of the questions raised regarding ESLI.

Even though the HGP has ended, researchers continue to improve DNA sequencing. Specifically, they continue to advance the bioinformatics and computational biology tools that are used in biomedical informatics. However, as Butte (2008) laments, "There is an absolute paucity of people trained to make use of these resources, to build the infrastructure, to ask these novel questions, and to even answer these questions" (p. 173).

These three projects were pivotal in genomics. The HGP focused on the DNA sequence from a single individual, the HapMap project focused on variation in the genome and on human populations, and the Cancer Genome Atlas Project is concerned with how cancer affects the genomes. As a result of these seminal projects and a unique culture of data sharing previously unknown among biological researchers, molecular data and measurement tools are now publicly available. Two examples of publicly available databases are the Gene Expression Omnibus, which is maintained by the National Center for Biotechnology Information at the National Library of Medicine, and Array-Express, which is maintained by the European Bioinformatics Institute (Butte, 2008). As new researchers with both biology and computational expertise emerge, bioinformatics and computational biology projects will contribute new insights into disease mechanisms and therapeutic interventions.

## What Does the Future Hold?

We have seen numerous advances ranging from possible treatments for Parkinson's diseases, unprecedented detail of the genetics of type 2 diabetes, the NIH creating

## BOX 24-2 ESLI QUESTIONS RAISED BY THE HUMAN GENOME PROJECT

- Who should have access to personal genetic information, and how will it be used?
- Who owns and controls genetic information?
- How does personal genetic information affect an individual and society's perceptions of that individual?
- How does genomic information affect members of minority communities?
- Do healthcare personnel properly counsel parents about the risks and limitations of genetic technology?
- How reliable and useful is fetal genetic testing?
- What are the larger societal issues raised by new reproductive technologies?
- How will genetic tests be evaluated and regulated for accuracy, reliability, and utility? (Currently, there is little regulation at the federal level.)
- How do we prepare healthcare professionals for the new genetics?
- How do we prepare the public to make informed choices?
- How do we as a society balance current scientific limitations and social risk with long-term benefits?
- Should testing be performed when no treatment is available?
- Should parents have the right to have their minor children tested for adult-onset diseases?
- Are genetic tests reliable and interpretable by the medical community?
- Do people's genes make them behave in a particular way?
- Can people always control their behavior?
- What is considered acceptable diversity?
- Where is the line between medical treatment and enhancement?
- Are genetically modified foods and other products safe to humans and the environment?
- How will these technologies affect developing nations' dependence on the West?
- Who owns genes and other pieces of DNA?
- Will patenting DNA sequences limit their accessibility and development into useful products?

Data from Human Genome Program. (2008). Human Genome Project information: Ethical, legal, and social issues. Retrieved from http://www.ornl.gov/sci/techresources/Human_Genome/elsi/elsi.shtml

an atlas of human malformation syndromes in diverse populations, NIH researchers identifying striking genomic signatures shared by five types of cancer, and NIH scientists discovering the genetic cause of rare allergy to vibration (NHGRI, 2016). However, it will take many more years of researching and applying bioinformatics and computational biology before the information in the human genome is understood in detail. Because these applications have the ability to allow one to analyze and interpret complex biological processes, researchers are on the path to understanding the etiology of disease and of treatment interventions at the molecular level.

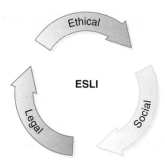

**Figure 24-2** Ethical, Social, and Legal Implications (ESLI)

Consider a typical day on any clinical unit. The advanced practice nurse who wants to prescribe a drug for a patient begins by reviewing the patient's genetic test results. The advanced practice nurse knows that this information must be assessed before prescribing so that a drug that will treat the patient's illness successfully without producing harmful side effects can be selected. The patient will receive only the medication that he or she needs, and one that is designed to interfere with or enhance the specific molecular processes that are the signature for the patient's particular health challenge. The advances that bioinformatics and biomedical informatics promise will dramatically impact healthcare delivery as it is known. As explained by Rajappa, Sharma, and Saxena (2004):

> *Understanding molecular mechanisms leads to better classification of disease and better management. A drop of blood from a hypertensive patient gives gene expression profile by cDNA microarray analysis. It may reveal SNPs [singlenucleotide polymorphisms] related to hypertension and others which predispose a patient to diabetes mellitus or myocardial infarction and the clinician can determine which drugs are beneficial and which are harmful. This scenario has a whale of difference from the current "trial and error" method of matching a patient with antihypertensives. (p. 128)*

This vision from 2004 has become a reality and the scope of treatments and interventions continues to expand. Our expectations and hopes are being met and surpassed.

Nurses can be involved in bioinformatics in many ways, including as nurse researchers helping to map molecular processes and as educators and advocates helping patients and families to understand these complex biological processes. For more information about the roles of nurses in this exciting new field, visit the website of the International Society of Nurses in Genetics (www.isong.org).

## Summary

The focus of this text is on nursing informatics, but one can clearly see the connection between biomedical informatics and nursing informatics. The discipline of bioinformatics and its use in biomedical informatics epitomize the integration of computer science, information science, computational biology, and health care. These new applications deal with the resources, devices, strategies, and methods needed to optimize the acquisition, processing, storage, retrieval, generation, and use of information in health and biomedicine. Biomedicine and its applications of bioinformatics support and manage all healthcare behaviors. They affect how clinicians deliver health care to the infirmed, prevent disease, promote health, conduct research, and provide formal education for entry-level practitioners and continuing education for those who are currently practicing. The field of biomedical informatics—that is, bioinformatics capabilities coupled with health care—includes informatics and computational biology algorithms and tools and clinical guidelines. This knowledge can be applied to the areas of nursing, pharmacy, laboratory, dentistry, medicine, and public health. Those living the profession of nursing know that the practice of nursing is intertwined with the management and processing of information including the new knowledge being generated by biomedical informatics.

On the biomedical side of informatics, one must be cognizant of the fact that medical data typically are extracted from personal, confidential, and legally protected medical records. The protection of human subjects must be paramount and all ESLI issues must be addressed.

Biomedical informatics provides knowledge about the effects of DNA disparities among individuals. Being able to study human genomes and biological processing at the molecular level will revolutionize how conditions are diagnosed and care is provided. It is helping to prevent disease. If one can better understand an organism's biological processes and genetic coding, one can better prevent or treat medical conditions. Clinical care as it is known will change; it will become genomics based.

## THOUGHT-PROVOKING QUESTIONS

1. After reading this chapter, you know that the study of genomics is helping clinicians to understand better the interaction between genes and the environment. This new information and knowledge will continue to help clinicians find ways to improve health and prevent disease. How do you envision patient care will change based on genomics in 10 years, 20 years, or 50 years in the future?

2. Review the ethical, social, and legal issues (ESLI) raised by the Human Genome Project presented in Box 24-2. Prepare a similar list of ESLI questions to apply to the public health databases being developed for health information exchanges. Can you appreciate how these ESLI questions are widely applicable to protecting information gathered from human subjects?

# References

Bioinformatics Organization. (2011). Bioinformatics. Retrieved from http://www.bioinformatics.org/wiki/bioinformatics

Butte, A. (2008). Translational bioinformatics: Coming of age. *Journal of the American Medical Informatics Association, 15*(6), 709–714. Retrieved from CINAHL database.

Human Genome Program (HGP). (2008). Human Genome Project information: Ethical, legal, and social issues. Retrieved from https://ghr.nlm.nih.gov/primer#hgp

Human Genome Program (HGP). (2010). Human Genome Project information. Retrieved from http://web.ornl.gov/sci/techresources/Human_Genome

International HapMap Project. (2006). About the International HapMap Project. Retrieved from https://www.genome.gov/10001688/international-hapmap-project

Kelly, R. (2008). What are "omics" technologies? Retrieved from http://www.reagank.com/2007/03/what_are_omics_technologies.php

Mulligen, E., Cases, M., Hettne, K., Molero, E., Weeber, M., Robertson, K., & Maojo, V. (2008). Training multidisciplinary biomedical informatics students: Three years of experience. *Journal of the American Medical Informatics Association, 15*(2), 246–254. PMCID: PMC2274784. doi: 10.1197/jamia.M2488

National Center for Biotechnology Information (NCBI). (2004). Bioinformatics. Retrieved from http://www.csub.edu/~psmith3/teaching/505-1.pdf

National Human Genome Research Institute (NHGRI). (2015). Bioinformatics: Finding genes. Retrieved from https://www.genome.gov/25020001/online-education-kit-bioinformatics-finding-genes

National Human Genome Research Institute (NHGRI). (2016). Newsroom: Current news releases. Retrieved from https://www.genome.gov/10000475/current-news-releases

National Institutes of Health (NIH). (2016a). The Cancer Genome Atlas (TCGA) Project. Retrieved from https://cancergenome.nih.gov

National Institutes of Health (NIH). (2016b). NIH Biomedical Information Science and Technology Initiative: About BISTI. Retrieved from https://www.bisti.nih.gov/Pages/Home.aspx

National Public Radio. (2010). Where the word *genome* came from. Retrieved from http://www.npr.org/templates/story/story.php?storyId=128410577

Network Science (NetSci). (2009). Terms and definitions in bioinformatics. Originally retrieved from http://www.netsci.org/Sciebce/Bioinform/definitions.html and currently preserved at http://petang.cgu.edu.tw/Bioinfomatics/MANUALS/Terms%20and%20Definitions%20in%20Bioinformatics.htm

Ohio State University Medical Center. (2010). College of Medicine, School of Biomedical Science: Biomedical informatics. Retrieved from https://medicine.osu.edu/bmi/Pages/index.aspx

Oregon Health & Science University (OHSU). (2016). What is biomedical informatics? Retrieved from http://www.ohsu.edu/xd/education/schools/school-of-medicine/departments/clinical-departments/dmice/about/what-is-biomedical-informatics.cfm

Rajappa, M., Sharma, A., & Saxena, A. (2004). Bioinformatics and its implications in clinical medicine: A review. *International Medical Journal, 11*(2), 125–129. Retrieved from CINAHL database.

University of Minnesota. (2012). What is bioinformatics? Retrieved from http://www.binf.umn.edu/about/whatsbinf.php

University of Texas at El Paso. (2010). College of Science: Bioinformatics. Retrieved from http://bioinformatics.utep.edu

Vanderbilt University. (2016). Department of Biomedical Informatics. Retrieved from https://medschool.vanderbilt.edu/dbmi

# Imagining the Future of Nursing Informatics

**You might wonder why we are including a chapter on caring as we discuss the future of nursing informatics.** The authors believe that nurses are taught to care and hone their ability to care for patients as they practice; however, in light of technologies that can sometimes be disruptive, the art of caring can become compromised or lost. We want to refocus nurses on the art of caring, while enhancing the science of nursing using informatics tools.

We challenge you to reflect on what you know and what you are learning and to think of where you are going in relation to your own practice and nursing informatics knowledge. Just as our professional and personal lives overlap at times, so do our social and professional informatics and networking experiences. We cannot assume that what we do or use in our personal lives is appropriate or even useful in our professional practice. This section begins with a chapter (*The Art of Caring in Technology-Laden Environments*) that considers the heart of what nurses do—caring.

The section ends with a chapter on *Nursing Informatics and the Foundation of Knowledge*. In this chapter you will examine emerging technologies that will impact the future of health care. The generation and management of organizational knowledge will be described in relation to quality implications. Although not explicitly at each point addressing the four key areas of the Foundation of Knowledge model, the sections of this chapter do consider how emerging technologies may address the four areas of (1) knowledge acquisition, (2) knowledge processing, (3) knowledge generation, and (4) knowledge dissemination and feedback. We also do not focus explicitly on changes in health care and nursing technologies, but rather on the more general changes that might be adapted or adopted for use by nurses or within health care.

The information in this chapter refocuses what you have learned about the many facets of nursing informatics and the interfacing of nurse knowledge workers and technology. The Foundation of Knowledge model provides a framework for examining the dynamic interrelationships among data, information, and knowledge used to meet the needs of healthcare delivery systems, organizations, patients, and nurses. The importance of knowledge management in nursing is emphasized by taking this one last opportunity to ensure that the reader understands and appreciates the value of knowledge management in the nursing profession and the role that technology has in knowledge acquisition, knowledge generation, knowledge dissemination, and knowledge processing.

The nursing informatics specialty is the synthesis of nursing science, information science, computer science, and cognitive science for the purpose of managing, disseminating and enhancing healthcare data, information, knowledge, and wisdom to improve collaboration and decision making, provide high quality patient care and advance the profession of nursing.

After reading the first six sections of this book, you should have a good idea of the current state of the science of nursing informatics. Now this final section challenges you to think about the future. Each reader should envision his or her current practice setting and the nursing informatics applications he or she uses. What will come next? What should come next?

The material within this text is placed within the context of the Foundation of Knowledge model (**Figure VII-1**) to meet the needs of healthcare delivery systems, organizations, patients, and nurses. The first chapter in this text, *Nursing Science and the Foundation of Knowledge*, provides a thorough overview of the Foundation of Knowledge model—a framework that embraces knowledge so that readers can develop the wisdom necessary to apply what they have learned. Wisdom is the application of knowledge to an appropriate situation. In the practice of nursing science, one expects action or actions directed by wisdom. Wisdom uses knowledge and experience to heighten common sense and insight, allowing one to exercise sound judgment in practical matters. Wisdom is developed through knowledge, experience, insight, and reflection. Wisdom is sometimes thought of as the highest form of common sense resulting from accumulated knowledge or erudition (deep, thorough learning) or enlightenment (education that results in understanding and the dissemination of knowledge). Wisdom is the ability to apply valuable and viable knowledge, experience, understanding, and insight while being prudent and sensible. Knowledge and wisdom are not synonymous. Knowledge abounds with others' thoughts and information, whereas wisdom is focused on one's own mind and the synthesis of one's own experience, insight, understanding, and knowledge.

Reflect on the model while reading through this final section. You are challenged to ask, "How can I use my wisdom to help create the theories, tools, and knowledge of the future?"

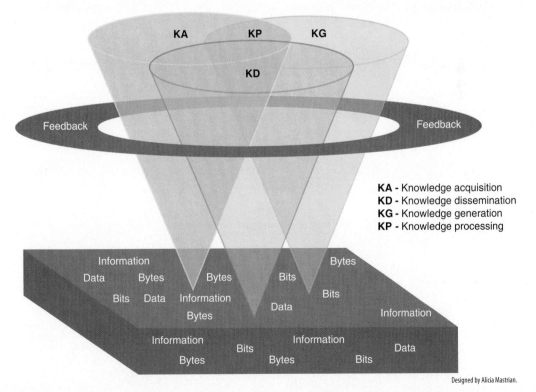

KA - Knowledge acquisition
KD - Knowledge dissemination
KG - Knowledge generation
KP - Knowledge processing

Designed by Alicia Mastrian.

**Figure VII-1** Foundation of Knowledge Model

# CHAPTER 25

# The Art of Caring in Technology-Laden Environments

Kathleen Mastrian and Dee McGonigle

## Introduction

Nursing is hard work. Depending on the site of practice, it can be both physically and mentally taxing. Nurses are masters at multitasking—that is, performing several caring functions simultaneously during a patient encounter. Some nursing interventions are readily apparent and easily described, such as collecting vital signs data and changing dressings, while others are less visible yet equally important, such as interpreting the vital signs data, generating knowledge about the patient's situation, and then using that knowledge to inform practice. Equally invisible, yet important to the therapeutic caring environment, are the little things that nurses say, project, and do in the caring episode. In this chapter, we pause to reflect on the art of caring. We emphasize the need to preserve this central and unique function of nursing and suggest ways that nurses can ensure that the caring functions do not become a lost art as technologies are introduced into patient care environments.

We derive a definition of nursing science from the American Nurses Association's definition of nursing. Nursing science is the ethical application of knowledge acquired through education, research, and practice to provide services and interventions to patients to maintain, enhance, or restore their health, and to acquire, process, generate, and disseminate nursing knowledge to advance the nursing profession. Caring functions, such as therapeutic communication, listening, touch, and mindfulness, are an integral part of nursing science, as they also help patients to maintain, enhance, or restore their health. While the new technologies such as smart pumps, bar-code medication administration systems, electronic health records (EHRs), wearables, and smartphones being introduced into our practice environments are designed to increase efficiency, promote safety, and streamline the work of nursing, we need to ask: To what extent do these technologies disrupt the nurse–patient caring encounter? How can we continue to care effectively for our patients and promote a healing environment while incorporating the advantages and efficiencies that technologies provide?

# Caring Theories

Anne Boykin and Savina Schoenhofer (2015) defined caring as an "altruistic, active expression of love and. . .the intentional and embodied recognition of value and connectedness" (p. 343). In their framework, theory of nursing as caring, caring is created from each moment the nurse is committed to nurture the person. Regardless of the challenges presented to a nurse, such as technology, time restraints, staffing issues, or difficult patients, a nurse needs to reach deep inside him/herself to make the commitment to know the person as caring. A nurse needs to be able to enter into each nursing situation with the intentional commitment to fully care for the person.

Let us also explore **caring** as a concept with the seminal work of Jean Watson. As Dr. Watson described:

> The Theory of Human Caring was developed between 1975 and 1979 while I was teaching at the University of Colorado. I tried to make explicit that nursing's values, knowledge, and practices of human caring were geared toward subjective inner healing processes and the life world of the experiencing person. This required unique caring–healing arts and a framework called "carative factors," which complemented conventional medicine but stood in stark contrast to "curative factors." (Watson, 2015, p 322)

It is important to remember that Watson developed her theory during a time when the nursing profession was struggling to define itself and identify the unique contributions of nursing to patient care. In the theory of human caring, Watson defined caring as "healing consciousness and intentionality to care and promote healing" and caring consciousness as "energy within the human–environmental field of a caring moment" (Watson, 2015, p. 323). Think about the use of the word "energy" in these definitions and pause to appreciate the level of cognitive energy that nurses expend as they care for patients. Nursing is hard work!

Watson further described the evolution of her theory from the original 10 carative factors to what she now calls **caritas processes**. As her work expanded, she recognized the need for "love and caring to come together for a new form of deep transpersonal caring." In the evolving theory, she has emphasized that the "relationship between love and caring connotes inner healing for self and others" (Watson, 2015, p. 324). The 10 caritas processes enumerated by Watson are summarized here:

1. The practice of loving kindness and equanimity within the context of caring consciousness
2. Being authentically present and enabling and sustaining the deep belief system and subjective life world of self and one being cared for
3. Cultivation of one's own spiritual practices and transpersonal self, going beyond ego self, opening to others with sensitivity and compassion
4. Developing and sustaining a helping–trusting, authentic caring relationship
5. Being present to, and supportive of, the expression of positive and negative feelings as a connection with deeper spirit of self and the one being cared for

6. Creative use of self and all ways of knowing as part of the caring process; to engage in artistry of caring–healing practices

7. Engaging in genuine teaching–learning experience that attends to unity of being and meaning, attempting to stay within others' frames of reference

8. Creating a healing environment at all levels (a physical and nonphysical, subtle environment of energy and consciousness, whereby wholeness, beauty, comfort, dignity, and peace are potentiated)

9. Assisting with basic needs, with an intentional caring consciousness, administering "human care essentials," which potentiate alignment of mind–body–spirit, wholeness, and unity of being in all aspects of care, tending to both embodied spirit and evolving spiritual emergence

10. Opening and attending to spiritual–mysterious and existential dimensions of one's own life–death; soul care for self and the one being cared for (Watson, 2015, p. 325)

Think about a recent patient encounter. Were you fully present in the moment and conscious of the individual and his or her uniqueness? Did you smile and greet the patient by name and acknowledge visitors? Did you place your tablet to the side, lean forward, and attentively listen to the concerns of the patient and family and offer them the opportunity to ask questions? Did you explain what you were doing with and for the patient, and why? (See **Figure 25-1.**) Conversely, did you focus your attention on the tablet and talk at the screen as you clicked on the drop-down menus to

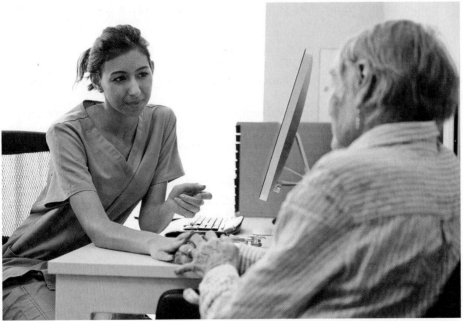

© Monkey Business Images/Shutterstock

**Figure 25-1** Active Listening

document the patient encounter? Did the technology create a barrier between you and the patient and his/her family? Did you depend solely on monitoring technologies to create your interpretation of the patient's experience? Was your assessment of the patient's current situation colored by the objective representation of the person created by the monitoring technologies present in the room (O'Keefe-McCarthy, 2009)? "The overwhelming presence of technology at the clinical bedside has the power to become the strongest reference point that nurses use to inform, direct, interpret, evaluate, and understand nursing care" (O'Keefe-McCarthy, p. 787). We must remember that "Technology, however, does not take into consideration the specific symptom presentation unique to the person experiencing the illness. Technology's use is not meant to replace the person-to-person interaction that is essential in any nurse–patient encounter" (p. 792).

Patient-centered care (PCC) is another way of describing the need for practitioners to focus on the subjective experience of patients with health challenges. Liberati et al. (2015) defined patient centeredness as "a collective achievement that is negotiated between patients and multiple health providers, comprising of social practices and relationships that are woven together through the material and immaterial resources available in specific organizational contexts" (p. 47). They suggest that a focus on PCC may have three specific outcomes:

- Patients can provide their subjective experience as an input to improve several, often undermined, aspects of healthcare delivery.
- Care providers might develop their capacity for reflexivity, which could improve their understanding of the implications of their actions.
- Patients and practitioners can thus provide insights into the overall health organization on how to innovate processes and facilities to better respond to local needs.

We will examine reflection on practice in more detail later in the chapter.

Central to the caritas processes described by Watson and the discussion about technology-mediated care by O'Keefe-McCarthy is the concept of a caring presence. Strategies for developing and enhancing caring presence are discussed in the latter part of this chapter.

The humanistic nursing theory developed by Paterson and Zderad also offers some insight into the less visible aspects of nursing care (Kleiman, 2010). These authors suggested that the basis of nursing is the response to the call for help in solving health related concerns.

> This call, a foundational concept of humanistic nursing, can be heard where nursing is offered, coming to our attention as a subtle murmur of pain, sorrow, anxiety, desperation, joy, laughter, even silence, that expresses the state-of-being of the protagonists in the drama of health-care delivery, our patients and ourselves. (Kleiman, 2010, p. 338)

Nurses hear the call and respond with their entire being. Their knowledge, experiences, ethics, and competencies shape the interaction with the patient as they respond.

> In humanistic nursing we say that each person is perceived as existing "all-at once." In the process of interacting with patients, nurses interweave professional identity, education, intuition, and experiences, with all their other

*life experiences, creating their own tapestry which unfolds during their re-*
*sponses. (Kleiman, 2010, pp. 341–342)*

Pause to reflect on how you create your own tapestry during patient interactions. Nursing care requires conscious awareness of self and the uniqueness of each of our patients. It requires emotional energy expenditure as we seek to find ways to meet the calls of our patients. We need to be aware of the potential for inadvertently dehumanizing the patient experience in our technology-laden practice environments. According to Kleiman (2010), "The context of Humanistic Nursing Theory is humans. The basic question it asks of nursing practice is: Is this particular intersubjective–transactional nursing event humanizing or dehumanizing?" (p. 349). We must be fully present and self-aware in every patient encounter, seeking to deliver exactly what is needed in every situation. Yes, nursing is hard work, but when we are able to respond with our whole being, we may find that our patients and families are more satisfied with the care we provide and that we also experience personal satisfaction and find joy in our profession.

# Presence

Presence is the act of being there and being with our patients—fully focusing on their needs. "Presence is an interpersonal process that is characterized by sensitivity, holism, intimacy, vulnerability and adaptation to unique circumstances" (Finfgeld-Connett, 2008, p. 528). Paterson and Zderad explained presence as establishing a relationship by fully being available and open to the experiences of another (Penque & Snyder, 2014). Penque and Snyder (2014) defined three types of presence: physical presence, full presence, and transcendent presence. A nurse who is physically present is largely competent in carrying out care, efficient with interventions, but inattentive to communication and nonverbal cues projected by the patient and family. When fully present, a nurse will greet the patient by name, communicate appropriately with the patient, and pay attention to what is being said and not said during the encounter. When nurses practice transcendent presence, they will first center themselves, clearing their mind of all potential distractions, and then use the patient's name and gentle touch to convey interest and responsiveness while carrying out the necessary physical interventions.

Paterson and Zderad felt presence was a vital element of their theory of humanistic nursing (Penque & Snyder, 2014). Presence requires one to be open and responsive to the situations around them. If a nurse is fully present to the patient in front of them, they will be able to notice the subtle changes that may not be evident if the nurse would only be physically present. The connection loss may cause the patient to feel that the nurse is detached from the situation. Penque and Snyder (2014) gave an example of presence from the book *Tuesdays with Morrie* by Mitch Albom (1997):

> *I believe in being fully present. That means you should be with the person you're with. When I'm talking with you now, Mitch, I try to keep focused only on what going on between us. I am not thinking about something we said last week.*
>
> *I am not thinking about what's coming up this Friday. I am not thinking about doing another Koppel show, or about medications I'm taking. I am talking to you; I am thinking about you. (pp. 135–136)*

## Strategies for Enhancing Caring Presence

Our patients have complex problems and needs. They may be scared, angry, resistant to change, or happily oblivious to the extent of their health challenges. We, too, have complex personal lives with many competing roles and issues that consume our energies. Our workplace may be short-staffed, resulting in care assignments that stretch us to our maximum. We may be struggling to learn to use the new technologies that are introduced nearly daily into our practice environments. As a result, we may feel disorganized, tired, angry, and emotionally spent.

We need to take care of ourselves first so that we can be effective in our patient and family care. Caring for ourselves involves conscious attention to our health and health practices. In addition, nurses have a "responsibility to model health behaviors" (Leonard, 2014, p. 17). Do we eat a balanced diet, get appropriate exercise, and get enough sleep? Do we have strategies to manage stress appropriately, and do we have adequate social support?

One approach to improving your health is to set goals and to keep track of your progress. As part of a concepts of health course, students are asked to develop a personal health plan and journal periodically during the semester about their ability to stick to the plan. Here is an example of a simple plan: "I will increase my intake of fruit and vegetables and walk outside for 30 minutes at least 3 times per week." As the students reflect on their ability to stick to the plan in the journal, caring for self is brought into conscious awareness. This simple self-reflective practice may be just the boost that is needed for a nurse to commit to self-awareness and self-care on a long-term basis (Figure 25-2). The following website gives information on well-being and a self-assessment tool, as well as tips on setting goals: www.takingcharge.csh.umn.edu/enhance-wellbeing (University of Minnesota, Center for Spirituality & Healing, 2013).

One additional strategy that we share with students is a breathing/meditative exercise from Tai Chi, Qi Gong, called the five-element breathing sequence. This meditative exercise, which can be performed in less than 10 minutes and can be very energizing and stress reducing, is described in Box 25-1.

The simplest and perhaps most effective strategy we can use to help us be fully present to our patients is to pause to take a few deep breaths to calm ourselves and clear

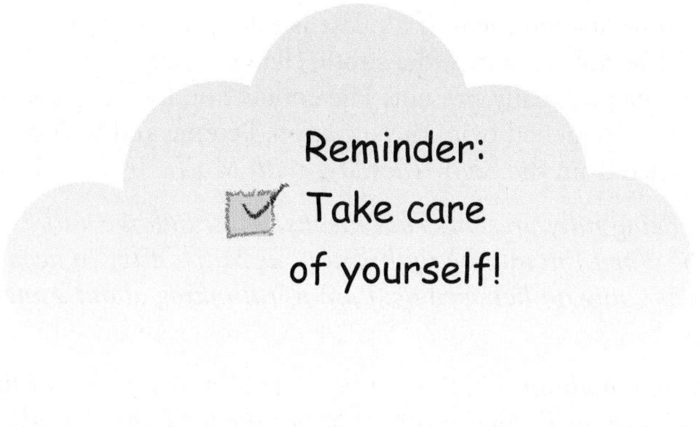

Reminder:
☑ Take care
of yourself!

**Figure 25-2** Reminder: Take Care of Yourself

## BOX 25-1 TAI CHI, QI GONG FIVE-ELEMENT BREATHING SEQUENCE

1. Stand with your feet shoulder-width apart. Relax your arms and shoulders.
2. Inhale slowly as you straighten and then move both arms slightly back and then up with palms facing up (as though you are gathering a giant ball of energy). Stretch to your full height as you inhale.
3. Exhale slowly as you press both palms down in front of you with hands slightly cupped and thumbs and index fingers nearly touching. Bend your knees slightly to sink down as you exhale.
4. Turn your hands over (palms up) just below the waist, and inhale slowly as you raise your hands in front of you, to chest height. Straighten your legs as you inhale. (Imagine lifting a ball of energy.)
5. Exhale slowly and extend the arms directly in front of you, chest high, and fan your hands open to release the energy in front of your chest. Bend the knees slightly to sink down as you exhale.
6. Inhale slowly, with palms facing you, to gather the energy back toward your chest. Straighten your legs as you inhale.
7. Press both arms straight out at shoulder height as you exhale. Pretend you are pushing on walls located on either side of you. Continue the exhalation as you bring your arms in front of you. Bend your knees slightly to sink down as you exhale.
8. Inhale slowly as you gather the energy to your chest. Straighten your legs as you inhale and stretch to your full height.
9. Exhale slowly as you raise your arms above your head to set the energy free. Bend your knees slightly to sink down as you exhale.
10. Transition your hands to the beginning to repeat the sequence by inhaling as you bring your hands halfway down and exhaling the rest of the way. (You can also end here by bringing your palms together in closure, first inhaling and then exhaling as you slowly move your hands down in front of you.)

the clutter from our minds before we address each patient. It also helps to repeat the patient's name silently a time or two before we enter the room. This practice, known as **centering**, enables the nurse to "be available with the whole self and be open to the personal and care needs of the patient" (Penque & Snyder, 2014, p. 31). When we are with a patient, we need to be certain that our mind is fully engaged in the interaction with this patient for the moment. We must be fully attentive to the patient, be both physically and mentally present, meet the patient where he or she is emotionally, listen actively to what the patient is saying, focus on the nonverbal cues the patient is projecting, touch the patient gently and reassuringly, and demonstrate acceptance (Penque & Snyder, 2014; Zerwekh, 2006). Being present can be used in any situation where the nurse is addressing the wants and needs of the patient. It is important not to force the encounter on the patient for the benefit of the nurse's agenda (Penque & Snyder, 2014).

Nurses may feel they do not have time to focus on caring presence. Caring opportunities are replaced by the time it takes to input all the information into the EHR and complete the measurable outcomes that are expected of nurses. The elimination of face-to-face interaction with the use of telephones, home monitoring, and other forms of telemedicine makes utilizing a caring presence more challenging. The theory of nursing as caring describes caring "as the end, rather than the means, of nursing, and that caring is the intention of nursing, rather than merely its instrument" (Boykin & Schoenhofer, 2015, p. 342).

A related and similar concept for practicing presence, caring between, is described in the nursing as caring theory (Boykin & Schonhofer, 2015). Consider, for example, that a nurse experienced in caring for elders with congestive heart failure will have expectations and preconceived ideas about what he or she will find in a patient situation. These expectations may not allow us to really "see" the whole patient and his experience of the illness. *Caring between* "is a loving relation into which nurse and nursed enter and which they cocreate by living the intention to care" (p. 344). The nurse needs to enter the situation knowing the person as a caring person. This knowledge will create an acceptance confirming the person as caring. The nurse's responsibility is not in determining what is wrong or needed in another, but to be present in the situation to know the person as caring and to foster a patient-specific caring environment. We need to come to know our patients both intuitively and scientifically. Our technologies provide an objective view of the patient, and the nurse synthesizes this view with his or her own perspective (wisdom) that is based on the nurse's experience, education, and intuition as applied to the patient's situation. This is the essence of caring. One of the first skills we were taught in our basic nursing education programs was **active listening**. We were taught to get down to the same level of the patient, make eye contact, touch gently (if culturally acceptable), listen attentively and nod appropriately, restate and clarify what we heard, ask questions to seek additional information, listen for feelings that are not being explicitly stated, and use silence to encourage the patient to think and provide additional information to us (Watanuki, Tracy, & Lindquist, 2014; Zerwekh, 2006). These communication skills are fundamental to caring. When was the last time you sat in a chair at a patient's bedside to get to the same level as the patient? Even a brief sit at the bedside can communicate volumes about your availability and willingness to listen, and it certainly feels good to get off of your feet for a moment. Have you ever experienced a patient who became emotional because you looked at them instead of your computer? We need to think carefully about the potential barriers to active listening that technology might present. Consider telephone encounters and e-health: Are you truly listening and present to a patient you cannot see? What are some of the ways that these caring presence skills could be adapted for use in a telehealth encounter? What are the challenges of communicating at a distance, yet being fully present for the patient?

We conclude our discussion of caring presence with a definition of the **art of nursing** provided by Finfgeld-Connett (2008):

> *The art of nursing is the expert use and adaptation of empirical and meta-physical knowledge and values. It is relationship-centered and involves sensitively adapting care to meet the needs of individual patients. In the face of uncertainty, creativity is employed in a discretionary manner. Artful*

*nursing promotes beneficent practice and results in enhanced mental and physical well-being among patients. It also results in professional satisfaction and personal growth among nurses. (p. 528)*

Let us all strive for beneficent practice that atones for the potential disruptions to the therapeutic nurse–patient relationship that our use of technology produces.

# Reflective Practice

As professionals, we should be constantly mindful of the need for practice improvement. Zande, Baart, and Vosman (2014) discussed ethical sensitivity as a type of practical wisdom. Ethical sensitivity is integral to high quality care and clinical decision making. They advocated for reflection on practice:

> *Taking daily practice of care as point of entry for reflection is a way to discern both explicit moral knowledge and tacit moral knowing. Nurses and other professionals can contribute to improvement on quality of care by creating opportunities to reflect on daily ethical concerns in an inter-professional team. (p. 75)*

Liberati et al. (2015) also advocated for the use of reflection to help professionals "observe their work from a different perspective. . . . Such an exploration may help providers to generate insights on how healthcare services, processes, and facilities could be modified to better respond to patients' needs" (p. 49).

One way to focus more specifically on our practice is to engage in reflective journaling (refer to **Figure 25-3**). In the concepts of health course, we ask students to complete a reflective practice assignment over a 6-week period. Students are directed to review concepts of caring presence and active listening and to commit to consciously using a strategy for 6 weeks. At 3 and 6 weeks, they are asked to complete the following reflective journal entry:

1. *Write a brief description* of the presence and therapeutic communication approaches you tried in your practice for the last 3 weeks. Provide specific examples of patient situations in which you tried the approach.
2. *Reflect* on the following:
   * What did you do well?
   * Which behaviors and skills do you need to improve?
   * How did you feel about the experience as it was happening? Did you plan thoroughly?
   * Did you achieve your objectives?
   * Which aspects of planning do you need to improve?
   * How will this experience affect your future practice?
3. Which personal professional development needs have you identified after reflecting on your performance? Which strategies will you use to address these needs?

Our students frequently report that they enjoy this experience and that the exercise helps to remind them why they were originally attracted to nursing. They describe experiences where they felt an authentic connection to the patient. They also report that after 6 weeks of consciously practicing the strategy, it becomes a part of their daily practice. Centering is the most frequent strategy that the students choose to practice.

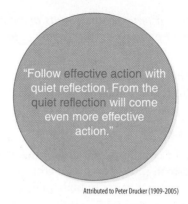

"Follow effective action with quiet reflection. From the quiet reflection will come even more effective action."

Attributed to Peter Drucker (1909-2005)

**Figure 25-3** Reflective Practice

## Summary

Nursing practice relies on information and communication technologies that receive inputs from the nurses as well as all of the patient care technologies. Computers, handheld devices, monitors, and other healthcare technologies are essential tools for nurses. Therefore, the nurse must have the ability to implement, monitor, and evaluate all of this equipment based on its inputs and outputs. The increased demands on the nurse make it easy to lose sight of the patient amid all of these technologies. Nurses must look at monitors, devices, and other gadgets to receive information; oftentimes, it is easy to forget the patient is at the core of our care.

We hope that this brief overview of caring presence prompts you to be more mindful of your practice and that you, too, will commit to employing strategies that enhance your caring presence in all patient encounters. We do not want our patients to feel that we are more focused on the machines that they are connected to or the workstations that we bring with us to the patient encounter. Yes, technology is great and it does help us collect meaningful data and generate knowledge about our patient situations, but equally important is the need to collect the human-to-human data that become available only when we step away from the technology and interact authentically with our patients.

When you save a person's life—they call you a hero

When you blend science with caring—they call you an expert

When you share your compassion—they call you a friend

When you do all three—they call you a nurse

—Author Unknown

**THOUGHT-PROVOKING QUESTIONS**

1. Examine each of the 10 caritas processes developed by Watson. Describe an example of a patient encounter that demonstrates the use of each caritas process.
2. Reflect on your personal health. Are you a role model for your patients? Which aspects of your personal health do you need to improve? Which strategies will you adopt to improve your health?
3. Choose a caring presence strategy to implement in your practice and use the reflective journal template provided in the chapter to reflect on your practice.

# References

Boykin, A., & Schoenhofer, S. O. (2015). Anne Boykin and Savina O. Schoenhofer's nursing as caring theory. In M. Smith & M. Parker (Eds.), *Nursing theories and nursing practice* (4th ed., pp. 341–356.). Philadelphia, PA: F. A. Davis.

Finfgeld-Connett, D. (2008). Qualitative convergence of three nursing concepts: Art of nursing, presence and caring. *Journal of Advanced Nursing, 63*(5), 527–534. doi: 10.1111/j.1365-2648.2008.04622.x

Kleiman, S. (2010). Josephine Paterson and Loretta Zderad's humanistic nursing theory. In M. Parker & M. Smith (Eds.), *Nursing theories and nursing practice* (3rd ed., pp. 337–350). Philadelphia, PA: F. A. Davis.

Leonard, B. (2014). Complementary therapies: Nurse's self-care. In M. Snyder, R. Lindquist, & M. Tracy (Eds.), *Complementary and alternative therapies in nursing* (7th ed., pp. 17–26). New York, NY: Springer.

Liberati, E. G., Gorli, M., Moja, L., Galuppo, L., Ripamonti, S., & Scaratti, G. (2015, May). Exploring the practice of patient centered care: The role of ethnography and reflexivity. *Social Science & Medicine*, 13345–13352. doi:10.1016/j.socscimed.2015.03.050

O'Keefe-McCarthy, S. (2009). Technologically-mediated nursing care: The impact on moral agency. *Nursing Ethics, 16*(6), 786–796.

Penque, S., & Snyder, M. (2014). Presence. In M. Snyder R. Lindquist & Tracy, M (Eds.), *Complementary and alternative therapies in nursing* (7th ed., pp. 27–37). New York, NY: Springer.

University of Minnesota, Center for Spirituality & Healing (2013). Taking charge of your health and wellbeing. Retrieved from http://www.takingcharge.csh.umn.edu/enhance-wellbeing

Watanuki, S., Tracy, M. F., & Lindquist, R. (2014). Therapeutic listening. In M. Snyder, R. Lindquist, & M. Tracy (Eds.), *Complementary and alternative therapies in nursing* (7th ed., pp. 39–53) New York, NY: Springer.

Watson, J. (2015). Jean Watson's theory of human caring. In M. Smith & M. Parker (Eds.), *Nursing theories and nursing practice* (4th ed., pp. 321–339). Philadelphia, PA: F. A. Davis.

Zande, M., Baart, A., & Vosman, F. (2014). Ethical sensitivity in practice: finding tacit moral knowing. *Journal of Advanced Nursing, 70*(1), 68–76. doi:10.1111/jan.12154

Zerwekh, J. (2006). Connecting and caring presence. In *Nursing care at the end of life: Palliative care for patients and families* (pp. 113–130). Philadelphia, PA: F. A. Davis Company.

# Nursing Informatics and the Foundation of Knowledge

Dee McGonigle and Kathleen Mastrian

## Introduction

Throughout this text, the reader has learned about the many facets of **nursing informatics (NI)** and the interfacing of nurse knowledge workers and technology. The Foundation of Knowledge model (**Figure 26-1**) has provided a framework for examining the dynamic interrelationships among **data, information,** and **knowledge** used to meet the needs of healthcare delivery systems, organizations, patients, and nurses. The importance of knowledge management in nursing and health care is emphasized by taking this one last opportunity to ensure that the reader understands and appreciates the value of knowledge management in the nursing profession and the role that technology has in supporting knowledge acquisition, knowledge generation, knowledge dissemination, and knowledge processing. We will also look at the characteristics of a learning healthcare organization and how information technology is integral to promoting and supporting learning organizations.

## Foundation of Knowledge Revisited

A review of the Foundation of Knowledge model that provides a framework for the development of this text is useful. At its base, the model has bits, bytes (computer terms for chunks of information), data, and information in a random representation. Growing out of the base are separate cones of light that expand as they reflect upward and represent **knowledge acquisition, knowledge generation,** and **knowledge dissemination**. At the intersection of the cones and forming a new cone is knowledge processing. Encircling and cutting through the knowledge cones is feedback, which acts on and may transform any or all aspects of knowledge represented by the cones.

Now, imagine the model as a dynamic figure with the cones of light and the feedback rotating and interacting rather than remaining static. Knowledge acquisition, knowledge generation, knowledge dissemination, knowledge processing, and feedback are constantly evolving for nurse scientists.

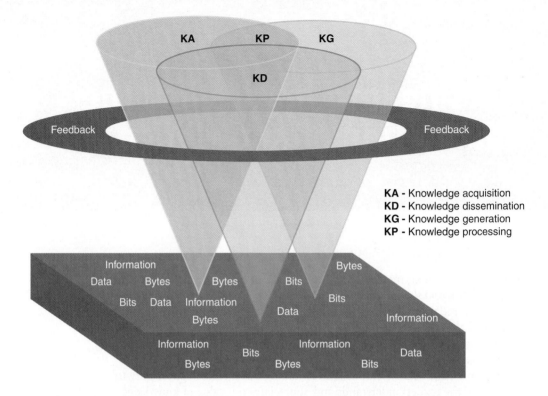

**Figure 26-1** Foundation of Knowledge Model
Designed by Alicia Mastrian.

The transparent effect of the cones is deliberate and is intended to suggest that as knowledge grows and expands, its use becomes more transparent; that is, the user is not even consciously aware of which aspect of knowledge he or she is using at any given moment during her or his practice.

If you are an experienced nurse, think back to when you were a novice. Did you feel like all you had in your head were bits of data and information that did not form any type of cohesive whole? As the model depicts, the processing of knowledge as an individual in professional practice begins a bit later (imagine a timeline applied vertically), with early experiences on the bottom and expertise growing as the processing of knowledge kicks in. Early on in nursing education, conscious attention is focused mainly on knowledge acquisition, and learners depend on their instructors and others to process, generate, and disseminate knowledge. As learners become more comfortable with the science of nursing, they begin to take over some of the other knowledge functions. However, to keep up with the explosion of information in nursing and health care, one must continue to rely on the knowledge generation and dissemination of others. In this sense, nurses are committed to lifelong learning and the use of knowledge in the practice of nursing science.

Knowledge management and transfer in healthcare organizations are likely to be studied in greater depth as our understanding of professional knowledge increases and processes to capture and codify it improve. The Foundation of Knowledge model is not perfect, and others have developed models of knowledge that are more complex. For example, Evans and Alleyne (2009) constructed the **knowledge domain process (KDP)** model to represent knowledge construction and dissemination in an organization. Yet, they caution:

> [T]he KDP model, like all models, is an abstraction aimed at making complex systems more easily understood. While the model presents knowledge processes in a structured and simplified form, the nature and structure of the processes themselves may be open to debate. (p. 148)

As we will learn later in the chapter, getting the knowledge to the user and creating a culture where new knowledge is seamlessly integrated into health care remains a challenge. Mason (2016) offered this insight:

> Simply put, knowledge management undertakes to identify what is in essence a human asset buried in the minds and hard drives of individuals working in an organization. Knowledge management also requires a system that will allow the creation of new knowledge, a dissemination system that will reach every employee, with the ability to package knowledge as value-added in products, services and systems. (para. 1)

**Figure 26-2** depicts knowledge management in an organization. Note the informatics tools that are integral to KM, particularly in the knowledge dissemination, knowledge development, and knowledge processing aspects of KM.

For nurse knowledge workers, information is their primary resource, and when one deals with information it is done in overlapping phases. That is, the nurse is continually acquiring, processing or assimilating, retaining, and using this information to generate and disseminate knowledge. However, it is not a sequential phasing; instead, there is a constant gleaning of data and information from the environment, with the data and information massaged into knowledge bases so that they can be applied and shared (disseminated).

## The Nature of Knowledge

Knowledge may be thought of as either explicit or tacit. Explicit knowledge is the knowledge that one can convey in letters, words, and numbers. It can be exchanged or shared in the form of data, manuals, product specifications, principles, policies, theories, and the like. Nurses can disseminate and share this knowledge publicly or on the record and scientifically or methodically. A nursing model or theory that is well developed and easily explained and understood is an example of explicit knowledge. Tacit knowledge, in contrast, is individualized and highly personal or private, including one's values or emotions. Knowing intuitively when and how to care is an example of tacit knowledge. This type of knowledge is difficult to convey, transmit, or share with others because it consists of one's own insights or slant on things, perceptions, intuitions, sense, hunches, or gut feelings. Tacit knowledge reflects skills and beliefs, which is why it is difficult to explain or communicate it to others. Lake (2005) stated:

> From close examination of and reflection on the literature it is possible to infer nursing prioritization of the patient need for care as it is initially taught to nursing students and is then developed in practice and influenced by practice setting. The process of nursing prioritization of the patient need for care involves discretionary judgment and ongoing assessment throughout

*and between unfolding patient situations. It is best understood from studies addressing clinical decision-making in nursing through the interpretive paradigm and in the plain language descriptions of nurse decision-making. The principles of such decision-making are discussed only in very general terms and the rationale remains the tacit knowledge of nursing. (p. 152)*

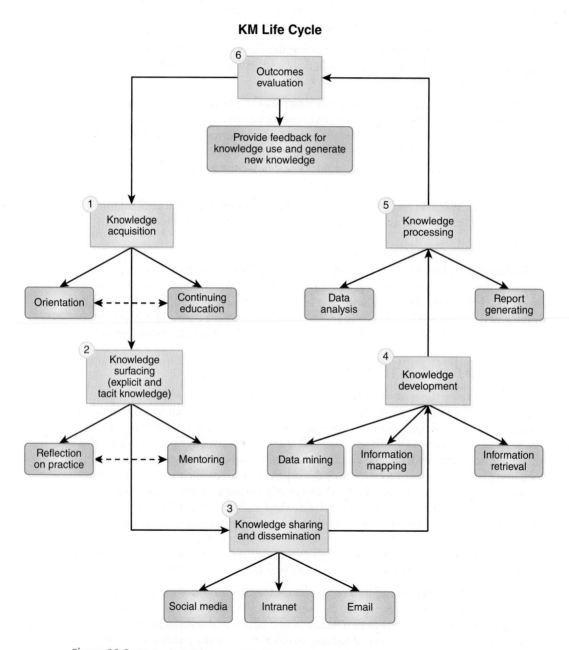

**Figure 26-2** The Knowledge Management Lifecycle

More recently, Farr and Cressy (2015) used grounded theory methodology to study how professionals perceive the quality of their performance and found that intangible, tacit knowledge was just as important to the perception of quality of performance as more standardized rational measures of quality based on organizational policy.

*This paper illuminates the importance of the tacit, intangible and relational dimensions of quality in actual practice. Staff values and personal and professional standards are core to understanding how quality is co-produced in service interactions. Professional experience, tacit clinical knowledge, personal standards and values, and conversations with patients and families all contributed to how staff understood and assessed the quality of their work in everyday practice. (p. 8)*

Along these same lines, references to co-creation of knowledge are beginning to surface in the literature. Bagayogo, Lapointe, Ramaprasad, and Vedel (2014) suggested that knowledge co-creation is increasingly important to innovation in organizations, and that knowledge is co-created as individuals collaborate on a shared task and share their experiences and perceptions. They reported on the use of social media support for breast and prostate cancer patients: "Individuals work together and co-create knowledge through a process that evolves temporally and is embedded in a web of interactions. Both temporal and interactional dimensions have been considered in the study of knowledge co-creation" (p. 627).

How nursing students and practicing nurses learn is directly affected by their practice experiences within their own personal frame of reference. The quality of clinical decision making is directly related to experience and knowledge. Knowledge is situational. Explicit and tacit knowledge are used to conduct assessments, diagnoses, intervention implementation, and evaluation of nursing actions for each individual patient. **Knowledge management systems (KMSs)** must blend these knowledge needs and provide knowledge bases and decision support systems to inform clinical decision making. Each person processes and assimilates knowledge in a unique way influenced by his or her unique perspective. What is needed is an explicit way of surfacing these nuggets of knowledge so that they can be shared among practitioners.

## Knowledge Use in Practice

One way to capture and codify tacit knowledge is to engage in reflection and reflective practice. Schutz (2007) believed that

*reflection is both a way of learning about practice and a basis for changing practice. One must engage in reflective practice because this approach can enable a practitioner to find a means in which to put this personal or experiential knowledge into words and to find a way of considering why the situation turned out as it did and whether future practice might be different. (p. 27)*

Some healthcare organizations are encouraging reflective practice to codify tacit knowledge and thus to build an organization's knowledge base. Sharing experiences in a Nursing Practice Council is one means to encourage collaboration and knowledge sharing among professionals. Joining a LISTSERV, creating a blog, or participating in a community of practice (CoP; see **Box 26-1** for more information) are other

**BOX 26-1 COMMUNITIES OF PRACTICE**

*Glenn Johnson and Jeff Swain*

*Revised by Dee McGonigle and Kathy Mastrian*

Developing and sustaining a community of practice in the work environment is beyond the main scope of this text. However, educators (in particular) and nurses need to understand how the effective collaboration skills that learners acquire in learning communities during their formal education may translate to and promote the development of CoPs in their professional lives. As the Web-based tools for collaboration continue to evolve, they are supporting online CoPs, also known as virtual communities of practice. The following is a brief overview of this important and emerging trend for work in the knowledge era.

Wenger (2006) defined a CoP as follows: "Communities of practice are groups of people who share a concern or a passion for something they do and learn how to do it better as they interact regularly" (para. 3). He suggests that CoPs have three important characteristics: (1) the domain, (2) the community, and (3) the practice. Wenger defines a domain as a shared interest about which people are passionate and for which they possess some related competence. The community aspect relates to the joint activities that are undertaken by the group to build relationships and knowledge about the domain. The practice aspect denotes that the members of the community are practitioners of something and through the CoP develop and share resources, knowledge, and solutions to problems. The recent improvement of Internet-based communications technologies has the potential to promote the global expansion of CoPs.

Nursing is a profession that is particularly well-suited to the development of CoPs, especially in light of the new knowledge generated and disseminated every day. The many nursing LISTSERVs are evidence of the growing trend toward sharing knowledge in a CoP. An early informatics LISTSERV was utilized by Caring (now ANIA), a nursing informatics organization. Members posted questions to other members and requested information and experiences related to informatics. For example, a member of the LISTSERV might ask others about their experiences related to a specific issue in implementing a bar-code medication administration system or about training procedures for implementing an electronic health record. Other members posted replies to the query. All members had the opportunity to view the question and the responses. One of the difficulties of using a LISTSERV as a CoP is that the discussion is not moderated; many threads could be running simultaneously.

Blogging is slowly replacing the LISTSERV as a collaboration tool. An advantage of blogging is that when one wants information, one seeks it out directly rather than working through the continuous feed to email that was common when using a LISTSERV as a collaboration tool (although it is also possible to subscribe to a blog feed). An example of a well-organized and global CoP is the Cochrane Collaboration (www.cochrane.org), an international organization that promotes and supports collaboration among healthcare professionals to develop evidence-based practice recommendations for healthcare interventions. A nursing practice council within a healthcare organization is another example of a CoP. In the future, it is hoped that the use of CoPs in nursing will grow beyond knowledge sharing and promote more knowledge discovery and sense making.

## REFERENCE

Wenger, E. (2006). Communities of practice: A brief introduction. Retrieved from https://web.archive.org/web/20130704222806/http://www.ewenger.com/theory/communities_of_practice_intro.htm

examples of collaboration to build knowledge. Watson (2007) described knowledge audits, narratives, and storytelling as means of surfacing tacit knowledge and assessing the knowledge resources of personnel within an organization. He described the use of **information technology (IT)** tools for knowledge management in an organization, such as intranets, extranets (shared intranets among several like organizations), knowledge directories, blogs, and wikis. Research suggests that organizations that embrace and encourage knowledge transfer among workers not only sustain and build professional competence and organizational engagement, but also enhance the quality of the work life for professionals (Leiter, Day, Harvie, & Shaughnessy, 2007). Mason (2016) suggested that, in order to facilitate knowledge co-creation, organizations must put "mechanisms of socialization, mentorships, apprenticeships, and opportunities for face-to-face communication in place" (para. 7). It is also clear that organizations must create and support a knowledge culture and user-friendly knowledge management infrastructure to offset the potential resistance to using knowledge management tools. Figure 26-3 depicts some of the issues associated with knowledge management that create knowledge management challenges.

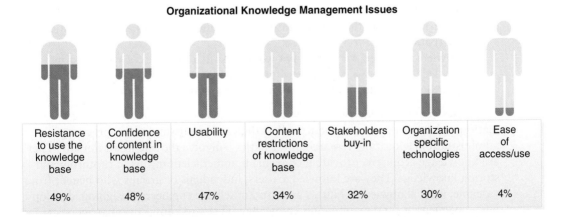

**Organizational Knowledge Management Issues**

| Resistance to use the knowledge base | Confidence of content in knowledge base | Usability | Content restrictions of knowledge base | Stakeholders buy-in | Organization specific technologies | Ease of access/use |
|---|---|---|---|---|---|---|
| 49% | 48% | 47% | 34% | 32% | 30% | 4% |

**Figure 26-3** Organizational Knowledge Management Issues
Data from UBM Tech. (2016). Knowledge management for the support center. Retrieved from http://www.thinkhdi.com/knowledge-management

# Characteristics of Knowledge Workers

According to Gent (2007), there are three types of **knowledge workers:** (1) knowledge consumers, (2) knowledge brokers, and (3) knowledge generators. This breakdown of knowledge workers is not mutually exclusive; instead, people transition between these states as their situations and experience, education, and knowledge change.

- Knowledge consumers are mainly users of knowledge who do not have the expertise to provide the knowledge they need for themselves. Novice nurses can be thought of as knowledge consumers who use the knowledge of experienced nurses or who search information systems for the knowledge necessary to apply to their practice. As responsible knowledge consumers, they must also question and challenge what is known to help them learn and understand. Their questioning and challenging facilitate critical thinking and the development of new knowledge.
- Knowledge brokers know where to find information and knowledge; they generate some knowledge but are mainly known for their ability to find what is needed. More experienced nurses and nursing students become knowledge brokers out of necessity, needing to know.
- Knowledge generators are the "primary sources of new knowledge" (para. 2). They include nursing researchers and nursing experts—the people who know. They are able to answer questions, craft theories, find solutions to nursing problems or concerns, and innovate as part of their practice.

Dixon (2012) blogged about knowledge work and knowledge workers and provides these insights:

- Knowledge workers need to acquire new knowledge every 4–5 years or else they become obsolete (para. 4).
- Knowledge work is invisible, interdependent, and constantly changing (para. 5).
- Knowledge workers, whether they are scientists, engineers, marketers, accountants, or administrators, must continuously read the situation in front of them and then, based on that interpretation, determine the appropriate next action to take (para. 5).
- Knowledge workers view their knowledge as their personal possession. The knowledge they possess is in their minds so when they leave the organization, the means of production leaves with them (para. 6).

Nurses are knowledge workers, working with information and generating information and knowledge as a product. All of the various nursing roles—practice, administration, education, research, informatics—involve the science of nursing. They are knowledge acquirers, providing convenient and efficient means of capturing and storing knowledge. They are knowledge users, individuals or groups who benefit from valuable, viable knowledge. Nurses are also knowledge engineers, designing, developing, implementing, and maintaining knowledge. They are knowledge managers, capturing and processing collective expertise and distributing it where it can create the largest benefit. They are knowledge developers or generators, changing and evolving knowledge based on the tasks at hand and information available.

The healthcare industry, the nursing profession, and patients all benefit as nurses develop nursing intelligence and intellectual capital by gaining insight into nursing science and its enactment, practice. NI applications of databases, knowledge management systems, and repositories where this knowledge can be analyzed and reused facilitate this process, enabling knowledge to be disseminated and reused.

## Knowledge Management in Organizations

To be able to enhance the acquisition, processing, generation, dissemination, and reuse of nursing knowledge, nurses must **codify** or be able to articulate knowledge structures so that they can be captured within the KMSs. According to Markus (2001), an early and prolific writer about organizational knowledge management:

> *Synthesis of evidence from a wide variety of sources suggests four distinct types of knowledge reuse situations according to the knowledge reuser and the purpose of knowledge reuse. The types involve shared work producers, who produce knowledge they later reuse; shared work practitioners, who reuse each other's knowledge contributions; expertise-seeking novices; and secondary knowledge miners. Each type of knowledge reuser has different requirements for knowledge repositories. (para. 1)*

Markus referred to **knowledge repositories** as "organizational memory systems" (para. 1). These memory systems gained popularity among help desk personnel who could access and reuse the knowledge of solutions when clients sought help for similar problems. Health care is an arena in which KMSs or knowledge repositories are clearly valuable. Hsia, Lin, Wu, and Tsai (2006) recognize that nurses are "knowledge-intensive" (para. 4) professionals who are "required to take new nursing knowledge and experience that can be acquired through various net-enabled applications or the Internet. Nursing professionals are being asked to do more with less in such contexts, while their nursing care responsibilities have increased" (para. 4). Today, information technology capabilities are expanding to develop and support a "**knowledge-centric** [boldface added] view rather than simply a **data-centric** [boldface added] view" (para. 4). Nurse knowledge workers must be able to access, use, and share these new informatics tools because "a well-designed IT-based knowledge management system (KMS) has become an ever more central force in improving the quality of care in competitive e-health environments" (para. 4). Capturing the explicit and tacit forms of knowledge is paramount to truly harness nursing knowledge. As knowledge repositories evolve to enhance sharing and repurposing of knowledge, nurses will be able to easily access, process, evaluate, reuse, generate, and disseminate knowledge.

Consider the retirement of a healthcare professional who has worked in a system for 40 years. What types of uncaptured, uncodified, tacit knowledge walk out the door on the day of the retirement? Can you appreciate the value of well-constructed knowledge repository? Interestingly, Dixon (2012) suggested that supervisors need to first recognize and acknowledge the tacit knowledge of seasoned professionals and find ways to make them feel valued by the organization. Using seasoned professionals as mentors to new professionals is a good way to help them surface tacit knowledge and share their wisdom. Nursing science is dependent on knowledge generation, and NI should facilitate all aspects of nursing, especially in the generation of knowledge, and support translational research, where we attempt to bridge the gap between what we know (research) and what we do (practice). Just like we emphasized earlier, Swan, Lang, and McGinley (2004) described NI and a common nursing language as important vehicles to access stores of clinical information that can be used as the basis for research and to help answer the question, "What do nurses do?" "Embedding nursing language within informatics structures is essential to make the work of nurses visible and articulate evidence about the quality and value of nursing in the care of patients, groups, and populations" (para. 27). In this text, it has been established that NI is a vital tool for evidence-based clinical decision making, especially when one is able to demonstrate how nurses structure and process information. An important direction for the future is to study the impact of NI on nursing science. As the HITECH Act has been implemented, the use of electronic health records (EHRs) has become more commonplace in the United States. Such records must be designed to enhance patient outcomes through content enrichment and improved caregiver decision making. As bioinformatics and computational biology continue to evolve, their integration into the EHR is inevitable. Nurse informaticists must facilitate the inclusion of computational tools and algorithms to help handle the collection, organization, analysis, processing, presentation, and dissemination of biological data to help address biological questions and unravel biological mysteries. It is imperative that current research strategies, such as those used to search for biomarkers, and new pharmacologic treatments be included in the EHR. In this bioinformatics era, one must be able to delineate biomarkers and have the necessary alerts, follow-ups, and reminders built into the system to make all caregivers aware of the bioinformatics information, such as the analysis of genes causing hypertension, cardiovascular disease, and diabetes. Bioinformatics and computational biology will complement all of the current methods and aid in the analysis of populations and tracking of selected diseases' progression. Consequently, nurse informaticists must be proactive in the development of policies and ethically based solutions to safeguard the genetic data contained in EHRs, manage the patient care implications of bioinformatics, and wisely use computational biology in this bioinformatics era. Visit www.nursingworld.org to access a document co-authored by Greco, Tinley, and Seibert (2011) for the ANA, *Essential Genetic and Genomic Competencies for Nurses with Graduate Degrees*.

NI can also be used to facilitate nursing administration and managerial studies of the work of nursing. Numerous opportunities for data mining in NI have been described in this text. Some larger healthcare systems store all of the clinical information from their affiliated hospitals and clinics in a central data warehouse. General data scans and analyses looking for patterns may, for example, suggest a trend toward better outcomes for patients with congestive heart failure in one of the affiliate hospitals. This identification of such a trend clearly begs for further analyses. A nurse researcher or administrator could ask, "Which factors contribute to these better outcomes and how can they be put into practice across the system?" Other research studies might focus on assessing the effectiveness of strategic planning and organizational goal setting or studying workflow, communication processes, and interprofessional collaboration in an organization.

## Managing Knowledge Across Disciplines

Interprofessional collaboration is emerging as a key to better quality outcomes for patients. This collaboration is supported by the EHR and other technologies that facilitate communication among health professionals. Stichler (2014), in a discussion of collaboration on the design of healthcare facilities, describes interprofessional collaboration as "magic at the intersection"; that is, "true interprofessional practice intersects and positive outcomes can be achieved as a result of the synergy that occurs among different professionals who come together with a common purpose and goal" (p. 10). Her words can also be applied to interprofessional collaboration in patient situations. Consider the ways that NI tools and technologies can help to ensure that the perspectives of all professionals are heard and valued to create this "magic at the intersection."

Another way for professionals to share perspectives and knowledge on patient situations is the HUDDLE (Healthcare, Utilizing, Deliberate, Discussion, Linking, Events) method, described in a review of the literature by Glymph et al. (2015). As they describe:

> *The huddle is a team-building tool that increases effective communication among healthcare providers. It is a quick meeting of healthcare members to share information. This brief meeting or huddle takes place at the start of the workday. It is also a time where groups plan for contingencies, express concerns, address conflicts, or reassign resources. (p. 184)*

Can you think of ways that the HUDDLE could be facilitated electronically in the future?

Research studies aimed at advancing the state of the science of NI are becoming more commonplace as the benefits of a robust NI system for managing knowledge are recognized. We will explore a few here. Rochefort, Buckenridge, and Forster (2015) explored the use of an algorithm to mine the EHR for the detection of three key adverse events (AEs): hospital-acquired pneumonia, catheter-associated bloodstream infections, and in-hospital falls. Prior to their work, the hospitals used discharge diagnostic codes for adverse event detection, which they believed resulted in both under- and overestimation of AEs. Their algorithm was designed to be more comprehensive and mine a combination of various types of data in the EHR. "To move this field forward, as well as to maximize the accuracy of AE detection, there is a need for comprehensive automated AE detection algorithms that integrate the information from all the available data sources (e.g., microbiology and laboratory results, free-text radiology reports and progress notes and electronic vital signs)" (para. 10). Evans, Yeung, Markoulakis, and Guilcher (2014) studied the use of an online CoP to promote the creation and sharing of knowledge related to manual therapies among physiotherapists. They demonstrated that the CoP approach promoted a social learning environment with a strong component of engagement, sharing, and co-creation of knowledge applicable to practice. Brown and colleagues (2013) demonstrated the use of a wiki platform to promote international collaboration for developing and maintaining evidence-based nutrition guidelines for adults with head and neck cancers. During the 4-month monitoring process, they reported over 2,000 page views from 33 different countries. Key to this process was the opportunity for international stakeholder feedback that was used to modify and update the practice guidelines. They conclude, "The use of this technology is expected to continue to rise as the advantages of maintaining a live current document for optimal clinical practice are realized" (p. 189).

We invite you to search the scholarly nursing literature for other examples of the use of information technologies to generate, share, and manage professional knowledge.

## The Learning Healthcare System

The Learning Healthcare System is a relatively new concept that is being implemented in some of the larger healthcare systems and is being developed in collaborative partnerships among groups of hospital systems. A learning healthcare system was defined in the 2013 Institute of Medicine (IOM) report, *Best Care at Lower Cost: The Path to Continuously Learning Health Care in America* as follows:

> *The foundation for a learning health care system is continuous knowledge development, improvement, and application. Although unprecedented levels of information are available, patients and clinicians often lack access to guidance that is relevant, timely, and useful for the circumstances at hand. Overcoming this challenge will require applying computing capabilities and analytic approaches to develop real-time insights from routine patient care, disseminating knowledge using new technological tools, and addressing the regulatory challenges that can inhibit progress. (p. 2)*

Some literature also refers to this concept as a rapid-learning healthcare system (Greene, Reid, & Larson, 2012): "The hallmarks of the rapid-learning health system are the vital partnership between research and clinical operations and a shared commitment to leverage scientific knowledge and evaluation for rapid, point-of-care improvements" (p. 209). These learning healthcare systems take advantage of informatics analytics concepts and processes for data mining the rich clinical data in the EHRs. Using both structured and unstructured data, these data are mined for new clinical understandings that are rapidly implemented to improve patient outcomes. The system depends on data sharing, rather than data hoarding that was part of the earlier competitive culture healthcare environment. As Greene and colleagues explain, "By blending research evidence with daily experiences of a frontline workforce, a learning organization leverages evidence about "what works" in the context of its own setting, population, available resources, and organizational culture" (p. 208). Figure 26-4 provides a schematic overview of knowledge management in a learning healthcare system.

The IOM (2013) report provides the following description of the characteristics of a Learning Healthcare System, which includes the use of science and informatics,

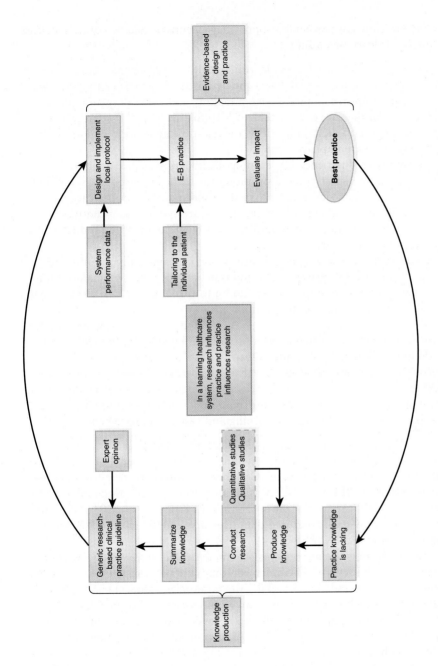

**Figure 26-4** The Learning Healthcare System

Data from Greene, S. M., Reid, R. J., & Larson, E. B. (2012). Implementing the learning health system: From concept to action. *Annals of Internal Medicine, 157*(3), 207.

encourages patient–clinician partnerships, provides incentives, and promotes a culture shift to a continuous learning culture:

- Real-time access to knowledge—A learning healthcare system continuously and reliably captures, curates, and delivers the best available evidence to guide, support, tailor, and improve clinical decision making and care safety and quality.
- Digital capture of the care experience—A learning healthcare system captures the care experience on digital platforms for real-time generation and application of knowledge for care improvement.
- Engaged, empowered patients—A learning healthcare system is anchored on patient needs and perspectives and promotes the inclusion of patients, families, and other caregivers as vital members of the continuously learning care team.
- Incentives aligned for value—A learning healthcare system has incentives actively aligned to encourage continuous improvement, identify and reduce waste, and reward high-value care.
- Full transparency—A learning healthcare system systematically monitors the safety, quality, processes, prices, costs, and outcomes of care, and makes information available for care improvement and informed choices and decision making by clinicians, patients, and their families.
- Leadership-instilled culture of learning—A learning healthcare system is stewarded by leadership committed to a culture of teamwork, collaboration, and adaptability in support of continuous learning as a core aim.
- Supportive system competencies—A learning healthcare system constantly refines complex care operations and processes through ongoing team training and skill building, systems analysis and information development, and creation of the feedback loops for continuous learning and system improvement. (p. 18)

Technologies that provide support for the collection and analysis of clinical data are also evolving. New infrastructures will need to be deployed. For example, Mandl et al. (2014) described the Scalable Collaborative Infrastructure for a Learning Healthcare System (SCILHS) architecture to support data collection and analysis from a group of 10 healthcare organizations. Similarly, Kaggal et al. (2016) described an infrastructure for mining unstructured data (free text entries) in the EHR using natural language processing (NLP) tools.

As learning healthcare systems concepts are implemented more widely, we will experience more rapid knowledge dissemination than was previously possible with more traditional forms of research, especially the randomized clinical trial. Research samples will no longer be limited by the researcher's access to subjects. Clearly, though, these new research paradigms will also necessitate new ethics considerations for the use of clinical data and the protection of human subjects. For more information about learning healthcare systems, track developments at The Learning Healthcare Project (www.learninghealthcareproject.org/index.php).

## Summary

In the future, there will be many more attempts to capture, represent, and explain knowledge processes in professional practice. It is hoped that the reader is convinced that for the nursing profession to evolve, knowledge must be dynamically generated, disseminated, and assimilated. This ever-changing interplay means that as knowledge is generated, disseminated, and assimilated, new questions about the impact of NI that will help new knowledge to be generated, assimilated, and so on will arise. The assimilation of new knowledge in a profession is a multifaceted approach of individual perception, challenges, and collective thought applied to the practice of nursing. Nurses challenge what is known and want to acquire, process, generate, and disseminate knowledge to improve patient outcomes.

As a result of reading this text, you should have a deeper understanding of knowledge and informatics, as well as the power they have to inform the science of nursing. It is hoped that you also gained valuable insights into the core principles of NI and the NI practice specialty. We hope that we have motivated you to continue to learn more and perhaps delve into the science of NI in a nursing research role. Readers are invited to become active participants in molding the future of both nursing and informatics sciences.

---

**THOUGHT-PROVOKING QUESTIONS**

Become informatics savvy and ask yourself the following questions:
1. How can I apply the knowledge I gain from my practice setting to benefit my patients and enhance my practice?
2. How can I help my colleagues and patients embrace, understand, and use technologies to manage health?
3. How can I use and communicate my wisdom to help create the theories, tools, and knowledge of the future?

---

# References

Bagayogo, F., Lapointe, L., Ramaprasad, J., & Vedel, I. (2014). Co-creation of knowledge in healthcare: A study of social media usage. Paper presented at the 47th Hawaii International Conference on System Sciences. Jan. 6, 2014 to Jan. 9, 2014. 626-635. doi:10.1109 /HICSS.2014.84

Brown, T., Findlay, M., Dincklage, J., Davidson, W., Hill, J., Isenring, E., . . . Bauer, J. (2013). Using a wiki platform to promote guidelines internationally and maintain their currency: Evidence-based guidelines for the nutritional management of adult patients with head and neck cancer. *Journal of Human Nutrition & Dietetics, 26*(2), 182–190. doi:10.1111 /jhn.12036

Dixon, N. (2012, October 10). Improving knowledge worker productivity. [Blog post.] Retrieved from http://www.nancydixonblog.com/2012/10/improving-knowledge-worker -productivity.html

Evans, C., Yeung, E., Markoulakis, R., & Guilcher, S. (2014). An online community of practice to support evidence-based physiotherapy practice in manual therapy. *Journal of Continuing Education in the Health Professions, 34*(4), 215–223. doi:10.1002/chp.21253

Evans, M., & Alleyne, J. (2009). The concept of knowledge in KM: A knowledge domain process model applied to inter-professional care. *Knowledge and Process Management, 16*(4), 147–161. Retrieved from ABI/INFORM Global. Document ID: 1890423631.

Farr, M., & Cressey, P. (2015). Understanding staff perspectives of quality in practice in healthcare. *BMC Health Services Research, 15*(1), 1–11. doi:10.1186/s12913-015-0788-1

Gent, A. (2007, October 17). Three types of knowledge workers. [Blog post.] Retrieved from http://incrediblydull.blogspot.com/2007/10/three-types-of-knowledge-workers.html

Glymph, D. C., Olenick, M., Barbera, S., Brown, E. L., Prestianni, L., & Miller, C. (2015). Healthcare Utilizing Deliberate Discussion Linking Events (HUDDLE): A systematic review. *AANA Journal, 83*(3), 183–188.

Greene, S. M., Reid, R. J., & Larson, E. B. (2012). Implementing the learning health system: From concept to action. *Annals of Internal Medicine, 157*(3), 207–210.

Hsia, T., Lin, L., Wu, J., & Tsai, H. (2006). A framework for designing nursing knowledge management systems. *Interdisciplinary Journal of Information, Knowledge and Management.* Retrieved from http://www.ijikm.org/Volume1/IJIKMv1p013-022_Hsia02.pdf

Institute of Medicine (IOM). (2013). *Best care at lower cost: The path to continuously learning health care in America.* Washington, DC: National Academies Press.

Kaggal, V. C., Elayavilli, R. K., Mehrabi, S., Pankratz, J. J., Sohn, S., Wang, Y., . . . Liu, H. (2016). Toward a learning health-care system: Knowledge delivery at the point of care empowered by big data and NLP. *Biomedical Informatics Insights, 8*(Suppl 1), 13. doi:10.4137/BII.S37977

Lake, S. (2005). Nursing prioritisation of the patient need for care: Tacit knowledge of clinical decision making in nursing. Retrieved from http://researcharchive.vuw.ac.nz/bitstream /10063/22/6/thesis.pdf

Leiter, M., Day, A., Harvie, P., & Shaughnessy, K. (2007). Personal and organizational knowledge transfer: Implications for worklife engagement. *Human Relations, 60*(2), 259–283. Retrieved from ABI/INFORM Global. Document ID: 1260239891.

Mandl, K. D., Kohane, I. S., McFadden, D., Weber, G. M., Natter, M., Mandel, J., . . . Murphy, S. N. (2014). Scalable collaborative infrastructure for a learning healthcare system (SCILHS): Architecture. *Journal of the American Medical Informatics Association, 21*(4), 615–620. doi:10.1136/amiajnl-2014-002727

Markus, M. (2001). Toward a theory of knowledge reuse: Types of knowledge reuse situations and factors in reuse success. *Journal of Management Information Systems, 18*(1), 57–94.

Mason, M. (2016). Knowledge management: The essence of the competitive edge. Retrieved from http://www.moyak.com/papers/knowledge-management.html

Rochefort, C. M., Buckeridge, D. L., & Forster, A. J. (2015). Accuracy of using automated methods for detecting adverse events from electronic health record data: A research protocol. *Implementation Science, 10*(1), 150–165. doi:10.1186/s13012-014-0197-6

Schutz, S. (2007). Reflection and reflective practice. *Community Practitioner, 80*(9), 26–29. Retrieved from ProQuest Nursing & Allied Health Source. Document ID: 1331520781.

Stichler, J. F. (2014). Interprofessional practice: Magic at the intersection. *Health Environments Research & Design Journal, 7*(3), 9–12.

Swan, B., Lang, N., & McGinley, A. (2004). Access to quality health care: Links between evidence, nursing language, and informatics. *Nursing Economics, 22*(6), 325–332. Retrieved from Health Module database. Document ID: 768191851.

Watson, M. (2007). Knowledge management in health and social care. *Journal of Integrated Care, 15*(1), 27–33. Retrieved from ProQuest Nursing & Allied Health Source. Document ID: 1221495781.

# Abbreviations

**3D** Three-dimensional
**ABC** Alternative billing codes
**ACLS** Advanced cardiac life support
**ADT** Admission, discharge, and transfer system
**AHRQ** Agency for Healthcare Research and Quality
**AI** Artificial intelligence
**ALA** American Library Association
**Alt** Alternate key on the computer keyboard
**ALU** Arithmetic logic unit
**AMIA** American Medical Informatics Association
**AMOLED** Active matrix organic light-emitting diode
**ANA** American Nurses Association
**ANGEL** A New Global Environment for Learning
**ANIA** American Nursing Informatics Association
**ANSI** American National Standards Institute
**API** Application programming interface
**APMs** Alternative Payment Models
**ARG** Augmented-reality game
**ARRA** American Recovery and Reinvestment Act
**ATSDR** Agency for Toxic Substances and Disease Registry
**b** Bit
**B** Byte
**BCMA** Bar Code Medication Administration
**BI** Bioinformatics
**BIOS** Basic input/output system
**BMP** Bitmap image
**bps** Bits per second
**BRFSS** Behavioral Risk Factor Surveillance System
**CAI** Computer-assisted instruction
**CASE** Computer-aided software engineering
**CBIS** Computer-based information system
**CCC** Clinical care classification
**CD** Compact disk
**CD-R** Compact disk—recordable
**CD-ROM** Compact disk—read-only memory
**CD-RW** Compact disk—recordable and rewritable
**CDC** Centers for Disease Control and Prevention
**CDS/CDSS** Clinical decision support/clinical decision support system
**CHESS** Comprehensive Health Enhancement Support System
**CHF** Congestive heart failure
**CHI** Consolidated health informatics

**CHIP** Children's Health Insurance Program
**CI** Cognitive informatics
**CINAHL** Cumulative Index to Nursing and Allied Health Literature
**CIO** Chief information officer
**CIS** Clinical information systems
**CMIS** Case management information system
**CMP** Civil monetary penalties
**CMS** Course management system; content management system; Centers for Medicare and Medicaid Services
**CNPII** Committee for Nursing Practice Information Infrastructure
**COPD** Chronic obstructive pulmonary disease
**CPGs** Clinical practice guidelines
**CPOE** Computerized physician/provider order entry
**CPU** Central processing unit
**CRA** Community risk assessment
**CRT** Cathode ray tube
**CSS** Cascading style sheets
**CTA** Cognitive task analysis
**CTO** Chief technical officer; chief technology officer
**Ctrl** Control key on the computer keyboard
**CWA** Cognitive work analysis
**DBMS** Database management system
**DDR SDRAM** Double data rate synchronous dynamic random-access memory
**DHIS** Division of Health Informatics and Surveillance
**DHR** Digital health record
**DPI** Dots per inch
**DRAM** Dynamic random-access memory
**DSDM** Dynamic system development method
**DSS** Decision support system
**DVD** Digital versatile disk; digital video disk
**DVD-R** Digital video disk—recordable
**DVD-RW** Digital video disk—recordable and rewritable
**DW** Data warehouse
**EB** Exabyte
**EBP** Evidence-based practice
**EDI** Electronic data interchange
**EEPROM** Electronically erasable programmable read-only memory
**EHR** Electronic health record
**ELSI** Ethical, legal, and social issues

**eMAR** Electronic mediation administration record

**EMR** Electronic medical record

**EPROM** Erasable programmable read-only memory

**ERD** Entity–relationship diagram

**ERIC** Education Resources Information Center

**ESC** Escape key

**ESLI** Ethical, social, and legal implications

**F key** Function key on the computer keyboard

**F/OSS or FOSS** Free/open source software

**FHIE** Federal Health Information Exchange

**FMEA** Failure modes and effects analysis

**FPROM** Field programmable read-only memory

**FPU** Floating-point unit

**GAO** Government Accountability Office

**GB** Gigabyte

**GDC** Genomic Data Commons

**GHz** Gigahertz

**GLBA** Gramm-Leach-Bliley Act

**GUI** Graphical user interface

**HCI** Human–computer interaction

**HCT** Human–computer technology

**HDMI** High-definition multimedia interface

**HGP** Human Genome Project

**HHA** Home health agency

**HIE** Health information exchange

**HIPAA** Health Insurance Portability and Accountability Act

**HIS** Hospital information system

**HIT** Health information technology

**HITECH** Health Information Technology for Economic and Clinical Health Act

**HL7** Health Level 7

**HMIS** Health management information system

**HMO** Health maintenance organization

**HTI** Human–technology interaction

**HTML** Hypertext Markup Language

**IaaS** Infrastructure as a service

**I/O** Input/output

**ICNP** International Classification of Nursing Practice

**IDE** Integrated drive electronics

**IEEE** Institute of Electrical and Electronics Engineers

**IHI** Institute for Healthcare Improvement

**IHIE** Indiana Health Information Exchange

**IM** Instant message

**IN** Informatics nurse

**INS** Informatics nurse specialist

**IP** Internet Protocol

**IPS LCD** In-plane switching liquid crystal display

**IS** Information system

**ISO** International Standards Organization or International Organization for Standardization

**IT** Information technology

**KB** Kilobyte

**KMS** Knowledge management system

**LAN** Local area network

**LCD** Liquid crystal display

**LOINC** Logical Observation Identifiers Names and Codes

**LOS** Length of stay

**LTC** Long-term care

**MACRA** Medicare Access and Summary CHIP Reauthorization Act

**MAN** Metropolitan area network

**MB** Megabyte

**MCIS** Managed care information system

**MHDC** Massachusetts Health Data Consortium

**MHz** Megahertz

**MIPS** Millions of instructions per second; Merit-based Incentive Payment System

**MMIS** Medicaid management information systems

**MMORPG** Massive multiplayer online role-playing game (sometimes shortened to MMO)

**Modem** Modulator–demodulator

**MOO** Object-oriented multiuser dungeon

**Moodle** Modular object-oriented dynamic learning environment

**MoSCoW** Must have, Should have, Could have, and Would have

**MP3** MPEG-1 Audio Layer-3

**MPEG** Moving Picture Experts Group

**MPI** Master patient index

**MRI** Magnetic resonance imaging

**MU** Meaningful use

**MUD** Multiuser dungeon

**MUSH** Multiuser shared hack, habitat, holodeck, or hallucination

**NANDA-I** NANDA International, Inc.

**NCPHI** National Center for Public Health Informatics

**NGC** National Guideline Clearinghouse

**NGI** Next-generation Internet

**NHANES** National Health and Nutrition Examination Survey

**NHII** National Health Information Infrastructure

**NHIN** National Health Information Network

**NHQR** National Healthcare Quality Report

**NI** Nursing informatics

**NIC** Nursing Intervention Classification; network interface card

**NIDSEC** Nursing Information and Data Set Evaluation Center

**NIS** Nursing information system

**NIST** National Institute of Standards and Technology

**NLS** National language support

**NMDS** Nursing Minimum Data Set

**NMMDS** Nursing Management Minimum Data Set

**NOC** Nursing outcome classification

**NPC** Nonplayer character

**NPI** National provider identifier

**OASIS** Outcomes and Assessment Information Set

**OCR** Office of Civil Rights

**ONC** Office of the National Coordinator for Health Information Technology

**OS** Operating system

**OSI** Open systems interconnection

**OWL** Web ontology language

**PaaS** Platform as a service

**PACS** Picture archiving and communication system

**PADS** Planned accelerated discharge protocols

**PB** Petabyte

**PBL** Problem-based learning

**PC** Personal computer

**PCA** Patient-controlled analgesia

**PCI** Peripheral component interconnection

**PCIS** Patient care information system

**PDA** Personal data assistant; personal digital assistant

**PEDA** Pre-brief/enactment/debrief/assessment

**PERS** Personal emergency response system

**PHI** Protected health information; public health informatics

**PHR** Personal health record

**PNDS** Perioperative Nursing Data Set

**POSIX** Portable Operating System Interface for UNIX

**PPS** Prospective payment system

**PROM** Programmable read-only memory

**PrtSc or Prnt Scrn** Print screen key

**PS/2** Personal System/2

**PT/INR** Prothrombin time/international normalized ratio

**QA** Quality assurance

**QCDR** Qualified Clinical Data Registry

**QPP** Quality Payment Program

**QRPH** Quality, research, and public health

**RAD** Rapid application development

**RAM** Random-access memory

**RATS** Readiness assessment tests

**RCT** Randomized controlled trial

**RDBMS** Relational database management system

**RDF** Resource description framework

**RFI** Radiofrequency identifier

**RFID** Radio frequency identification

**RHIO** Regional health information organization

**RIS** Radiology information system

**ROM** Read-only memory

**RSS** Really simple syndication

**RSVP** Rapid Syndromic Validation Project

**RU** Research utilization

**SaaS** Software as a service

**SCSI** Small Computer System Interface

**SDLC** Systems development life cycle

**SDO** Standards developing organization

**SDRAM** Synchronous dynamic random-access memory

**SGML** Standard Generalized Markup Language

**SNOMED CT** Systematic Nomenclature of Medical Clinical Terms

**SOX** Sarbanes-Oxley Act

**SPRC** Suicide Prevention Resource Center

**SQL** Structured English Query Language

**STEM** Science, technology, engineering, and math

**TB** Terabyte

**TCP** Transmission Control Protocol

**TELOS** Technological and systems, economic, legal, operational, and schedule feasibility

**TPO** Treatment payment operations

**URL** Uniform resource locator

**USB** Universal serial bus

**VNA** Visiting Nurse Association

**VoIP** Voice-over-Internet Protocol

**VR** Virtual reality

**W3C** World Wide Web Consortium

**WAN** Wide area network

**WMC** Web-based medical chart

**WWW** World Wide Web

**XML** Extensible Markup Language

**YB** Yottabyte

**YRBSS** Youth Risk Behavior Surveillance System

**ZB** Zettabyte

# Glossary

**A New Global Environment for Learning (ANGEL)** A course management system designed to support classroom learning in academic settings.

**Acceptable use** A corporate policy that defines the types of activities that are acceptable on the corporate computer network, identifies the activities that are not acceptable, and specifies the consequences for violations.

**Access** To obtain or retrieve data in order to process it.

**Accessibility** Ease of accessing the information and knowledge needed to deliver care or manage a health service; the extent to which a system is usable by as many users as possible.

**Acquisition** The act of acquiring; to locate and hold. We acquire data and information.

**Active listening** A therapeutic communication technique in which the nurse employs conscious attention to what a patient is saying, reflects back feelings and phrases, and asks questions to clarify meaning.

**Acuity systems** Systems that calculate the nursing care requirements for individual patients based on severity of illness, specialized equipment and technology needed, and intensity of nursing interventions; and determine the amount of daily nursing care needed for each patient in a nursing unit.

**Administrative processes** The processes used by administration, such as the electronic scheduling, billing, and claims management systems including electronic scheduling for inpatient and outpatient visits and procedures, electronic insurance eligibility validation, claim authorization and prior approval, identification of possible research study participants, and drug recall support.

**Admission, discharge, and transfer (ADT) systems** Systems that provide the backbone structure for the other types of clinical and business systems; they contain the groundwork for the other types of healthcare information systems because they include the patient's name, medical record number, visit or account number, and demographic information such as age, sex, home address, and contact information. They are the central sources for collecting this type of patient information and communicating it to the other types of healthcare information systems, including clinical and business systems.

**Advanced cardiac life support (ACLS)** Protocol for a set of knowledge, skills, and clinical interventions for the immediate or initial treatment of life-threatening medical emergencies such as cardiac arrest or stroke.

**Adverse events** Any undesirable experiences or outcomes in a patient related to the use of a medical treatment or product.

**Advocate** Someone who represents another person's interests; to act in patients' best interest; to act and/or speak on patients' behalf; to make the healthcare delivery system responsive to patients' needs.

**Advocate/policy developer** A nurse informatics specialist who is key to developing the infrastructure of health policy. Policy development on the local, national, and international levels is an integral part of this role.

**Agency for Healthcare Research and Quality (AHRQ)** An agency within the U.S. Department of Health and Human Services that supports health services research initiatives.

**Agency for Toxic Substances and Disease Registry (ATSDR)** A federal agency that acts as a repository for research and data regarding hazardous materials that serves the public by using the best science, taking responsive public health actions, and providing trusted health information to prevent harmful exposures and diseases related to toxic substances.

**Aggregate data** Any types of data that can be referenced as a single entity, but that also consist of more than one piece of data; collected, gathered, and reported data that are related and kept together in a way that addresses their relationship. For example, the population of a state is an aggregate of the populations of its cities, counties, and regions.

**Alarm fatigue** Multiple false alarms by smart technology that cause workers to ignore or respond slowly to them.

**Alert** Warning or additional information provided to clinicians to help with decision making; the action of the clinician or system triggers the generation of an alert. For example, an alert could be generated if the patient's serum potassium level is high and he is on potassium chloride; the system would alert the nurse on the screen (soft copy alert) with or without audio and/or by a printed (hard copy alert) warning. Also known as a trigger.

**Algorithms** Step-by-step procedures for problem solving or calculating; sets of rules for problem solving. In data mining, an algorithm defines the parameters of the data mining model; it is the recipe or method with which the data mining model is developed.

**Alleles** Members of a pair or series of genes that occupy a specific position on a specific chromosome.

**Alternative payment models (APMs)** The Reauthorization Act of 2015 (MACRA) reformed Medicare payments by making changes that created a quality payment program (QPP) to replace the hodgepodge system of Medicare reporting programs. The MACRA QPP has two paths—merit-based payment system (MIPS) or alternative payment models (APMs)—that will be in effect through 2021 and beyond. The APMs are not just incentives, but fundamental changes in how we pay for health care in the United States. It is these models, particularly those dealing with total cost of care, that have the potential to fundamentally alter the value we receive from health care.

**Alternatives** Choices between two or more options.

**American Library Association** A U.S.-based organization that promotes libraries and library education internationally.

**American National Standards Institute (ANSI)** An organization dedicated to promoting consensus on norms and guidelines related to the assessment of health agencies.

**American Recovery and Reinvestment Act (ARRA)** An economic stimulus package enacted in February 2009 that was intended to create jobs and promote investment and consumer spending during the recession. This act has also been referred to as the Stimulus or Recovery Act. There was a push for widespread adoption of health information technology, and Title XIII of ARRA was given a subtitle: Health Information Technology for Economic and Clinical Health (HITECH) Act. Through this act, healthcare organizations can qualify for financial incentives based on the level of meaningful use achieved; the HITECH Act specifically incentivizes health organizations and providers to become meaningful users.

**AMOLED (active matrix organic light-emitting diode)** Smartphone display with individual pixels being lit separately (active matrix); the next generation super AMOLED type includes touch sensors. With the active matrix, you have crisp, vivid colors and darker blacks.

**Analysis** Separating a whole into its elements or component parts; examination of a concept or phenomena, its elements, and their relations.

**Analytical model** A method, process, and structure for analyzing and examining a dataset.

**Antiprinciplism** Theory that emerged with the expansive technological changes in recent years and the tremendous rise in ethical dilemmas accompanying these changes. Opponents of principlism include those who claim that its principles do not represent a theoretical approach and those who claim that its principles are too far removed from the concrete particularities of everyday human existence; the principles are too conceptual, intangible, or abstract; or the principles disregard or do not take into account a person's psychological factors, personality, life history, sexual orientation, religious, ethnic, and cultural background.

**Antivirus software** A computer program that is designed to recognize and neutralize computer viruses—that is, malicious codes that replicate over and over and eventually take over the computer's memory and interfere with its normal functioning.

**Application** The implementation software of a computer system. This software allows users to complete tasks such as word processing, developing presentations, and managing data.

**Applications (apps)** Software used on a smartphone or other mobile device.

**Archetype** Broad or general, idealized model of an object or concept from which similar instances are derived, copied, patterned, or emulated; the original model after which other similar things are patterned; the first form from which varieties arise or imitations are made.

**Arithmetic logic units** Essential building blocks of the processor of a computer that digitally perform arithmetic and logical functions.

**Art of nursing** The relationship-centered aspects of nursing care, in which the focus is on communicating caring and providing emotional support and comfort to the patient.

**Artificial intelligence** The field that deals with the conception, development, and implementation of informatics tools based on intelligent technologies. This field attempts to capture the complex processes of human thought and intelligence.

**Assessment** The simulation stage in which student performance is rated or graded. The student should be provided with a detailed explanation of how they will be assessed and graded that relates to the goal, educational outcomes, and, if applicable, course/program outcomes. Detailed rubrics are recommended.

**Asynchronous** That which is not synchronous; not in real time, or does not occur or exist at the same time, having the same period or time frame. Learning anywhere and at any time using Internet and World Wide Web software tools (e.g., course management systems, e-mail, electronic bulletin boards, webpages) as the principal delivery mechanisms for instruction.

**Attribute** Quality or characteristic; field or element of an entity in a database.

**Audiopod** Traditional, audio-based podcast or utility to download podcasts.

**Augmented-reality games (ARGs)** Games in which a device, such as a smartphone, is used to overlay on the real world and bring people together physically and virtually to solve a series of challenges.

**Authentication** Processes to serve to authenticate or prove who is accessing the system.

**Autonomy** The right of an individual to choose for himself or herself.

**Avatar** Image on the Internet that represents the user in virtual communities or other interactions on the Internet; three-dimensional or two-dimensional image representing one user on the Internet.

**Bagging** The use of voting and averaging in predictive data mining to synthesize the predictions from many models or methods or for using the same type of a model on different data; it deals with the unpredictability of results when complex models are used to data mine small datasets.

**Baiting** Tricking a user to load an infected physical device onto their computer by leaving it in a public area such as a copy room. The user loads the device to try to identify its owner.

**Bar-code medication administration (BCMA)** A system using bar-code technology affixed to the medication, the patient ID bracelet, and the nurse ID badge to support the five rights of medication administration.

**Basic input/output system (BIOS)** Binary input/output system, basic integrated operating system, or built-in operating system; a system that resides or is embedded on a chip that recognizes and controls a computer's devices.

**Behavioral Risk Factor Surveillance System (BRFSS)** An assessment system initially designed to collect information on the movement of mentally impaired persons from state-operated facilities into community settings. The assessments have since been expanded to include other populations and are designed to determine the effectiveness of programs in meeting the healthcare needs of at-risk populations.

**Beneficence** Actions performed that contribute to the welfare of others.

**Big data** Voluminous amounts of datasets that are difficult to process using typical data processing; huge amounts of semistructured and unstructured data that are unwieldy to manage within relational databases. Unstructured big data residing in text files represent more than 75% of an organization's data.

**Binary system** System used by computers; a numeric system that uses two symbols: 0 and 1.

**Bioethics** The study and formulation of healthcare ethics. Bioethics takes on relevant ethical problems experienced by healthcare providers in the provision of care to individuals and groups.

**Bioinformatics** The application of computer science, information science, and cognitive science principles to biological systems, especially in the human genome field of study; an interdisciplinary science that applies computer and information sciences to solve biological problems.

**Biomedical informatics** Interdisciplinary science of acquiring, structuring, analyzing, and providing access to biomedical data, information, and knowledge to improve the detection, prevention, and treatment of disease.

**Biometrics** Study of processes or means to uniquely recognize individual users (humans) based on one or more intrinsic physical or behavioral attributes or characteristics. Authentication devices that recognize thumb prints, retinal patterns, or facial patterns are available. Depending on the level of security needed, organizations will commonly use a combination of these types of authentication.

**Bioterrorism** The use of pathogens or other potentially harmful biological agents to sicken or kill members of a targeted population. Informatics database applications are used to track strategic indicators, such as emergency room visits, disease case reports, frequency and type of lab testing ordered by physicians and/or nurse practitioners, missed work, and over-the-counter medication purchases, that may indicate an outbreak that can be attributed to bioterrorism.

**Bit** Unit of measurement that holds one binary digit, 0 or 1. The smallest possible chunk of data memory used in computer processing, making up the binary system of the computer.

**Blended** An approach to education that combines traditional face-to-face instruction with technology-based (online) instruction. *See also* hybrid.

**Blogs** Interactive, online weblogs. Typically a combination of what is happening on the Web as well as what is happening in the blogger's or creator's life. A blog is as unique as the blogger or person creating it. Thought of as a diary and guide.

**Blogger** Someone who creates and maintains a blog; a person who blogs.

**Boosting** Increasing the power of models by weighting the combinations of predictions from those models to create a predicted classification; an iterative process using voting or averaging to combine the different classifiers.

**Borrowed theory** Theories borrowed or made use of from other disciplines. As nursing began to evolve, theories from other disciplines (e.g., psychology, sociology) were adopted to try to empirically describe, explain, or predict nursing phenomena. As nursing theories continue to be developed, nurses are now questioning whether these borrowed theories were sufficient or satisfactory in their relation to the nursing phenomena they were used to describe, explain, or predict.

**Brain** The central information processing unit of humans. An organ that controls the central nervous system, it is responsible for cognition and the interpretation, processing, and reaction to sensory input.

**Browser** Software used to locate and display webpages. Also known as a web browser or Internet browser.

**Brushing** A technique whereby the user manually chooses specific data points or observations or subsets of data on an interactive data display; these data can be visualized in two-dimensional or three-dimensional surfaces as scatterplots. Also known as graphical exploratory data analysis.

**Brute force attack** A technique where software creates many possible combinations of characters in an attempt to guess passwords to gain access to a network or a computer.

**Building blocks** Basic elements or parts of nursing informatics such as information science, computer science, cognitive science, and nursing science.

**Bus** Subsystem that transfers data between a computer's internal components or between computers.

**Byte** Unit of memory equal to eight bits or eight informational storage units, which represents one keystroke (e.g., any push of a key on a keyboard such as pressing the space bar, a lowercase "a" or an uppercase "T"). It is considered the best way to indicate computer memory or storage capacity.

**Cache memory** Smaller and faster memory storage used by a computer's processor to store copies of frequently used data in main memory.

**Call centers** Registered nurse–staffed facilities at which nurses typically act as case managers for callers or perform patient triage.

**Care ethics** An ethical approach to solving moral dilemmas encountered in health care that is based on relationships and a caring attitude toward others.

**Care plan** A set of guidelines that outline the course of treatment and the recommended interventions that will achieve optimal results.

**Caring** The nontechnical aspects of nursing interventions that communicate acceptance and concern for a patient.

**Caritas processes** Nursing interventions that communicate loving concern for the unique humanity of every patient.

**Case management information systems** Computer programs and information management tools that interact to support and facilitate the practice of case managers.

**Case study** An account of a nursing informatics activity, event, or problem containing some of the background and complexities actually encountered by a nurse. The case is used to enhance one's learning about nursing informatics principles, practices, and trends. Each case describes a series of events that reflect the nursing informatics episode as it actually occurred.

**Casuist approach** An approach to ethical decision making that grew out of the concern for more concrete methods of examining ethical dilemmas. Casuistry is a case-based ethical reasoning method that analyzes the facts of a case in a sound, logical, and ordered or structured manner. The facts are compared to the decisions arising out of consensus in previous paradigmatic or model cases.

**Centering** The act of taking a moment to clear one's mind of clutter and focus one's attention exclusively on a patient prior to engaging in a therapeutic encounter.

**Centers for Disease Control and Prevention (CDC)** An agency of the U.S. Department of Health and Human Services that works to protect public health and safety related to disease control and prevention.

**Centers for Medicare and Medicaid Services** The largest health insurer in the United States, particularly for home healthcare services, and for the elderly, for healthcare services.

**Central processing unit (CPU)** An old term for processors and microprocessors that execute computer programs, thought of as the brain controlling the functioning of the computer; the computer component that actually executes, calculates, and processes the binary computer code instigated by the operating system and other applications on the computer. It serves as the command center that directs the actions of all other components of the computer and manages both incoming and outgoing data.

**Central stations** Multifunctional telehealthcare platforms for receiving, retrieving, and/or displaying patients' vital signs and other information transmitted from telecommunications-ready medical devices.

**Certification** System for validating that a nurse possesses certain skills and knowledge or is competent to complete a task. Competence and skill level are determined by or based on an external review, assessment, examination, or education.

**Certified EHR technology** An electronic health record (EHR) that meets specific governmental standards for the type of record involved, either an ambulatory EHR used by office-based healthcare practitioners or an inpatient EHR used by hospitals. The specific standards to be met are set forth in federal regulations.

**Change** A transition to something different.

**Chat** Real-time electronic communications; users type what they want to say, and their messages are displayed on the screens of all participants in the same chat. Internet Relay Chat (IRC) is the Internet protocol for chat.

**Chief information officers** People involved with the information technology infrastructure of an organization. This role is sometimes called chief knowledge officer.

**Chief technical officers** People focused on organizationally based scientific and technical issues and responsible for technological research and development as part of the organization's products and services.

**Chief technology officers** Another name for chief technical officers.

**Chronic disease** Long-term disease, such as congestive heart failure, diabetes, and respiratory ailments.

**Civil monetary penalties** Fines laid out by the Social Security Act, which the Secretary of Health and Human Services can assess for many types of noncompliant conduct.

**Classification** The technique of dividing a dataset into mutually exclusive groups.

**Classification and regression trees (CART)** A decision tree method that is used for sorting or classifying a dataset. A set of rules that can be applied to a new dataset that has not been classified; the set of rules is designed to predict which records will have a specified outcome.

**Clinical analytics** Process of analysis by which clinical data are used to help make decisions and develop predictive analytics.

**Clinical databases** Collections of related patient records stored in a computer system using software that permits a person or program to query the data to extract needed patient information.

**Clinical decision support (CDS)** A computer-based program designed to assist clinicians in making clinical decisions by filtering or integrating vast amounts of information and providing suggestions for clinical intervention. May also be called a clinical decision support system (CDSS).

**Clinical documentation systems** Arrays or collections of applications and functionality; amalgamations of systems, medical equipment, and technologies working together that are committed or dedicated to collecting, storing, and manipulating healthcare data and information and providing secure access to interdisciplinary clinicians navigating the continuum of client care. Designed to collect patient data in real time and to enhance care by putting data at the clinician's fingertips and enabling decision making where it needs to occur—at the bedside. Also known as clinical information systems (CISs).

**Clinical guidelines** Recommendations that serve as a guide to decisions and provide criteria for specific practice areas.

**Clinical informatics** Application of informatics and information technology to deliver healthcare services. It is also referred to as applied clinical informatics or operational informatics.

**Clinical information systems** Arrays or collections of applications and functionality; amalgamations of systems, medical equipment, and technologies working together that are committed or dedicated to collecting, storing, and manipulating healthcare data and information and providing secure access to interdisciplinary clinicians navigating the continuum of client care. Designed to collect patient data in real time and to enhance care by putting data at the clinician's fingertips and enabling decision making where it needs to occur—at the bedside. Also known as clinical documentation systems.

**Clinical outcomes** Patients' results and consequences from clinical interventions.

**Clinical practice council** Group that uses the information generated by the clinical information systems to design clinical education programs. Also called nursing practice council.

**Clinical practice guidelines** Informal or formal rules or guiding principles that a healthcare provider uses when determining diagnostic tests and treatment strategies for individual patients. In the electronic health record, they are included in a variety of ways such as prompts, pop-ups, and text messages.

**Clinical research informatics** The use of informatics in the discovery and management of new knowledge relating to health and disease. It includes management of information related to clinical trials and also involves informatics related to secondary research use of clinical data. Clinical research informatics and translational bioinformatics are the primary domains related to informatics activities to support translational research,

**Clinical transformation** The complete alteration of the clinical environment; widespread change accompanies transformational activities, and clinical transformation implies that the manner in which work is carried out and the outcomes achieved are completely different from the prior state, which is not always true in the case of simply implementing technology. Technology can be used to launch or in conjunction with a clinical transformation initiative; however, the implementation of technology alone is not justifiably transformational ability. Therefore, this term should be used cautiously to describe redesign efforts.

**Cloud computing** Web browser–based login-accessible data, software, and hardware; could link systems together and reduce costs.

**Cloud storage** Data storage provided by networked online servers that are typically outside of the institution whose data are being housed.

**Coded terminology** Nursing terminologies that are given a specific and standardized designation so that they can be easily entered into computerized nursing documentation systems, searched for, and easily retrieved.

**Codify** To classify, reduce to code, or articulate.

**Cognitive** That which uses one's capacity to think. The process of cognition is important to generate knowledge. Conscious intellectual or mental activity such as thinking, reasoning, and remembering, it includes imagination or the ability to imagine and the ability to learn.

**Cognitive activity** Any process or task (activity) that involves the capacity to think, reason, imagine, and learn.

**Cognitive informatics** Field of study made up of the disciplines of neuroscience, linguistics, artificial intelligence, and psychology. This multidisciplinary study of cognition and information sciences investigates human information-processing mechanisms and processes and their engineering applications in computing.

**Cognitive science** Interdisciplinary field that studies the mind, intelligence, and behavior from an information processing perspective.

**Cognitive task analysis (CTA)** Examination of the nature of a task by breaking it down into its component parts and identifying the performers' thought processes.

**Cognitive walkthrough** A technique used to evaluate a computer interface or a software program by breaking down and explaining the steps that a user will take to accomplish a task.

**Cognitive work analysis (CWA)** A multifaceted analytic procedure developed specifically for the analysis of complex, high-technology work domains.

**Collaboration** The sharing of ideas and experiences for the purposes of mutual understanding and learning.

**Columns** Fields or attributes of an entity in a database.

**Communication science** Area of concentration or discipline that studies human communication.

**Communication software** Technology programs used to transmit messages via e-mail, telephone, paging, broadcast (such as MP3), and Internet (such as instant messaging, Voice-over-Internet Protocol, or Listservs).

**Communication systems** Collections of individual communications networks and transmission systems. In health care, they include call light systems, wireless phones, pagers, e-mail, instant messaging, and any other devices or networks that clinicians use to communicate with patients, families, other professionals, and internal and external resources.

**Communications hub** A device that captures and assists in the transmission of information from peripheral equipment. A processor organizes the data, appropriately encrypts the data to assure confidentiality, and transmits the encrypted data to appropriate decision makers. Data can be transmitted via traditional phone lines, through the Internet, or over wireless networks. Typically the hub will be a small box, to which peripheral equipment is connected.

**Community risk assessment (CRA)** A comprehensive examination of a community to identify factors that potentially affect the health of the members of that community. Often used in public health program planning.

**Compact disk read-only memory (CD-ROM)** Disk that can hold approximately 700 megabytes of data accessible by a computer.

**Compact disk-recordable (CD-R)** Compact disk that can be used once for recording.

**Compact disk-rewritable (CD-RW)** Compact disk that can be recorded onto many times.

**Compatibility** The ability to work with each other or other devices or systems; for example, software that works with a computer.

**Competency** A statement or description of goals, skills, or behaviors to be achieved.

**Compliance** Conforming or performing in an acceptable manner; correctly following the rules.

**Comprehensive Health Enhancement Support System (CHESS)** A computer-based system designed to help underserved breast cancer patients manage their disease.

**Computational biology** The action complement of bioinformatics and, therefore, biomedicine; it is the actual process of analyzing and interpreting data.

**Computer** A machine that stores and executes programs; a machine with peripheral hardware and software to carry out selected programming.

**Computer-aided software engineering (CASE)** Systematic application of computer software tools and techniques to facilitate engineering practice.

**Computer-assisted instruction (CAI)** Any instruction that is aided by the use of a computer.

**Computer-based** That which uses the computer to interact; the computer is the base tool.

**Computer-based information systems** Combinations of hardware, software, and telecommunications networks that people build and use to collect, create, and distribute useful data, typically in organizational settings.

**Computer science** Branch of engineering (application of science) that studies the theoretical foundations of information and computation and their implementation and application in computer systems. The study of storage/memory, conversion and transformation, and transfer or transmission of information in machines—that is, computers—through both algorithms and practical implementation problems. Algorithms are detailed, unambiguous action sequences in the design, efficiency, and application of computer systems, whereas practical implementation problems deal with the software and hardware.

**Computerized physician (provider) order entry systems** Systems that automate the way that orders have traditionally been initiated for patients. Clinicians place orders within these systems instead of using traditional handwritten transcription onto paper. These systems provide major safeguards by ensuring that physician orders are legible and complete, thereby providing a level of patient safety that was historically missing with paper-based orders. They provide decision support and automated alert functionality that was previously unavailable with paper-based orders.

**Computerized provider order entry (CPOE)** An electronic process or system that automates the way that orders have traditionally been initiated for patients. It allows a healthcare provider to enter orders electronically and to also manage the results of those orders.

**Conceptual framework** Framework used in research to chart feasible courses of action or to present a desired approach to a study or analysis; built from a set of concepts that are related to a proposed or existing system of methods, behaviors, functions, relationships, and objects. A relational model. A formal way of thinking or conceptualizing about a phenomenon, process, or system under study.

**Conferencing software** Electronic communications system or software that supports and facilitates two or more people meeting for discussion. High-end systems offer telepresence (a lifelike experience allowing people to feel as if they were present in person—it would be as though the nurse were physically there with the patient—so people can work, learn, and play in person over the Internet or have an effect at a remote location).

**Confidentiality** The mandate that all personal information be safeguarded by ensuring that access is limited to only those who are authorized to view that information.

**Connectionism** A component of cognitive science that uses computer modeling through artificial neural networks to try to explain human intellectual abilities.

**Connectivity** Ability to hook up to the electronic resources necessary to meet the user's needs. The ability to use computer networks to link to people and resources. The unbiased transmission or transport of Internet Protocol packets between two end points.

**Consequences** Outcomes or products resulting from one's decision choices.

**Consolidated health informatics (CHI)** A collaborative effort to adopt health information interoperability standards, particularly health vocabulary and messaging standards, for implementation in federal government systems.

**Consultant** A person hired to provide expert advice, opinions, and recommendations based on his or her area of expertise.

**Context of care** The setting, services, patient, environment, and professional and social interactions surrounding the delivery of patient interventions.

**Continuing education** Coursework or training completed after achievement of a baccalaureate degree, often for the purpose of recertification.

**Continuous learner** Person who gleans lessons or learns from success as well as failures, or who constantly searches for information to add to his or her knowledge base.

**Copyright** A legal term used by many governments around the world that gives the inventor or designer of an original product sole or exclusive rights to that product for a limited time; the same laws that cover physical books, artwork, and other creative material are still applicable in the digital world.

**Core business systems** Systems that enhance administrative tasks within healthcare organizations. Unlike clinical information systems, whose aim is to provide direct patient care, these systems support the management of health care within an organization. They provide the framework for reimbursement, support of best practices, quality control, and resource allocation. There are four common types of core business systems: (1) admission, discharge, and transfer (ADT); (2) financial; (3) acuity; and (4) scheduling systems.

**Core sciences** The branches of study and knowledge that form the foundation of nursing informatics, including nursing, computer, and information sciences. Some, including the editors of this text, believe that cognitive science should also be included in the list of NI core sciences.

**Courage** The strength to face difficulty.

**Course management system (CMS)** Software system designed for both faculty and students that supports educational episodes, including tools for grading, learner assessment, content presentation/interaction, and communication. These systems provide for the support of learning activities throughout course delivery; proprietary examples include ANGEL, Blackboard, WebCT, Learning Space, and eCollege.

**Covered entity** A healthcare provider that conducts certain transactions in electronic form (a "covered healthcare provider"), a healthcare clearinghouse, or a health plan that electronically transmits any health information in connection with transactions (billing and payment for services or insurance coverage) for which the U.S. Department of Health and Human Services has adopted standards; identified in the Administrative Simplification regulations.

**Creativity software** Programs that support and facilitate innovation and creativity (an intellectual process relating to the creation or generation of new ideas, concepts, or new relationships between currently existing ideas or concepts); they allow users to focus or concentrate more on creating new things in today's digital age and less on the mechanics or workings of how they are created or developed.

**Crowdsourcing** Information generated by individuals on social media.

**Culture broker** Person who can translate between science and clinical care and between science and the self-caring citizen.

**Cumulative Index to Nursing and Allied Health Literature** A comprehensive nursing and allied health literature database.

**Data** Raw facts that lack meaning.

**Data-centric** Data are the central focus.

**Data dictionary** Software that contains a listing of tables and their details, including field names, validation settings, and data types.

**Data file** A collection of related records.

**Data gatherer** One involved in the direct procurement of raw facts (data); raw facts (data) collector.

**Data mart** Collection of data focusing on a specific topic or organizational unit or department created to facilitate management personnel making strategic business decisions. Could be as small as one database or larger, such as a compilation of databases; generally smaller than a data warehouse.

**Data mining** A process of utilizing software to sort through data so as to discover patterns and ascertain or establish relationships. This process may help to discover or uncover previously unidentified relationships among the data in a database.

**Data warehouse** An extremely large database or repository that stores all of an organization's or institution's data and makes this data available for data mining. A combination of an institution's many different databases that provides management personnel flexible access to the data.

**Database** A collection of related records stored in a computer system using software that permits a person or program to query the data so as to extract needed information; it may consist of one or more related data files or tables.

**Database management system (DBMS)** Software program/s and the hardware used to create and manage data.

**Datasets** Collections of interrelated data.

**Debrief** The simulation stage comprised of a student-centered discussion, during which the participants and observers reflect on performance during the scenario and make recommendations for future practice.

**Decision making** Output of cognition; outcome of our intellectual processing.

**Decision support** Recommendations for interventions based on computerized care protocols. The decision support recommendations may include such items as additional screenings, medication interactions, or drug and dosage monitoring.

**Decision support/outcomes manager** Person charged with reviewing the effects of interventions suggested by the computerized decision support system.

**Decision support system** Computer applications designed to facilitate human decision-making processes. Usually are rule based, using a specified knowledge base and a set of rules to analyze data and information and provide recommendations to users.

**Decision tree** A set of decisions represented in a tree-shaped pattern; the decisions produce the rules for the classification of a dataset.

**Degradation** Loss of quality; for example, in telecommunications, it is the loss of quality in the electronic signal.

**Desktop** Computer's interface that resembles the top of a desk, where the user keeps things he or she wants to access quickly, such as paper clips, pens, and paper. On the computer's desktop, the user can customize the look and feel to have easy access to the programs, folders, and files on the hard drive that the individual uses the most.

**Digital divide** The gap between those who have and those who do not have access to online information.

**Digital health record (DHR)** An electronic record of patient assessments that are collected over time, typically by a telemonitoring device. For example, daily assessments of weight and blood pressure can be captured electronically and graphically displayed to allow for the detection of subtle trends.

**Digital pen** A writing implement that can also digitally capture handwriting or drawings. This device is battery operated and generally comes with a universal serial bus (USB) cradle that permits uploading captured materials to a desktop, laptop, or palmtop computer. The user can use it as a ballpoint pen and write on regular paper just as he or she would with a normal pen or can capture the output digitally after writing on digital paper.

**Digital video disk/digital versatile disk (DVD)** Optical disk storage format that can generally hold or store more than six times the amount of data that a compact disk can.

**Digital video disk–recordable (DVD-R)** Disk on which a user can record once.

**Digital video disk–recordable and rewritable (DVD-RW)** Disk on which a user can record many times.

**Dimension** A collection of related attributes that provide information about the data or the context of the facts. In a multidimensional database, a set of similar entities is known as a dimension; in a relational database, each field is considered a dimension.

**Dissemination** A thoughtful, intentional, goal-oriented communication of specific, useful information or knowledge.

**Distance education** Education provided from a remote location.

**Document** To capture and save information for later use.

**Documentation** Communication in the form of written or typed text, audio, video, graphics, photographs, pictures, or any blending of these means used to describe some characteristics or elements of an object, system, or practice. For example, nursing documentation generates information about a patient (individual, family, group, community, populations) that describes the care and/or services that have been provided and allows for the

communication necessary between nurses and other healthcare providers.

**Domain name** A series of alphanumeric characters that forms part of the Internet address or URL (e.g., psu.edu denotes Pennsylvania State University's address).

**Dots per inch (DPI) switch** An actual switch on a computer mouse that allows you to adjust the mouse's sensitivity to movement to result in faster or slower mouse pointer speeds. Slowing the speed can enhance precision while speeding it up can facilitate large data transfers.

**Double data rate synchronous dynamic random-access memory (DDR SDRAM)** A chip that allows for greater bandwidth and twice the transfers per the computer's internal clock's unit of time; one of the transfers occurs at the start of the new unit of time and the other transfer occurs at the end of the unit of time.

**Drill down** A means of viewing data warehouse information by going down to lower levels of the database to focus on information that is pertinent to the user's needs at the moment.

**Duty** One's feeling of being bound or obligated to carry out specific tasks or roles based on one's rank or position.

**Dynamic random-access memory (DRAM)** Type of RAM chip requiring less space to store the same amount on a similar static RAM (SRAM) chip; however, DRAM requires more power than SRAM because DRAM needs to keep its charge by constantly refreshing.

**Dynamic system development method (DSDM)** An agile software development strategy based on the rapid application development model, which is iterative and used in the system development life cycle and project management.

**Dynamic webpage shells** Webpages that can be custom scripted to provide realistic case scenarios during a simulation experience.

**E-brochure** Electronic brochure. Patient education material that is typically tied to an agency website and may include such information as descriptions of diseases and their management, medication information, or where to get assistance with a healthcare issue.

**E-health** Healthcare initiatives and practice supported by electronic or digital media. The most typical use is for patient and family education where information is communicated electronically.

**E-learning** Electronic learning or learning that is facilitated by electronic means such as computers and the Internet. E-learning, online, and Web-based education has caused a significant shift in student–teacher relationships in nursing education.

**Email** Electronic mail. To compose, send, receive, and store messages in electronic communication systems.

**Email client** Program that manages email functions.

**E-portfolio** Personalized collections of evidence from coursework, experiences outside of the classroom, and reflective commentary related to this evidence that can be shared with others electronically; categorized electronic presentation of one's skills, education, and examples of work and/or career achievements.

**Earcons** Auditory tones that are combined to represent relationships among data elements, such as the relationship of systolic blood pressure to diastolic blood pressure.

**Educational Resources Information Center** A comprehensive educational resources database. An international database of educational literature.

**Educator** Sage, leader, and/or guide who assists in the process or practice of learning.

**Edutainment** Learning while having fun; an activity where the learner is engaged and entertained while they learn; a combination of "education" and "entertainment."

**eHealth Initiative** Initiative developed to address the growing need for managing health information and to promote technology as a means of improving health information exchange, health literacy, and healthcare delivery.

**Electronic communication** Any exchange of information that is transmitted electronically.

**Electronic data interchange (EDI)** Specific set of standards for exchanging information between or among computers (computer to computer).

**Electronic health records (EHRs)** Computer-based data warehouses or repositories of information regarding the health status of a client, which are replacing the former paper-based medical records; they are the systematic documentation of a client's health status and health care in a secured digital format, meaning that they can be processed, stored, transmitted, and accessed by authorized interdisciplinary professionals for the purpose of supporting efficient, high-quality health care across the client's healthcare continuum. Also known as electronic medical records (EMRs).

**Electronic mailing list** Automatic mailing list server such as LISTSERV that sends an e-mail addressed to the list to everyone who has subscribed to the list automatically. Similar to an electronic bulletin board or news forum.

**Electronic medical records (EMRs)** See electronic health records (EHRs).

**Electronic medication administration record (eMAR)** A system that uses bar-coding technology in order to submit and fill prescriptions. Typically, handheld scanners read bar codes and transmit them to the pharmacy.

**Electronically erasable programmable read-only memory (EEPROM)** A nonvolatile storage chip used in computers and other devices to store small amounts of volatile data (e.g., calibration tables or device configuration).

**Embedded devices** Specialized devices that contain an operating system designed to perform a dedicated function or special purpose. Smart devices can connect to the Internet, while dumb devices cannot. Embedded devices have extensive applications in the consumer, business, and healthcare marketplaces. Examples of embedded devices are banking ATMs, appliances such as dishwashers, security systems, answering machines, vehicular navigation systems, portable music players, cable TV boxes, routers, glucometers, and portable EKG machines.

**Emerging technologies** New technologies that are likely to impact health care in a significant way, such as nanotechnology or biotechnology.

**Empiricism** Knowledge that is derived from our experiences or senses.

**Empowerment** Promotion of self-actualization; achievement of power or control over one's own life.

**Enactment** The simulation stage in which a student enacts an assigned role during the established timeframe in a prepared simulation area.

**End users** Target users or consumers of software and computer technology. Software or computing applications should be designed for the end user, the person who will ultimately be using them.

**Engage** To capture the attention of the student and motivate or energize them to actively participate in the educational activity.

**Enterprise integration** Electronically linking healthcare providers, health plans, government, and other interested parties to facilitate electronic exchange and use of health information among all stakeholders.

**Entities** See covered entity.

**Entity–relationship diagram (ERD)** Diagram that specifies the relationships among the entities in the database. Sometimes the implied relationships are apparent based on the entities' definitions; however, all relationships should be specified as to how items relate to one another. There are typically three relationships: one to one, one to many, and many to many.

**Entrepreneur** Person who assumes the risks of beginning an enterprise or business and accepts responsibility for organizing and managing the organization.

**Enumerative approach** Nursing terminology in which words or phrases are represented in a list or a simple hierarchy; gives an explicit and exhaustive listing of all the objects that fall under the concept or term in question.

**Epidemiology** The field of study identifying things that come upon the people. Incidence, prevalence, and control of disease. Case finding.

**Epistemology** Study of the nature and origin of knowledge; what it means to know.

**Erasable programmable read-only memory (EPROM)** Type of computer memory chip that retains its data when its power supply is switched off and can be erased with ultraviolet light.

**Ergonomics** In the United States, this term is used to describe the physical characteristics of equipment—for example, the optimal fit of a scissors to a human hand. In Europe, it is synonymous with human factors—that is, the interaction of humans with physical attributes of equipment or the interaction of humans and the arrangement of equipment in the work environment.

**Ethical decision making** The process of making informed choices about ethical dilemmas based on a set of standards differentiating right from wrong. The decision making reflects an understanding of the principles and standards of ethical decision making, as well as philosophical approaches to ethical decision making. It requires a systematic framework for addressing the complex and often controversial moral questions.

**Ethical dilemma** A difficult choice or issue that requires the application of standards or principles to solve. Issues that challenge us ethically.

**Ethical, social, and legal implications** Consideration and understanding of the ethical, social, or legal connections or aspects of an issue that relate to a moral question of right and wrong.

**Ethicists** Experts in the arbitrary, ambiguous, and ungrounded judgments of other people. Ethicists know that they make the best decision they can based on the situation and stakeholders at hand.

**Ethics** A process of systematically examining varying viewpoints related to moral questions of right and wrong.

**Eudaemonistic** A system of ethical evaluation that involves consideration of which actions lead to being an excellent and happy person.

**Events** Occurrences that might be significant to other objects in a system or to external agents; for example, creating a laboratory request is an example of a healthcare event in a laboratory application. An event is defined and could be a triggering event for the task or workflow; a task or workflow can have several triggering events.

**Evidence** Artifacts, productions, attestations, or other examples that demonstrate an individual's knowledge, skills, or valued attributes.

**Evidence-based practice (EBP)** Nursing practice that is informed by research-generated evidence of best practices.

**Exabytes (EB)** Units of measure for computer memory equal to one quintillion bytes of computer memory.

**Executes** Carries out software's or a program's instructions.

**Exome** The part of the genome formed by exons.

**Exome sequencing** The reading of changes in the genes of the genome to identify mutations relating to a trait or illness.

**Exon** A section of a gene that is transcribed into RNA and translated into protein.

**Expert systems** Decision support systems that implement the knowledge of one or more human experts.

**Exploratory data analysis (EDA)** Approach or philosophy that uses mainly graphical techniques to gain insight into a dataset. It identifies the most important variables. Conducted during the exploratory phase, EDA provides guidance into the complexity or general nature of the various models that should be considered for implementation during pattern discovery.

**Extensibility** System design feature that allows for future expansion without the need for changes to the basic infrastructure.

**Extensible Markup Language (XML)** Computer language that began as a simplified subset of Standard Generalized Markup Language (SGML). Its major purpose is to facilitate the exchange of structured data across different information systems, especially via the Internet. XML is considered an extensible language because it permits its users to define their own elements, allowing customization to enable purpose-specific development.

**Face-to-face** Most widely used teaching method among nurse educators, where the teacher and the learners meet together in one location at the same time.

**Failure modes and effects analysis (FMEA)** A systematic evaluation of a process to determine how and why it failed to produce the desired results.

**Fair use** Doctrine that permits the limited use of original works without the copyright holder's permission; an example would be quoting or citing an author in a scholarly manuscript.

**Federal Health Information Exchange (FHIE)** A federal information technology healthcare initiative that enables the secure electronic one-way exchange of patient medical information from the Department of Defense's legacy health information system, the Composite Health Care System (CHCS), for all separated service members to the Veterans Affairs' (VA) VistA Computerized Patient Record System (CPRS). The point of care in veterans affairs.

**Feedback** Input in the form of opinions about or reactions to something such as shared knowledge. In an information system, feedback refers to information from the system that is used to make modifications in the input, processing actions, or outputs.

**Fidelity** The extent to which a simulation mimics the processes of a real environment; in the context of ethics, the right to what has been promised.

**Fields** Columns or attributes of an entity in a database.

**Field study** Study in which end users evaluate a prototype in the actual work setting prior to its general release. Also called field test, alpha test, or beta test.

**Financial systems** Systems used to manage the expenses and revenues accrued while providing health care. The finance, auditing, and accounting departments within an organization most commonly use financial systems. These systems determine the direction for maintenance and growth for a given facility. Financial systems often interface to share information with materials management, staffing, and billing systems to balance the financial impact of these resources within an organization. These systems report the fiscal outcomes so that these outcomes can be tracked against the organizational goals of an institution. Financial systems are one of the major decision-making factors as healthcare institutions prepare their fiscal budgets. They often play a pivotal role in determining the strategic direction for an organization.

**Firewall** A tool commonly used by organizations to protect their corporate networks when they are attached to the Internet. A firewall can be either hardware or software, or a combination of the two. It examines all incoming messages or traffic to the network. The firewall can be set up to allow only messages from known senders into the corporate network; it can also be set up to look at outgoing information from the corporate network.

**FireWire** Apple Computer's version of a high-performance serial bus used to connect devices to a computer.

**Firmware** Hardware and software programs or data written onto ROM, PROM, and EPROM.

**Flash drives** Small, removable storage devices.

**Flash memory** Special type of EEPROM that can be erased and reprogrammed in blocks instead of one byte at a time. Many modern PCs have their BIOS stored on a flash memory chip so that it can easily be updated if necessary.

**Folksonomies** Organization and classification of online content by users; derived from "folk" and "taxonomy." Users tag information with key words to make it easier to index and search vast amounts of information.

**Foundation of Knowledge model** Model proposing that humans are organic information systems constantly acquiring, processing, generating, and disseminating information or knowledge in both their professional and personal lives. The organizing framework of this text.

**Futurologist** Guru who is a forward thinker and looks to the future.

**Game** A structured activity undertaken for enjoyment.

**Game mechanics** The rules, instructions, directions, and constructs that the player or learner interacts with while playing the game. It is imperative that the rules are clearly stated in the instructions or directions so the player knows what is expected of them and the game itself has rules that it too must obey. The mechanics determine how the players or learners interact with the rules and how the game responds to the player's or learner's moves or behaviors within the game, thus connecting the player's or learner's actions to the purpose of the game.

**Gameplay** How the player or learner interacts with or plays the game.

**Genome** A body of genes. Hans Winkler is credited with merging "genesis" and "soma" (genome) to create this term.

**Genomic data commons (GDC)** The data-sharing platform promoting precision medicine in oncology.

**Genomics** The study of the genome.

**Gigabyte (GB)** Unit of measure used to express bytes of data storage and capability in computer systems; 1 gigabyte equals 1,000 megabytes.

**Gigahertz** Unit of measure used to express speed and power of some components such as the microprocessor; 1 gigahertz equals 1,000 megahertz.

**Good** Favorable outcome in ethics.

**Google Glass** A wearable computer from Google that can take pictures, play video, and display text messages without anyone else knowing. Currently, it costs approximately $1,500.

**Government Accountability Office (GAO)** The highest audit institution of the federal government that provides auditing, evaluation, and investigative services for the U.S. Congress.

**Gramm-Leach-Bliley Act** Federal legislation in the United States that controls how financial institutions handle the private information they collect from individuals.

**Graphical user interface (GUI)** (pronounced "gooey") Software that provides a user-friendly desktop metaphor interface that is made up of the input and output devices as well as icons that represent files, programs, actions, and processes.

**Graphics card** A board that plugs into a personal computer to give it display capabilities.

**Gray gap** A term used to reflect the age disparities in computer connectivity; there are fewer persons older than age 65 who use computer technology than members of younger age groups.

**Gulf of evaluation** The gap between knowing one's intention (goal) and knowing the effects of one's actions.

**Gulf of execution** The gap between knowing what one wants to have happen (the goal) and knowing what to do to bring it about (the means to achieve the goal).

**Hackers** Computer-savvy individuals most commonly thought of as malicious people who hack, or break, through security to steal or alter data and information; can also be any of a group of computer aficionados who band together in clubs and organizations or who use their skills as a hobby.

**Half-life of knowledge** The time span from when knowledge is gained to when it becomes obsolete.

**Handheld devices** Computers that are small enough to be used while holding in one's hand or easily carried in a pocket; synonymous with PDA (personal digital assistant).

**Haplotypes** Sets of closely linked alleles on a chromosome that tends to be inherited together.

**HapMap** Describes the common patterns of human DNA sequence variation and is expected to be a key resource for researchers to use to find genes affecting health, disease, and responses to drugs and environmental factors.

**Haptic** Sense of touch; The science of applying tactile sensation or touch to human-computer interactions allowing for users to use special input/output devices such as joysticks, data gloves, etc. to feel or sense and manipulate or control a virtual, three-dimensional object's attributes of texture, shape, surface, temperature, and/or weight.

**Hard disk** Magnetic disk that stores electronic data.

**Hard drive** Permanent data storage area that holds the data, information, documents, and programs saved on the computer, even when the computer is shut off. The actual physical body of the computer and its components.

**Hardware** Physical or tangible parts of the computer. Computer parts that one can touch and that are involved in the performance or function of the computer, such as the keyboard and monitor.

**Harm** Physical or mental injury or damage. Unfavorable outcome in ethics.

**Health disparities** The health status differences between different groups of people, especially minorities and nonminorities; the gaps between the health status of minorities and nonminorities in the United States are ongoing even with the advances in technology and healthcare practices.

**Health information exchange (HIE)** Organization that prepares and organizes people and resources to manage healthcare information electronically across organizations within a community or region.

**Health Information Portability and Accountability Act (HIPAA)** Law signed by President Bill Clinton in 1996 addressing the need for standards to regulate and safeguard health information and making provisions for health insurance coverage for employed persons who change jobs.

**Health information technology (HIT)** Hardware, software, integrated technologies or related licenses, intellectual property, upgrades, or packaged solutions sold as services that are designed for or support the use by healthcare entities or patients for the electronic creation, maintenance, access, or exchange of health information.

**Health Information Technology for Economic and Clinical Health (HITECH) Act** Title XIII of the American Recovery and Reinvestment Act, which was enacted in February 2009. Under this act, healthcare organizations can qualify for financial incentives based on the level of meaningful use achieved; the HITECH Act specifically incentivizes health organizations and providers to become "meaningful users."

**Health Level 7** An accredited standards-developing organization that is committed to developing standard terminologies for information technology that support interoperability of healthcare information management systems.

**Health literacy** The acquisition of knowledge that promotes the ability to understand and to manage one's health.

**Health management information system (HMIS)** An information system that is specially intended to support and help with the planning, resource allocation, and management of health programming to make healthcare more effective and efficient; an information system that plans and manages health programs, rather than the actual delivery of health care.

**Healthcare-associated infections** Infections that patients acquire while being treated in a healthcare facility.

**Healthcare information** Information that is related to health and well-being of a person, especially information related to therapeutic (care) interactions between people and healthcare providers.

**Healthcare provider** A qualified person delivering appropriate health care professionally to an individual, group, family, community, or population in need of healthcare services; includes hospitals, skilled nursing facilities, nursing homes, long-term care facilities, home health agencies, hemodialysis centers, clinics, community mental health centers, ambulatory surgery centers, group practices, pharmacies and pharmacists, laboratories, physicians, and therapists.

**HealthVault** Microsoft's online personal health record system.

**Heuristic evaluation** An evaluation in which a small number of evaluators (often experts in relevant fields such as human factors or cognitive engineering) evaluate the degree to which an interface design complies with recognized usability principles (the "heuristics").

**High-definition multimedia interface (HDMI)** An adapter that has expanded connectivity and transfer. HDMI is replacing analog video standards as an audio/video interface that can transfer compressed and uncompressed video and digital audio data from any device that is HDMI compliant to compatible monitors, televisions, video projectors, and audio devices.

**High-fidelity** A high level of realism generated by the equipment used in simulations.

**High-hazard drugs** Drugs known to cause significant adverse side effects when administered inappropriately; drugs subject to frequent administration errors.

**Home health agency (HHA)** Organization that delivers part-time and intermittent skilled services, including nursing and other therapeutic services, in the patient's home.

**Home health care** An alternative site for healthcare services typically focusing on post–hospital discharge patient needs.

**Home telehealth care** Home healthcare clinical and educational services provided via telecommunications-ready tools.

**HONcode** One of the two most common symbols that power users look for to identify trusted health sites.

**Hospital information system (HIS)** An information system intended to manage the clinical, financial, and administrative needs of the hospital; refers to the paper-based as well as computer-based information processing that manages the functional aspects (administrative, financial, and clinical) of a hospital.

**Human factors engineering** Recognizing the limitations of human performance and developing products to overcome these limitations.

**Human Genome Project (HGP)** A 13-year project designed to identify all of the 20,000–25,000 genes in human DNA; determine the sequences of 3 billion chemical base pairs in human DNA; create databases to store this information; and address the resultant ethical, legal, and social issues.

**Human Mental Work Load (HMWL)** Mental processing or cognitive demands placed on a person when he or she is interacting with technology.

**Human–computer interactions** How people use and interact with computers; the study of how people use computers and software applications and the ways that computers influence people.

**Human–computer interface** The hardware and software through which the user interacts with the computer.

**Human–technology interaction (HTI)** How users interact with technology. The study of that interaction.

**Human–technology interface** The hardware and software through which the user interacts with any technology (e.g., computers, patient monitors, telephone).

**Hybrid** A descriptor for individual courses in which instruction is delivered using multiple formats such as online, face to face, print based, or audio or videoconference (e.g., PicTel).

**Hypertext** Clickable words that allow users to access another document at a remote location.

**Indiana Health Information Exchange** A collaborative effort among institutions in Indiana to provide high-quality patient care and enhance the safety and efficiency of health care.

**Industrial Age** Late 18th and early 19th centuries, when major changes occurred in manufacturing, farming, and transportation; inventions and innovations led these changes.

**Informaticists** People with specialized training or certification in informatics; specialists in using technology to manage health data and information.

**Informatics** A field that integrates a specialty's science, computer science, cognitive science, and information science to manage and communicate data, information, knowledge, and wisdom in a specialty's practice.

**Informatics innovator** One who makes enhancements or improvements and creative, novel, and inventive solutions in the informatics specialty.

**Informatics nurse** A nurse with specialized skills, knowledge, and competencies in informatics. A registered nurse with an interest or experience working in an informatics field. A generalist in the field of informatics in nursing.

**Informatics nurse specialist** A registered nurse with formal, graduate education in the field of informatics or a related field, who is considered a specialist in the field of nursing informatics.

**Informatics solution** A generic term used to describe the product that an informatics nurse specialist recommends after identifying and analyzing an issue. Informatics solutions may encompass technology and nontechnology products such as information systems, new applications, nursing vocabulary, or informatics curricula.

**Information** Data that are interpreted, organized, or structured. Data processed using knowledge or data made functional through the application of knowledge.

**Information Age** Period at the end of the 20th century, when information was easily accessible using computers, networks, and the Internet.

**Information literacy** Recognizing when information is needed and having the ability to locate, evaluate, and effectively use the needed information. An intellectual framework for finding, understanding, evaluating, and using information.

**Information mediator** A new nursing role arising out of the need for technology to support immediate access to up-to-date knowledge anywhere and anytime.

**Information science** The science of information, studying the application and usage of information and knowledge in organizations and the interfacings or interaction between people, organizations, and information systems. An extensive, interdisciplinary science that integrates features from cognitive science, communication science, computer science, library science, and social sciences.

**Information systems** The manual and/or automated components of system of users or people, recorded data, and actions used to process the data into information for a user, group of users, or an organization.

**Information technology (IT)** Use of hardware, software, services, and supporting infrastructure to manage and deliver information using voice, data, and video, or the use of technologies from computing, electronics, and telecommunications to process and distribute information in digital and other forms. Anything related to computing technology, such as networking, hardware, software, the Internet, or the people who work with these technologies. Many hospitals have IT departments for managing the computers, networks, and other technical areas of the healthcare industry.

**Information user** The person who accesses and makes use of information made available to her/him.

**Informatique** French term referring to the computer milieu.

**Infrastructure** Structural elements that provide the framework supporting a system. In the case of information technology, infrastructure refers to the architecture of the computer system, its operating system, and various other systems that are fundamental to its operation.

**Infrastructure as a service (IaaS)** Cloud-based services that provide a rentable backbone to companies enabling the scalable, on-demand infrastructure they need to support their dynamic workloads; the user pays what they use and they do not have to invest in hardware, including networks, storage, and data center space.

**Input** Data and information entered into a computer system.

**Input devices** Hardware and software used to enter data and information into a computer.

**Input/output system (I/O)** (Pronounced "eye-oh.") Any program, operation, or device that transfers data to or from a computer and to or from a peripheral device.

**Instant message (IM)** Form of real-time communication between two or more people based on typed text conveyed via computers connected over a network.

**Integrated drive electronics (IDE)** Technology where the drive controller is located on the drive itself instead of being a separate controller connected to the motherboard of a computer.

**Integration** Assimilating or combining to make whole; in computer terminology, the process through which different technologies—software and hardware components—are synchronized and combined to make a functional and structural system.

**Integrity** Quality and accuracy. Employees need to have confidence that the information they are provided is, in fact, true. To accomplish this, organizations need clear policies to clarify how data are actually input, to determine who has the authorization to change such data, and to track how and when data are changed.

**Intelligence** Mental ability to think logically, reason, prepare, ideate, assess alternative solutions to problems, problem solve by choosing a proposed solution, think abstractly, comprehend and grasp ideas, understand and use language, and learn.

**Interactions** Interfacing with users commonly using tasks or notifications.

**Interactive technologies** Technologies that promote or support user communication with other persons (e.g., e-mail) or technologies that depend on a user response (e.g., games).

**Interdisciplinary knowledge team** A team composed of members of various disciplines in a healthcare organization, each of whom contributes unique knowledge to the team in problem-solving or management situations.

**Interfaces** Mechanisms or systems used by separate things to interact. For example, if one wants to change a CD in a CD player, one could use a remote; the human user is not related to the CD player but can interact with it using the remote control. Therefore, the remote control becomes the interface that enables that person to tell the CD player which CD to play.

**International Organization for Standardization (ISO)** An international network supporting collaboration among the standards-developing agencies of numerous countries for the development of consistent standards in a multitude of industries to support a global economy. ISO is best known in the technology industries for the ISO 9000 standards. *See* International Standards Organization.

**International Standards Organization** A nongovernmental group that connects and bridges the public and private sectors to develop and publish international standards that assimilate the latest expert knowledge, with the goal being to provide practical tools for tracking economic, environmental, and societal challenges. Also known as International Organization for Standardization.

**Internet** A global system of computer networks whose connectivity promotes worldwide communications via computers.

**Internet2** A nonprofit consortium that develops and deploys advanced network applications and technologies, for education and high-speed data transfer purposes. Led by 212 universities, it is also known as University Corporation for Advanced Internet Development.

**Internet browser** Software used to locate and display webpages. Also known as web browser or browser.

**Internet of Things (IoT)** Electronic devices that connect with each other to provide real-time data and interpretation of data without human intervention

**Interoperability** Ability of various systems and organizations to work together to exchange information.

**Intranet** A computer network that is contained within an enterprise and that has restricted access; it has the look and feel of the Internet and often provides links to the Internet. The purpose of an intranet varies but can include provision of employee and departmental directories, policies and procedures, internal and external resources, schedules, and updates on programs and business. The benefits are browsing capabilities and the ability to maintain contact information and phone numbers in a central location, with easy dissemination.

**Introns** The sections of a gene that are transcribed but are removed before being translated into protein.

**Intrusion detection devices** Both hardware and software that allow an organization to monitor who is using its network and which files that user has accessed.

**Intrusion detection system** Method of security that uses both hardware and software detection devices as a system that can be set up to monitor a single computer or an entire network. Corporations must diligently monitor for unauthorized access of their networks.

**Intuition** A way of acquiring knowledge that cannot be obtained by inference, deduction, observation, reason, analysis, or experience.

**Iowa model** A model that facilitates the translation of research evidence into clinical practice. Also known as the Iowa model of evidence-based practice.

**iPod** The name given to a family of portable MP3 players from Apple Computer.

**IPS LCD (in-plane switching liquid crystal display)** Smartphone display using polarized light passing through a color filter and all of the pixels are backlit. The liquid crystals control the brightness and which pixels are on or off. With the active matrix, you have crisp, vivid colors and darker blacks.

**Iteration** Replication and refinement of a method until it meets a goal or provides the desired result; each repetition is referred to as an iteration.

**Jump drives** Small, removable storage devices.

**Just culture** An atmosphere of trust. In a just culture, everyone understands what is acceptable and unacceptable behavior and they are urged and rewarded for supplying vital safety-related information.

**Justice** Fairness. Treatment of everyone in the same way.

**Key field** Within each database record, one of the fields identified as the primary key. It contains a code, name, number, or other bit of information that acts as a unique identifier for that record. In a healthcare system, for example, a patient is assigned a patient number or ID that is unique for that patient.

**Keyboard** Set of keys resembling an actual typewriter that permits the user to input data into a computer.

**Know–do gap** Situation that exists because solutions to global health problems are available but are not implemented in a timely fashion because of the lack of access to important health information. The Internet connections in developing countries are widely scattered, for example, and may not be efficient or sufficient for viewing healthcare information.

**Knowledge** The awareness and understanding of a set of information and ways that information can be made useful to support a specific task or arrive at a decision; abounds with others' thoughts and information. Information that is synthesized so that relationships are identified and formalized. Understanding that comes through a process of interaction or experience with the world around us. Information that has judgment applied to it or meaning extracted from it. Processed information that helps to clarify or explain some portion of our environment or world that we can use as a basis for action or upon which we can act. Internal process of thinking or cognition. External process of testing, senses, observation, and interacting.

**Knowledge acquisition** The act of getting knowledge.

**Knowledge brokers** People who know where to find information and knowledge. They generate some knowledge but are mainly known for their ability to find what is needed. More experienced nurses and nursing students become knowledge brokers out of necessity—needing to know.

**Knowledge builder** Person who examines, interprets, and compares clinical data and trends with an eye toward improving clinical practice based on the available evidence.

**Knowledge-centric** Knowledge is the central focus.

**Knowledge consumers** Users of knowledge who do not have the expertise to provide the knowledge they need for themselves.

**Knowledge dissemination** Distribution and sharing of knowledge.

**Knowledge domain process (KDP) model** Model that represents knowledge construction and dissemination in an organization.

**Knowledge exchange** The product of collaboration when sharing an understanding of information promotes learning to make better decisions in the future.

**Knowledge generation** The creation of new knowledge by changing and evolving knowledge based on one's experience, education, and input from others.

**Knowledge generators** Nursing researchers and nursing experts—the people who know; they are able to answer questions, craft theories, find solutions to nursing problems or concerns, and innovate practice.

**Knowledge management systems (KMSs)** Repositories of information that contain the latest collective expertise based on experience and research. The knowledge is typically stored in a computerized system that promotes easy access for use.

**Knowledge processing** The activity or process of gathering or collecting, perceiving, analyzing, synthesizing, saving or storing, manipulating, conveying, and transmitting knowledge.

**Knowledge repositories** Collections of information made available to an organization's workers to support and inform their work.

**Knowledge user** Individual or group who benefits from valuable, viable knowledge.

**Knowledge workers** Those who work with information and generate information and knowledge as a product.

**Lab-on-a-chip device** A nanotechnology device designed to perform blood analyses.

**Laboratory information systems** Systems that report on blood, body fluid, and tissue samples along with biological specimens that are collected at the bedside and received in a central laboratory. These systems provide clinicians with reference ranges for tests indicating high, low, or normal values so that they can make care decisions. Often the laboratory system provides result information directing clinicians toward the next course of action within a treatment regimen.

**Laptop** Portable battery-powered computer that the user can take with him or her. Also known as a notebook.

**Latex-based simulation** Simulation using manikins and/or other training devices made of latex.

**Legacy system** Old computer systems or programs that are not replaced because the institution does not want to expend the resources; they can cause problems, especially in interfacing with newer systems.

**Liberty** The independence from controlling influences.

**Library science** An interdisciplinary science that integrates law, applied science, and the humanities to study issues and topics related to libraries (collection, organization, preservation, archiving, and dissemination of information resources).

**Local area network (LAN)** Organizationally based network; joined together locally.

**Logic** A system of thinking that uses principles of inference and reasoned ideas to govern action.

**Logical Observation Identifiers Names and Codes (LOINC)** A database, universal standards, structured names, and coding system for identifying medical laboratory tests, measurements, and observations. Created and maintained by the Regenstrief Institute, a U.S. nonprofit medical research organization.

**Long-term care facility** A healthcare institution designed to support the needs of those who need ongoing care, especially the aged.

**Longevity** Usability beyond the immediate clinical encounter. Long-term value.

**Machine learning** A subset of artificial intelligence that permits computers to learn either inductively or deductively. Inductive machine learning is the process of reasoning and making generalizations or extracting patterns and rules from huge datasets—that is, reasoning from a large number of examples to a general rule. Deductive machine learning moves from premises that are assumed true to conclusions that must be true if the premises are true.

**Main memory** A computer's internal memory.

**Mainframes** Extremely high-performance computers that are smaller than a supercomputer, used for high-volume, processor-intensive computing. Computers used by some large businesses and/or for scientific processing purposes.

**Malicious code** Software that includes spyware, viruses, worms, and Trojan horses.

**Malicious insiders** Insiders or employees who sabotage or add malicious code or hacks into systems to cause damage or to steal data and information.

**Malware** Malicious software; an evil, malicious program that infects a device and is intended to steal information, take control of, irritate, damage, or destroy data, information, or the device.

**Managed care information systems** Information systems that cross organizational boundaries so that data can be obtained at any and all of the patient areas; these information systems make it possible for nurses and physicians to make clinical decisions while being mindful of their financial ramifications.

**Mapping** How environmental facts (e.g., the order of light switches or variables in a physiologic monitoring display) are accurately depicted by the information presentation.

**Mask** Method that a proxy server uses to protect the identity of a corporation's employees while they are surfing the World Wide Web. The proxy server keeps track of which employees are using which masks and directs the traffic appropriately.

**Massachusetts Health Data Consortium** A consortium of regional healthcare organizations that collects data, publishes comparative information, supports and promotes electronic standards, educates, and researches.

**Massive multiplayer online role-playing games** Games using the Internet to provide a shared, simultaneous experience for dozens or even hundreds of players.

**Master patient index** A tool that identifies, compares, removes duplicate entries, combines, and cleans patient records so that they can be added to a master index; it provides a comprehensive and single view of a patient via that person's record while establishing a master index of all patients.

**Meaningful use** The American Recovery and Reinvestment Act of 2009 specifies three main components of meaningful use: (1) the use of a certified electronic health record (EHR) in a meaningful manner, such as e-prescribing; (2) the use of certified EHR technology for electronic exchange of health information to improve quality of health care; and (3) the use of certified EHR technology to submit clinical quality and other measures. The criteria for meaningful use will be staged in three steps. Stage 1 (2011–2012) set the baseline for electronic data capture and information sharing. Stage 2 (2013) and Stage 3 (expected to be implemented in 2015) continue to expand on this baseline and be developed through future rule making.

**Medicaid management information system (MMIS)** An integrated group of procedures and computer processing operations (subsystems) developed at the general design level to meet Medicaid's principal objectives of control and administrative costs; service to recipients, providers, and inquiries; operations of claims control and computer capabilities; and management reporting for planning and control.

**Medical home/health information exchange** An information technology platform that enables the seamless exchange of important patient information among many providers in a healthcare system. Typically the primary care physician (medical home) initiates the collection of patient data, coordinates the care of the patient, and helps to maintain the accuracy of such data. Other care providers access the information and add to it as they provide services to patients.

**Medical informatics** A specialty that integrates medical science, computer science, cognitive science, and information science to manage and communicate data, information, knowledge, and wisdom in medical practice.

**Medicare Access and Summary CHIP Reauthorization Act of 2015 (MACRA)** An act that reformed Medicare payment by making changes that created a quality payment program (QPP) to replace the hodgepodge system of Medicare reporting programs.

**Medication management devices** Range of telecommunications-ready medication devices to remind or otherwise alert patients to medication compliance needs.

**MEDLINE** A database that contains more than 22 million records, maintained and produced by the National Library of Medicine.

**Megabyte (MB)** Unit of measure used to express the amount of data storage and capability in computer systems; 1 megabyte equals 1,000 kilobytes.

**Megahertz** Unit of measure used to express the speed and power of some components such as the microprocessor.

**Memory** Data stored in digital format; generally refers to random-access memory (RAM).

**Merit-Based Incentive Payment System (MIPS)** The Reauthorization Act of 2015 (MACRA) reformed Medicare payments by making changes that created a quality payment program (QPP) to replace the hodgepodge system of Medicare reporting programs. The MACRA QPP has two paths—Merit-based Payment System (MIPS) or Alternative Payment Models (APMs)—that will be in effect through 2021 and beyond. As a consolidation and refinement of various incentive programs, MIPS is an important program, but it neither aspires to nor will drive change in the value of health care at anywhere near the levels of change that the retirement of the baby boomer generation will force upon Medicare and society.

**Meta-analysis** A form of systematic review that uses statistical methods to combine the results of several research studies.

**Meta-learning** Learning that combines the predictions from several data mining models with the goal of synthesizing these predicted classifications to generate a final best predicted classification; also known as stacking.

**Metadata** Data about data; in data mining, data contained in the data mining model that describes other data. For example, metadata would describe the patterns, trends, and relationships of the mined data.

**Metrics** Measurements or a set of measurements to quantify performance; they provide understanding about the performance of a process or function. Typically, within clinical technology projects, one identifies and collects specific metrics about the performance of the technology or metrics that capture the level of participation or adoption. Equally important is the need for process performance metrics. Process metrics are collected at the initial stage of a project or problem identification. Current-state metrics are then benchmarked against internal indicators. When there are no internal indicators to benchmark against, a suitable course of action is to benchmark against an external source, such as a similar business practice within a different industry.

**Microprocessor** Chip that integrates the processor onto one circuit, incorporating the functions of the computer's central processing unit or processor. Microprocessors continue to evolve in terms of their processing capacity.

**Microsoft Surface** Windows-based tablet computers featuring touch screens and interactive whiteboards.

**Milestones** Predetermined planned occurrences that indicate the completion or achievement of a deliverable.

**Millions of instructions per second (MIPS)** The number of machine instructions that a computer can execute in one second; in this case, millions per second.

**Mind** The brain's conscious processing; encompasses thought processes, memory, imagination and creativity, emotions, perceptions, and inner drive or will.

**Mobile devices** Handheld computers, such as smartphones or tablets.

**Mobile e-health (mobile health, m-health)** Health-related uses of mobile technologies including mobile phones (and increasingly, Internet-enabled, wireless-connected smartphones), personal digital assistants, tablet computers and subnotebook microcomputers, remote diagnostic and monitoring devices, and global positioning system (GPS)/geographic information system mapping equipment.

**Model of terminology use** A domain content model that is optimized for the management of particular entities within an informational and/or operational context.

**Modem** Hardware that allows a user to send and receive information over the phone or cable lines, for example, with a computer. It enables Internet connectivity via a telephone line or cable connection through network adaptors situated within the computer apparatus.

**Monitor** Computer display that allows the user to view text and graphic images.

**Moral dilemmas** Situations for which there is no clear evidence that one of several alternatives is morally right or wrong.

**Moral rights** Ethical privileges.

**Morals** Social conventions about right and wrong human conduct that are socially constructed and tacitly agreed upon as good or right.

**MoSCoW** Must have, Should have, Could have, and Would have; an approach where a team works with stakeholders to develop a prioritized requirements list and a development plan.

**Motherboard** A key foundational computer component. All other components are connected to it in some way (either via local sockets, attached directly to it, or connected via cables). The essential structures of the motherboard include the major chipset, super I/O chip, BIOS, read-only memory, bus communications pathways, and a variety of sockets that allow components to plug into it.

**Mouse** A small device that one can roll along or scroll to control the movement of the pointer or cursor on a display and click to search for and/or execute features.

**MP3 aggregator** A program that can facilitate the process of finding, subscribing to, and downloading podcasts. A commonly known aggregator is Apple Computer's iTunes, which is a free program available as a download from apple.com. Using a program such as iTunes gives the user the ability to search for podcasts based on many criteria, including category, author, or title. iTunes provides access to audio downloads, which may be either songs or podcasts.

**MPEG-1 Audio Layer-3 (MP3)** Digital or electronic audio programming format.

**Multidimensional databases** Databases that combine data from numerous data sources and are optimized for online analytical processing applications; they use multidimensional structures to organize the data, and each data attribute is considered as a separate dimension.

**Multimedia** A computer-based technology that incorporates traditional forms of communication to create a seamless and interactive learning environment.

**Multispatial** Relating to the need for educators in the age of technology to account for both physical and virtual spaces and their relationship to the learning process.

**Multiuser dungeon** A computer program, usually running over the Internet, that allows multiple users to participate in virtual-reality role-playing games.

**Multiuser shared hack, habitat, holodeck, or hallucination (MUSH)** A computer program that allows the user to extend a virtual-reality "world" by adding new rooms, objects, and features.

**NANDA International, Inc. (NANDA-I)** A standardized nursing terminology consisting of a taxonomy of nursing diagnoses.

**Nanotechnology** Microscopic technology on the order of one billionth of a meter.

**National Center for Public Health Informatics (NCPHI)** Center created in 2005 by the Centers for Disease Control and Prevention to provide leadership in the field of public health informatics.

**National Guideline Clearinghouse (NGC)** A comprehensive database of clinical practice guidelines developed as a result of research. The NGC website allows users to browse for clinical guidelines, view abstracts and full-text links, download full-text clinical guidelines to personal digital assistive devices, obtain technical reports, and compare guidelines.

**National Health and Nutrition Examination Survey (NHANES)** A survey sponsored by the Centers for Disease Control and Prevention that combines both questionnaires and physical examinations to collect data on the health and nutritional status of adults and children in the United States.

**National Health Information Infrastructure** An initiative intended to improve the effectiveness, efficiency, and overall quality of health and health care in the United States. A comprehensive knowledge-based network of interoperable systems of clinical, public health, and personal health information that would improve decision making by making health information available when and where it is needed. The set of technologies, standards, applications, systems, values, and laws that support all facets of individual health, health care, and public health. The NHII is voluntary and not a centralized database of medical records or a government regulation.

**Nationwide Health Information Network (NHIN)** An agency of the U.S. Department of Health and Human Services charged with the development of a safe, secure, interoperable health information infrastructure.

**National Healthcare Quality Report (NHQR)** A report that explores the quality of health care in the United States; it has been issued by the Agency for Healthcare Research and Quality every year since 2003.

**National Institute of Standards and Technology** A nonregulatory federal agency within the U.S. Department of Commerce that was founded in 1901; its mission is to promote U.S. innovation and industrial competitiveness by advancing measurement science, standards, and technology in ways that enhance economic security and improve the quality of life. From automated teller machines and atomic clocks to mammograms and semiconductors, innumerable products and services rely in some way on technology, measurement, and standards provided by NIST.

**National provider identifier (NPI)** A standard 10-position unique identifier (code) mandated by HIPAA legislation and designed to replace previous provider identifiers.

**Negligence** A departure from the standard of due care—prudent, reasonable care—toward others, including intentionally posing risks that are unreasonable as well as unintentionally, but carelessly, imposing risks.

**Negligent insider** A well-meaning, but careless employee who unintentionally exposes a network to security vulnerabilities by ignoring or forgetting about proper security procedures

**Net generation** Students used to surfing the Web and interacting online.

**Networks** Connections of computers that can be local and/or organizationally based, joined together into a local area network, on a wider area scope (such as a city or district) using a metropolitan area network, or from an even greater distance (e.g., a whole country or continent or the Internet in general) using a wide area network configuration.

**Network accessibility** The ability of the network to be accessed by the right user to obtain what that person needs when he or she needs it.

**Network availability** The state in which network information is accessible when needed.

**Network security** The specific precautions taken to ensure that the integrity of a network is safe from unauthorized entry and that the data and information stored on the network are accessible only by authorized users.

**Neural network** A nonlinear predictive model. Such models learn by training and resembling the structure of biological neural networks. Neural networks model the neural behavior of the human brain and are a way to bridge the gap between computers and humans.

**Neuroscience** The study of the nervous system.

**Never events** Events that should never occur, such as wrong-site surgeries and retained surgical objects. While rare, over 4,000 patients per year have the wrong site operated on or have retained surgical objects.

**New England Health EDI Network** An example of an implementation model for building regional health information organizations that are functional, sustainable, and growing while reducing administrative costs.

**Next-Generation Internet** A government project to develop new, faster technologies to enhance research and communication.

**Nicomachean** An approach to ethical thinking based on the work of Aristotle.

**Nonmaleficence** Doing no harm.

**Nonplayer character (NPC)** An individual in a simulation, virtual world, or game that is controlled by the program, not another person.

**Nonsynchronous** That which is not in real time or does not occur or exist at the same time, having the same period or time frame. Occurring anywhere and anytime using Internet and World Wide Web software tools (e.g., course management systems, e-mail, electronic bulletin boards, webpages) as the principal delivery mechanisms.

**Nursing informatics (NI)** Traditional definition: A specialty that integrates nursing science, computer science, and information science to manage and communicate data, information, knowledge, and wisdom in nursing practice. Our definition: The synthesis of nursing science, information science, computer science, and cognitive science for the purpose of managing, disseminating, and enhancing healthcare data, information, knowledge, and wisdom to improve collaboration and decision making; provide high quality patient care; and advance the profession of nursing. NI is the specialty that integrates nursing science with multiple information management and analytical sciences to identify, define, manage, and communicate data, information, knowledge, and wisdom in nursing practice. NI supports nurses, consumers, patients, the interprofessional healthcare team, and other stakeholders in their decision making in all roles and settings to achieve desired outcomes. This support is accomplished through the use of information structures, information processes, and information technology.

**Nursing informatics competencies** A set of essential skills related to informatics deemed appropriate for various levels of nursing practice.

**Nursing interventions classifications (NIC)** A comprehensive, standardized classification of interventions that nurses perform. It is research-based and useful for clinical documentation and communicating care provided across settings and integrating data across systems and various practice settings. These classifications aid in conducting effectiveness research, measuring productivity, and evaluating competencies. The NIC is also used for reimbursement as well as aiding in designing curriculums.

**Nursing knowledge** A body of facts accumulated over time from experience, education, and research that are used to make nursing decisions.

**Nursing outcomes classifications (NOC)** A comprehensive, standardized classification of measurable patient outcomes that was developed for use in all settings and with all patient populations. Standardized outcomes are used in information systems and electronic health records and are critical to the advancement of nursing knowledge and the practice of nursing education.

**Nursing science** The ethical application of knowledge acquired through education, research, and practice to provide services and interventions to patients so as to maintain, enhance, or restore their health; to advocate for health; and to acquire, process, generate, and disseminate nursing knowledge to advance the nursing profession.

**Nursing terminology** Body of the terms used in nursing.

**Nursing theory** Concepts, propositions, and definitions that represent a methodical viewpoint and provide a framework for organizing and standardizing nursing actions.

**Object-oriented multiuser dungeon** Similar to a multiuser dungeon—a computer program, usually running over the Internet, that allows multiple users to participate in virtual-reality role-playing games—but with more advanced programming features.

**Office of Civil Rights** Part of the U.S. Department of Health and Human Services and responsible for enforcing the Health Insurance Portability and Accountability Act. It provides significant information and guidance to clinicians who must comply with the Privacy and Security Rules. It has been tracking complaints and investigating violations since 2003.

**Office of the National Coordinator (ONC) for Health Information Technology** An office within the U.S. Department of Health and Human Services that was established through the HITECH Act. The ONC is headed by the national coordinator, who is responsible for overseeing the development of a nationwide health information technology infrastructure that supports the use and exchange of information.

**Office suite** Software that is generally distributed together with a consistent user interface that is designed for knowledge workers and clerical personnel. These software packages can interact with each other to enhance productivity and ease of use.

**Online** Something accomplished while connected to or using a computer.

**Online analytic processing (OLAP)** A fast analysis of shared data stored in a multidimensional database that allows the user to easily and selectively extract and view data from different points of view. OLAP and data mining complement each other even though they are quite different.

**Online chats** Synchronous interactions with another person facilitated by an Internet connection technology.

**Ontological approach** Theory that considers ontology development (domain analysis) and its mapping to object models (specification of infrastructure). Based on enumerating all concepts used in a domain and in providing their formal definitions according to suitable formalisms (usually logic based).

**Ontology** Study of that which is compositional in nature and a partial representation of the entities within a domain and the relationships that hold between them. An explicit specification of a conceptualization.

**Open Access Initiative** A worldwide movement to make a library of knowledge available to anyone with Internet access.

**Open source** Computer software where the source code is made available for use and/or modification without charge. The developers share code in the hopes that the software will evolve as others modify and improve upon the base.

**Open source software** Software that enables users to freely copy and reuse or repurpose the software by providing access to the source code; free and open use of software source code.

**Open Systems Interconnection (OSI)** A model of standardization for communications in a network developed to ensure that various programs would work efficiently with one another.

**Operating system (OS)** The most important software on any computer. It is the very first program to load on computer start-up and is fundamental for the operation of all other software as well as the computer's hardware.

**Order entry management** A program that allows a clinician to enter medication and other care orders directly into a computer, including orders for laboratory, microbiology, pathology, radiology, nursing, and medicine; supply orders; ancillary services; and consults.

**Order entry systems** Systems that automate the way that orders are initiated for patients. Clinicians place orders within these systems instead of using traditional handwritten transcription onto paper. Such systems provide major safeguards by ensuring that physician orders are legible and complete, thereby providing a level of patient safety that was historically missing with paper-based orders. They also provide decision support and automated alert functionality that was previously unavailable with paper-based orders.

**Outcome** Changes, results, and/or impacts from inputting and processing.

**Output** Changes that exit a system and that can activate or modify processing.

**Palm computers** Miniature or small computers that fit in the palm of the hand.

**Parallel port** Interface for connecting an external device that is capable of receiving more than one bit at a time.

**Password** A code established by the user to identify himself or herself when the user enters the system. Most organizations today enforce a strong password policy. Strong password policies include using combinations of letters, numbers, and special characters such as plus (+) signs and ampersands (&). Policies typically include the enforcement of changing passwords every 30 or 60 days.

**Patient care information system (PCIS)** Patient-centered information systems focused on collecting data and disseminating information related to direct care. Several of these systems have become mainstream types of systems used in health care. The four types of systems most commonly found in healthcare organizations include (1) clinical documentation systems, (2) pharmacy information systems, (3) laboratory information systems, and (4) radiology information systems.

**Patient care support system** System of components that make up each of the specialty disciplines within health care and their associated patient care information systems. The four types of systems most commonly found in healthcare organizations include (1) clinical documentation systems, (2) pharmacy information systems, (3) laboratory information systems, and (4) radiology information systems.

**Patient-centered** Focused on the patient/person (rather than on the illness/healthcare professional), with patients becoming active participants in their own healthcare initiatives. Patients as active participants receive services designed to meet their individual needs and preferences, under the guidance and counsel of their healthcare professionals. Data, observations, interventions, and outcomes focused on direct patient care.

**Patient-centered care** Care that is responsive to and cognizant of patient preferences, values, and needs.

**Patient informed consent** A document that a patient signs to agree to treatment. A document that a home healthcare patient signs to agree to receive telehealthcare services in addition to conventional home health care.

**Patient outcomes** Measurable effects resulting from best practice treatment interventions that improve or stabilize the course of health over time.

**Patient support** The total array of tools and software that can be used to provide information and assistance to help meet the healthcare needs of consumers.

**Payer organization** An organization that contracts with healthcare agencies and service providers to attempt to manage healthcare costs.

**PEDA** Pre-brief, enactment, debrief, and assessment: the four major components of simulations; see individual term definitions.

**Perception** The process of acquiring knowledge about the environment or situation by obtaining, interpreting, selecting, and organizing sensory information from seeing, hearing, touching, tasting, and smelling. Sensory experience foundational to formulating knowledge.

**Performance improvement** Enhancement of performance. A quality indicator.

**Performance improvement analyst** Person who analyzes performance improvement initiatives. Person who is intimately involved in the design of the system used by nursing.

**Peripheral biometric (medical) devices** A variety of telecommunications-ready measurement devices, such as blood pressure cuffs and blood glucose meters, that typically use the household telephone jack to transmit patient data to a central server location.

**Peripheral component interconnection (PCI)** Mechanism for attaching peripheral devices to a motherboard via computer bus, expansion slots, or integrated circuits.

**Peripheral devices** Devices with a digital readout typically used in home telehealth and whose output is capable of being captured by computer. Generally this equipment is self-administered by the patient or family caregiver. Examples of commonly used peripheral devices include a weight scale, blood pressure monitor, pulse oximeter, thermometer, glucometer, spirometer, prothrombin/International Normalized Ratio meter, digital camera (to capture images of wounds), and a personal digital assistant–based or telephonic self-reporting device.

**Personal computer (PC)** Computer made for individual use or directly used by an end user.

**Personal digital assistant (PDA)** A handheld device, miniature or small computer, or palmtop that uses a pen for inputting data instead of a keyboard. Also called a hand-held computer. Also known as personal digital assistive.

**Personal emergency response systems** Signaling devices that enable patients to access emergency and other care needs.

**Petabytes (PB)** Units of information or computer storage equal to 1 quadrillion bytes, or 1,000 terabytes.

**Pharmacy information systems** Information systems that facilitate the ordering, managing, and dispensing of medications for a facility. They also commonly incorporate allergy and height/weight information for effective medication management; they streamline the order entry, dispensing, verification, and authorization process for medication administration while often interfacing with clinical documentation and order entry systems so that clinicians can order and document the administration of medications and prescriptions to patients while having the benefits of decision support alerting and interaction checking.

**Phishing** An attempt to steal information by manipulating the recipient of an e-mail or phone call to provide passwords or other private information.

**Picture archiving and communication system (PACS)** System that is designed to collect, store, and distribute medical images such as computed tomography (CT) scans, magnetic resonance images, and X-rays; it replaces traditional hard copy films with digital media that are easy to store, retrieve, and present to clinicians. This system may be a stand-alone system, separate from the main radiology system, or it can be integrated with a radiology information system and a computer information system. The benefit of PACSs is their ability to assist in diagnosis and to store vital patient care support data.

**Platform as a service (PaaS)** Cloud computing service that provides everything needed to support the cloud application's building and delivering lifecycle, enabling users to develop and launch custom Web applications rapidly to the cloud.

**Plug and play** The ability to add new devices to a computer easily without having to manually install and reconfigure the computer to accept the device.

**Podcast** A digital media file or collection of related files that are distributed over the Internet using syndication or subscription feeds for playback on portable media players such as MP3 players, laptops, and personal computers; the subscription relies on RSS feeds. Online media delivery. Enhanced podcasts contain slides and pictures; vodcasts contain videos.

**Policies** Basic principles that guide behavior and performance and are enforced. For example, in a corporation, corporate policy would be enforced by corporate administration; the U.S. government enforces public policy.

**Population health management** A term adopted by healthcare management companies to express their goal of achieving optimal health outcomes at a reasonable cost. The management process involves data collection and trend analyses that are used to predict clinical outcomes in a group of people.

**Port** Interface between a computer and other devices or other computers.

**Portability** Ability to be transported easily. For example, users can easily take handheld computers wherever they go.

**Portable Operating System Interface for UNIX (POSIX)** A uniform set of standards adopted by the Institute of Electrical and Electronics Engineers and the International Standards Organization that define an interface between programs and operating systems. The standardization ensures that software can be easily ported to other POSIX-compliant operating systems.

**Portals** Tools for organizing information from webpages into simple menus on one's desktop. Also, multifunctional telehealthcare platforms for receiving, retrieving, and/or displaying patients' vital signs and other information transmitted from telecommunications-ready medical devices.

**Portfolio** A collection of evidence used to demonstrate knowledge and skill achievement. A nursing portfolio provides the opportunity for a student to document a variety of sometimes unquantifiable skills, such as creativity, communication, and critical thinking.

**Power supply** A device that supplies electrical energy or power; the device that provides the electrical energy or power to the computer. A battery can be a source of energy or power.

**Pre-brief** The simulation stage in which the student receives the simulation information: goal, educational outcomes, and related course/program outcomes. The simulation is explained and focused for the student. He or she should know how to prepare for the activity; told what is expected of him or her; provided with the background necessary to be able to fully enact his or her role in the activity; and given specifics about how he or she will be assessed. The student must also be provided with the timeframe within which the simulation must be completed.

**Precision medicine** An evolving approach for disease treatment and prevention that considers individual variability in genes, environment, and lifestyle for each patient.

**Presence** The act of being fully there and being fully with patients; exclusively focusing on patients and their unique needs.

**Presentation** Act of presenting or showing; typically uses presentation software in a slide show format. The most commonly used presentation software in the United States is Microsoft PowerPoint.

**Primary key** A field within a record (also known as the key field) that contains a code, name, number, or other bit of information that acts as a unique identifier for that record. In a healthcare system, for example, a patient is assigned a patient number or ID that is unique for that patient.

**Principlism** A foundation for ethical decision making. Principles are expansive enough to be shared by all rational individuals, regardless of their background and individual beliefs.

**Privacy** An important issue related to personal information, about the owner or about other individuals, that focuses on sharing this information with others electronically and the mechanisms that restrict access to this personal information.

**Private cloud** Cloud space operated for a single organization with the infrastructure being managed and/or hosted internally or outsourced to a third party; it provides added control and avoids multi-tenancy.

**Problem-based** Typically refers to a type of student-centered instructional strategy where students collaboratively solve problems and reflect on their experiences.

**Problem solving** Cognitive process of critically thinking through a problem or issue to determine a course of action.

**Process analysis** Breaking down the work process into a sequential series of steps that can be examined and assessed to improve effectiveness and efficiency; explains how work takes place, gets done, or how it can be done.

**Process map** A visual depiction of the output of workflow analysis process.

**Process owners** Those persons who directly engage in the workflow to be analyzed and redesigned and have the ultimate responsibility for the performance of the process. These individuals can speak about the intricacy of the process, including process variations from the normal. When constructing a team, it is important to include individuals who are able to contribute information about the exact current-state workflow and offer suggestions for future-state improvements.

**Processing** Acting on something by taking it through established procedures so as to convert it from one form to another. Examples include the processing of information into data and the processing of a credit application to get a loan.

**Processor** Newer term for central processing unit (CPU); the component that executes computer programs, thought of as the brain controlling the functioning of the computer; the computer component that actually executes, calculates, and processes the binary computer code instigated by the operating system and other applications on the computer. It serves as the command center that directs the actions of all other components of the computer and manages both incoming and outgoing data.

**Product developer** One who designs, creates, and builds a product, such as a computer program, network, and/ or system. One who employs productivity software to create a product.

**Productivity software** Programs or software that help us compose, create, or develop. An example is the Microsoft Office suite of productivity tools, which offers word processing, spreadsheet, database, presentation, and Web tools to help us complete both professional and personal tasks.

**Professional development** Acquisition of skills required for maintaining a specific career path or general skills offered through continuing education, including the more general skills area of personal development. It can be seen as training to keep current with changing technology and practices in a profession or as part of the concept of lifelong learning.

**Professional networking** Connecting with other professionals in a field with a predetermined and focused purpose as well as an identified target audience in mind.

**Programmable read-only memory (PROM)** Form of digital memory where the setting of each bit is locked on a chip by a fuse or antifuse. PROM is used to store programs permanently, so it is useful in applications where the programming needs to be permanent. The device cannot be erased, so it must be replaced if changes are deemed necessary in the system.

**Project manager** Person responsible for the success of a project, who manages the planning and enactment of the project.

**Protected health information** Any and all information about a person's health that is tied to any type of personal identification.

**Prototype** Original mockup or first model; original form that is studied, tested, and processed before duplication.

**Proxy server** Hardware security tool to help protect an organization against security breaches.

**Psychology** The field that studies the mind and behavior.

**PsycINFO** A comprehensive database in the field of education and psychology.

**Public cloud** Cloud space owned and operated by companies offering public access to computing resources. It is believed to be more affordable and economically sound than private clouds because the user does not need to purchase or maintain the hardware, software, or supporting infrastructure, as these are managed and owned by the cloud provider.

**Public health** The science of protecting the well-being of communities and the population through education, research, intervention, and prevention.

**Public health informatics (PHI)** An aspect of informatics focused on the promotion of health and disease prevention in populations and communities.

**Public health interventions** Actions taken to promote and secure the well-being of a population or a community.

**Publishing** The process of production and dissemination of information.

**Qualified Clinical Data Registries (QCDRs)** Introduced for the Physician Quality Reporting System (PQRS) beginning in 2014, a QCDR will complete the collection and submission of PQRS quality measures data on behalf of individual eligible professionals (EPs) and PQRS group practices. For 2016, a QCDR is a Centers for Medicare and Medicaid Services–approved entity that collects medical and/or clinical data for the purpose of patient and disease tracking to foster improvement in the quality of care provided to patients.

**Qualified electronic health record** An electronic record containing health-related information on an individual, which consists of the individual's demographic and clinical health information, including medical history and a list of health problems, and supports entry of physician orders. A qualified electronic health record can capture and query information relevant to healthcare quality and exchange electronic health information with and assimilate such information from other sources to provide support for clinical decision making.

**Qualitative studies** Types of research design that focus on the human experience of a phenomenon using words, concepts, language, and meanings rather than numbers to capture the essence of the subject under study. Subjective studies.

**Quality** A level or grade of excellence; relative merit; a distinct or essential characteristic, attribute, or property.

**Quality assurance (QA)** The systematic process of assessing and testing to verify that a product or service being developed or used is meeting its specified requirements; focuses on discovering and correcting defects before they become part of the final product.

**Quantitative studies** Research that looks at the *what*, *where*, and *when* to provide understanding of phenomena based on quantifying data and using statistical measures; depending on the research, they may ascertain cause-and-effect relationships. Objective studies.

**Quantum bits (qubits)** Three-dimensional arrays of atoms in quantum states.

**Quantum computer** A proposed machine that is not based on the binary system, but instead performs calculations based on the behavior of subatomic particles or qubits. It is estimated that if quantum computing is ever realized, we will be able to execute millions of instructions per second (MIPS) due to the qubits existing in more than one state at a time or having the ability to simultaneously execute and process.

**Quantum computing** Using a quantum computer.

**Query** A form of questioning. A request for information; an example would be a database query.

**QWERTY** Name given to the typical computer keyboard layout, derived from the six letters in the first row below the numeric or number row.

**Radio frequency identification (RFID) chip** An identification chip that stores information for retrieval.

**Radio frequency identifier (RFI)** A reprogrammable chip that communicates with a reader to aid in identifying an object.

**Radiology information system (RIS)** Information system designed to schedule, report, and store information as it relates to diagnostic radiology procedures. One common feature found in most radiology systems is a picture archiving and communication system (PACS). The benefit of RISs and PACSs is their ability to assist in diagnosing complex cases and storing vital patient care support data.

**Random-access memory (RAM)** Volatile, temporary storage system that allows a computer's processor to access program codes and data while working on a task. RAM is lost once the system is rebooted, shut off, or loses power.

**Randomized controlled trial (RCT)** A study design that randomly assigns participants into an experimental group or a control group. As the study is conducted, the only expected difference between the control and experimental groups in an RCT is the outcome variable being studied.

**Ransomware** A specific type of malware or malicious code that cripples the computer network until a ransom is paid by the organization whose network was compromised.

**Rapid application development (RAD)** A method using prototyping and reiteration to develop products faster and of superior quality.

**Rapid Syndromic Validation Project** System where local healthcare professionals report cases such as influenza. Data are analyzed centrally, and the resulting information is shared with appropriate local authorities in an attempt to identify outbreaks early and prevent the spread of contagious diseases.

**Rationalism** An ethical position that contends knowledge is derived from deductive reasoning and not from the senses.

**RDF site summary** Resource description framework site summary. *See* Really simple syndication (RSS).

**Read-only memory (ROM)** Essential permanent or semi-permanent, nonvolatile memory that stores saved data and is critical in the working of the computer's operating system and other activities. ROM is primarily stored in the motherboard but may also be available through the graphics card, other expansion cards, and peripherals.

**Real environment data** Patient data collected in the home during telehealth monitoring. These data are typically more reflective of the true patient situation because they are collected in the real environment and not the artificial environment of a healthcare agency.

**Real time** Human time; occurs live, with users or learners interacting at the same time.

**Real-time telehealth** Live interactions between two or more clinicians, usually performed with videoconferencing equipment.

**Really simple syndication (RSS)** A form of web feed used to publish frequently updated content in podcasts, blog entries, or even news headlines. Subscribers receive update notices whenever new content is added or a site is updated. Also known as RDF site summary (RSS 1.0 and RSS 0.90) and rich site summary (RSS 0.91).

**Reasoning** Way of thinking, calculating, interpreting, or introspectively rethinking or critically thinking through an issue; reflective thought to analyze or think through one's ideas and alternatives.

**Records** Rows in a relational database representing individual patients, for example; also called tuples. Groups of related fields in a database. Captures audio and video using specific devices.

**Reflective commentary** Narrative comments that focus on why an individual thinks specific evidence is important, the ways in which the individual values what he or she has learned, or why the individual thinks the evidence is important for his or her profession.

**Regional health information exchanges** *See* regional health information organization.

**Regional health information organization (RHIO)** A regional network of healthcare organizations and providers who exchange information related to the health of the population. The goal is to work together without duplication to provide cost-effective health care and promote community well-being.

**Relational database** A database that can store and retrieve data very rapidly. "Relational" refers to how the data are stored in the database and how they are organized.

**Relational database management system (RDBMS)** A system that manages data using the relational model. A relational database could link a patient's table to a treatment table, for example, by a common field such as the patient ID number field.

**Reporting** The act of using of documents or information system outputs to convey information to stakeholders.

**Reporting and population health management** The data collection tools to support public and private reporting requirements, including data represented in a standardized terminology and machine-readable format.

**Report** Document that contains data or information based on a query or investigation designed to yield customized content in relation to a situation and a user, group of users, or an organization. Designed to inform, reports may include recommendations or suggestions based on programming and other embedded parameters.

**Repository** Central place where data are collected, stored, and maintained. Central location for multiple databases or files that can be distributed over a network or directly accessible to the user. Location for files and databases so that the data can be reused, analyzed, explored, or repurposed.

**Research utilization** The process of moving new understandings generated in research into practice.

**Research validity** A conclusion that can be drawn about the conduct of research based on an analysis of the research design and methods (internal validity) and the applicability of the findings to the general population (external validity).

**Researcher** A person who performs systematic inquiries of a topic in order to develop knowledge on that topic; a person who does research.

**Resource description framework (RDF)** A structure of consistent semantics adopted by the World Wide Web Consortium (W3C) to promote encoding, exchange, and reuse of metadata.

**Results management** An approach to evaluating the outcomes of a process to determine whether that process was useful or valuable.

**Reusability** The extent to which software or other work-related artifacts can be used in more than one computing program or software system.

**Rights** Privileges; include the right to privacy, confidentiality, and so on.

**Risk assessment** Determination of risk or danger, such as assessing for risk factors related to heart disease.

**Robotics** The design, development, and implementation of robots or machines to carry out tasks typically performed by people.

**Role playing** Situation that allows students to try on real-life scenarios by filling either pre-scripted or ad-libbed roles (e.g., doctor, nurse, patient, clinician) without the fear or pressure of putting another's life at risk while trying to determine the best course of action or find a solution to a fictitious patient's health issue.

**Root-cause analysis** Similar to failure modes and events analysis; analysis to discover why a process is faulty or produces an undesired result.

**Rows** Records in a database; also known as tuples.

**Safety culture** An organizational commitment to patient safety and the prevention of medical errors.

**Sarbanes-Oxley Act** Legislation that was put in place to protect shareholders as well as the public from deceptive accounting practices in organizations.

**Scaffolding** Adding initial support for a task and then gradually removing that support over time.

**Scareware** An e-mail designed to scare the user into believing that their computer has been infected. The hacker seeks to gain remote access to the computer to "fix" it.

**Scenario** Mock description of a situation or series of events.

**Scheduling systems** Systems designed to track resources within a facility while managing the frequency and distribution of those resources. For example, resource scheduling systems provide information about operating room utilization, or availability of intensive care unit beds and regular nursing unit beds.

**Scoring** The data mining process of applying a model to new data.

**Second Life** A proprietary virtual reality tool that allows users to create virtual communities.

**Secure information** Information that is protected from error, unauthorized access, and other threats that can compromise its integrity and safety.

**Security** Protection from danger or loss. In informatics, one must protect against unauthorized access, malicious damage, and incidental and accidental damage and enforce secure behavior and maintain security of computing, data, applications, information, and networks.

**Security breaches** Any security violations.

**Self-control** Self-discipline. Strength of will.

**Sensor and activity monitoring systems** Systems for tracking activities of daily living of seniors and other at-risk individuals in their places of residence. For example, applications use sensors to detect anomalies or problems such as faucets and stoves left turned on.

**Serial port** An interface for connecting an external device that is capable of receiving only one bit at a time, such as a mouse, a modem, and some printers.

**Serious game** A game that has as its main purpose something other than entertainment; for example, an educational game, designed for learning, that is a subset of both education and fun.

**Server** A computer or a group of computers that link computers together or provide services to a group of computers.

**Shoulder surfing** Watching over someone's back as he or she is working on a computer. This is still a major way that confidentiality is compromised.

**Simulated documentation** A replicated documentation system that nursing students can use to learn how to access electronic health records and document nursing care.

**Simulation scenario** A case or situation developed in a simulation setting to mimic an actual practice situation.

**Simulations** Imitations of real-life events or circumstances; in nursing education, replications of clinical scenarios developed to provide an opportunity for practice in a mock situation. Simulations can be web-based, latex-based, or virtual in a virtual world.

**Simulator** A mechanical or electronic device that provides an environment in which a simulation can occur. Some of these may be quite large.

**Situational awareness** The ability to detect, integrate, and understand critical information that leads to an overall understanding of a problem or situation.

**Six Sigma/Lean** Business management tactic that seeks to improve the quality of process outputs by identifying and removing the causes of imperfections (errors) and reducing inconsistency and variability in processes; Lean and Six Sigma are a complementary combination of activities that focus on doing the right steps and actions (Lean) and doing them right the first time (Six Sigma).

**Small Computer System Interface (SCSI)** Set of standards for physically connecting and transferring data between computers and peripheral devices. The SCSI standards define commands, protocols, and electrical and optical interfaces. Standardization among commercial products helps to ensure that devices will interface with many different systems.

**Smart pump** Machine used to infuse medication that includes dose-checking technology and safeguards designed to help avert medication errors.

**Smart rooms** Patient rooms that are equipped with technologies to increase patient safety and improve patient care.

**Smartphone** A cell phone that has limited personal digital assistant capabilities. Smartphones have limited personal computer functionality; they have an operating system and facilitate the use of e-mail and other applications.

**SNOMED CT** One of a suite of designated standards for use in U.S. Federal Government systems for the electronic exchange of clinical health information; a required standard in interoperability specifications of the U.S. Healthcare Information Technology Standards Panel. The clinical terminology is owned and maintained by the International Health Terminology Standards Development Organisation (IHTSDO), a not-for-profit association.

**Social bookmarking** Saving bookmarks or Internet URLs to a public website instead of on the user's private computer. The purpose is to share and grow the list of websites related to a specific topic. As users add bookmarks, they also typically add keyword tags that aid in search and organization processes.

**Social engineering** The manipulation of a relationship based on one's position in an organization. For example, someone attempting to access a network may pretend to be an employee from the corporate information technology office, who then simply asks for an employee's digital ID and password. Another example of social engineering is a hacker impersonating a federal government agent. After talking an employee into revealing network information, the hacker basically has an open door to enter the corporate network.

**Social media** Communication tools such as Twitter and Facebook that promote real-time information exchange.

**Social networking** Subscribing to and utilizing Web-based applications for the purpose of sharing personal information with others.

**Social sciences** Collection of academic/scientific fields or disciplines concerned with the study of the human aspects of our world/environment.

**Software** Anything that can be stored electronically. Software is divided into two types: system software (includes the operating system and other software necessary for the computer to function) and application software (allows users to complete specific tasks, such as word processors, spreadsheet software, presentation software, database managers, and media players).

**Software as a service (SaaS)** Cloud-based applications with the following benefits: the ability to quickly start using innovative or specific business apps that are scalable to your needs, any connected computer can access the apps and data, and data are not lost if your hard drive crashes because the data are stored in the cloud.

**Sound card** A computer expansion card that facilitates the input and output of audio signals to and from a computer under control of computer programs. Also known as an audio card.

**Spear phishing** A targeting phishing scheme that takes advantage of specific information provided in an organization's directory, thus allowing for a personalized scam e-mail.

**Spreadsheet** Text and numbers located in cells on a grid and the software necessary to process formulas and other computations such as creating graphs and charts.

**Spyware** A program that may contain malicious code that may attack or attempt to "take over" a computer. Spyware may also be nonmalicious in intent and monitor the user's behavior in an attempt to gain information about the user for targeted advertising.

**Stacking** The process of synthesizing the predictions from several models.

**Staff development** The process of providing opportunities for professional growth and skills development. Computer information systems are frequently used to assist with the ongoing education and development of nursing staff members, as this medium can embed prompts, information, and related questions in the nursing documentation system with a link to an appropriate clinical protocol.

**Stakeholders** Individuals or groups with the responsibility for completing a project and influencing the overall design, and those who are most impacted by success or failure of the system implementation.

**Standard Generalized Markup Language (SGML)** Meta-language; markup language for documents. Extensible Markup Language (XML) began as a simplified subset of SGML.

**Standardized nursing terminology** A body of terms used in nursing that is in some ways approved by an appropriate authority or by general consent.

**Standardized plan of care** A plan that presents clinicians with treatment protocols to maximize their outcomes and support best practices.

**Standards** Benchmarks. Criteria. Rules. Norms. Principles.

**Standards-developing organizations** Organizations that create guidelines, standards, and rules to help healthcare entities collect, store, manipulate, dispose of, and exchange secure protected health information.

**Static medium** Something that cannot be updated; for example, a print-based brochure may be outdated almost as soon as it is printed.

**STEM (science, technology, engineering, and math)** A curriculum based on an interdisciplinary and applied approach to educating students in science, technology, engineering, and mathematics. STEM integrates these subjects and learning occurs through authentic or real-world applications.

**Store-and-forward telehealth transmission** An application of telehealth care in which images and other clinical data are captured and transmitted to specialist clinicians.

**Structured English Query Language (SQL)** (pronounced "sequel") A database querying language, rather than a programming language. SQL is a standard language for accessing and manipulating databases. It simplifies the process of retrieving information from a database in a functional or usable form while facilitating the reorganization of data within the database.

**Suicide prevention community assessment tool** Risk assessment method that addresses general community information, prevention networks, and the demographics of the target population as well as community assets and risk factors.

**Summaries** Condensed versions of the original designed to highlight its major points.

**Supercomputers** The fastest computers; designed to run special applications that require numerous calculations.

**Surveillance** The act of watching for trends in health-related data for early detection of health threats.

**Surveillance data system** A networked computer system designed to use health-related data trends to predict the probability of an outbreak of a contagious or infectious disease or to detect morbidity and mortality trends in a geographic area as a precursor to public health planning or response.

**Synchronous** Real time or occurring at the same time; having the same period or time frame. Learning anywhere and anytime in real time using delivery modalities such as traditional face-to-face, Internet, and World Wide Web software tools (e.g., course management systems, chat, e-mail, electronic bulletin boards, audio– video communication tools).

**Synchronous dynamic random-access memory (SDRAM)** The most common type of dynamic random-access memory found in personal computers.

**Syndromic surveillance** A specialized system of data collection that seeks to detect trends in the incidence and severity of a specific disease or health-related syndrome and plan the public health response.

**Synthesis** Combining parts of existing material or ideas into a new entity or concept.

**Systems development life cycle (SDLC)** Stages involved in the life of a system, typically an information system; a model used in the project management of a system's development effort, spanning from feasibility to its demise.

**Systems engineering** An approach where technology manufacturers partner with organizations to identify risks to patient safety and promote safe technology integration.

**Table** A collection of related records in a database.

**Tags/tag clouds** A collection of keywords (tags) that describe the contents of websites related to a topic of interest, which are then organized by importance using differing colors and font sizes and styles (cloud). Many tag clouds are navigable; that is, the tags are hyperlinks to webpages.

**Task analysis** Analytic technique that focuses on how a task must be accomplished, including detailed descriptions of task-related activities, task characteristics and complexity, and the environmental conditions required for a person to perform a given task.

**Tasks** Actions that are value added and necessary. For example, some tasks come about because of workarounds or for other unsubstantiated reasons. Tasks that are considered non–value added and are not necessary for the purpose of compliance or regulatory reasons should be eliminated from the future-state process.

**Technologist** Person skilled in the use of technology.

**Technology** Method by which people use knowledge and tools. Knowledge used to solve problems, control and adapt to our environment, and extend human potential. Generally people use technology to refer to machines or devices such as computers and the infrastructure that supports them. For example, cell phones and planes are technologies that are tangible—one can see and touch them—but cannot see and touch the vast infrastructures supporting them, such as the wireless communications between the device (cell phone) and the cell towers, and the electronic guidance used by the device (plane) to navigate the skies.

**Telecommunications** Broadcasting or transmitting signals over a distance from one person to another person or from one location to another location for the purpose of communication.

**Telehealth** Telecommunication technologies used to deliver health-related services or to connect patients and healthcare providers to maximize patients' health status. A relatively new term in the medical/nursing vocabulary, referring to a wide range of health services that are delivered by telecommunications-ready tools such as the telephone, videophone, and computer.

**Telehealth care** Health services delivered by telecommunications-ready tools, usually supervised by a nurse or other clinician.

**Telehealth hardware** Equipment that captures objective vital signs data. Some systems use interactive self-reporting devices to capture subjective information on how a patient feels as well. The values obtained from the patient are then collected and transmitted by a communication hub. Peripheral devices used in home telehealth can include any item with a digital readout. Generally this equipment is self-administered by the patient or family caregiver.

**Telehealth software** Computer programs designed to collect and interpret health data gathered remotely via a telehealth communications system.

**Telemedicine** Health services delivered by telecommunications-ready tools, supervised or directed by a physician.

**Telemonitoring** Remote measurement of patients' vital signs and other necessary data.

**Telenursing** Health services delivered by telecommunications-ready tools, supervised or directed by a nurse.

**Telepathology** Use of telecommunications technology to facilitate the transmission and transfer of pathology data for the purposes of diagnosis, education, and research. Transmission and exchange of image-rich pathology data between remote locations.

**Telephony** Telephone monitoring of patients at their residences by off-site telenurses.

**Teleradiology** Use of telecommunications technology to electronically transmit and exchange radiographic patient images with the consultative text or radiologist reports from one location to another.

**TELOS strategy** An approach that provides a clear picture of the feasibility of a project; TELOS stands for "technologic and systems, economic, legal, operational, and schedule feasibility."

**Terabytes (TB)** Units of measurement for data storage capacity. One terabyte equals 1,024 gigabytes.

**Term** At its simplest level, a word or phrase used to describe something concrete (e.g., *leg*) or abstract (e.g., *plan*).

**Terminology** Vocabulary of technical terms used in a particular field, subject, science, or art; concerned with the collection, description, processing, and presentation of terms belonging to specialized areas of usage of one or more languages; nomenclature.

**Thick (fat) client** A computer connected to a network designed primarily for data processing and not communications or storage.

**Thin client** A computer that conveys input and output from the user to the server and back, but does no processing.

**Three-dimensional (3D)** A geometric model of the physical universe in which we live; the three dimensions are typically length, width, and depth (or height), although any three directions can be chosen, as long as they do not lie in the same plane.

**Three-dimensional (3D) computer graphics** Graphics that use three-dimensional representations of geometric data stored in the computer for the purposes of performing calculations and rendering images. These images may be stored for later viewing or displayed in real time.

**Throughput** The amount of work a computer can do in a given time period; a measure of computer performance that can be used for system comparison.

**Thumb drives** Small, removable storage devices.

**TIGER initiative** The work of the Technology Informatics Guiding Education Reform team. This team of nursing leaders developed a vision for utilizing information technology to transform nursing practice.

**Touch pad** An alternative to using a mouse. A device that senses the pressure of the user's finger along with the movement of the finger on the touch pad to control input positioning.

**Touch screen** A display used as an input device for interacting with or relating to the display's materials or content. The user can touch or press on the designated display area to respond, execute, or request information or output.

**Transistor** Solid-state semiconductors that resulted in the second generation of computers. Digital devices much smaller and faster than analog computers.

**Translational bioinformatics** The development of storage, analytic, and interpretive methods to optimize the transformation of increasingly voluminous biomedical and genomic data into proactive, predictive, preventive, and participatory information.

**Translational informatics** The application of research informatics to translational research in order to close the gap from research to the bedside to improve the health of patients and the community.

**Translational research** Research that is conducted with a vision toward transforming clinical nursing practice (translating the results into practice).

**Transparent** Done without conscious thought.

**Transparent technology** Technology that is not visible or recognizable by the user, therefore allowing the user to focus on the function or output and not the challenges of the technology itself.

**Transparent wisdom** Applying knowledge in a practical way or translating knowledge into actions without conscious thought.

**Transput** Input and output activities, collectively.

**Treatment/payment/operations** The treatment of patients, the payment for services, or the operations of the entity. Providers and other covered entities were not originally required to include in the accounting any disclosures that were made to facilitate the treatment of patients, the payment for services, or the operations of the entity (the "TPO exception"); this exception ended in January 2011 for providers that recently implemented electronic health record (EHR) systems. For those providers with EHR systems that were implemented before passage of the HITECH Act, the TPO exception ended in January 2014. It is easy to understand why this exception ended: Because all providers must implement comprehensive EHR systems, it will be very easy to generate an electronic record with an accounting of anyone who accessed a patient's record.

**Trend** General movement; a line of development. The process of getting others to emulate one's actions.

**Trending** The process of collecting patient data and analyzing those data collected over time via telehealth technology. Trending analysis provides a more accurate picture of health status than the analysis of episodic data collected during an agency visit.

**Triage** The process of assessing patients who are ill or injured and determining the need for intervention based on the severity of the health issue. Some software programs used in telehealth monitoring systems provide this function by comparing actual data with a preset standard and then alerting clinicians that an intervention is necessary.

**Trojan horses** Malicious code, capable of replicating within a computer, that is hidden in data or a program that appears to be safe.

**Trust-e** One of the two most common symbols that power users look for to identify trusted health sites.

**Truth** Fact. Certainty. Sincere action, character, and fidelity.

**Tuples** Records in a database; also known as rows.

**Tutorial** Learning materials available to the learner, who must then be self-directed to study the specific topical area presented.

**U-health** *See* ubiquitous health.

**U-nursing** Based on the concept of ubiquitous computing, the concept that nurses will provide care to anyone, anytime, anywhere using emerging transparent (ubiquitous) technologies and devices that support nursing care and practice.

**Ubiquitous** Existing or being everywhere at the same time; widespread.

**Ubiquitous health** The concept of health care that is so present in one's daily life that it seems invisible or in the background. Based on the concept of ubiquitous computing, wherein technologies become increasingly invisible as they are incorporated into everyday use—so much so that they are not even thought of while being used.

**Ubiquity** State of being everywhere at once (or seeming to be everywhere at once). Presence in many places especially simultaneously. With changing models of healthcare delivery, information and knowledge should be available anywhere.

**Uncertainty** Ambiguity. Insecurity. Vagueness.

**Universal serial bus (USB)** A means of connecting a myriad of plug-in devices, such as portable flash drives, digital cameras, MP3 players, graphics tablets, light pens, and so on, using a plug and play connection without rebooting the computer.

**Unstructured data** Data that are not contained in a database; data residing in text files, which can represent more than 75% of an organization's data; data that are not organized or that lack structure.

**Usability** The ease with which people can use an interface to achieve a particular goal. Issues of human performance during computer interactions for specific tasks within a particular context.

**USB flash drive** A portable memory device that uses electronically erasable programmable ROM to provide fast permanent memory. The USB flash drive is typically a removable and rewritable device that includes flash memory and an integrated universal serial bus (USB) interface. They are portable, due to their small size; durable; dependable; and obtain their power from the device they are connected to via the USB port.

**User friendly** Programs and peripherals that make it easy to interact or use computers. Design of a program to enhance the ease with which the user can utilize and maximize the productivity from computer programs.

**User interface** Mechanisms or systems used by users to interact with programs.

**Value** Relative worth of an object or action, such as aesthetic beauty or ethical value.

**Values** Important and lasting beliefs that provide principles and guidance for behaviors and beliefs.

**Veracity** Right to truth.

**Video adapter card** A board or card that is inserted or plugged into a computer to provide display capabilities.

**Videopod** A podcast that provides video in addition to audio functionality; self-contained system with a video transmitter.

**Virtual memory** The use of hard disk space on a temporary basis when the user is running many programs simultaneously. This temporary use frees up RAM to allow programs to run simultaneously and seamlessly.

**Virtual peers** Virtual populations of individuals who are genetically and behaviorally alike.

**Virtual reality** Technology that simulates reality in a virtual medium.

**Virtual simulation** Simulation using a three-dimensional virtual world or environment resembling the real-world setting and activities being simulated.

**Virtual world** A world that exists in cyberspace where people can establish avatars, purchase land, and interact with others. Emerging virtual worlds such as Second Life are changing the meaning of social networking. It is a live, online, interactive three-dimensional environment in which users interact using speech or text via a personalized avatar. Access requires a modern computer and Internet connection.

**Virtue** A certain ideal toward which we should strive that provides for the full development of our humanity. Attitude or character trait that enables us to be and to act in ways that develop our highest potential; examples are honesty, courage, compassion, generosity, fidelity, integrity, fairness, self-control, and prudence. Like habits, virtues become characteristics of a person. The virtuous person is the ethical person.

**Virtue ethics** Theory that suggests individuals use power to bring about human benefit. One must consider the needs of others and the responsibility to meet those needs.

**Viruses** Malicious codes that attach to an existing program and execute its harmful script when opened.

**Visiting Nurse Association (VNA)** A nonprofit home healthcare agency.

**Voice recognition** A type of software that allows the user to input data or to navigate the Web using voice commands. Voice interactivity should help to reduce the disparity associated with those who have limited keyboard or mousing skills.

**Waterfall model** An early systems development life cycle model that is linear in nature; when one phase ends, you move onto the next phase and do not go back, unlike in its modern counterparts that stress iterative development.

**Wearable computing** Devices that a person can don or put on like other articles of clothing or watches, jewelry, and other accessories. Wearable devices are being used to provide remote monitoring of physiologic parameters in care settings, including patients' own homes.

**Wearable technology** The study or practice of inventing, designing, building, or using miniature body-borne computational and sensory devices. Wearable computers may be worn under, over, or in clothing, or may actually be the clothes themselves.

**Web 2.0** Developing tools for social networking. The implications of the social networking technologies that are major elements of Web 2.0 will have significant impacts on the amount of information and knowledge that are generated and the ways in which they are used.

**Web publishing** The design and development of webpages that include links to digital files that are uploaded to web servers, thereby making these files accessible to others via web browsers.

**Web quests** Searches of the World Wide Web for information.

**Web servers** Multifunctional telehealthcare platforms for receiving, retrieving, and/or displaying patients' vital signs and other information transmitted from telecommunications-ready medical devices.

**Web-based** Originating from the World Wide Web.

**Web-based simulation** Simulation using the Internet or Web to resemble the real-world setting and activities being simulated.

**Web-enhanced** That which uses the World Wide Web to enhance or promote functions or tasks such as effective learning and skill acquisition.

**Webcast** Media distributed over the Internet as a broadcast, which relies on streaming media technology to facilitate downloading and participation. Such broadcasts could be distributed in real time, live, or recorded for asynchronous interaction.

**Webinar** Web-based seminar. Web conferencing that allows a presenter to share his or her computer screen/files and collaborate with the audience; attendance is controlled by an access code.

**Weblog** A website that contains the contributions of single or multiple users about a particular topic or issue. Similar in nature to a threaded discussion board or a personal diary, weblogs (also known as blogs) can provide insight into the perceptions of the contributors about the topic.

**Wetware** Direct body–brain interfaces. A reference to the human mind or central nervous system when interfaced with a computer; derived from computer terminology such as "software" and "hardware."

**Wi-Fi** A wireless technology brand owned by Wi-Fi Alliance, which is used to improve the interoperability of wireless networking devices.

**Wiki** Server software that allows users to create, edit, and link webpage content from any web browser. Server software that supports hyperlinks. The simplest online database; used to develop collaborative websites.

**Wisdom** Knowledge applied in a practical way or translated into actions; the use of knowledge and experience to heighten common sense and insight so as to exercise sound judgment in practical matters. Sometimes thought of as the highest form of common sense, resulting from accumulated knowledge or erudition (deep, thorough learning) or enlightenment (education that results in understanding and the dissemination of knowledge). Wisdom is the ability to apply valuable and viable knowledge, experience, understanding, and insight while being prudent and sensible. It is focused on our own minds; it is the synthesis of our experience, insight, understanding, and knowledge. Wisdom is the appropriate use of knowledge to solve human problems. It is knowing when and how to apply knowledge.

**Word processing** Creating documents using a word processing software package such as Microsoft Word.

**Work process** See workflow.

**Workarounds** Ways invented by users to bypass the system to accomplish a task; usually indicate a poor fit of the system or technology to the workflow or user. Devised methods to beat a system that does not function appropriately or is not suited to the task it was developed to assist with. For example, a nurse might remove the armband from the patient and attach it to the bed if the bar-code reader fails to interpret bar codes when the bracelet curves tightly around a small arm.

**Workflow** A progression of steps (tasks, events, and interactions) that constitute a work process; involve two or more persons; and create or add value to the organization's activities. In a sequential workflow, each step depends on the occurrence of the previous step; in a parallel workflow, two or more steps can occur concurrently. The term "workflow" is sometimes used interchangeably with "process" or "process flow," particularly in the context of implementations. A sequence of connected steps in the work of a person or team of people—that is, the process or flow of work within an organization; a virtual illustration of the "real" work or steps (flow) that workers enact to complete their tasks (work). The purpose of examining and redesigning workflow is to streamline the work process by removing any unnecessary steps that do not add value or might even hinder the flow of work.

**Workflow analysis** Not an optional part of clinical implementations, but rather a necessity for safe patient care fostered by technology. The ultimate goal of workflow analysis is not to "pave the cow path," but rather to create a future-state solution that maximizes the use of technology and eliminates non–value-added activities. Although many tools and methods can be used to accomplish workflow redesign (e.g., Six Sigma, Lean), the best method is the one that complements the organization and supports the work of clinicians.

**World Wide Web (WWW)** An international network of computers and servers that offers access to stored documents written in HTML code, and access to graphics, audio, and video files.

**Worms** Forms of malicious code. Self-replicating computer programs that use a network to send multiple copies of itself to other computers, subsequently tying up bandwidth and incapacitating networks.

**Yottabytes (YB)** Units of information or computer storage equal to 1 septillion bytes.

**Youth Risk Behavior Surveillance System (YRBSS)** An epidemiologic survey conducted by the Centers for Disease Control and Protection to identify and track the most common health risk behaviors that lead to illnesses and mortality among youth.

**Zero day attack** A technique where a hacker searches for and exploits software vulnerabilities before the vendor is able to release a patch or a fix.

**Zettabyte (ZB)** Unit of information or computer storage equal to 1 sextillion bytes.

# Index

Note: Page numbers followed by *b*, *f* and *t* indicate material in boxes, figures and tables respectively.

## A

AAACN. *See* American Academy of Ambulatory Care Nursing
AAAI. *See* Association for the Advancement of Artificial Intelligence
AACN. *See* Association of Colleges of Nursing
Academic Center for Evidence-Based Practice (ACE), 502*t*
Academic Competencies, 267
access, 160, 472
accessibility, 24, 113*b*
Accountable Care Organizations (ACOs), 285
accurate information, 24
ACE Star model, 504*t*
ACOs. *See* Accountable Care Organizations
acquisition, 35. *See also* knowledge acquisition
action games, 448–449
active listening, 527*f*, 532
Active Matrix Organic Light-Emitting Diode (AMOLED), 53
activity-monitoring systems, 377
actual users, surveys of, 219
acuity systems, 193
administrative information systems
    aggregating patient and organizational data, 197–202
    case management information systems, 190
    communication systems, 190–191
    core business systems, 191–193
    department collaboration and exchange of knowledge and information, 202–203
    healthcare organization information systems, types of, 190
    interoperability, 195–196
    order entry systems, 193–194
    patient care support systems, 194–195
administrative processes, 272
admission, discharge, and transfer (ADT) systems, 192
ADT systems. *See* admission, discharge, and transfer systems
Advanced Audio Coding (AAC), 418*b*
advanced cardiac life support (ACLS), 435
adventure games, 449
adverse events, 294
advocates, 422
    policy developer, 131
adware software, 234, 238
Affordable Care Act, 385. *See also* Patient Protection and Affordable Care Act
Agency for Healthcare Research and Quality (AHRQ), 150, 153, 234, 251, 274, 294, 332, 384, 501
    role of informatics, 502*t*

safety culture, 295
    strategies for developing safety culture, 296
Agency for Healthcare Research and Quality Patient Safety Network, 193
Agency for Toxic Substances and Disease Registry (ATSDR), 345, 349
AHIMA. *See* American Health Information Management Association
AHRQ. *See* Agency for Healthcare Research and Quality
AI. *See* artificial intelligence
alarm fatigue, 297
alert, 31
algorithms, 486
alleles, 515
Alliance for Nursing Informatics (ANI), 139, 140*b*
Alliance for Patient Safety, 294
Allison, 91–92, 93
    alternatives, 92
alphabetic data, 22
alphanumeric data, 22
Alternative Payment Models (APMs), 247
alternatives, 92
Amazon's S3, 284*b*
American Academy of Ambulatory Care Nursing (AAACN), 380
American Association for Justice, 245
American Association of Colleges of Nursing (AACN), 405
American Association of Critical-Care Nurses (AACN), 372
American Association of Health Plans, 501
American Health Information Management Association (AHIMA), 140*b*, 267
American Library Association (ALA), 463
American Medical Association, 501
American Medical Informatics Association (AMIA), 107, 134, 138–139, 140*b*, 497
American National Standards Institute (ANSI), 157*b*, 201*b*
American Nurses Association (ANA), 8, 107, 108, 380, 436
    Code of Ethics for Nurses, 162
    definition of nursing informatics, 108–109
    *Nursing Informatics: Scope and Standards of Practice*, 128, 251
    recognized terminologies supporting nursing practice, 116*b*
    standardized terminologies, use of, 279
American Nurses Credentialing Center (ANCC), 133, 426
American Nursing Association of Occupational Health Nurses, 424
American Nursing Informatics Association (ANIA), 139, 140*b*, 424
American Psychological Association (APA), 427, 466
American Recovery and Reinvestment Act (ARRA), 149, 246, 268, 284